# FOOT AND ANKLE
# R A D I O L O G Y

# FOOT AND ANKLE
# RADIOLOGY

**Robert A. Christman, DPM**

Director of Radiology
Associate Professor, Department of Medicine
Director of Online Learning
Temple University School of Podiatric Medicine
Philadelphia, PA
Fellow, American College of Podiatric Radiology (FACPR)
Diplomate, American Board of Podiatric Orthopedics and Primary Podiatric Medicine (ABPOPPM)

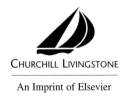

CHURCHILL LIVINGSTONE

An Imprint of Elsevier

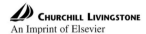
**Churchill Livingstone**
An Imprint of Elsevier

11830 Westline Industrial Drive
St. Louis, Missouri 63146

---

**NOTICE**

Radiology is an ever-changing field. Standard safety precautions must be followed, but as new research and clinical experience broaden our knowledge, changes in treatment and drug therapy may become necessary or appropriate. Readers are advised to check the most current product information provided by the manufacturer of each drug to be administered to verify the recommended dose, the method and duration of administration, and contraindications. It is the responsibility of the licensed prescriber, relying on experience and knowledge of the patient, to determine dosages and the best treatment for each individual patient. Neither the publisher nor the author assumes any liability for any injury and/or damage to persons or property arising from this publication.

---

**Library of Congress Cataloging-in-Publication Data**

Christman, Robert A.
  Foot and ankle radiology / Robert A. Christman.
    p. ; cm.
  Includes bibliographical references and index.
  ISBN 0-443-08782-2
    1. Foot--Radiography. 2. Ankle--Radiography. 3. Foot--Diseases--Diagnosis. 4.
 Ankle--Diseases--Diagnosis. I. Title.
    [DNLM: 1. Foot--radiography. 2. Ankle--radiography. 3. Foot Diseases--radiography.
  WE 880 V555f 2003]
  RC951 .C477 2003
  617.5'8507572--dc21

                                                   2002034871

*Managing Editor:* Christie M. Hart
*Project Manager:* Joy Moore
*Designer:* Julia Dummitt
*Cover Art:* Sheilah Barrett

GW-MVY

Printed in the United States of America
Last digit is the print number:   9   8   7   6   5   4   3   2

*To my wife, Irene, for her love and support.*
*To my daughter, Jessica, for providing occasional (and necessary) distraction.*
*To my students, past, present, and future, for their encouragement and inquisitiveness.*
*To the Lord God, for all His provisions and blessings.*

**Robert L. Baron, DPM, FACPR, FACFAOM**
Professor and Chair, Department of Radiology
William M. Scholl College of Podiatric Medicine
Finch University of Health Sciences / The Chicago
    Medical School
Private Practice
Chicago, IL
Fellow, American College of Podiatric Radiology
Fellow in Primary Podiatric Medicine, ABPOPPM
Fellow in Podiatric Orthopedics, ABPOPPM

**Philip J. Bresnahan, DPM, DABPS, FACFAS**
Past Assistant Professor, Department of Orthopedics
Temple University School of Podiatric Medicine
Philadelphia, PA
Past President, American College of Foot and Ankle
    Pediatrics
Diplomate, American Board of Podiatric Surgery
Fellow, American College of Foot and Ankle Surgeons
Private Practice, Souderton, PA

**Randy E. Cohen, DPM, FACFR**
Professor and Chairman, Radiology Department
New York College of Podiatric Medicine, New York
Diplomate of American Board of Podiatric Orthopedics
Private Practice
Staten Island, NY

**Youseff Kabbani, DPM**
Northeastern Hospital
Philadelphia, PA

**Bambino Martins, PhD**
Westville, NJ

**David Mayer, MD, MS, FACR**
Chairman, Department of Radiology
Mercy Health System
Darby, PA

**Mary C. Oehler, RT**
Radiology Supervisor
Radiology Department
Temple University School of Podiatric Medicine
Philadelphia, PA

**Lawrence S. Osher, DPM, BS**
Director of Radiology
Full Professor
Ohio College of Podiatric Medicine
Cleveland, OH
University Hospitals East
St. Vincent Charity Hospital
Cleveland, OH

**Robin C. Ross, DPM, FACFAS, FACFAOM**
Diplomate, American Board of Podiatric Surgery
Diplomate, American Board of Podiatric Orthopedics and
    Primary Podiatric Medicine
Private Practice
Southold and Shelter Island, New York

**William H. Sanner, DPM**
Chairman
Podiatry Department
Ochsner Clinic Foundation
Baton Rouge, LA

**Jeffrey E. Shook, DPM**
Director Residency Training
Huntington Podiatric Surgical Residency
St. Mary's Hospital
Huntington, WV
Scott Orthopedics Center, Inc.
Huntington, WV

**Frank Spinosa, DPM, FACFAS, FACFAOM,
FACPR, FAAHP, FASPM**
Diplomate, American Board of Podiatric Surgery
Diplomate, American Board of Podiatric Orthopedics and
    Primary Podiatric Medicine
Diplomate, American Board of Podiatric Public Health
Diplomate, American Board of Quality Assurance and
    Utilization Review Physicians
Former Associate Professor
Department of Radiology
New York College of Podiatric Medicine
Past President, New York State Podiatric Medical Association
Private Practice
Shelter Island, NY

**Casimir F. Strugielski, RT (R), ASRT**

Instructor and Supervisor
Department of Radiology
Dr. William M. Scholl College of Podiatric Medicine
Finch University of Health Sciences / The Chicago
    Medical School
Chicago, IL
American Registry of Radiologic Technologists
American Society of Radiologic Technologists

**Marie L. Williams, DPM**

Director of Podiatric Surgical Residency Parkway Regional
    Medical Center
Diplomate American Board of Podiatric Surgery
Adjunct Professor Barry University School of Podiatric
    Medicine
Private Practice
North Miami Beach, FL

**David E. Williamson**

Sr. Technical Representative
Planning and Technical Manager
District Manager
Photo Products Department
Medical Products Division
E.I. DuPont de Nemours & Company, Inc.
Wilmington, DE

# FOREWORD

Dr. Robert Christman has provided us, in his unique text, insights into his personal approach to evaluating radiographs of the foot. How to logically analyze the cardinal radiographic findings seen in a radiograph and its most appropriate list of differential diagnoses is made easy. In his chapter dealing with joint disease, the reader is led step by step into constructing practical and concise differential diagnoses. This approach is rare in most texts dealing with this important subject. Dr. Christman's emphasis on radiographic anatomy and variants are truly appreciated. In most texts this section is only skimmed. Also, sections dealing with radiographic biomechanical analysis correlating radiographic positional finding to foot structure and function as well as fracture and dislocation classifications using actual radiographs are included. An entire section is also dedicated to dealing with the radiologic sciences. Dr. Christman has succeeded in including everything necessary for a podiatric student to learn as well as practice podiatric radiology and radiologic interpretation.

The book should serve as a reference for all podiatrists, students, and podiatric assistants.

**Harvey Lemont, DPM**

The purpose of *Foot and Ankle Radiology* is threefold: to introduce the podiatric medical student to the scope of diagnostic radiology applicable to podiatric medicine, to prepare the podiatric medical student to apply podiatric radiography and radiographic interpretation in practice, and to provide the podiatric practitioner with a comprehensive base of knowledge to make informed decisions.

Radiology is an important diagnostic tool useful for the evaluation of foot and ankle pathology. However, because of the potential risks associated with ionizing radiation, those involved in its production must have knowledge of the radiologic sciences in order to provide protection and safety to all involved. The Doctor of Podiatric Medicine is responsible for the practice of proper radiography in the office setting, whether by himself or herself or by an appropriate assistant/technologist. The doctor must also be familiar with all special imaging studies applicable to imaging of the foot and ankle so that they are ordered as warranted.

The podiatric physician encounters numerous pathologic conditions radiographically that are either intrinsic to the foot or represent manifestations of extrinsic disease. Therefore the student must not only learn specific radiologic pathology of the foot and ankle, but must acquire an understanding of general diagnostic radiology and pathologic correlation. Furthermore the student must learn how to analyze a radiograph systematically and acquire a basic knowledge of bone radiology to interpret radiographs and establish differential diagnoses.

To these ends, this text includes sections on plain film radiography (radiologic science, radiation protection and safety, principles of radiography, and foot and ankle radiography); radiographic anatomy (normal and variant presentations of the adult and developing foot and ankle); systematic approach to bone and joint abnormalities (how to select appropriate views and a using a fundamental process to analyze the radiographic study); radiographic biomechanical analysis (correlating the clinical and radiographic presentations of both the adult and child); special imaging procedures (emphasizing indications and cross-sectional imaging); and bone and joint disorders (including systematic approaches to interpreting skeletal pathology rather than simply description by disease).

Podiatric radiology textbooks have come and gone over the years; at this writing, not one is in print. A scattering of foot and ankle radiology texts written by radiologist or orthopedist is presently available; however, they are geared to the practicing physician and not the student. As a result, they are devoid of sections pertinent to the podiatrist in training, in particular radiologic science and systematic assessment of skeletal abnormalities. Furthermore this textbook devotes serious attention to plain film radiographic anatomy and radiographic biomechanical analysis. An entire chapter is devoted to fracture and dislocation classification systems, classically found not in radiology textbooks but orthopedic texts. Also unique to this text is the inclusion of a chapter on podiatric radiography equipment.

*Foot and Ankle Radiology* will also serve as a valuable reference source to the podiatric assistant, radiologic technologist, and limited license extremity technologist. Also, the radiologist and orthopedist may find this text to be a valuable addition to their library.

This text was written with the following goals in mind. Specifically, that the podiatric student and practitioner be able to:

- Describe the principles of radiation physics and biology.
- Practice appropriate radiation protection and safety.

- Describe lower extremity radiography equipment and accessories.
- Discuss the formation of the radiographic image.
- Assess film quality.
- Perform radiologic positioning techniques of the foot and ankle.
- Apply the principles of film interpretation to any given radiograph.
- Identify normal and variant radiographic anatomy of the foot and ankle.
- Identify normal and variant development of the foot and ankle.
- Systematically assess bone and joint abnormalities in a radiograph.
- Identify and describe the radiologic features of pertinent pathology, including the following:
  - Positional abnormalities
  - Congenital anomalies
  - Skeletal dysplasias
  - Fractures and related disorders
  - Arthritis
  - Infection
  - Tumors, tumor-like processes, and soft tissue abnormalities
  - Metabolic, endocrine, circulatory, and nutritional disorders
  - Soft tissue abnormalities
- Discuss special imaging techniques applicable to foot and ankle imaging.
- Discuss indications and alternatives for prescribing special imaging procedures.

## ACKNOWLEDGMENTS

Stephen D. Weissman, DPM, for providing the opportunity to pursue a personalized two-year podiatric radiology fellowship program. Harvey Lemont, DPM, for his professional and personal mentorship as my chair and friend. Carol Romano, for assisting whenever needed and for words of comfort. Jean Martino, for invaluable last-minute assistance. Temple University School of Podiatric Medicine, for appreciating my talents and gifts.

# CONTENTS

## SECTION 1
## Plain Film Radiography

# SECTION 2
# Radiographic Anatomy

# SECTION 3
# Systematic Approach to Bone and Joint Abnormalities

# SECTION 4
## Radiographic Biomechanical Analysis

# SECTION 5
# Special Imaging Procedures

# SECTION 6
# Bone and Joint Disorders

# SECTION 1

# Plain Film Radiography

# CHAPTER 1

# Radiation Physics, Biology, and Safety

BAMBINO MARTINS

## ◼ THE PHYSICS OF DIAGNOSTIC IMAGING

An *image* may be defined as a likeness of an object produced on photographic material. A *diagnostic image* is one that contains information that may be useful in medical diagnosis. Although many modern diagnostic imaging procedures may involve neither x rays nor photographic film, most diagnostic imaging of the foot and ankle is done with x rays and photographic film. This section describes the nature of radiation and matter, how x rays are produced, and how they interact with matter. Other aspects of the physics of diagnostic radiology, such as characteristics of photographic film and image quality, are discussed in Chapter 5.

### Radiation and Matter

*Radiation* is defined as energy in motion. Radiation may be classified as follows:

1. *Particulate/nonparticulate.* When radiation (e.g., electrons and protons) acts primarily as a particle or corpuscle, it is considered particulate radiation; if the radiation (e.g., x rays) interacts primarily as a wave, then it is nonparticulate.
2. *Charged/uncharged.* When radiation carries a positive (+) charge (e.g., alpha particles) or negative (−) charge (e.g., electrons), then it is charged radiation, if it is neutral (e.g., photons) then it is uncharged radiation.
3. *Ionizing/nonionizing.* Ionization is the formation of positively or negatively charged particles or ions. If the radiation has enough energy to cause ionization, then it is considered to be ionizing radiation; otherwise, it is nonionizing radiation. Only those radiations having energy exceeding the ionization potential, which varies from 4.3 eV (electron volt) to 17.4 eV (average about 13 eV) for biologically significant atoms, can cause

ionization. In the electromagnetic spectrum, this includes radiations with energy exceeding that of UV light (i.e., x rays and gamma rays). In Sweden, the dividing line between ionizing and nonionizing electromagnetic radiations is set at 12.4 eV. Particulate radiations such as alpha rays and beta rays, neutrons, and heavy ions are also ionizing radiations. Nonionizing radiations include ultraviolet, visible, and infrared light, microwaves, television and radio waves, and low-frequency electric and magnetic fields, as well as acoustic and ultrasound waves. Ionizing radiation may be directly ionizing or indirectly ionizing. Directly ionizing radiation includes charged particles such as electrons and alpha particles, which have sufficient kinetic energy to cause ionization by collision. Indirectly ionizing radiation includes uncharged particles such as x rays, gamma rays, and neutrons, which release directly ionizing particles or initiate nuclear transformation.

### The Structure of Matter

When a philosopher was asked what *mind* is, she said, "Doesn't matter" and when asked what *matter* is, she replied, "Never mind." Fortunately, physicists have come a long way in their understanding of matter. All matter is made of atoms. An atom is the smallest part into which matter can be divided while still retaining the properties of that material.

### The Structure of an Atom

In its simplest form, an atom may be visualized as a solar system, with the nucleus being the sun and the electrons representing the orbiting planets (Figure 1-1). The primary subatomic particles constituting the nucleus are the neutron, which has no electrical charge, and the proton, which has a positive charge. The nucleus, as a whole, has a positive charge, which in a neutral or nonionized atom is balanced by the negative charge on the orbiting electrons. The electrons are in specific orbits, the innermost orbit being the K-shell;

the subsequent shells are L, M, N, and O. The maximum number of electrons in each shell is governed by specific laws and the inner shells are filled in before electrons enter outer shells. Electrons in each shell have a specific energy level, and when an electron from an inner shell is knocked out, its place is taken up by an electron from an outer shell with release of electromagnetic radiation. An atom is about $10^{-10}$ m in size, whereas the nucleus is only $10^{-15}$ m.

An atom is symbolized by $^{A}_{Z}X$, where $A$ is the mass number, which is the number of nucleons (neutrons +

protons), $Z$ is the atomic number, which is the number of protons (and also the number of orbital electrons in a neutral atom), and $X$ is the chemical symbol for the atom. For example $^{3}_{1}H$ represents tritium, an atom of hydrogen with a mass of 3, and $^{235}_{94}Pu$ is the atom of plutonium, with a mass of 235.

## Dual Nature of Matter

Physicists recognize that matter and energy are interchangeable, as given by Einstein's famous equation: $E = mc^2$, where $E$ = energy in joules (J), $m$ = mass in kilograms (kg), and $c$ = velocity of light, which is $3 \times 10^8$ meters per second (m/s). Matter also has a dual nature, particulate and wavelike, as postulated by de Broglie.

X rays are a form of electromagnetic radiation. Electromagnetic radiation is characterized by the simultaneous transfer of energy through both electric and magnetic fields. It covers the spectrum from low-frequency electromagnetic fields through visible light to cosmic rays (Table 1-1). Electromagnetic radiation often propagates like waves in water. The velocity of propagation, in a vacuum, is always the same and is equal to $3 \times 10^8$ m/s. The wavelength and frequency of propagation are related by $c = \lambda \nu$, where $c$ is the velocity in meters per second, $\lambda$ is the wavelength in meters, and $\nu$ is the frequency in Hertz. From this relationship, it is obvious that the longer the wavelength, the lower is the frequency. Electromagnetic radiation also behaves as though it were made of discrete particles or bundles of energy called *photons* or *quanta*. The energy carried by a photon is given by $E = h\nu$, where $E$ is the energy in Joules, $h$ is the Planck constant (= $6.63 \times 10^{-34}$ J-s), and $\nu$ is the frequency in Hertz. Combining the two relationships, it can be shown that $E$ (in kiloelectron volts, keV) = $12.4/\lambda$ (in angstrom units, Å,

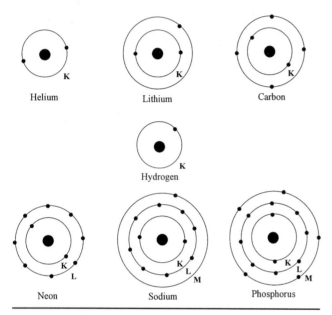

Figure 1-1  Schematic diagram showing electrons in orbit around the nuclei of hydrogen, $_1$H; helium, $_2$He; lithium, $_3$Li; carbon, $_6$C; neon, $_{10}$Ne; sodium, $_{11}$Na; and phosphorous, $_{15}$P.

| TABLE 1-1 The Electromagnetic Spectrum | | | |
|---|---|---|---|
| Radiation Type | Frequency (Hz) | Wavelength (m) | Photon Energy (eV) |
| Low-frequency electromagnetic fields | $<10^5$ | $>3 \times 10^3$ | $<4.1 \times 10^{-10}$ |
| Radio waves | $10^5$ to $3 \times 10^{10}$ | $3 \times 10^3$ | $4.1 \times 10^{-10}$ |
| | | $10^{-2}$ | $1.24 \times 10^{-4}$ |
| Infrared | $3 \times 10^{12}$ to $3 \times 10^{14}$ | $10^{-4}$ | $1.24 \times 10^{-2}$ |
| | | $10^{-6}$ | $1.24$ |
| Visible | $3 \times 10^{14}$ to $7.5 \times 10^{14}$ | $10^{-6}$ | $1.24$ |
| | | $4 \times 10^{-7}$ | $3.1$ |
| Ultraviolet | $3 \times 10^{15}$ | $10^{-7}$ | $12.4$ |
| X rays | $3 \times 10^{16}$ to $3 \times 10^{23}$ | $10^{-8}$ | $124$ |
| | | $10^{-15}$ | $1.24 \times 10^9$ |
| Gamma rays | $3 \times 10^{18}$ to $3 \times 10^{21}$ | $10^{-10}$ | $1.24 \times 10^4$ |
| | | $10^{-13}$ | $1.24 \times 10^7$ |
| Cosmic rays | $3 \times 10^{21}$ to $3 \times 10^{22}$ | $10^{-13}$ | $10^7$ |
| | | $10^{-14}$ | $10^8$ |

Note that in Sweden, radiations with energy above 12.4 eV are considered ionizing and radiations below 12.4 eV are considered nonionizing. Adapted from Shleien B: *The health physics and radiological health handbook*, Silver Spring, Md., 1992, Scinta.

which equals $10^{-10}$ m). Thus we see that high-energy radiations, such as x rays, have a high frequency and short wavelength, whereas long-wavelength radiations, such as television and radio waves, have low energy and a short frequency (see Table 1-1).

## Production of X Rays

The production of x rays is an example of the conversion of one form of energy into another. In an x-ray tube, when fast-moving electrons produced by heating a tungsten filament strike a tungsten target, a very small fraction of energy is converted into x rays. The filament is the cathode (– terminal), and the target is the anode (+ terminal). The cathode and anode are enclosed in an evacuated glass bulb (Figure 1-2).

The number of electrons passing from the cathode to the anode in 1 second is a measure of the x-ray tube current and is usually expressed in milliamperes (mA). The voltage, usually expressed in kilovolts (kV), is the potential difference across the anode and the cathode.

There are several types of x-ray generators, and depending on the circuitry producing the high voltage, these may be classified as single-phase, three-phase, or constant potential. The maximum or peak potential difference applied across the cathode and anode is the kVp. The kVp determines the quality of the x rays, and the mA is a measure of the quantity of x rays produced.

When electrons from the cathode hit the anode, most (99%) of the energy is converted into heat and only about 1% goes into the production of x rays. The efficiency of x-ray production is the ratio of the energy put out as x rays to the energy deposited onto the anode by the electrons. It is given by $E = 9 \times 10^{-10} \, ZV$, where $E$ is the efficiency, $Z$ is the atomic number of the target, and $V$ is the tube voltage in volts.

There are two processes by which energy of the electrons is converted into x rays: bremsstrahlung and characteristic x rays.

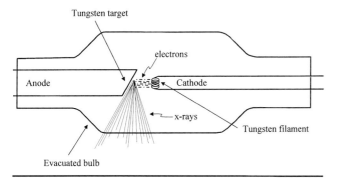

Figure 1-2    Schematic diagram of an x-ray tube.

## Bremsstrahlung

Bremsstrahlung is a German word meaning "braking radiation." When the negatively charged electrons approach the vicinity of a positively charged nucleus, the electron may be deflected from its path. This sudden change in velocity causes the electron to lose part of its energy as x rays. The efficiency of bremsstrahlung production increases with the square of the atomic number. Bremsstrahlung radiation has a broad range of energies up to a peak energy determined by the kVp.

## Characteristic X Rays

An electron may also interact with an orbiting electron, ejecting it from the atom. The vacancy created in that orbit is filled up by an electron from a higher orbit. In this process, electromagnetic radiation is released. The energy of the radiation is characteristic of the target material and is sharply defined in energy. For high-$Z$ targets and inner shell transitions, the escaping radiation has energy in the range of the x-ray spectrum.

## Quality of X Rays

Whereas characteristic x rays have discrete energies, bremsstrahlung radiation has a broad range of energies, and therefore the photons produced by an x-ray generator are heterogeneous in energy. Because of the heterogeneous nature of the photons produced by an x-ray machine, one needs a quantity to characterize a photon beam.

Several factors, such as kVp, average keV, half value layer (HVL), and equivalent keV, are used for this purpose; but each has its limitations. The kVp is a measure of the maximum energy in keV of the x rays produced. The average keV is about one third of the maximum keV and is a better measure of x-ray quality. The HVL is the thickness of a given material (usually aluminum or copper) that will reduce the intensity of the photon beam to half. Unfortunately, the HVL for a heterogeneous beam is not constant but increases with each succeeding HVL because of the preferential absorption of low-energy x rays by the initial HVLs and the consequent hardening of the beam. To account for this, a homogeneity coefficient has been defined as the ratio of the second HVL to the first HVL. The higher the homogeneity coefficient, the more homogeneous is the beam. The equivalent keV is the keV of a homogeneous beam that has the same HVL as the given heterogeneous beam.

Note that low-energy photons do not contribute to a diagnostic image, because these photons do not reach the film but are absorbed by the patient, unnecessarily increasing patient dose. Even though some very low-energy x rays are absorbed by the tube housing (inherent filtration), the National Council on Radiation Protection and Measurements (NCRP) recommends and state regulations require the use of added filters (usually made of aluminum)

| TABLE 1-2 | Minimum Total Filtration and HVLs Recommended by the NCRP | |
|---|---|---|
| kVp | Total Filtration (mm Al) | HVL (mm Al) |
| 49 | 0.5 | 0.5 |
| 50 | 1.5 | 1.2 |
| 60 | 1.5 | 1.3 |
| 70 | 1.5 | 1.5 |
| 71 | 2.5 | 2.1 |
| 80 | 2.5 | 2.3 |
| 90 | 2.5 | 2.5 |

to harden the beam. The minimum amount of total filtration (inherent plus added) and the recommended HVLs are given in Table 1-2.

## Heel Effect

Beams produced by an x-ray machine have nonuniform angular distributions, with the intensity on the cathode side being greater than on the anode side. This is called the heel effect (Figure 1-3), and it is more evident for large field sizes and shorter source to film distances. One way to exploit this apparent disadvantage is to position thicker parts being examined toward the cathode. Thus the thinner forefoot should be placed under the anode and the thicker rearfoot under the cathode.

## Tube Rating

As mentioned earlier, about 99% of the energy of electrons hitting the anode is converted into heat. Provisions must be made to dissipate this heat, lest the anode melts. Notwithstanding the design features built into the tube to dissipate heat, in actual use of the tube one must consider

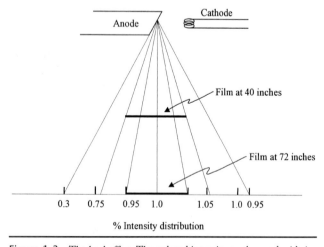

Figure 1-3   The heel effect. The reduced intensity on the anode side is particularly evident for large field sizes and at large film-to-focus distances.

the tube rating, which is given in heat units (HU) and is a measure of the maximum load (kVp, mA, and exposure time) that can be applied to an x-ray tube. To prolong the life of an x-ray tube and to avoid permanent damage to it, always operate an x-ray unit so that the tube rating is not exceeded.

## Collimation

Regulatory agencies require that the beam striking a patient be limited to the area of clinical interest and not exceed the size of the film within strict limits. This is because neither x-ray photons outside the area of clinical interest, nor photons that strike outside the film, contribute any diagnostic information. Also, the larger the field size, the greater is the scatter radiation reaching the film and contributing to noise. There are several ways to restrict the size of an x-ray beam, all involving the use of lead absorbers. The method used in most modern x-ray units is the light-limiting variable collimator (LLVC), which allows for stepless adjustment of x-ray field size over a large range and also permits visualization of the field size on the patient. An x-ray unit often has an automatic collimating system called positive beam limitation (PBL), which automatically adjusts the x-ray field size to the size of the film.

## Grids

To cut down on the amount of scatter that reaches the film and contributes to image degradation, grids are used. These are strips of lead foil alternating with aluminum or other material that absorbs scattered x rays. Grids improve contrast.

## Interaction of X Rays With Matter

Now that we have given some idea of what matter is and what x rays are, it is time to explain how x rays interact with matter. There are five types of interactions:

1. *Elastic scattering.* When a photon passes near an electron, the electric field associated with the moving photon accelerates the electron, which radiates energy. The photon changes direction, and the atom returns to its initial state. There is no transfer of energy and no ionization. This interaction is unimportant in diagnostic radiology and is a small fraction (<5%) of the total number of interactions.

2. *Photoelectric effect.* In this interaction, the incoming x-ray photon interacts with one of the inner-shell electrons, knocking it out. The total energy of the photon is dissipated in this process, with some going to overcome the bidding energy of the electron and the rest providing kinetic energy to the ejected electron. The void created in the inner shell when an

electron is ejected is filled up by an electron from a higher shell, producing characteristic x rays. For the photoelectric process to occur, the energy of the incoming photon must exceed the biding energy of the electron. It has the greatest likelihood of occurrence when the photon energy just exceeds the binding energy. The probability of photoelectric interaction is directly proportional to the cube of the atomic number ($Z^3$) and inversely proportional to the cube of the photon energy ($E^{-3}$).

3. *Compton scattering.* Compton scattering can be considered as an interaction between two billiard balls (the incoming photon and an outer loosely bound or free electron). The photon is deflected in one direction, and the electron recoils in another direction. The laws of conservation of energy and momentum determine the energy and direction of the scattered photon and electron. The probability of Compton scattering decreases with increasing energy and is directly proportional to the number of electrons per gram, which is approximately the same in most materials.

4. *Pair production.* In pair production, a photon with energy above 1.02 MeV interacts with the nucleus and disintegrates into an electron and a positron (positively charged electron). The total energy is split equally between the two particles, which travel in opposite directions. The positron soon combines with an electron and is annihilated with the production of x rays. The probability of pair production depends on Z and increases with increasing energy above the threshold of 1.02 MeV.

5. *Photonuclear disintegration.* In photonuclear disintegration an x-ray photon interacts with the nucleus, resulting in the disintegration of the nucleus, with ejection of one or more nuclear particles. The threshold for this interaction is about 7 MeV.

In the energy range of interest in foot and ankle radiology, the dominant interactions are the photoelectric effect and Compton scattering. That is why there is very little soft tissue contrast, whereas bone contrasts with soft tissue.

## ■ BIOLOGICAL EFFECTS OF IONIZING RADIATION

In the beginning is energy and at the end is death; what is in between is the subject of this section. It is mind-boggling to consider how much ionizing radiation energy is required to kill a cell or to transform a normal cell into a cancer cell. The first consequence of the interaction of ionizing radiation with matter is ionization, that is, the formation of positively and negatively charged ions. A single ionization has the potential to cause the death of a cell, which in itself may not be too bad, considering that there may be several such cells in an organism. What is worse is that instead of killing a cell, the ionization may lead to the transformation of a normal cell into a cancer cell with potentially unlimited capacity for growth, leading to the eventual death of the organism.

It is believed that the dose required to kill half the people exposed to radiation (the mean lethal dose, or MLD) is about 4.5 to 6 Sv (450 to 600 rem). (*Note:* The units of dose measurement are defined in the section on radiation protection later in this chapter and in Table 1-3.) Considering that 1 Sv is the absorption of 1 J of energy per kilogram of material, it can be shown that 5 Sv will raise the temperature of tissue by only 0.0012° C, yet half the people exposed to that much radiation will die within about 30 days ($LD_{50}^{30}$). Or from another viewpoint, the energy absorbed from drinking a cup of coffee is more than the energy absorbed from a whole-body dose of 5 Sv.

### Molecular Effects

There are two distinct mechanisms through which an ionization can lead to biological damage: direct and indirect. The term *direct effect* refers to lethal damage caused through direct ionization of a crucial molecule, which in most cases

---

| TABLE 1-3 | Quantities and Units in Radiation Protection | |
|---|---|---|
| Quantity | Old Unit | Système International (SI) Unit |
| Exposure | Roentgen (R) | Coulomb per kilogram (C/kg) |
| Absorbed dose | Radiation absorbed dose (rad) | Joule per kilogram (J/kg) *Special name:* gray (Gy) |
| Dose equivalent or equivalent dose | Rad equivalent mammal (rem) | Joule per kilogram (J/kg) *Special name:* sievert (Sv) |
| Effective dose equivalent of effective dose | Rad equivalent mammal (rem) | Joule per kilogram (J/kg) *Special name:* sievert (Sv) |

is assumed to be deoxyribonucleic acid (DNA) or some lipoproteins in the nuclear or cytoplasmic membrane. This effect accounts for only a small fraction of damage caused by low-LET (linear energy transfer—defined later) radiation but accounts for most of the damage caused by high-LET radiations.

The term *indirect effect* refers to lethal damage to crucial molecules caused by free radicals. Given that about 80% of biological material is water, it is easy to see that most of the initial ionization will consist of a water molecule forming an aqueous (solvated) electron, or an ionized water molecule breaking up into hydrogen ion and a hydroxyl radical. Also, a water molecule could be raised to an excited state and then split apart to form a hydrogen and a hydroxyl radical. The hydrogen and hydroxyl radicals are free radicals. A free radical has a free or unpaired electron and is therefore highly reactive. These free radicals and the aqueous electron react with crucial molecules. The indirect effect is dominant for low-LET radiations.

Because a free radical is extremely reactive and has a very short life span, on the order of a few microseconds, most damage at the molecular level occurs within a few seconds. It is the amplification of this damage through biological processes that takes days and years and that may eventually cause death.

## Cellular Effects

The study of the biological effects of radiation at the cellular level was advanced considerably by the technique of growing single mammalian cells in culture, developed by T. T. Puck in 1955.

### Survival Curves

A survival curve (Figure 1-4) is a plot, on semilogarithmic paper, of the relationship between dose and survival. The dose is plotted on the linear $x$-axis, and the survival is plotted on the logarithmic $y$-axis. Survival curves are assumed to be either exponential or sigmoidal, based on the multitarget, multihit theory, which is often used to fit data points and to interpret the survival curves. This theory assumes that cell death results from damage to one or more targets, with each target requiring one or more hits for inactivation.

An exponential survival curve (see Figure 1-4, *curve A*) results when there is only a single target and it takes only one hit to inactivate it. This is a single-hit, single-target model. Mathematically, the survival is given by the following equation:

$$S = e^{-D/D_0}$$

where $S$ = survival

$e$ = base for the natural logarithms

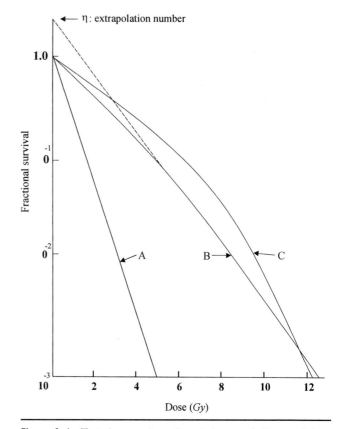

Figure 1-4    Typical mammalian cell survival curves. **A,** Exponential; **B,** single-hit, multitarget (sigmoidal); **C,** linear quadratic.

$D$ = dose

$D_0$ is the dose that reduces survival to 37% of the initial value.

A sigmoidal survival curve (see Figure 1-4, *curve B*) is observed when one hit is required to inactivate a target and there is more than one target per cell. The equation for a multitarget single-hit survival curve is as follows:

$$S = 1 - (1 - e^{-D/D_0})^n$$

where $n$ = number of targets.

For doses that are large compared to $D_0$, the preceding equation becomes

$$S = ne^{-D/D_0}$$

A sigmoidal survival curve is characterized by a shoulder, or curved portion at low doses, and an exponential part at high doses. The target number, $n$, is called the extrapolation number and is the number on the $y$-axis, obtained by extrapolating the straight line portion of the curve to the $y$-axis. The $D_0$ applies only to the linear portion of the curve.

For high-LET radiations, the survival curve is usually exponential, and for low-LET radiations the survival curve is sigmoidal.

For several years, single-cell mammalian survival data fitted or was force-fitted to the target theory, which held the fort. Then someone threw a curve, and in recent years more and more radiobiologists have come to believe that the survival curve has a continuous downward concave curvature. Today survival curves are fitted to the linear-quadratic model, which assumes that radiation damage results from interaction between two separate lesions. The equation for this model is

$$S = e^{-(\alpha D + \beta D2)}$$

where $D$ = dose

α is the probability that both lesions are caused by the same ionization track

β is the probability that the two lesions are produced independently

This model results in a curve that is continuously concave downward (see Figure 1-4, *curve C*).

## Protectors and Sensitizers

Some substances influence the response of cells to radiation. Those substances that reduce radiation-induced damage are called *protectors*. Substances with the −OH and −SH groups, such as alcohol and cysteine, usually act as protectors. Substances that enhance the effects of radiation are called *sensitizers*. Oxygen is a sensitizer of radiation, and the drug metronidazole (Flagyl) is an example of *hypoxic sensitizers*, that is, substances that sensitize hypoxic cells but not normal or oxic cells. It is believed that protectors act as scavengers soaking up the free radicals before these radicals can damage critical molecules. In contrast, sensitizers increase the number of free radicals. Therefore protectors and sensitizers can be expected to be less effective in those situations where the direct effect is dominant, as with high-LET radiations. Experimental evidence shows that protectors and sensitizers are, indeed, effective with low-LET radiations and not with high-LET radiations.

## Dose Rate Effect and Dose Fractionation

An interesting observation of the effect of radiation on cells is that when radiation is delivered at low dose rates, it is less effective than when exposure is at acute dose rates. This is confirmed experimentally when a given total dose is delivered in two fractions, with a time interval between fractions; that is, a fractionated dose is found to be less effective than the same total dose when given at one time. The dose-rate effect and loss of effectiveness of a fractionated dose have been explained by assuming that radiation causes sublethal damage (see next section). Given that most occupational and environmental exposures are at chronic or low dose rates, it may be assumed that such exposures are less damaging than indicated from data obtained at high dose rates.

## Sublethal and Potentially Lethal Damage

Besides causing lethal damage, radiation also induces sublethal and potentially lethal lesions. A sublethal lesion, is a lesion, which if not repaired, can interact with another sublethal lesion causing lethal damage. A potentially lethal lesion is a lesion that, if not repaired, will lead to lethal damage. Enzymes responsible for repair of sublethal and potentially lethal damage have been identified in cells.

## LET, RBE, and OER

Linear energy transfer (LET) is a measure of the amount of energy transferred along the track or path of radiation. It is measured in energy loss per unit length (keV/μ). X and gamma rays are low-LET radiations, neutrons are medium-LET, and alpha particles and heavy ions are high-LET radiations. High-LET radiations usually cause direct damage. The effectiveness of one form of radiation compared to another (usually x rays are taken as the reference radiation) is the relative biological effectiveness (RBE). It is usually calculated as the ratio of the dose that causes a certain effect for a given radiation, to the dose for the reference radiation that causes the same effect. The RBE depends on various factors, such as the end point, but in general high-LET radiations have high RBE values.

As mentioned earlier, oxygen is a sensitizer, which means that oxic cells are more sensitive to radiation than are anoxic cells. The ratio of the dose that kills a certain fraction of cells under anoxic conditions to the dose that kills the same fraction of cells under oxic conditions is the oxygen enhancement ratio (OER). The OER is about 3 for low-LET radiations and close to 1 for high-LET radiations. OER plays a very significant role in radiation therapy.

## Cell Cycle Effect

A cell in the process of growing and dividing goes through a cycle made up of several stages. In $G_0$, the cell is in the resting stage; $G_1$ phase follows the mitotic (M) or dividing phase and precedes the S-phase during which a cell synthesizes DNA. This is followed by the $G_2$ phase. The sensitivity of a cell to radiation varies with the phase, being maximum in the mitotic and $G_2$ phases and minimum at the S-phase. This variation in sensitivity is less evident for high-LET radiation.

The amount and structure of DNA varies with the cell cycle, and this variability is used not only to explain the variation in cell sensitivity through the cell cycle but also to support the view that the DNA molecule is the crucial molecule in radiation-induced damage.

## Mechanism of Cell Death

Considerable experimental evidence indicates that the crucial molecule involved in radiation-induced damage is DNA. Some of the evidence is derived from experiments where only part of a cell (nucleus or cytoplasm) is irradiated using alpha particles. The variation in the response of a cell during the cell cycle also supports the hypothesis that DNA is the crucial molecule. Nevertheless, some believe that at least some cell death results from primary damage to cell membranes, specifically lipoproteins in nuclear membranes.

## Effects on Tissues

The effects of radiation on tissues are best described by the law of Bergonie and Tribondeau, which states that the sensitivity of tissues to radiation depends on two factors: proliferative capacity and differentiation. Tissues that are rapidly dividing are more sensitive to radiation than are tissues in which cells are dividing slowly or are dormant. Tissues, in which cells are differentiating are more sensitive to radiation than are tissues with fully differentiated cells.

Based on the law of Bergonie and Tribondeau, the bone marrow is considered the most sensitive tissue, with lymphocytes being very sensitive, followed by the gastro-intestinal tract. The central nervous system is the most resistant to radiation.

Doses around 0.15 Sv (15 rem) cause a reduction in the white blood cell count, which becomes evident within about 2 weeks. Higher doses, of about 1 Sv (100 rem), will cause nausea and vomiting, because of damage to the gastro-intestinal tract. The central nervous system is resistant to radiation and can withstand a dose of several hundred Sv.

## Whole-Body Effects

The biological effects of ionizing radiation on the organism as a whole may be classified in the following three different ways.

### Somatic/Genetic Effects

Somatic effects are the effects observed in the individual exposed to radiation, whereas genetic effects are effects observed in the progeny born to individuals exposed to radiation. Included in somatic effects are the effects observed in children exposed in utero.

**Somatic.**   The MLD (mean lethal dose) or $LD_{50}^{30}$ (lethal dose to kill 50% in 30 days) for humans is estimated to be about 4.5 to 6 Sv and may be higher if autologous bone marrow transplants are done. The primary cause of radiation-induced death is inability to fight infection because of damage to the bone marrow and bleeding through the GI tract.

*Fetal Exposure.*   It is not true that all fetal exposure to radiation is fatal. During the first 2 weeks following conception, when the mother may not even be aware of her pregnancy, radiation exposure has an all-or-none effect. If the dose is high, then the fetus aborts spontaneously;

otherwise, the child is usually born without any abnormalities. During the first trimester (particularly 8 to 15 weeks), the fetus is specially sensitive to radiation. Three consequences of in utero exposure are (1) childhood cancer, mainly leukemia, which becomes evident within 2 to 15 years following exposure; (2) reduced IQ; and (3) microcephaly, or reduced head size. Box 1-1 shows the

| BOX 1-1 | Risks to the Embryo Fetus From Radiation and From Other Factors |
|---|---|

|  | Per 1000 births |
|---|---|
| I.  Radiation Risks |  |
| A.  Childhood cancer: |  |
| Risk from natural causes | 1.4 |
| Excess risk from 1000 mrem received before birth | 0.6 |
| B.  Small head size (microcephaly) |  |
| Risk from natural causes | 40 |
| Excess risk from 1000 mrem received 4-7 weeks after conception | 5 |
| Excess risk from 1000 mrem received 8-11 weeks after conception | 9 |
| C.  Mental retardation (reduced IQ) |  |
| Risk from natural causes | 4 |
| Excess risk from 1000 mrem received 8-15 weeks after conception | 4 |
| II.  Nonradiation Risks |  |
| A.  Occupation |  |
| 1.  Stillbirth or spontaneous abortion |  |
| Risk from natural cause | 200 |
| Excess risk from work in in high-risk occupations | 90 |
| B.  Alcohol consumption |  |
| 1.  Fetal alcohol syndrome |  |
| Risk due to natural causes | 1-2 |
| Excess risk from 2-4 drinks/day | 100 |
| Excess risk from more than 4 drinks/day | 200 |
| Excess risk from chronic alcoholism (>10 drinks/day) | 350 |
| 2.  Perinatal infant death |  |
| Risk from natural causes | 23 |
| Excess risk from chronic alcoholism (>10 drinks/day) | 170 |
| C.  Smoking |  |
| 1.  Perinatal infant death |  |
| Risk from natural causes | 23 |
| Excess risk from < 1 pack/day | 5 |
| Excess risk from > 1 pack/day | 10 |

Adapted from NRC Regulatory Guide #8.13, USNRC: Instruction concerning prenatal radiation exposure, December 1987.

magnitude of these risks and compares the risk of fetal exposure to radiation to the risk to the fetus from other factors.

**Genetic.** Genetic effects have not been observed in humans, but based on animal studies, these are expected to occur at a rate of about 50 per million live births for 0.01 Sv (1 rem) of exposure over a 30-year generation period. This is very small compared to the spontaneous risk of serious genetic damage of 6 to 9 per 100 live births. The dose required to double the mutation frequency in humans is assumed to be about 1 Sv (100 rem)

**Genetically Significant Dose (GSD).** The GSD (genetically significant dose) is a dose that, if received by every individual in a population, would result in the same amount of genetic damage as caused by the sum of the doses actually received by exposed members of the population. It is a measure of the risk that an exposed population has of genetic risk. For a foot examination, the mean gonadal dose for a male is 0.15 mSv (15 mrem) and the GSD is 0.0125 mSv (1.25 mrem); for females the mean gonadal dose and the GSD are less than 0.01 μSv (1 μrem).

## Early (Prompt)/Late (Delayed) Effects

The effects of radiation can become evident as early as a few hours following exposure but generally are expressed several years later. Early effects are those that become evident within hours to a year following exposure, whereas late effects become evident after a year.

White blood cell depletion, nausea, vomiting, loss of hair, and erythema are examples of prompt effects, whereas cataract and cancer are delayed effects. The latent period, which varies considerably, is about 2 years for childhood leukemia following exposure in utero. It is about 5 years for soft tissue cancers and is more than 10 years for bone and lung cancers. The latent period for development of radiation-induced cataract is about 5 years.

## Stochastic/Nonstochastic (Deterministic) Effects

Stochastic effects are those effects in which the probability of occurrence, but not its severity, increases with dose. These effects generally do not have a threshold dose. An example of stochastic effects is cancer. The term *stochastic* is a Greek word meaning "chance." Being exposed to radiation is like buying lottery tickets. One individual could buy a few hundred lotteries and not win anything, whereas another individual could buy a single lottery and win a few million dollars. In the same manner, one individual may be exposed to a very large dose of radiation and develop no cancer, whereas another individual may be exposed to very little radiation and develop cancer. Just as with lotteries, there is no guarantee of anybody getting or not getting cancer, no matter what the dose. But the *risk* goes up directly with the magnitude of the dose.

Nonstochastic (deterministic) effects, in contrast, have a threshold dose, which must be exceeded before the effects become evident. Once the threshold, which is different for different effects, is exceeded, the severity of the effect is proportional to the dose. An example of a nonstochastic (deterministic) effect is cataract, the threshold for which is about 2 Sv.

## Radiation-Induced Risk of Cancer

Presently, no data are available to determine what the risk of cancer is when doses and/or dose rates are low, such as one encounters from environmental and occupational exposures. It is also unlikely that such data will become available in the near future. So risks are based on data at high doses (above 0.2 Sv or 20 rem) and acute dose rates (above 100 mSv/hr or 10 rem/hr). Extrapolation from high to low doses is based on theoretical models (Figure 1-5). The linear model *(curve B)* assumes that one can extrapolate linearly from high to low doses. In fact, its proponents prefer this model, because it gives conservative estimates of the risks. The linear-quadratic model *(curve C)* assumes that low doses are less effective, and the supralinear model *(curve A)* assumes that low doses are more effective than high doses, whereas the linear-with-threshold model *(curve D)* assumes that there is a threshold for cancer induction. The risk estimates, of course, differ significantly, depending on the model.

The Biological Effects of Ionizing Radiations (BEIR) committees set up by the National Academy of Sciences have, in several reports over the years, estimated the increased risk of mortality from all radiation-induced cancers to an individual in the U.S. population. The latest report, *BEIR V*, was published in 1990.

The *BEIR V* estimate of excess (above spontaneous rates) radiation-induced cancer mortality rates, is 800 per 100,000 people, each exposed to 0.1 Sv (10 rem). This risk is

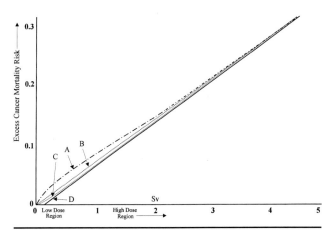

**Figure 1-5**  Dependence of cancer risk on model. **A**, Supralinear; **B**, linear; **C**, linear quadratic; **D**, linear with threshold.

averaged over all ages and sites (organs) and assumes equal number of males and females.

Note that the excess risk of 800 for 10,000 person-Sv (*person-sievert*—sometimes abbreviated to *pervert*—is a unit of collective dose equivalent and is the product of the average dose, in Sv, to which a group is exposed and the total number of individuals in that group) does not consider low-dose and low-dose-rates effects. For low doses and low dose rates, the excess cancer mortality risk is about 270 per 10,000 person-Sv (about 3 excess cancer deaths for every 100 perverts), depending on the dose-rate effectiveness factor (DREF). The risk is significantly different for specific groups and types of cancers. Specific risks, by site and age, for men and women are available from the BEIR reports. NCRP Report No. 116 gives a risk of $5.0 \times 10^{-2}$/Sv for fatal cancers, $1.3 \times 10^{-2}$/Sv for serious genetic damage, and $1.0 \times 10^{-2}$/Sv for nonfatal cancers to give a total detriment of $7.3 \times 10^{-2}$/Sv.

## Probability of Causation (PC)

To the Mad Hatter, words mean no more and no less than what he wants them to mean. To many of us, PC is just a personal computer: to others, PC stands for "political correctness." However, in the context of cancer and radiation, PC is probability of causation. It is impossible, at the present time, to prove or disprove that a specific cancer was caused by a specific exposure. PC is an estimate of the probability that a specific malignancy was caused by a specific radiation exposure. The National Institutes of Health have developed probability-of-causation tables. The concept of probability of causation is discussed in Statement No. 7 issued by the NCRP.

## Comparison of Radiation Risks With Risks From Other Detrimental Factors

Despite what one hears and reads, radiation is not the only source of all ills that befall humankind. In fact, radiation may not even be the worst culprit. At least, radiation and its effects has been studied more thoroughly than the effects of any other environmental factor that is a scourge to us.

Man is not immortal, and in this respect women enjoy equality with men, although not full equality, because women in general live a little longer. But that aside, eventually we all die. So the yardstick for comparing the risks of radiation with the risks from other sources should not be the magnitude of the risk of cancer mortality, but the effect on life as a whole. Unfortunately, there are no objective criteria to judge the quality of life. One criterion that is used to compare risks from different factors is loss of quality-adjusted life years (QALY). A cruder criterion is longevity, or more specifically, the number of days (or years) of life expectancy lost, following exposure to a given factor. Box 1-2 shows one such set of data. You can see that if one

| BOX 1-2 | Comparison of Risks From Various Causes |
|---|---|

| RISK | DAYS OF LIFE EXPECTANCY LOST |
|---|---|
| Smoking (one or more packs/day) | |
| Male | 2400 |
| Female | 1400 |
| Passive smoking | 50 |
| Cardiovascular disease | 2050 |
| Cancer | 1250 |
| All accidents | 300 |
| Motor accidents | 200 |
| Overweight by 25% | 300 |
| Alcohol consumption (U.S. average) | 130 |
| Radiation: | |
| Continuous exposure to 10 mSv/yr from age 18 to 65 | 50 |
| Natural background (0.94 mSv/yr, excluding radon) | 6 |
| Radon (average in U.S. homes: 37 Bq per cubic meter) | 30 |
| Medical diagnostic (0.63 mSv/yr) | 9 |

Adapted from Cohen BL: *Health Phys*, 61(3):317-335, 1991.

worked with radiation for 30 years (an average working life) and during each of those years was exposed to the maximum permissible dose of 0.05 Sv (5 rem) per year (hardly likely, because the average yearly exposure for radiation workers in the United States is about 3.5 mSv or 350 mrem), then the total number of days of life expectancy lost would be about 250. If that is not comforting, note that smoking or being overweight by 25% exacts a heavier toll, with auto accidents and alcohol consumption close behind.

It is puzzling how the public is made to perceive risks. When sexuality researchers Masters and Johnson stated that under certain circumstances, one could get infected with the human immunodeficiency virus (HIV) from using public toilets, a large number of scientists pounced on them. But the "as low as reasonably achievable" (ALARA) philosophy, which is the cornerstone of the radiation safety program, is based on protecting people from stochastic effects, whose minuscule probabilities of occurrence are calculated from dubious assumptions and theories derived from confounding data. Why then, I wonder, is it alright to warn people that behind every millirem there lurks a bogeyman, but foolhardy to alert them to the possibility that they might "catch" HIV while sitting on the "throne"?

## ■ RADIATION PROTECTION

Now that we have some idea of what radiation is, how it interacts with matter and what it can do to biological systems, we have to learn how and why to protect ourselves from this colorless, odorless energy that is all around us and even within us.

The NCRP states that the specific objectives of radiation protection are to prevent occurrence of deterministic effects by limiting doses to below-threshold levels for such effects and to limit risk of stochastic effects, cancers, and genetic effects, giving due consideration to economic factors and to the needs and benefits of society.

Any exposure to radiation must be justified, optimized to comply with the ALARA principle, and limited so that individuals are not subjected to unacceptable risks. The fatal accident rate, in what are considered as safe industries, is about $10^{-4}$ per year, whereas the maximum annual fatal accident rate that workers will tolerate is about $10^{-3}$.

## Quantities and Units

There are four different but related quantities that are important in the field of radiation protection (see Table 1-3).

### Exposure

Exposure is a measure of the amount of ionization that is produced when radiation passes through matter. The old unit for exposure is the roentgen (R). The Système International (SI) unit is coulomb/kilogram (C/kg). 1R = $2.58 \times 10^{-4}$ C/kg.

### Absorbed Dose

The absorbed dose is a measure of the amount of energy that is absorbed in matter when radiation passes through it. The old unit for absorbed dose is rad (radiation-absorbed dose). It is equivalent to the absorption of 100 ergs of energy per gram of material. The SI unit is the gray (Gy). It is equivalent to the absorption of 1 joule of energy per kg; 1 Gy = 100 rad.

### Dose Equivalent

The dose equivalent is a measure of the biological damage caused by radiation. It is equal to the absorbed dose multiplied by a quality factor (Q) that accounts for the observation that for the same amount of absorbed radiation, different types of radiation cause different amounts of biological damage. Q is related to the RBE of that radiation. The old unit for dose equivalent is the rem (radiation equivalent mammal); 1 rem = rad × Q. The SI unit is the sievert (Sv). 1 Sv = 1 Gy × Q. It follows that 1 Sv = 100 rem.

Q differs for different types of radiation and for different end points. It is 1 for x rays, gamma rays, and beta particles. It varies from 2 to 20 for neutrons, depending on neutron energy, is 10 for high-energy protons and 20 for alpha particles and heavy ions.

For all practical purposes, when dealing with x rays, the roentgen, the rad, and the rem may be considered equivalent. For radiation safety purposes, the dose equivalent is often expressed in millirems (a mrem is one thousandth of a rem), or in millisieverts (a mSv is one thousandth of a Sv; 1 mSv = 100 mrem).

Dose equivalent has now been replaced by equivalent dose, which is defined as the product of the average absorbed dose in a tissue or organ from a radiation and a radiation weighting factor ($w_R$) for that radiation. $w_R$ accounts for differences in the RBE of different types of radiations. $w_R$ is given the value of 1 for x and gamma rays and electrons. It varies from 5 to 20 for neutrons, depending on energy; 2 for protons of energy less than 2 MeV; and 20 for alpha particles, fission fragments, and heavy ions. The units for equivalent dose are the same as for dose equivalent.

### Effective Dose Equivalent

Very often, we have to deal with exposures to only a part of the body. In such situations, the effective dose equivalent is used. It is the dose equivalent multiplied by the weighting factor. The weighting factor is a measure of the risk from exposure to that organ compared to the risk from whole-body exposure to the same dose. The unit for the effective dose equivalent is the sievert (the rem, for the oldies). The entrance skin exposure (ESE) for a radiograph of an extremity is about 30 to 100 mrem, and the effective dose equivalent is about 0.01 mSv (1 mrem).

Effective dose equivalent has been replaced by effective dose, which is defined as the sum of the products of the equivalent dose received by a tissue and the tissue weighting factor ($w_T$), which represents the proportionate risk of stochastic effects for that tissue compared to the risk when the whole body is irradiated uniformly. $w_T$ varies from 0.01 for bone surfaces and skin through 0.05 for breast and 0.12 for lung to 0.20 for gonads. The units for effective dose are the same as for effective dose equivalent.

## Sources of Radiation: Natural and Man-Made

There is radiation everywhere around us, and even within us. It is primarily natural, but some exposure is to man-made radiation. Natural radiation is terrestrial or cosmic in origin. Exposure to man-made radiation is mostly from medical procedures such as diagnostic x-rays and nuclear medicine tests, with some contribution from occupational exposure, consumer products (such as televisions, some types of wrist watches, smoke detectors, optical glasses, and Fiesta dinnerware), and radiation released from nuclear reactors or fallout from nuclear bomb tests.

It has been estimated that, on an average, an individual in the United States is exposed to about 3.6 mSv (360 mrem) per year, that is, about 1 mrem per day. Most (3 mSv) is from natural background radiation, including about 2 mSv from radon. Radon is the radioactive gas that is found in homes (particularly in basements) and is supposedly responsible for about 13,000 or 10% of the lung cancer deaths per year in the United States.

Diagnostic medical procedures contribute about 0.5 mSv per year. Consumer products make up the remaining 0.1 mSv. Contributions from nuclear power plants, fallout, and occupational exposures are negligible.

Note that we are exposed to radiation not only from outside of us but also from within us. Radionuclides such as K-40, H-3, C-14, and Po-210 are integral parts of our body, and as with external exposure may be natural in origin or man-made. Internal exposure may be as much as 10% of the yearly background exposure we receive.

Also, note that natural background radiation levels vary considerably from place to place. Moving from Philadelphia to Denver will increase the yearly dose equivalent by about 0.5 mSv. And in some parts of the world. background radiation levels may be as high as 50 mSv/yr, which is the maximum permissible dose for the whole body for a radiation worker per year.

## Regulatory Agencies and Standards for Radiation Protection

State and federal agencies license and or regulate the use of radiation in the United States. National (NCRP) and international groups (ICRP, International Commission on Radiological Protection) provide the scientific basis and recommendations for radiation protection.

To reduce patient exposure, the U.S. government, through the Center for Devices and Radiological Health (CDRH) has established regulations for the design and manufacture of x-ray equipment. Thus both the equipment and its use are regulated. Federal and state agencies conduct inspections to check compliance with the regulations.

Current (1987, 1993) recommendations from the NCRP are given in Box 1-3. These are usually adopted by state and federal agencies.

---

**BOX 1-3**    **Maximum Permissible Doses (MPD)**

The yearly maximum permissible doses for radiation workers, from occupational exposure are as follows:

1. *Whole body:* 0.05 Sv (5 rem), with a limit equal to age × 10 mSv (1 rem), i.e., an average of 10 mSv/yr (1 rem/yr)
2. *Lens of eye:* 0.15 Sv (15 rem)
3. *All other organs:* 0.5 Sv (50 rem)

---

Note that these limits do not include exposure to background radiation or any exposure while undergoing diagnostic or therapy procedures. Also, doses from internal exposure through inhalation or ingestion are at present treated separately, whereas the limits given in Box 1-3 include internal and external exposure.

The NCRP states that its average annual occupational dose limit of 10 mSv/yr results in a cumulative lifetime risk of between $10^{-4}$ and $10^{-3}$ from each year's exposure. However, the cumulative lifetime risk to an average radiation worker is estimated to be between $2 \times 10^{-5}$ and $2 \times 10^{-4}$ for each year.

The MPD for the general public is 5 mSv (500 mrem) per year for infrequent exposure, and 1 mSv (100 mrem) per year, if exposure is on a regular basis. The limit for the lens of the eye is 15 mSv (1500 mrem), and for skin, hands, and feet it is 50 mSv (5000 mrem).

Minors—that is, individuals under 18 years—should be restricted to an annual effective dose less than 1 mSv (100 mrem), an annual dose equivalent of less than 15 mSv (1500 mrem) to the lens of the eye and less than 50 mSv (500 mrem) to the skin, hands, and feet.

In view of the increased sensitivity of the fetus, it is recommended that if a radiation worker declares her pregnancy, the exposure to the fetus not exceed 0.5 mSv (50 mrem) per month. The NCRP (1993) estimates a risk of $1.0 \times 10^{-1}$/Sv for fatal cancers following fetal exposure. For exposures from lower extremity–specific x-ray units, even if the mother were exposed to the maximum permissible dose of 50 mSv/yr, the fetal dose should not exceed 0.5 mSv per month provided exposure was at a reasonably uniform rate during the pregnancy. This is because of the shielding provided to the fetus by the intervening abdominal tissue.

### Ten-Day Rule

The increased sensitivity of the fetus has also led to what is called the *Ten-Day Rule*. It has been suggested that radiological procedures, on women of childbearing age, involving the abdomen and the pelvis, where there is potential for increased exposure to the fetus, should be performed only during the first 10 days following the onset of menstruation.

## How to Protect Oneself From Radiation

There are three ways by which one can protect oneself from radiation: (1) time, (2) distance, and (3) shielding.

### Time

The less time one spends in a radiation area, the less exposure one will receive. The dose is directly proportional to the time in the radiation area.

## Distance

Radiation exposure falls off inversely as the distance squared. For example, if at 1 meter the exposure is 4 mR/h, then at 2 meters the exposure will be 1 mR/h.

## Shielding

Any material interspersed between a source of radiation and an individual could protect that individual from radiation. The effectiveness of the shielding material depends on the type and energy of the radiation and the type and thickness of the shielding material. For example, the layer of dead cells on the skin provides 100% protection from the low-energy beta particles emitted by tritium ($^3$H), and a lead apron (0.5-mm Pb-equivalent) cuts off about 95% of the low kVp (below about 70 kVp) x rays in a diagnostic x-ray department or from a lower extremity–specific x-ray unit, but it is ineffective when working with high-energy x rays.

Because of the preceding calculations, to achieve maximum protection only essential people should be present when x-ray exposures are being made. These individuals should wear appropriate protective clothing and stay as far as possible from the source of radiation.

## Room Shielding

In its Report No. 49 (1976) and its adjunct report, the NCRP establishes criteria for structural shielding design of rooms or areas where radiation is used. Technique factors (kVp, mAs), amount of usage, location of the x-ray unit, and occupancy of surrounding areas determine the amount of shielding required. For most podiatric installations, minimal shielding is required. It is essential that a radiation survey be conducted after the equipment and shielding have been set up, to determine compliance with regulations.

## Principles of Radiation Protection: As Low As Reasonably Achievable (ALARA), Below Regulatory Concern (BRC) or De Minimus, and Hormesis

There are three different schools of thought regarding radiation protection, as follows.

### ALARA

Federal and state regulatory agencies require that all radiation users today operate under the as low as reasonably achievable (ALARA) principle. The objective is to ensure that exposure to radiation, of the user and of other individuals, is kept as low as is reasonably achievable. This is because of stochastic effects, particularly cancer. Any discussion of ALARA has to include a risk–benefit analysis. However, not only is it not always possible to make value judgments about the costs of the risks and benefits involved, but very often the benefits accrue to one group, whereas the risks are borne by another group. What is even more pathetic, is that even reasonable people don't always agree as to what is reasonable! Despite that, ALARA is the law of the land.

### De Minimus or Below Regulatory Concern (BRC)

Natural background radiation levels vary substantially. Few people would think twice about living in or moving to Denver, Colorado, because of the 0.5 mSv (50 mrem) extra exposure there per year, nor would most people give up traveling by air because of the extra 0.002 mSv (0.2 mrem) exposure for each hour of flight. Even more interestingly, no positive correlation has been found between high background radiation levels and incidence of cancer or other ill effects. In fact, some studies indicate that areas of high radiation levels may have lower incidence of cancer and of other ill effects.

Therefore, it has been suggested that regulatory agencies should not be concerned with levels of radiation below a certain level—the so-called de minimus or below regulatory concern (BRC) level. It has been recommended that the BRC level should be set within the range of variation of natural background radiation or, at least, at about 0.1 mSv/yr (10 mrem/yr). The Nuclear Regulatory Commission (NRC) attempted to apply this principle, but some groups raised a hue and cry and Congress advised the NRC to shelve the idea for the time being.

The NCRP considers a risk of $10^{-7}$ per year as a negligible individual risk level (NIRL) and the corresponding annual effective dose of 0.01 mSv (1 mrem) as a negligible individual dose (NID) for each source or practice.

### Hormesis

It is sad that there is more than one side to everything. It is sad because that makes life miserable to those who feel compelled to straddle the fence. Things are not always what they seem, nor are they always black or white. The same may be true of radiation. Contrary to prevailing opinion, some people believe that radiation may have hormetic (stimulatory or beneficial) effects.

Some studies indicate that people living in high-radiation areas have a lower incidence of cancer. Also, some experiments in animals and plants indicate that small amounts of radiation may extend the life span and have other stimulatory effects, particularly on the immune system. This is consistent with the observation of pharmacologists that certain substances, such as trace elements, are essential for survival at low concentrations, but are detrimental to health at high concentrations. So don't be surprised if in the not-too-distant future, the maximum permissible dose (MPD) of radiation is replaced by the recommended daily allowance (RDA) of radiation.

## ▇ CRITIQUE

The physics of radiation is well understood and not controversial. Much is known about how to obtain excellent diagnostic images with considerably less exposure to patient and technologist than was the case a decade ago. What is required is the establishment of a good quality assurance program and a commitment by the user of radiation to that program. The biological effects of radiation have been studied in great detail. Unfortunately, there is much controversy about the effects of low doses of radiation, particularly when exposure is spread over several years at low dose rates. This is because there is nothing distinctive about the biological damage, including cancer, caused by radiation. Any number of other factors can and do cause the same effects, and because several years may elapse between an exposure to radiation and the observed effect, any cause–effect relationship becomes tenuous, at best.

If the field of biological effects of low doses and of low dose rates is controversial, the field of radiation protection is a minefield, where nevertheless many have dared to set foot. The interpretation of what little scientific data there are is mired in the quagmire of pseudoscience. Obsession with wanting to be politically correct often determines what is permitted and what is prohibited. Mark Twain, with his own inimitable wit, once remarked, "There is something fascinating about science. One gets such wholesale returns of conjecture from such a trifling investment of fact."

Imbibing *BEIR I* may have whetted our appetite for information on the risks of radiation. *BEIR II, III,* and *IV* may have got us intoxicated, and *BEIR V* may have quenched our thirst for knowledge. Even then, I am confident many more committees will be set up in the future to deal with this issue. But I am not sure how many years it will be before we are set free of this crisis.

---

### Suggested Readings

*Radiation Physics*

Curry III TS, Dowdey JE, Murry Jr. RC: *Christensen's physics of diagnostic radiology,* ed 4, Philadelphia, 1990, Lea & Febiger.

Johns HE, Cunningham JR: *The physics of radiology,* ed 4, Springfield, Ill. 1983, Charles C Thomas.

*Radiation Biology*

Hall EJ: *Radiobiology for the radiologist,* ed 2, Hagerstown, Md, 1978, Harper & Row.

Pizzarello DJ: *Radiation biology,* Boca Raton, Fla, 1982, CRC Press.

National Council on Radiation Protection and Measurements:

NCRP Report Nos. 49 (1976), 53 & 54 (1977), 82 (1985), 91, 93, 94, & 95 (1987), 99 (1988), 100 & 101 (1989), 116 (1993), and NCRP Statement No. 7 (1992). NCRP Publications, Bethesda, Md.

*Radiation Protection\**

Shapiro J: *Radiation protection,* Cambridge, Mass, 1972, Harvard University Press.

Shleien B: *The health physics and radiological health handbook,* rev. ed., Silver Spring, Md, 1992, Scinta.

U.S. National Academy of Sciences: *Biological Effects of Ionizing Radiations (BEIR) Committee reports I through v.* Washington, DC, National Academy Press.

---

\*Individual states have rules and regulations with which users of lower extremity–specific x-ray units must comply.

# CHAPTER 2

# Radiography Equipment Considerations and Accessories

ROBERT A. CHRISTMAN • MARY OEHLER

Foot and ankle radiographic studies are performed with a variety of x-ray units, from general-purpose high-voltage units to wall-mounted modified dental x-ray machines. Lower extremity–specific units are available for foot and ankle radiography and are especially useful for weight-bearing pedal studies. The advantages and disadvantages of these units will be discussed, as will other considerations for selecting an extremity x-ray unit. In addition, positioning devices and aids, film and screens, darkroom and processing equipment, film identification devices, and other miscellaneous accessories for lower extremity application will be discussed.

## ■ LOWER EXTREMITY–SPECIFIC X-RAY UNITS

Diagnostic lower extremity–specific x-ray units are available either from dealers or directly from the manufacturer. All are shockproof and plug into a standard 110-volt outlet. The kilovoltage (kVp), milliamperage (mA), and source-to-image distance (SID) may either be fixed or variable. Three types of lower extremity x-ray units are available: stationary, wall mounted, and mobile.

The stationary lower extremity x-ray unit (Figure 2-1) is connected to a platform known as an orthoposer (described under the section heading "Positioning Equipment and Aids"). The tubehead is attached to the orthoposer by an arm or track and has a fixed SID. The fixed SID aids in preventing technical errors that can result in poor-quality films; repeat studies increase radiation exposure to the patient. The stationary unit is ideal for performing weight-bearing studies. The disadvantage of this unit is that non–weight-bearing studies may be difficult to perform;

they occasionally require awkward positioning of the patient who is seated in a chair. Non–weight-bearing antero-posterior and oblique ankle studies may be impossible to perform unless the patient stands on the platform. This poses a safety hazard to some patients, especially those with limited mobility, impaired balance, or muscle weakness.[1]

Two types of wall-mounted x-ray units are available: One has the tubehead secured to a flexible arm that extends from the wall; in the second, the tubehead is attached to a pulleylike device with a counterbalance and slides up or down along a track attached to the wall.

The flexible arm unit (Figure 2-2) can be used with either an orthoposer or an examination/radiographic table or chair, depending on the height it is mounted on the wall. A unit that is mounted for primary use with an orthoposer could possibly perform non–weight-bearing studies on a low examination/radiographic table or chair. However, the SID may be significantly reduced in the latter case, so this practice is not recommended. The length that the arm extends from the wall varies, depending on the unit selected. Some have short arms; others long arms. The arms of all units fold compactly against the wall.

Another variable is the size of tubehead used with the flexible arm unit. The larger, heavier tubehead has an mA of 10 or greater, and the smaller tubehead (typically a modified dental unit) is less than 10 mA. Flexible arm units with the larger tubehead are awkward to position; the arm design is not as flexible as that of the unit with a smaller tubehead. Also, the arm with a larger tubehead occasionally must be adjusted so the tubehead doesn't drift from the desired position. Although the unit with a lighter tubehead is more flexible, it operates at a lower mA setting and therefore requires a shorter SID or longer exposure time to obtain the same film density as do the higher mA units.

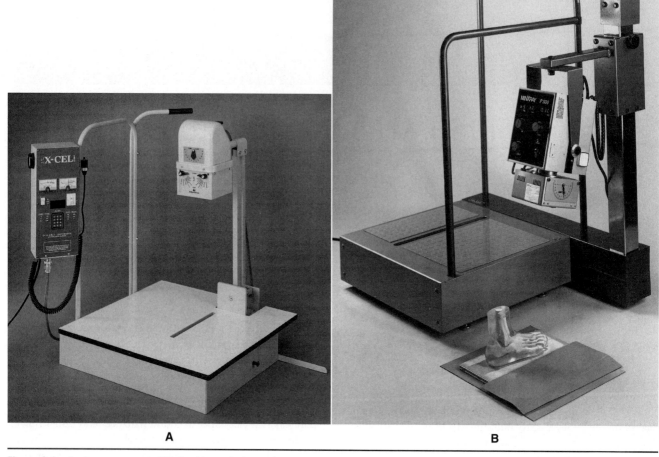

**A**                                                                 **B**

Figure 2-1    Stationary x-ray unit. Tubehead is attached to orthoposer at a fixed source-to-image distance. (**A**, Courtesy X-Cel X-Ray Corp., Crystal Lake, Ill; **B**, courtesy MinXray Inc., Northbrook, Ill.)

A disadvantage of all wall-mounted flexible arm units is the variable source-to-image distance. A measuring device, either a measuring tape or a telescoping antenna-like device, must be attached to the tubehead to determine the SID. (If a measuring device is not provided as original equipment, ask the manufacturer to supply one.) Positioning of the tubehead with the flexible arm unit is not a simple task compared to positioning the stationary units with fixed SID. Inconstant SID will have a profound effect on the quality of the final image if other technical factors are not calculated and adjusted accordingly.

The sliding wall-mounted x-ray unit is mounted to the wall and floor (Figure 2-3). It functions differently from the flexible arm unit: The tubehead slides along a track by means of a pulley and counterbalance mechanism. The arm of this unit is directed perpendicular to the track and wall. It pivots and, with the tubehead, can be turned toward the wall when not in use. The tubehead can be easily positioned at a predetermined SID by moving it along the track. This unit

can be used with an orthoposer or an examination/radiographic table or chair, but either must be positioned adjacent to the wall and in line with the tubehead.

Wall-mounted units must be securely installed. This is especially important for flexible arm units with a larger tubehead. Many dealers, as well as manufacturer representatives, will either assist in or recommend proper installation of a unit. If the unit is not properly installed, it will tear off the wall, damage the tubehead (if it hits the floor), and possibly injure the patient or radiographer.

The mobile x-ray unit (Figure 2-4) has a stand with wheels. The tubehead is attached to either a flexible arm or sliding track with counterbalance. They are essentially the same units as just described except they are mounted to a movable stand instead of a wall or an orthoposer. Mobile units can be moved easily from room to room. However, the wheels must lock to prevent movement during the exposure. Also, a measuring device must be attached to the tubehead to determine the source-to-image distance. Mobile units

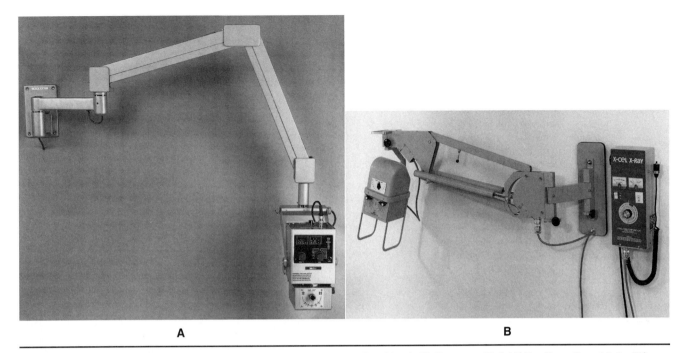

A          B

Figure 2-2    Flexible arm wall-mounted x-ray unit. (**A**, Courtesy MinXray Inc., Northbrook, Ill.; **B**, courtesy X-Cel X-Ray Corp., Crystal Lake, Ill.)

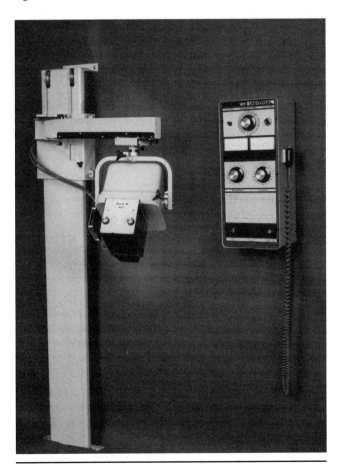

Figure 2-3    Sliding wall-mounted x-ray unit. (Courtesy Universal Imaging, Inc., Chicago Ill.)

can be used in conjunction with an orthoposer, an examination/radiographic table or chair, or both, depending on the design of the mobile unit. Appropriate radiation protection and safety procedures should be followed, because the unit is typically used in rooms not specifically designed for radiographic studies. A portable lead-shielded barrier, also on wheels, can be purchased and used by the operator and other personnel in the same room (Figure 2-5).

The lower extremity x-ray unit has the following components: tubehead, beam limitation device, arm, and control panel. Each will be discussed in turn. This discussion is followed by a guideline for selecting an x-ray unit.

## Tubehead

The housing for the x-ray tube has a lead lining and is filled with oil. The housing and the oil absorb off-focus or leakage radiation that does not contribute to the useful x-ray beam. This is known as inherent filtration. Another function of the oil is to disperse heat that is generated by the production of x rays from the tube.

The x-ray tube is a vacuum tube; its components are sealed within a glass envelope. The main components of the x-ray tube are the cathode and the anode (Figure 2-6).

The cathode is the negative electrode of the x-ray tube; it consists of a filament and a focusing cup. The filament heats up and glows similar to a light bulb filament. However, instead of producing light, the cathode filament produces electrons. The filament is usually made of tungsten and, because of its high melting point, will not melt at high

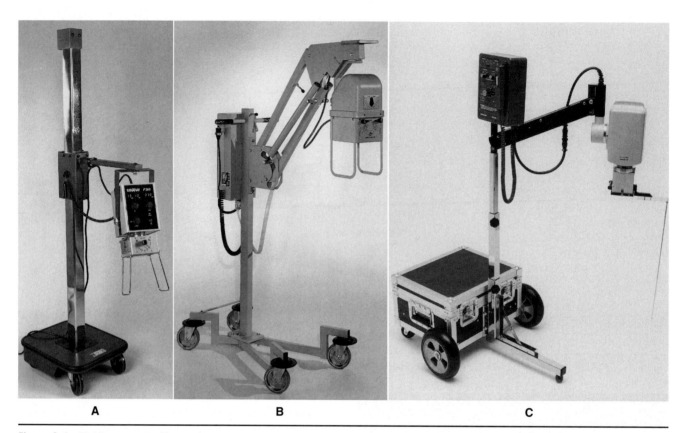

**A**            **B**            **C**

Figure 2-4   Mobile x-ray units. Freestanding units that may or may not be "packed away." (**A**, Courtesy MinXray Inc., Northbrook, Ill; **B**, courtesy X-Cel X-Ray Corp., Crystal Lake, Ill; **C**, courtesy M-DEC, Bellevue, Wash.)

temperatures under normal circumstances. The electrons that are emitted by the filament are then directed toward the anode by the focusing cup. The tube current, or the number of electrons produced by the cathode, is determined by the temperature of the filament and is measured in milliamperes (mA).[2]

The anode is the positive electrode of the x-ray tube. Electrons produced at the cathode are directed toward a small tungsten target on the anode. The area on the target from which x rays are emitted is known as the focal spot. The focal spot of lower extremity x-ray units is approximately 1 mm. Because a large amount of heat is generated by this bombardment of electrons and subsequent formation of x rays, the anode (except for the target) is made of copper for efficient heat dissipation.

Anodes can either be stationary or rotating. General-purpose x-ray units operate at high tube currents (up to 1200 mA) and produce excessive amounts of heat at the target. The targets of these particular units are therefore located on a disk that rotates at a high rate. Heat can then be transferred across a larger surface area, thereby reducing the chance of damage to the tungsten target. In contrast, lower extremity–specific x-ray units operate at low tube currents (between 7 and 30 mA). Therefore, the targets of

these units are attached to a less expensive fixed, or stationary, anode.

An aluminum filter is located in the path of the primary (useful) x-ray beam after it exits from the tube. This is known as added filtration. Its function is to absorb the low-energy x-ray photons that would otherwise be absorbed by the subject. It does not alter the quality of the radiographic image. Lower extremity x-ray units typically are supplied with 2.0- to 2.5-mm aluminum filters, meeting or exceeding the required total filtration for machines operating between 50 and 70 kVp. Occasionally an yttrium filter may be used in place of aluminum.

## Beam Limitation Device

Beam limitation devices shape the dimensions of the x-ray beam, exiting the tubehead so that only the area of interest is exposed to radiation. This process, known as collimation, also regulates scatter radiation that can fog the film or be absorbed by the patient. At the very least, the primary beam must be restricted to no more than the size of the x-ray film being exposed. Beam-limiting devices (collimators) come in three basic formats: cone, diaphragm, and variable aperture.

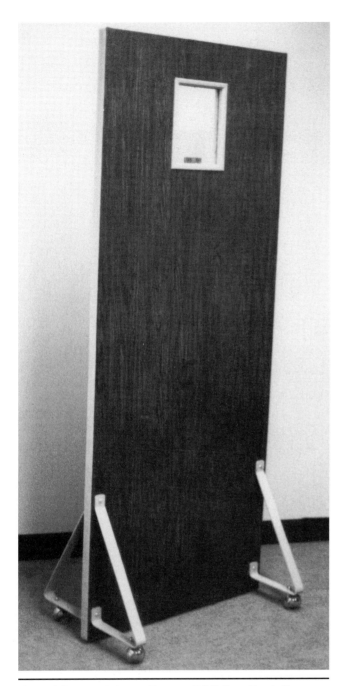

Figure 2-5    Portable barrier. (Courtesy Gill Podiatry Supply Co., Middleburg Heights, Ohio.)

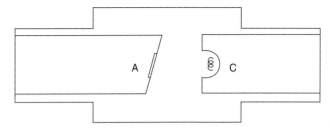

Figure 2-6    Components of an x-ray tube. Stationary anode *(A)*, cathode *(C)*.

flat sheets of lead or lead-lined metal with either circular, square, or rectangular openings. These are the simplest of all beam-limiting devices and are commonly used in combination with cones and variable-aperture collimators.

The opening in the aperture diaphragm must correspond to the size of the x-ray film in use or, more appropriately, to the area in question. For example, an aperture diaphragm made for 10- × 12-inch or smaller films must be used with a 10- × 12-inch x-ray film. However, if only a portion of the x-ray film is going to be exposed, such as when dividing the x-ray film into halves for individual foot exposures, a 5- × 12-inch aperture diaphragm should be used. Proper collimation of the x-ray beam will reduce scatter radiation; scatter radiation increases the patient radiation exposure and can impair the quality of the image on the film. Appropriately sized aperture diaphragms are available for exposure of even smaller areas, such as the toes. The manufacturer of applicable units includes interchangeable aperture diaphragms of different sizes as standard equipment or can be requested (Figure 2-8). Diaphragms that specify an exposure field (5 × 12 inches, for example) are accurate only at a predetermined SID. If the SID is changed, the field size denoted on the diaphragm will be inaccurate.

Diaphragm and variable-aperture collimators use a light source that defines the field of the x-ray beam, hence the name *light beam collimator*. Depressing a small button activates the light source that remains on for a preset period of time. The tubehead can then be positioned so that the x-ray beam is directed to the area in question. The area lit by the light source correlates to the area that will be exposed by the x-ray beam. The center of the light source is marked with crosshairs or a "bull's-eye" so that the central beam is accurately positioned.

Limiting the size of the x-ray beam is most easily and accurately accomplished with a variable-aperture collimator (Figure 2-9). The size of the x-ray beam is controlled by adjusting shutters, much like those of a photographic camera. Variable-aperture collimators made for lower extremity x-ray units usually consist of two sets of shutters or plates, oriented at 90 degrees to one another, and are controlled by two knobs. A light source projects onto the

Cones are primarily found on dental x-ray units. They come in various shapes and sizes and are made of metal or plastic. To reduce radiation exposure to the patient, plastic cones are lead lined. Some dental x-ray units can be modified for extremity use by adding a specially designed beam-limiting device (Figure 2-7).

Diaphragms, also known as aperture diaphragms, are provided with some lower extremity x-ray units. They are

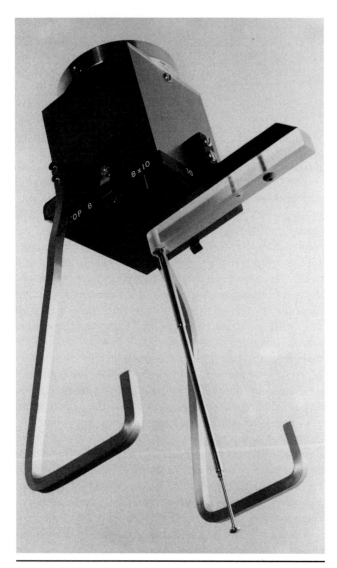

Figure 2-7    Beam-limiting device available to adapt dental units for lower extremity use. (Courtesy Margraf Corporation, Jenkintown, Pa.)

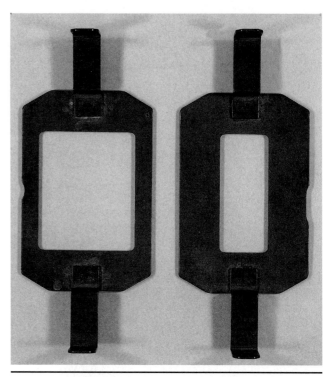

Figure 2-8    Diaphragm apertures.

patient so the operator can adjust the aperture size and direct the x-ray beam over the body part of interest. Variable-aperture collimators are standard equipment on most new lower extremity x-ray units. They are strongly recommended for use on all lower extremity units, if available.

## Arm

The arm's function is to hold the tubehead firmly in place. Any movement of the tubehead during the exposure could impair the quality of the final image. The arm or tubehead is never to be held in position by the patient.

Depending on the type of x-ray unit one owns or operates, the arm may originate from a plate or track

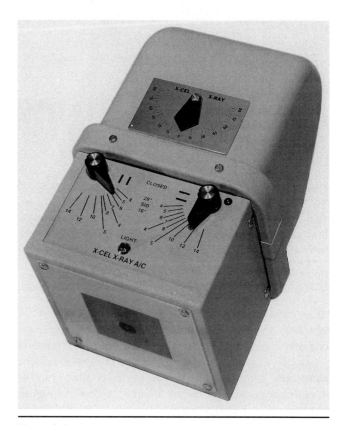

Figure 2-9    Variable-aperture collimator. (Courtesy X-Cel X-Ray Corp., Crystal Lake, Ill.)

attached to the wall, from an orthoposer, or from a mobile stand (see Figures 2-1, 2-2, 2-3, and 2-4). Arms that originate from an orthoposer are convenient to use because the distance between the x-ray tube and the subject is fixed. In contrast, this distance must be determined manually when using a mobile or wall-mounted unit. The latter case is prone to technical errors that can impair the quality of the final image. However, many of these units are equipped with either a measuring tape or a telescoping antenna-like device for determining the x-ray source-to-image distance. On mobile or wall-mounted x-ray units that do not come equipped with a measuring device as standard equipment, contact the manufacturer. Many states, if not all, require that units be equipped with a measuring device. The manufacturer may supply one at no charge.

## Control Panel

The x-ray unit's control panel can either be a separate box that is located inside or outside the x-ray room (see Figures 2-1, *A*, and 2-3), or it may be incorporated as part of the tubehead itself (see Figure 2-4). Three factors can be under the radiographer's control: milliamperage, kilovoltage, and time.

Milliamperage, or mA, represents the x-ray tube current. This is a measure of the number (quantity) of electrons that travel between the cathode and anode. As noted previously, the mA of lower extremity x-ray units is quite low, between 7 and 30 mA. Some units do not have optional tube currents and are preset at the factory. If a choice is available, select the highest mA offered (see section on mAs).

Kilovoltage peak, or kVp, is a unit of electric potential and relates to the energy (quality) of the x-ray beam. A kVp between 55 and 65 is typically used for most foot and ankle applications. One can select between 50 and 70 kVp on most lower extremity x-ray units; higher kVp units (up to 90) are also available. The kVp, if not fixed, can be adjusted by the turn of a knob. Some machines don't specify the actual kVp or mA value on the unit itself. Letters may identify predetermined techniques instead. Check with the manual or manufacturer to obtain the specifications.

A timer controls the length of exposure. A wide array of timer values can be selected, ranging from seconds to fractions of a second. The time selected (assuming that the mA is fixed) is dependent on the type of x-ray film used and whether or not intensifying screens are used. Timers may either be mechanical, synchronous, or electronic in nature.

The exposure switch is attached to the control panel by a long, coiled cord. It allows the operator to stand a minimum of 6 feet away from the x-ray source. The exposure button operates as a deadman's switch; the exposure only occurs as the button is depressed and will shut off at the selected time or if the button is released, whichever occurs first.

## Selecting a Lower Extremity X-Ray Unit

The style of lower extremity x-ray unit chosen will depend on personal preferences and room requirements. The ideal unit would be one that allows the radiographer to perform both weight-bearing and non–weight-bearing extremity studies with ease. This obviously requires two units in one. Stationary units are best for performing weight-bearing studies, but are quite limited and unsafe for performing some non–weight-bearing studies. Weight-bearing and non–weight-bearing studies can be performed with some flexible arm wall-mounted units by using an orthoposer and examination/radiographic table or chair, respectively. However, the SID may be significantly shortened for studies performed on a table or chair if the unit is mounted at the appropriate SID for an orthoposer. Also, flexible arm units with a large tubehead are not as easy to maneuver and position as other units. In contrast, the mA of flexible arm units with a smaller tubehead (modified dental x-ray units) is barely sufficient; long exposure times and/or shortened SIDs are necessary when using a similar film/screen combination as compared to higher mA units. A unit with a tubehead that slides along a long track offers the best of both worlds: Studies can be performed with both an examination/radiographic table and an orthoposer at an acceptable SID and with relative ease. A long sliding-track mechanism can be found on some wall-mounted and mobile units. Unfortunately, their availability is limited.

Another factor to consider that was briefly mentioned earlier is a unit's ease of use. It is strongly recommended that the radiographer try out different units before a purchase decision is made. Also, speak to radiographers and practitioners at offices or facilities that use lower extremity–specific x-ray units. They should best be able to explain the advantages and disadvantages of a particular unit.

After narrowing your selection to one type of radiography unit, whether mobile, wall mounted, or stationary, it is important to select a unit that has an appropriate focal spot size, mA, SID, kVp, and timer. All units are not created equal. Seriously consider purchasing a unit that meets the following recommendations:

1. *Smaller focal spot size.* Most lower extremity x-ray units have a focal spot approximating 1 mm. Avoid units with a larger focal-spot size. The larger the focal spot, the more geometric blurring of the image.
2. *Higher mA.* Although the cost of equipment increases with higher mA x-ray units, the advantage will be the use of shorter exposure time (assuming all other factors remain the same). Decreased exposure time can potentially improve image quality; patient movement, when present, will result in blurring of the image at longer exposure times. A misconception is that the use of higher mA with lower extremity units will result in

shortened tube life. This effect is negligible with the range available on lower extremity units. Furthermore, lowering the mA using the same film/screen combination will result in having to increase the time of exposure proportionately (mAs = mA × s). Therefore, the same number of electrons will still have to be produced by the x-ray tube. When using a lower extremity x-ray unit with varying mA selectivity, simply select the mA that is highest. (Be sure to adjust exposure time accordingly if all other factors remain unchanged.) The exception would be if a unit's mA selection is directly linked to the kVp setting. If so, select the highest available mA at a reasonable kVp. Some manufacturers compensate for a lower mA by reducing the source-to-image distance. Although this may reduce the exposure time for any particular study, a shorter SID will result in greater geometric blurring of the final image.

3. *Appropriate source-to-image distance.* A 40-inch source-to-image distance is commonly used for examination of extremities with general purpose x-ray units. These units typically operate at mA values much higher than that available with a lower extremity x-ray unit. The latter is affordable to the individual practitioner because of their lower tube current. However, to keep exposure time down and reduce the potential for blurring due to patient movement, the SID is shortened. The SID for lower extremity x-ray units is typically between 21 and 28 inches. Considered separately, a longer SID produces less geometric blurring than a shorter SID and, therefore, a sharper image. There is a tradeoff, however; a longer SID requires increased mAs to obtain a film of similar density.

4. *Appropriate kVp.* Because most exposures of the foot or ankle are best performed at a kVp between 55 and 65, select a unit that meets this need. Although higher kVp technique can reduce the overall exposure to the patient, subject contrast is sacrificed in the resultant image. Therefore, avoid selecting an x-ray unit that limits the kVp selection between 70 and 90. Other methods are available for reducing patient exposure dose, such as using a rare-earth intensifying screen/film system (described under the section heading Radiographic Film, Screens, and Cassettes) and practicing proper collimation.

5. *Synchronous or electronic timer.* Lower extremity x-ray units come equipped with either mechanical, synchronous, or electronic timers. Mechanical timers are not only the least accurate of the three, but cannot be set to times much less than one quarter second. Use of rare-earth film/screen combinations often requires setting the exposure time to a shorter period. Synchronous timers are frequently used; they are more

accurate than mechanical timers and can be set as low as one sixtieth of a second. Electronic timers are the most accurate of the three timers, to 1/100th of a second. The typical exposure range for foot and ankle studies using a high-detail rare-earth film/two-screen system at 15 mA, 62 kVp, and a 28-inch SID is between 12/60ths of a second and 1 second.

## X-Ray Equipment Quality Control

All newly acquired x-ray units should be tested before use. This examination is referred to as an acceptance test and should not be performed by a manufacturer representative but by someone else.[3] In addition, an x-ray unit should routinely be evaluated periodically (ideally every year) to assess its performance. Parameters tested include the kVp calibration, mA linearity, exposure timer accuracy, collimation alignment, effective focal-spot size, exposure reproducibility, and filtration (half-value layer). Any deviation from the norm must be corrected. Records should be kept regarding the results of these tests and any corrections made.

## Extremity Fluoroscopy Equipment

Compact real-time fluoroscopic units are available for evaluating the extremities (Figure 2-10). They use either a radioisotope (iodine-125) for the radiation source or a low-output x-ray tube. Units equipped with a radioisotope energy source must be registered with and licensed by the Nuclear Regulatory Commission. They must also be certified semiannually against leakage. The energy source is expensive and is replaced periodically. Some extremity fluoroscopic units are portable, hand-held units that can be used away from the office.

The fluoroscopic imaging screen is quite small (2 to 3 inches in diameter), but most units can be connected to a larger video monitor. "Spot" image hard copies can be obtained if the unit is so equipped. Another option may include radiographic capability. Compact real-time fluoroscopic units have been used primarily as an adjunct to foot surgery.[4,5] Other applications include identification and localization of foreign bodies and fractures and as an adjunct to performing contrast examinations (arthrography and tenography, for example).[6,7]

## ■ POSITIONING EQUIPMENT AND AIDS

### Orthoposer

An orthoposer is a platform designed for weight-bearing radiographic studies of the foot and ankle. It is built to support the weight of a patient. The platform height is typically 6 to 8 inches. The x-ray film can be placed either

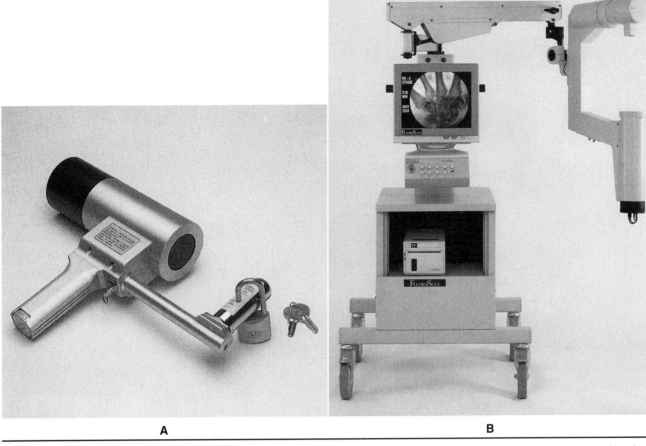

| A | B |

**Figure 2-10**    Compact real-time fluoroscopic units. (**A**, Courtesy Lixi, Inc., Downers Grove, Ill; **B**, Courtesy Dow Corning Wright, Arlington, Tenn.)

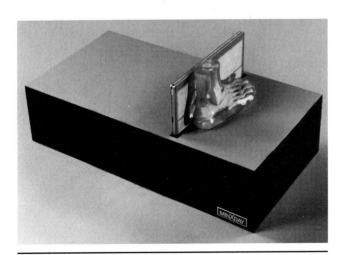

**Figure 2-11**    Orthoposer unit. (Courtesy MinXray Inc., Northbrook, Ill.)

flat (horizontal) on the orthoposer or vertical in a well, depending on which positioning technique is performed. Both the platform and well are lined with lead. Cassettes of 8- × 10-inch and 10- × 12-inch sizes fit into the well. The tube housing may be fixed to the orthoposer by an arm at a fixed SID, as noted previously (see Figure 2-1). A free-standing orthoposer (Figure 2-11) can be used with either a mobile or wall-mounted x-ray unit.

The orthoposer-mounted x-ray unit has handrails attached to it for patient safety. Freestanding orthoposers, however, may not have any patient support rails. In the latter case, the orthoposer should be placed adjacent to a wall, preferably near a corner at two intersecting walls. Handrails must be firmly mounted to these walls to ensure patient safety. Furthermore, handrails will help the patient feel safe, reducing imbalance and subsequent movement during the x-ray exposure.

## Podium

Weight-bearing radiographic studies of the foot or ankle cannot be safely performed on radiographic tables with general-purpose x-ray units found in hospitals and imaging centers. However, a platform, called the podium, has been designed by a medical center facility for use with suspended-head x-ray units[8] (Figure 2-12). The podium is similar to an

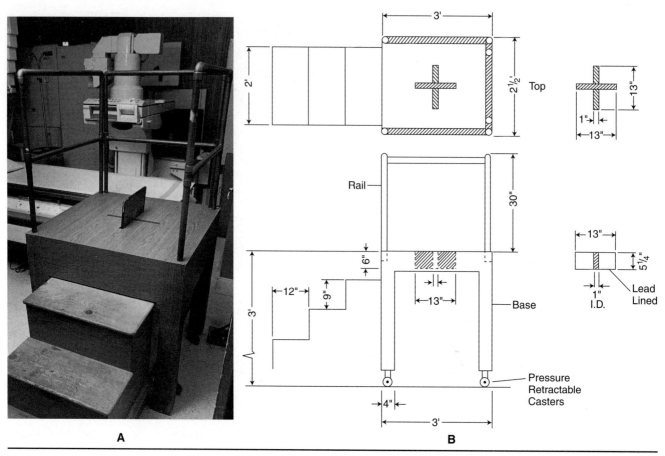

Figure 2-12    **A**, Podium; **B**, design specifications. (**A**, Courtesy St. Michael's Medical Center, NJ; **B**, from Estersohn HS, Wolf KL, Day JC: *J Am Podiatr Med Assoc* 71:222, 1981.)

orthoposer in construction; it has slots for positioning the cassette vertically during lateral positioning techniques. The podium is raised off the ground and is level with the radiographic table; the patient must climb steps to access the platform. Rails are attached along three of the four sides for patient support and safety. Casters are found along the bottom of both the steps and podium for storage. (The steps roll under the podium.)

## Cassette Holder

A cassette holder can be used to perform non–weight-bearing studies on a stretcher, examination bench, treatment chair, or operating table. It holds a cassette vertically for radiographic exposure, and has clamps to accommodate any size cassette (Figure 2-13). The cassette holder is especially useful for performing radiographic studies of a patient confined to a wheelchair. Another application is for performance of weight-bearing ankle or knee studies.

## Positioning Blocks

Positioning blocks or wedges are useful aids to position the foot or ankle for non–weight-bearing oblique techniques. They are made of a radiolucent material and are resilient, firm, durable, and washable. Positioning blocks will not slip when positioned properly under the patient. Wedges are available in a variety of shapes and sizes; a 45-degree triangular wedge accommodates most oblique positioning techniques.

## Sandbags

Motion unsharpness is a detrimental factor affecting radiographic quality. Sandbags provide a quick and safe means of immobilization. A sandbag is placed across or against the extremity, outside the area of interest. The sandbag is heavy enough to restrict and restrain the patient but not to cause harm. More than one sandbag may be needed to achieve the desired positioning and immobilization.

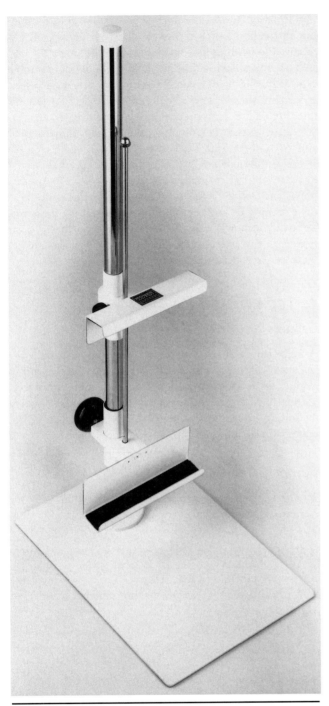

Figure 2-13    Cassette holder. (Courtesy Monee X-Ray Works, Monee, Ill.)

## Axial Sesamoid-Positioning Device

A device called the axial poser is valuable for performing a weight-bearing axial sesamoid-positioning technique. It is sold in pairs, for the left and right foot, and is made of radiolucent Styrofoam or plastic (Figure 2-14). The front and back of the device are angled superiorly to elevate the digits

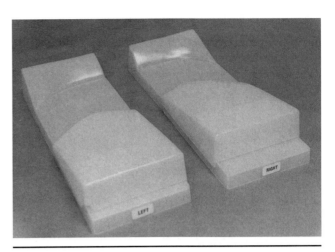

Figure 2-14    Sesamoid-positioning device. (Courtesy Gill Podiatry Supply Co., Middleburg Heights, Ohio.)

and rearfoot. This positioning causes the metatarsal heads to be positioned inferiorly relative to the remainder of the foot.

## Ankle-Specific Positioning Equipment

Ankle-specific positioning devices must be used on a radiographic table or bench that will safely support the unit and a recumbent patient. They cannot be used on an orthoposer. Also, the extremity does not have close contact with the cassette; the object-to-film distance is slightly increased compared to conventional positioning without the device. This results in slight magnification, and the image therefore may be less sharp. Three devices are available to assist in the performance of ankle studies, two for standard techniques and one for stress studies.

A device known as the Foot Fixator (AO Medical Products AB, Stockholm, Sweden) was developed to provide reproducible lower extremity studies (Figure 2-15). Although it is useful for ankle radiography, it cannot be used to image the foot. The foot rests on a radiolucent plate and is held in place by Velcro straps. A supporting cup holds the heel, and a smaller guide plate attaches along its medial border. The foot can be variably positioned in two planes, sagittal and transverse. The angle of the foot is easily adjusted, and values can be recorded for future reference if follow-up studies are performed.[9] The film cassette fits into guides along the bottom of the unit.

Another unit is the ALARM (Adjustable Leg and Ankle Positioning Mechanism) (M.C. Johnson Company, Leominster, Mass.). It was designed to provide positioning for lower leg and ankle studies. Foot studies can also be performed on the unit, although it is technically easier to perform them in the conventional manner without the device. It is composed of durable radiolucent plastic that can be disassembled for cleaning. The lower leg lies in a well for its entire length. The foot is secured onto a plate with a Velcro strap. The foot plate and leg can be rotated 45 degrees internally and externally; 13 degrees dorsiflexion and 30 degrees plantarflexion motions are also possible. The

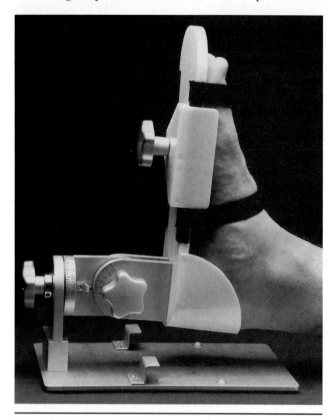

Figure 2-15   Ankle-positioning device, the Foot Fixator. (Courtesy AO Medical Products AB, Stockholm, Sweden.)

film is placed into a slot under or beside the ankle, depending on the positioning technique desired. The foot plate is removed to perform dorsoplantar foot projections.

The Telos ankle stress apparatus (Telos Corporation, Griesheim, Germany) is used to perform inversion, eversion, and lateral stress studies (Figure 2-16). It can also test the integrity of the dorsolateral calcaneocuboid ligament. The extremity is firmly held in place, and constant torque can be applied and measured so that the study is performed symmetrically bilaterally. Gradual application of the stress force minimizes pain and muscle guarding.[10] Another important feature of this unit: The examiner does not hold the extremity during the exposure and can leave the room. To avoid technical errors, care is necessary during positioning of the extremity in the Telos unit. The cassette lies on the table beneath the ankle.

### ◼ TECHNICAL AIDS

### Caliper

A caliper is a measuring device used to determine the thickness of the body part to be studied. A crossbar moves along a scale calibrated in both inches and centimeters (Figure 2-17). The dimensions are to be used with a technique chart to standardize technical factors for radiographic studies.

### Compensation Filter

The foot thickness is not the same in the forefoot as in the rearfoot. The film density of the dorsoplantar foot view,

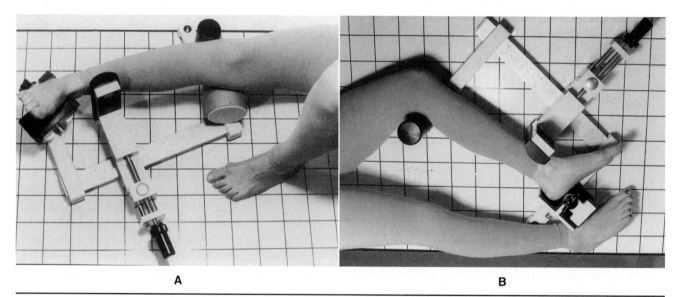

|    A    |    B    |

Figure 2-16   Ankle-positioning device, Telos ankle stress apparatus. **A**, Stress inversion test; **B**, lateral stress test. (Courtesy Austin & Associates, Inc., Fallston, Md.)

therefore, varies considerably between the toes and the tarsus. If a technique is selected to obtain an ideal film density for the toes, the tarsus will be underexposed (decreased film density) and unreadable. In contrast, a technique chosen to image the tarsus will overexpose the toes, which will appear dark (increased film density). A device known as a compensation filter compensates for the unequal subject thickness between the forefoot and rearfoot.[11,12] It is wedge shaped and made of a clear, lead-plastic material.

The compensation filter system has two components: a filter holder and the filter itself (Figure 2-18). The mounting plate is easily attached to most conventional collimators with two adhesive fasteners. The plate is made of radiolucent clear plastic and does not alter image quality. It can be left attached to the collimator permanently, or it can be easily removed and replaced again. Patient, film, and tubehead positioning and light beam collimation are performed before attaching the filter. The filter has two magnetic strips and is easily positioned onto the filter holder before exposure. Attention must be paid to initial installment of the filter holder and placement of the filter. The thick portion of the wedge must be positioned at the toe end of the light field so that the thinner portion of the wedge approaches the midfoot. To be certain the filter is positioned over the forefoot properly, light beam collimation should also be performed after attaching the filter. Technical factors should be the same as that used to image the tarsus. The radiographer must remember to remove the filter before performing other positioning techniques.

After use of the compensation filter, the toes are more visible and are a similar film density as the tarsus. But a word of caution: More attractive doesn't mean the image is as sharp as a film obtained without the filter. It is best to not use the filter if looking for subtle findings; a spot illuminator will suffice. Also, if the area of concern is limited to the digits, a collimated view of the toes alone is preferable; the adjustment of technical factors obviates the need for the compensation filter.

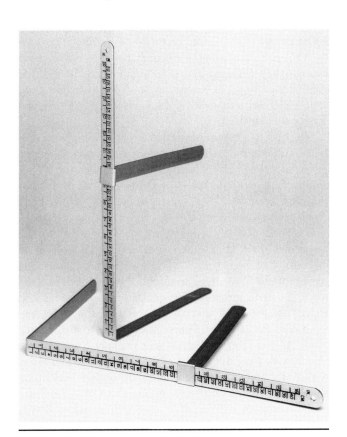

Figure 2-17   Thickness caliper. (Courtesy Providence Imaging Products, Inc., Providence, RI.)

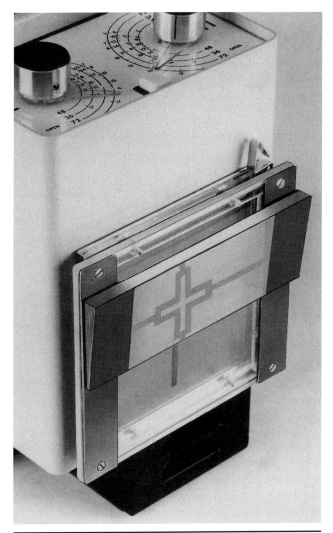

Figure 2-18   Compensation filter system. (Courtesy Nuclear Associates, Carle Place, NY.)

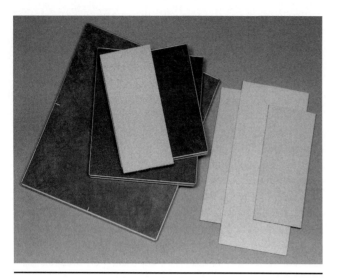

Figure 2-19    Lead blocker. (Courtesy Providence Imaging Products, Inc., Providence, RI.)

## Lead Blocker

A lead-impregnated, rubberized sheet is frequently used to divide a film in half for radiographic studies (Figure 2-19). It should not be used as a substitute for proper collimation.

## Technique Chart

A technique chart should be attached to the control panel of each x-ray unit. This chart can reduce the number of re-exposures resulting from improper technical factors and is required by many states. It should include the mA, kVp, and time of exposure for each positioning technique at the SID recommended by the unit's manufacturer. Also, your film vendor should be able to provide a technique chart for guidance.

## ■ PROTECTION AND SAFETY AIDS

### Radiation-Protective Clothing

During the radiographic study, the patient should wear radiation-protective clothing. Examples include the lead apron, diaper, and gonad shield. The radiographer, assistant, parent, or guardian must wear radiation-protective apparel if he or she must remain in the examination room during an exposure. To avoid damage to the protective lead lining, the apparel must be stored properly.

Personnel and patient protection apparel is designed for safety and comfort. Lead aprons (Figure 2-20) are available in numerous designs, sizes, shapes, and thicknesses. They are tied to the body by straps and fastened by buckle or Velcro closure. Also, back support and full-wrap aprons exist for special studies. Protective aprons come in both male and

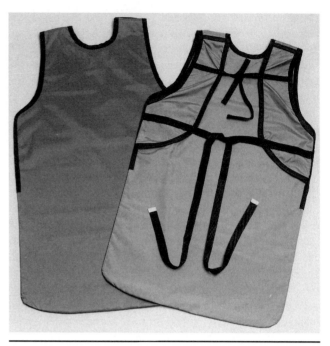

Figure 2-20    Lead protective clothing: apron. (Courtesy Providence Imaging Products, Inc., Providence, RI.)

female sizes, from small to extra large. It is important to choose the correct size to accommodate all staff members. At least two adult-size aprons should be available: one worn by the patient, and the second by the assistant or radiographer, if needed. A smaller apron should be available for children. Specific colors can be ordered so the apron coordinates with an office decor. Even monogrammed aprons are available.

The apron vinyl is impregnated with lead. An apron's lead equivalent thickness relates to its x-ray attenuation at a given kilovoltage (kVp) setting. For example, at 50 kVp, aprons with either a 0.25- or 0.50-mm lead equivalent thickness attenuate 97% or greater of the x rays. However, at 75 kVp the 0.25-mm lead equivalent thickness apron absorbs only 66% of the x-rays compared to 88% with the apron that offers a 0.50-mm lead equivalent thickness.[3]

Aprons of higher lead thickness are very heavy and uncomfortable if worn for an extended length of time. Keep in mind that an apron of 0.50-mm lead equivalent thickness weighs nearly twice that of an apron of 0.25-mm lead equivalent thickness (the latter can weigh anywhere between 3 to 10 pounds).[3] Geriatric patients may have extreme difficulty wearing the heavier apron, which presents a safety hazard for weight-bearing studies. A lighter lead apron should be available for these patients.

Lead aprons will crack if care is not taken during handling and storage, especially if aprons are folded. Radiation easily penetrates through the crack to the wearer. Always place a lead apron on an apron hanger between uses, to pre-

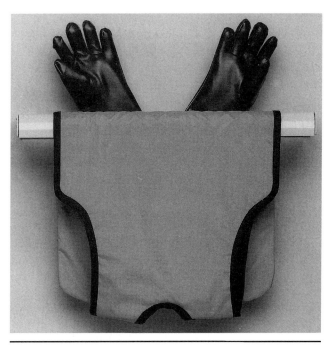

Figure 2-21    Apron and glove hanger. (Courtesy Providence Imaging Products, Inc., Providence, RI.)

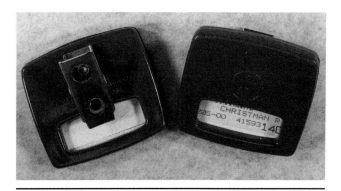

Figure 2-22    Film badge, showing clip on back.

vent damage to the radiation-protective material. Radiographs of all aprons should be made periodically to check for leaks. Records of such examinations should be kept on file.

A lead apron hanger functions like a coat hanger. It may be constructed of metal or wood and is designed to support a lead apron while hanging on a rack. The lead apron rack comes in two styles: It can either fully support a lead apron, or it will have prongs to hold an apron hanger. It may be wall mounted or mobile. A wall-mounted rack may need extra support if several aprons are to be stored on it. Another apron storage device is a bar or rail; the apron is draped over it (Figure 2-21). However, when using this device care must be taken to not wrinkle or crease the apron. Whatever hanger is used, lay the apron smooth; proper storage of a lead apron will extend its useful life.

Molded lead gloves are covered with vinyl or resilient leather for flexible use. They come in 0.25-mm and 0.5-mm lead equivalent thicknesses. Soft glove liners are provided with lead gloves; they can be removed and washed as needed or desired. A lead glove hanger should be used to support and store the glove when not in use. The glove hanger is available as a separate unit that can be mounted to the wall, or it may be purchased as a combination lead apron/glove hanger unit.

Gonad shields are useful for children who can't wear a lead apron during the exposure. An adult can also use them, especially for non–weight-bearing studies performed on a radiographic table, if an apron doesn't provide adequate protection. Gonad shields have 0.5- to 1-mm lead

equivalency and are held in place by straps. Shield sheets, measuring 18 × 24 inches, and triangular-shaped lead diapers with a lead thickness of 0.5 to 1 mm also can be placed over the patient's reproductive organs.

## Protective Barriers

A mobile protective barrier can be used in settings where limited protection is available. The barrier moves on casters and is lead lined. A lead glass window allows the radiographer to view the patient during exposure (see Figure 2-5). The typical size of the mobile barrier is 7 feet high × 30 inches wide.

## Radiation Dosimetry Badges

All personnel involved in radiography should be monitored to estimate their amount of radiation exposure. Film badges (Figure 2-22) must be obtained from a certified laboratory. They should be worn at waist or chest level and outside a protective apron, if applicable. A control badge is placed in an area where there is no ionizing radiation exposure. New film is received from the laboratory monthly. Each month the personnel-monitoring film and the control film are removed from the badges and sent back to the laboratory. The laboratory provides monthly reports, which should be filed for future reference.

## ■ RADIOGRAPHIC FILM, SCREENS, AND CASSETTES

The radiographic image is greatly influenced by the type of film and intensifying screen used. There are many different types of films and screens; they must be properly matched to one another and the study (in this case, extremity radiography). Inappropriately matched film/screen combinations can significantly impair the radiographic quality. The wrong film/screen combination can ultimately lead to missed diagnoses and increase radiation exposure to the patient if a study is repeated.

## Radiographic Film

The two primary types of radiographic film are direct exposure film and screen film. Direct exposure film provides a sharp image of thin body parts having high subject contrast. It was primarily employed to assess the extremities but has been widely replaced with high-detail film/screen combinations. Because direct exposure film is used without intensifying screens, it is composed of a thicker silver halide emulsion to enhance x-ray interaction and is usually processed manually. High-exposure techniques are required with direct exposure film. It may be individually wrapped or combined with a cardboard holder.

Many types of screen film are available from several manufacturers. This type of film is sensitive to light emitted from an intensifying screen as well as x-rays. Screen film is either single or double emulsion. Single-emulsion film is only coated on one side. It provides a sharper image when used with a single-emulsion, high-detail/fine-grain intensifying screen than does double emulsion film used with two screens. However, the former requires double the exposure. Also, attention must be paid to place the emulsion side of a single-emulsion film against the intensifying screen. Other film characteristics to consider include contrast, speed, and light absorption.[3] After selecting a film type, it must be matched to an appropriate intensifying screen.

The choices for film contrast are high, medium, and low. High-contrast film produces more blacks and whites on the radiograph. Medium-contrast film has more shades of gray than does high-contrast film. Low-contrast film demonstrates a long scale of grays, referred to as latitude. Latitude is inversely proportional to contrast. Medium- to high-contrast film is typically used for extremity radiography.

The term *film speed* refers to the time it takes to respond to an exposure. Faster film speed correlates to less radiation exposure for the patient. However, faster films are not as sharp as slower films. Slower speed, high-detail (high-resolution) films are primarily employed for extremity studies.

Each type of film has specific light absorption characteristics. There are blue-sensitive and green-sensitive (also known as orthochromatic) films. A blue-sensitive film must be used with an intensifying screen that emits blue light and a green-sensitive film with a screen that emits green light. Mismatched film/screen combinations require increased exposures, thereby increasing the patient dose.

Specific guidelines should be followed regarding storage and handling of radiographic film. Film should be stored in a cool, dry location. In a hot, humid environment, the film may stick together. Check the expiration date of each box of film; rotate the film accordingly, using older film first.

Expired film should not be used; film quality may be impaired. Film should be stored on its side or end, not flat. Pressure marks (artifacts) may develop if the film is stored flat. Handle films with clean, dry hands. Be careful not to bend or crease the film during handling.

## Intensifying Screens

Intensifying screens are composed of light-emitting phosphors that fluoresce when exposed to x rays. Because screen film is sensitive to light, fewer x rays are needed to expose the film, reducing the exposure technique. Intensifying screen selection traits include its speed and, more importantly, spectral qualities.[11]

Two types of intensifying screens are available: calcium tungstate and rare earth. Calcium tungstate screens emit light in the blue/blue-violet portion of the visible light spectrum; rare-earth screens primarily emit green light, although a few emit blue light. Green-sensitive (orthochromatic) film must be used with green-emitting intensifying screens, and blue-sensitive film with blue-emitting intensifying screens. Incorrect matching of the film and screen will result in a slower film/screen system speed. Rare-earth intensifying screens are faster than calcium tungstate film/screen systems and do not sacrifice resolution. They have, therefore, widely replaced calcium tungstate systems.

If they are cared for properly and not accidentally damaged, intensifying screens can last many years. They should be cleaned as recommended by the manufacturer. If

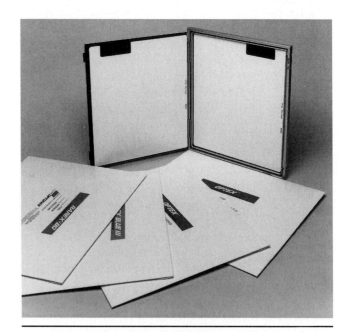

**Figure 2-23** Rigid cassette (opened, revealing intensifying screens and rectangular cutouts for identification imprinting). (Courtesy Providence Imaging Products, Inc., Providence, RI.)

spray chemicals are purchased from the manufacturer to clean the screen, do not spray the formula directly onto the screen; spray onto a cloth first. A drop of chemical could stain or damage the screen before it is wiped off. Exercise extreme care not to touch the screen except when cleaning. Scratches, for example, will permanently damage the screen.

## Cassettes

Cassettes are light-tight film and screen holders. They swing open on a hinge mechanism. The screens are permanently affixed inside the cassette, one on each side (if two screens are used). The film is "sandwiched" between the two screens; it must be loaded in the darkroom (unless one is using a daylight loading system). Most cassettes are rigid devices (Figure 2-23); other film/screen holders are made of a flexible vinyl. Some vinyl cassettes have a cardboard backing to provide some rigidity. The only advantage of vinyl cassettes is their cost; they are relatively inexpensive, compared to rigid cassettes. Major film manufacturers may provide cassettes at little or no cost if you agree to use their film. Screens are less likely to be damaged or worn in a rigid cassette; film-to-screen contact is also better achieved with a rigid cassette.

All cassettes have a backing material to absorb radiation that passes through the cassette. This prevents backscatter that could otherwise impair the image quality.

## ■ PROCESSING AND DARKROOM EQUIPMENT AND ACCESSORIES

A darkroom is used for several purposes: film storage, loading, processing, and duplication. Applicable equipment and furniture include a film storage box, workbench, processor unit (manual or automatic), and duplicator. The room must be properly lit with a white light while anyone is cleaning the work area and equipment and replacing or replenishing processing chemicals. A wash basin should also be in the room for cleaning purposes. An exhaust fan or other means of ventilation is necessary to prevent a buildup of noxious fumes in the darkroom. Any doors providing access to the darkroom must be light tight. The door should have a lock on the inside to prevent unauthorized access during safelight conditions. Safelights or light filters are used during film handling and processing. The workbench area must be kept clean and free from dust and spills. Careless handling of unprocessed film results in artifacts (discussed in Chapter 5) and poor-quality radiographs. Finally, a radiograph illuminator (viewbox) should be in mounted in the darkroom, especially for a manual processing setup or if using an automatic processor that discharges the film into the same room. Figure 2-24 shows a sample darkroom layout.

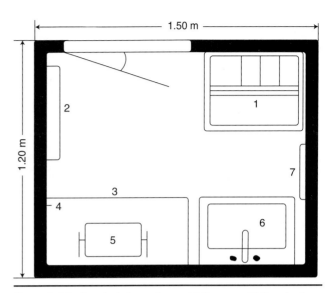

Figure 2-24  Sample darkroom layout. *(1)* Processor, *(2)* film-viewing box, *(3)* film storage, *(4)* film-loading area, *(5)* safe light, *(6)* wash basin, *(7)* air exhauster. (Courtesy Philips Medical Systems, Inc., Stamford, Conn.)

## Safelight

The type of x-ray film used determines the appropriate safelight filter for a darkroom. Two types of film are standard, each having its own spectral response to light. One is blue sensitive, the other is green sensitive. A red safelight filter must be used with green-sensitive (orthochromatic) film. Either an amber or red safelight filter can be used with blue-sensitive film. However, light passing through the amber filter will fog green-sensitive film.

Different types of safelight units are available. Generally speaking, a 15-watt bulb is used in the safelight lamp fixture with the filter placed in front of the safelight bulb. Units can be purchased that either screw into an existing light fixture or plug into an electrical outlet (Figure 2-25). The latter is mounted to the wall or ceiling. Fluorescent lights can also be adapted with a slip-on polycarbonate filter sleeve. The safelight must be located at least 4 feet from wherever the film is to be handled. Handle the film quickly and carefully, especially before processing the undeveloped, exposed film.

Examine safelight filters closely on a periodic basis. Any filter that has a crack or split should be replaced immediately.

## Film Storage

A film bin is a light-tight storage container for unexposed x-ray film. An economical unit is compact and sits on the countertop (Figure 2-26). For larger storage needs, a floor-standing cabinet is standard fare. This type of film bin has a hinged front door that tilts outward from the top; it is best positioned under the darkroom workbench. Film bins with

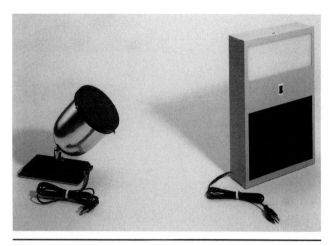

Figure 2-25   Safelight. Swivel wall- or ceiling-mounted and combination safelight/room light. (Courtesy Wolf X-Ray Co., West Hempstead, NY.)

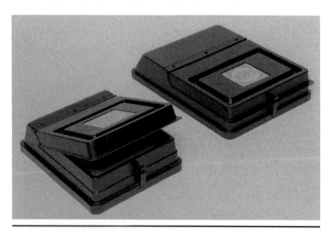

Figure 2-26   A compact x-ray film storage bin. (Courtesy Providence Imaging Products, Inc., Providence, RI.)

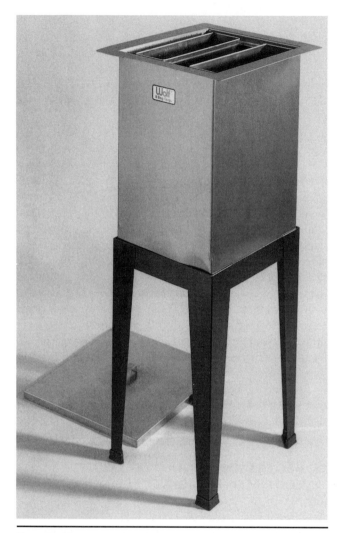

Figure 2-27   X-ray developing tank. (Courtesy Providence Imaging Products, Inc., Providence, RI.)

locking systems are available that can be only opened in safelight conditions.

## Film Carry Case

The transport of undeveloped, exposed films to a processing area away from the darkroom necessitates the use of a lightproof carrier. It looks like a briefcase and holds any size film up to and including 14 × 17 inches. An economical carrying case is made of plastic.

## Manual Processing Equipment

Manual processing tanks are stainless steel and resist corrosion (Figure 2-27). Hot and cold water plumbing must be accessible to the master tank to maintain the temperature of the chemicals for film processing. Two smaller stainless steel insert tanks fit inside the master tank for the developer

and fixer chemicals. The master tank is filled with water and functions as the stop bath between the developer and fixer and as the final wash bath after fixation. The main drain in the bottom of the master tank is used to empty the water and chemicals. An overflow drain is located along the back of the master tank. A plumber can properly install the inlet and outlet pipes and fixtures.

Periodic maintenance of the processing tanks is imperative to consistently maintain high-quality radiographs. The film processing chemicals age after several weeks and must be changed accordingly. Aged chemicals impair the film contrast, resulting in an overall gray, dull appearance. Also, the water in the master tank must be changed and the tank cleaned regularly to ensure proper film washing. Water is frequently contaminated by developer and fixer as the film is removed from the insert tanks and placed in the master tank.

The size of the master tank and the insert tanks can vary. Insert tanks can hold 2½ to 20 gallons. The smaller 2½- to 5-gallon insert tank can accommodate film sizes up to and including 10 × 12 inches and is most often used for office film processing of small to moderate volume.

Covers for the insert tanks are highly recommended. The developer is susceptible to aerial oxidation if left uncovered. This aerial oxidation will impair the radiographic quality. Also, the developer would have to be changed more often, an added and unnecessary cost. The fixer has a strong and unpleasant odor that can be contained if a lid is placed on the insert tank. A single cover may be available to enclose an entire tank system, especially for a small processing tank.

Two types of chemical mixing utensils are available: tank paddles and stirring rods. The tank paddle is made of hard rubber and the stirring rod is stainless steel. Both can be used to mix and agitate manual film-processing chemicals. There should be separate developer and fixer paddles so as not to contaminate the chemicals.

A timer is necessary to correctly time the processing cycles for film developing. Analog and electronic timers are available that operate by a spring mechanism, battery, or electricity. A loud, clear, long-ring timer is preferable.

The film-developing hanger is a solid, one-piece stainless steel frame. It has clips in all four corners to hold the film firmly and tightly in place to ensure complete surface film processing. The bottom clips are fixed (stationary), and the top clips are movable. Always clip the film onto the stationary clips first; then bring the movable suspension clips to the top of the film and attach them last. This will hold the film flat and firmly in place. Hangers are available for most film sizes.

A film-drying rack is a stainless steel device that is wall mounted (Figure 2-28). It holds the developing hangers at an angle while the films drip and air-dry. They should not be hung over the workbench nor in an area where unprocessed film is handled but over a basin or drip tray. A mobile cart that includes a drip tray is also available.

There are three types of thermometers used for manual processing: suspension, floating, and dial. The suspension thermometer is immersed in the tank. It is suspended from a spring clip that is attached to the edge of the tank. It can be easily removed for reading. The floating glass thermometer is a dual-scale, glass-enclosed hydrometer-type thermometer. It is weighted to float upright in a tank. This thermometer also must be removed from the chemicals to be read. The dial thermometer is a narrow thermometer with an attached circular dial at the top, similar to a meat thermometer. It can also be used to test the temperature of the chemicals in an automatic processor unit. Pertaining to all types of thermometers, be sure to wait an appropriate amount of time to allow the thermometer to reach the correct temperature.

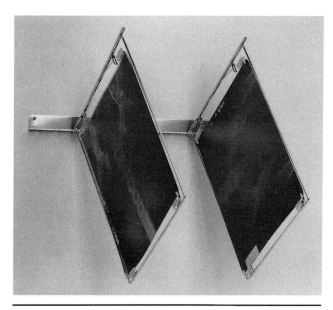

Figure 2-28    Film-drying rack. (Courtesy Providence Imaging Products, Inc., Providence, RI.)

An immersion heater can be used to raise the temperature of the water in the master tank. This is an alternative to draining some water and adding hot water to reach the desired temperature.

## Automatic Film Processors

There are two major designs for automatic film processors, full size and compact. They have functional systems for temperature control, transport, circulation, replenishment, and drying. The larger automatic film processor is designed to process all sizes of films up to and including 14- × 17-inch films. They have processing capacities of up to 250 sheets or more per hour, depending on the size of film used. The unit may occupy from 4 to 5 square feet. The full-size automatic film processor is usually installed so that the unprocessed film is loaded into the processor in the darkroom and the processed film will exit on the other side of the wall into a radiograph-viewing room. Large film processors are suitable for hospitals, large clinics, and high-volume film processing areas. Compact and economical, automatic cold water processors are also available. They have standby controls that reduce water and power consumption. The time cycles on the processor can vary from 90 seconds to 3 minutes. Thirty-second processors are available for use in emergency and surgical areas. The chemicals in 30-second processors are very concentrated, and the developer and fixer temperatures are very high.

Compact film processors require less than 3 square feet of space and sit on a stand, cart, or tabletop. They are designed for private offices and are ideal for low-volume film

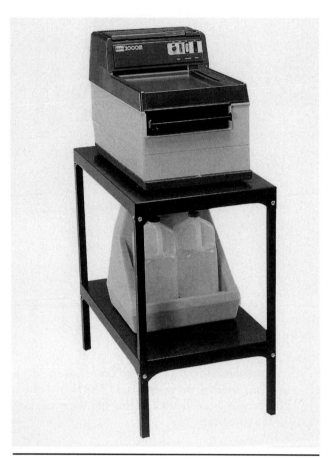

**Figure 2-29**  Compact automatic processor. (Courtesy All-Pro Imaging Corporation, Hicksville, NY.)

processing (Figure 2-29). Several different compact processors are available. Some can be installed with a through-the-wall kit so that the unprocessed film is loaded in the darkroom and the processed film exits into a viewing room. However, most compact film processors are designed for darkroom use only. The typical unit has front film feed and top return of the processed film. Others have top feed and front delivery. Some compact film processors have a light-tight feed tray that allows the operator to open the exit door and leave the darkroom during film feed.

The processing capacity of compact processors can range from 30 films per day to 125 films per hour. Smaller units may only accept film sizes up to 8 × 10 inches, but compact processors are available that accept 10- × 12-inch films, sufficient for office settings performing only foot and ankle studies. Like the larger processors, there is often the need for a plumber to install the compact processor. Access to cold water may be all that is necessary.

Plastic replenisher tanks for the developer and fixer are connected to automatic processor units by dispenser tubes. It is important that the tanks are accurately labeled as "developer" and "fixer." Tanks for large processor units may

hold between 14 and 55 gallons. These units are usually cleaned and replenished by a maintenance company. Replenishing systems for compact processors either can be small, plastic tanks that hold up to 8 gallons, or can be plastic 1-gallon bottles. Film-processing chemicals for compact automatic film processors are supplied in two forms, either as a concentrate that must be mixed with water or in a premixed, ready-to-use bottle.

A daylight loading system can be used with general-purpose automatic processors, as well as with some compact, low-volume automatic processors. However, it must be used with daylight cassettes and a daylight identification printer (unless radiopaque labeling tape is used during the exposure). A daylight loader eliminates the need for a darkroom. The film is automatically unloaded through a slot at one end of the cassette and fed into the processor. Some daylight loaders can reload the cassette with an unexposed film before returning it to the radiographer. The daylight film loader may be either built into a daylight automatic processing system or externally attached to a conventional automatic processor. The daylight system is designed for film processing only. Use of a total daylight loading system virtually eliminates film-handling artifacts. It also is an extremely efficient process, although relatively expensive compared to conventional processing equipment and accessories.

## Silver Recovery System

It is strongly recommended, for environmental safety reasons, that silver be recovered from the processor outflow before being discharged into a common drain. It may even be required at the local or state level (check with the applicable environmental protection agency). This safety measure can be achieved with a silver recovery unit.

## Processing Quality Control

Faulty processing produces films that are of poor quality and sometimes unreadable. This either results in potentially missed diagnoses or, if the study is repeated, increased radiation exposure to the patient. These scenarios are preventable in many instances if the processor is monitored daily. The goal is to maintain high-quality film processing and produce optimal diagnostic images. Uniform radiographic quality can be maintained by performing a simple procedure at the beginning of each working day. This procedure uses the methods of sensitometry and densitometry.

Processor quality control should be performed before processing any films. Equipment required for this procedure includes a box of control film, a sensitometer, a densitometer, and control charts. The control film should not be from the same box used for patient radiography; a separate, fresh box of film should be used for this purpose. The control film need not be 10 × 12 inches in size; to contain cost, a smaller size can be used.

The sensitometer is an instrument that exposes the control film to light. It precisely controls the intensity and duration of film exposure.[13] Light is projected through a neutral density step tablet that modulates the exposure received by the control film.[14] A 21-step density wedge is typically used. The individual performing this test must know the spectral sensitivity of the film being used (blue or green) before sensitometry is performed. The light source is set accordingly, usually by a switch on the instrument. Once exposed, the control film is then run through the warmed-up automatic processor or manual development tanks.

A densitometer is used to measure optical density, that is, light transmitted through the processed film.[15] The control film is placed in the densitometer, and the light passing through the exposed area on the film is measured. Density values can then be plotted to obtain a curve of film optical density versus log relative exposure (); this relationship is called a characteristic curve or the H & D curve, after Hurter and Driffield.[3] Measured parameters, including base plus fog, speed index, and contrast index, are plotted daily on a control chart.[16] The developer temperature is also recorded daily and plotted on the control chart.

Sensitometers and densitometers are available that are small, portable, and battery operated. Sensitometry, densitometry, and their relationship to film quality (including characteristic curves and control charts) are further discussed and illustrated in Chapter 5.

Other processor quality-control activities include cleaning and maintenance.[3] The transport and crossover racks, including rollers, should be removed and cleaned weekly or more frequently if sludge and debris build up. (Cleaning is necessary if particles are found on the processed film.) Routine assessment of all mechanical, moving parts should be observed weekly as part of a scheduled maintenance plan. And, replacement of parts before their failure (preventive maintenance) is necessary to prevent processor downtime.

Darkroom cleanliness should also be monitored. The room should be cleaned regularly and tasks and date documented.

## Polaroid Radiographic System

The Polaroid radiographic system (Polaroid Corporation, Cambridge, Massachusetts) is a dry processing method that requires a special type of film and cassette. It can be performed in daylight, eliminating the need for a darkroom. A positive radiograph (8 × 10 inches) is produced (in contrast to the negative produced by conventional radiography). The Polaroid cassette has a built-in, high-speed

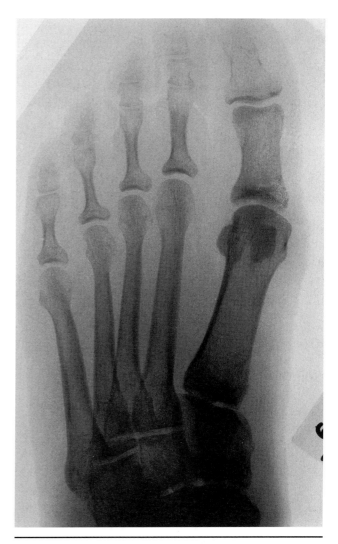

Figure 2-30   Polaroid positive radiograph.

intensifying screen processing orthochromatic spectral sensitivity and medium- to high-contrast properties.

Polaroid film has two major components. The first component is a light-sensitive negative sheet in a light-tight envelope that is loaded into the cassette and exposed. The second component is a transparent, blue-tinted polyester positive imaging sheet, not light sensitive, with a pod of processing chemicals attached. The image is transferred to the positive imaging sheet during film processing; the negative is discarded. The final film must be properly coated manually following processing. Improper coating will result in streaking; deterioration of the image will occur in uncoated areas.

The advantages of a Polaroid system are the 60-second daylight processing and absence of wet processing. A room need not be dedicated to film handling and processing, and the processing unit is reasonably priced. Bone detail is similar to that obtained with conventional films. However, with the advent of compact automatic processors comes an affordable, convenient means of film processing, similar to the speed of the Polaroid system. Also, the positive Polaroid radiograph has a completely different appearance from the negative conventional film. There is reversal of the black and the white densities; bones appear black and the background is radiolucent or clear (Figure 2-30). Furthermore, Polaroid film is considerably more expensive than conventional x-ray film.

## FILM IDENTIFICATION AND STORAGE

All radiographic films must be properly identified for medical and legal purposes. Identification should include the physician's name or facility where the radiographic study was performed, address (city and state), date of study, and the patient's name and age or birth date. Identification handwritten on or taped to an already processed radiograph is not admissible in a court of law.[17] Identification must be incorporated into the radiograph before processing. This may be performed with a film identification printer, radiographic labeling tape, or marker set.

### Film Identification Printer

Radiographic film is sensitive to light as well as x rays. The identification printer uses a light source and 3- × 5-inch index card to identify a radiograph (Figure 2-31). It also requires using a cassette that has been prepared by the manufacturer especially for this procedure. The cassette has

a rectangular lead blocker located in a corner or along an edge (Figures 2-32 and 2-33). That portion of the film beneath the lead blocker remains unexposed after the radiographic study. Before the study, patient information is typed or written onto the identification card. This card, ordered from a printer, includes standard information identifying the doctor's office or facility where the study is performed and provides a template for adding additional information, including the date and the patient's name and birth date or age. It is the easiest way to perform film identification and the most professional looking.

The following is an overview of the process: First, fill out the index card with the proper information. Perform the radiographic study. Be certain that the body part is not over the cassette's rectangular lead blocker. (The area is usually identified by a sticker.) In the darkroom, insert the identification card into the identification printer's slot, remove the film from the cassette, and slide the rectangular lead block area under the card. (Guides on the identification printer can be adjusted to aid in proper placement of the card and film.) The film will meet resistance and stop when aligned with the card. Press down on the exposure plate or button, and release when the light exposure is complete. The identification printer comes with an adjustment for light intensity and exposure. When the process is complete, the information will be displayed on the film in a rectangular area.

The procedure just described applies to the identification printer used in a darkroom. A daylight identification printer can also be used; the rectangular identification area is exposed while still inside the cassette. On its back side, the cassette has a rectangular slot that slides open inside the daylight printer for exposure (see Figure 2-33).

### Radiopaque Labeling Tape

Radiopaque label tape contains a semisoft strip of lead or tungsten mixture onto which is written or typed the pertinent information. It can be purchased in precut strips or as a long roll. The protective backing is peeled away from the adhesive tape that can then be placed on the cassette before the exposure. The label tape should be positioned such that it

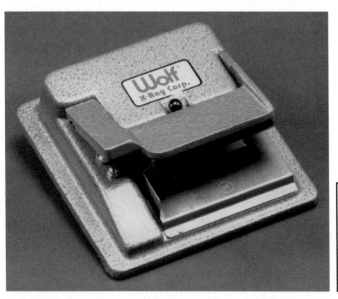

**THE FOOT & ANKLE INSTITUTE**
EIGHTH AT RACE ST., PHILA., PA 19107

Name                                                        Age

No.                                                          Date

Dr.

A                                                                                  B

Figure 2-31    **A,** Darkroom identification printer; **B,** index card. (**A,** Courtesy Wolf X-Ray Corp., West Hempstead, NY.)

will not be superimposed on the body part being studied. The patient's information then becomes part of the radiograph.

Identification labeling tape is usually combined with a holder device (Figure 2-34). The holder contains a density filter that blocks excessive radiation so that the information is visible radiographically. Choose a density filter that corresponds to the mAs and kVp settings typically used. The holder can be customized with the physician's or facility's name and address along its top and bottom edges. Some

holders have right (R) and left (L) indicators built in. The label tape with pertinent information is centered on top of the holder and is then placed on the cassette while positioning the patient, before exposure.

## Lead Character Marker Identification Sets

Another form of radiographic identification uses small lead characters (letters and numbers) that slide onto a holder.

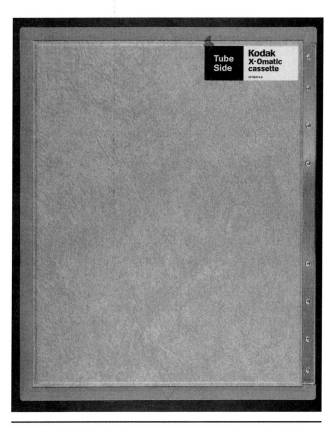

Figure 2-32    The location of the rectangular lead blocker (not visible) is marked by the identification sticker along the corner of this cassette.

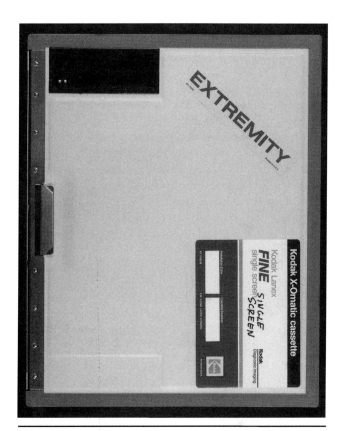

Figure 2-33    Daylight identification cassette. The black rectangular "window" in the corner of the cassette corresponds to the lead-blocked area. The window automatically slides open inside the identification camera and is exposed.

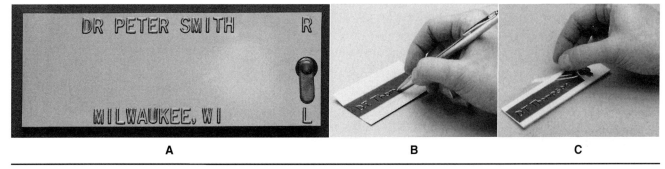

A    B    C

Figure 2-34    **A,** Radiopaque label tape holder; **B,** writing information on labeling tape; **C,** application of tape onto holder. (**A,** Courtesy Medical I.D. Systems Inc., Grand Rapids, Mich.; **B** and C, courtesy X-Rite, Inc., Grandville, Mich.)

The holder can be customized with the physician's or facility's name and address permanently affixed. The patient's name, age or birth date, and date of the study are added with the lead characters. The holder is then placed on the cassette during patient positioning outside the shadow of the subject image, especially in an area not superimposed by the area of concern. The information becomes a permanent part of the radiograph during the exposure.

## Right (R) and Left (L) Identification Markers

All extremity radiographs must be correctly identified as either right or left. This labeling must also be a permanent part of the radiograph.

The capital letters R and L are used to identify right and left extremities (Figure 2-35). The markers vary in size and are made of lead. Stainless steel "clip" markers are also available. This U-shaped device has an R and L punched out on either arm of the clip. The marker slides over the cassette's edge; the applicable letter is positioned over the front of the cassette. This device is especially useful for vertically positioned cassettes. The R or L will become a permanent part of the radiograph during the exposure.

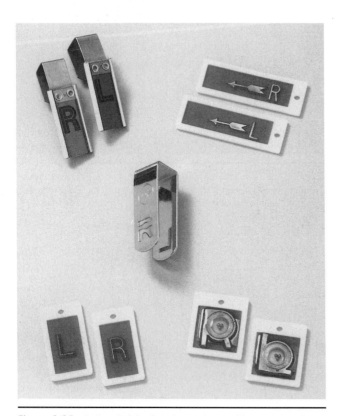

Figure 2-35    Left and right identification letters. (Courtesy Providence Imaging Products, Inc., Providence, RI.)

## ■ FILM-VIEWING TOOLS

Viewboxes (illuminators), spotlights, and magnifying glasses comprise the required viewing tools. Further information about these instruments and recommendations can be found in Chapter 6.

### Radiograph Illuminators

Bright and even illumination is essential to properly view a radiograph. Holding the radiograph up to a lamp or an overhead light fixture does not provide proper illumination. The viewing area on the illuminator should ideally be the size of the radiograph. Any ambient light that escapes from the margins of a film placed on a larger viewbox will impair visualization of the image. Illuminators should be selected based on the largest-size film used. Ideally, differently sized viewboxes should be available for each different size of radiograph. Fortunately, an office dedicated to performing only foot and ankle studies will use only one size of film.

Illuminators are available with 8- × 10-inch, 10- × 12-inch, and 11- × 14-inch viewing areas. An illuminator may have a single viewing area for a particular size of film, or a bank of multiple illuminators positioned side-by-side or in a double tier. It is strongly recommended that viewing areas of bank illuminators be separated by reflectors and have individual on/off switches. Surface-mounted, recessed wall-mounted, and desktop illuminators are available (Figure 2-36). A wet film illuminator has a plastic or stainless steel tray at the bottom; the film hanger with radiograph hooks along the top of the viewbox. This type of illuminator is ideal for a darkroom that uses manual processing.

Illuminators use either Circline or straight fluorescent tubes. A daylight or cool white fluorescent bulb provides the

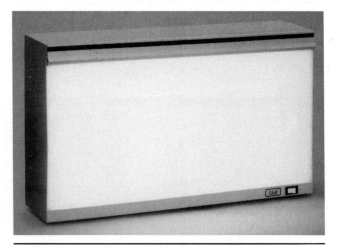

Figure 2-36    This 12- by 24-inch illuminator can either be wall mounted or set on a desk or countertop. (Courtesy Wolf X-Ray Corp., West Hempstead, NY.)

light source. Use the same type of bulb (cool white or daylight) in an illuminator with multiple bulbs. The two types have different light hues. Green fluorescent tubes are also available that, a manufacturer claims, enhance viewing of the radiograph and decrease eyestrain.

Film retainers are found along the top of an illuminator. Their purpose is to grip the film and hold it in place. The grip mechanism varies; try each and choose one that "feels" right to you. Optional film-activated microswitches can be ordered; the bulb turns on as a film is placed under the retaining clip.

The viewing panel is a white, radiolucent acrylic sheet. It is easily removed to service the light bulbs and fixtures. The viewing panel must be kept clean and free of dirt, marks, and scratches.

## Magnifiers

Magnifiers are useful aids for radiographic interpretation. They can be hand held or mounted on a moving arm attached to a viewbox.

## Spotlight Illuminators

A bright spotlight increases the illumination in a small area of the film and enhances visibility. It is not meant to be a replacement for technically overexposed or overdeveloped films. The typical spotlight is equipped with a standard incandescent lamp that should not exceed 75 Watts (check the manufacturer's recommendation). Films will easily be damaged with higher-wattage bulbs. An attached rheostat foot pedal allows the viewer to control gradients of

brightness (Figure 2-37). On more expensive units, an adjustable shutter can limit the viewing area to a smaller desired area of interest, and intensification can be adjusted accordingly. Use the light intermittently to avoid burning the film, which can occur quite quickly. A reflector surface surrounds the bulb; both must be kept clean.

## ■ FILM LABELING, FILING, AND DUPLICATION

### Film Envelopes/Preservers

Film preservers are constructed of heavy brown Kraft stock. The envelopes can be ordered with a preprinted template for patient identification, which may be either ruled or unruled. They come in many sizes, styles, and colors.

### X-Ray File Cabinets

Radiographs should be stored in a cabinet with firm, preferably metal, reinforced shelving. Wood shelves may warp under the weight of many files. Open and stackable film storage units are available, as are enclosed filing cabinets with pullout drawers. Steel drawer filing cabinets specific for storing radiographs are also available.

### Filing System

Radiographs can be filed with the medical chart or separately. If separate, it should be filed according to the system used for the medical file or chart. It is much easier to retrieve radiographs with matching case numbers or names.

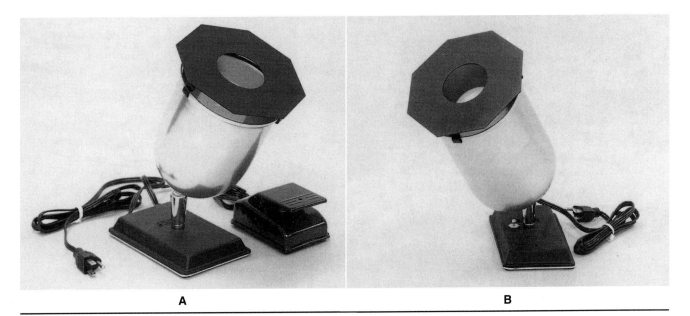

| A | B |

Figure 2-37    Spotlight illuminators with **(A)** and without **(B)** rheostat foot pedal. (Courtesy Wolf X-Ray Corp., West Hempstead, NY.)

## Film Label Tape

If a patient has or will have numerous radiographic studies, it is best to color-code the films and index the code on the film envelope. A color-coded tape system will expedite retrieval of radiographs performed on a specific date. The date is logged on the front of the patient's film envelope and a piece of colored label tape (approximately one inch in length) is placed adjacent to the date. A piece of the same color tape is then placed across the top edge of the film or films performed on that date. Films are stored with the top edge of the film (with the tape) at the top or open end of the envelope.

## Logbook

Many states require that an x-ray study logbook be maintained. Information should include the date of the examination, patient name and file number (if applicable), techniques performed, purpose of the study, technique (mA, kVp, SID, and time), type of film/screen system, and the name of any person holding the patient during an exposure. Even the radiation dose for the study (predetermined for each technique by a radiation physicist) could be included. All information should be recorded immediately following the study.

## Radiographic Film Duplicators

The radiograph is a vital component of a patient's medical history. Occasionally a patient, physician, insurance carrier, or attorney may request copies of radiographs. Or you may desire to send a study to another physician for consultation. Never let an original film leave the office unless a copy has been made first. It is strongly recommended to keep the original and send a copy.

Duplicating film, a direct reversal film, is used to copy radiographs. The emulsion is only coated on one side of the film. It is formulated to react to light sources with a high ultraviolet light output, such as a BLB (blacklight blue) fluorescent lamp, included with many commercially available duplicators.[18]

There are many types of film duplicators to choose from (Figure 2-38). Large, self-contained units include a BBL fluorescent lamp and operate in one of two fashions: Either the films are placed onto a glass plate (known as a box-type contact printer), or they are fed through a processor-like machine with a rotating cylinder.[19] Depending on the unit, there will be controls for the light intensity or the time of exposure. Exposure times are typically on the order of several seconds. An economical method of copying radiographs employs a cassettelike device known as a printing frame. It has a rigid frame with a clear glass or plastic plate front that uses overhead light fixtures or a viewbox as the light source. Homemade duplicating units can also be constructed.[20,21] The exposure time for duplication with an incandescent or a daylight or cool white fluorescent lamp is longer than those units using a BLB fluorescent lamp. (The fluorescent bulbs of a viewbox could be replaced with BLB bulbs for duplication purposes.) Experimentation is necessary to obtain copies of adequate exposure for all methods of duplication.

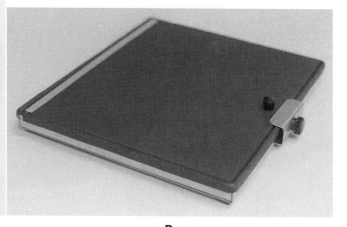

|  A  |  B  |

Figure 2-38  Duplicators. **A,** Self-contained unit (box-type contact printer); **B,** economical cassettelike unit (printing frame).  (**A,** Courtesy Star X-Ray Co., Inc., Amityville, NY; **B,** courtesy Gill Podiatry Supply Co., Middleburg Heights, Ohio.)

Radiographs are easily copied, but certain guidelines must be followed. The duplicating film should be the same size as the original radiograph. A specific order and placement of the two films is required: The original radiograph is positioned closest to the light source, and the emulsion side of the duplicating film is placed against the original radiograph. (Duplicating films have a notch in one corner that aids in film placement.) The two films (original and duplicating) are then placed in the copying device and covered tightly (if applicable). The copying process requires that both the original and duplicating films be held in close contact with one another. Poor film-to-film contact will result in blurring of the duplicate image. Variable light or timer controls allow a dark or light original film to be enhanced. The light intensity or time is increased to make a duplicate radiograph appear less dense than the original and is decreased to make it darker (increased film density). A standard fluorescent lamp will result in a duplicate that has higher contrast than the original.[22]

## References

1. Christman RA, Zulli LP: Radiologic aspects of aging in the foot, *Clin Podiatr Med Surg* 10:97, 1993.
2. *The fundamentals of radiography,* ed 12, Rochester, NY, 1980, Eastman Kodak.
3. Bushong SC: *Radiologic science for technologists,* ed 5, St Louis, 1993, Mosby.
4. *Portable hand-held x-ray instrument (Lixiscope),* Health Technology Assessment Series: Health Technology Assessment Report No. 15, Rockville, Md, 1985, National Center for Health Services Research and Health Care Technology Assessment.
5. George FW: The Lixiscope, *Clin Podiatry* 2:511, 1985.
6. Gorecki GA et al: Lixiscope: a podiatric evaluation, *J Am Podiatr Med Assoc* 72:304, 1982.
7. Tansey WJ: Low intensity x-ray imaging scope, *Am J Sports Med* 9:360, 1981.
8. Estersohn HS, Wolf KL, Day JC: The podium, *J Am Podiatr Med Assoc* 71:222, 1981.
9. Mattsson O: A foot-fixator for exact imaging reproducibility in lower extremity radiography, *Acta Radiologica* 30:335, 1989.
10. Christensen JC, Dockery GL, Schuberth JM: Evaluation of ankle ligamentous insufficiency using the Telos ankle stress apparatus, *J Am Podiatr Med Assoc* 76:527, 1986.
11. Geissberger H: Wedge-shaped filters for improved radiography of the thoracic vertebrae and the foot, *Med Radiogr Photogr* 42:6, 1966.
12. Block IH: Wedge-shaped filters for radiography of the foot, *J Am Podiatry Assoc* 58:182, 1968.
13. Lawrence DJ: A simple method of processor control, *Med Radiogr Photogr* 49:2, 1973.
14. *Sensitometric properties of x-ray films,* Rochester, NY, 1974, Eastman Kodak.
15. Groenendyk DJ: Densitometers and sensitometers in QC, *Radiol Technol* 65(4):249, 1994.
16. *Processor quality assurance: an informational guide to monitoring x-ray and cine film processors,* Grandville, Mich, 1990, X-Rite.
17. *Basic x-ray machine operator study guide,* Tallahassee, 1986, Florida Department of Health and Rehabilitative Services.
18. Christensen EE, Curry TS, Dowdey JE: *An introduction to the physics of diagnostic radiology,* ed 2, Philadelphia, 1978, Lea & Febiger.
19. *Kodak X-Omat duplicating film technic guide,* Rochester, NY, 1982, Eastman Kodak.
20. Josephs, RL: Technique for duplicating x-rays, *J Am Podiatry Assoc* 64:794, 1974.
21. Spencer RB, Bradley MB: Radiographic reproduction, *Podiatry Today,* February 1990, p. 45.
22. *The fundamentals of radiography,* ed 12, Rochester, NY, 1980, Eastman Kodak.

# CHAPTER 3

# Positioning Techniques and Terminology

ROBERT L. BARON • CASIMIR F. STRUGIELSKI • ROBERT A. CHRISTMAN

lain film radiography has played, and continues to play, an integral role in assessing foot and ankle disorders. Initially, views must be selected that will best image the part in question (see Chapter 11). The objective is to select positioning techniques that will yield the most information while minimizing radiation exposure. A firm knowledge of normal radiographic anatomy is a prerequisite.

A diversity of positioning techniques are available for foot and ankle radiography. The radiographer must clearly understand specific terminology used to describe positioning techniques before attempting to perform them. Unfortunately, discrepancy exists regarding use of the terms *view*, *position*, and *projection*. Even the word *lateral* can have two meanings. The following discussion of these terms, we hope, will clarify their application, especially as to the naming of positioning techniques.

## ■ VIEWS, PROJECTIONS, AND POSITIONS

Numerous techniques have been described for plain film radiography of the foot and ankle. They range from non–weight bearing to weight bearing, and have every possible aspect of the extremity positioned against the film. Oblique foot techniques can be especially confounding; they may be performed non–weight bearing, with the planto-medial, plantolateral, dorsomedial, or dorsolateral aspect of the foot positioned against the film, or weight bearing, with the central x-ray beam directed at 45 degrees toward either the dorsomedial or dorsolateral aspect of the foot. The result is confusion not only over to which positioning techniques to choose for a particular study but also over what to name them. The positioning techniques are described in this chapter; Chapter 11 discusses how to choose applicable techniques. The present chapter addresses the problems

regarding use of the terms *view*, *position*, and *projection* and provides a guide for standardizing their usage and application.

## The Predicament

Several factors contribute to the current disarray regarding terminology for positioning techniques and radiographs. They include whether positioning techniques are named as positions or projections and how people use the terms *projection*, *position*, and *view*.

Positioning techniques have historically been named by two methods: (1) according to the path or projection of the x-ray beam through the body part and (2) by that surface of the body positioned closer to the film. The former classically pertains to examination of the coronal anatomic plane (anteroposterior and posteroanterior projections). Position, in contrast, is used to describe oblique and lateral techniques.[1,2] Initially, positional terms alone were sufficient to specify oblique and lateral techniques. However, as specialized positioning techniques evolved, projectional terms were being used in conjunction with, and even in place of, positional terms to describe oblique and lateral techniques. Use of the term view further confounds the predicament.

The term *view* should pertain only to the final image or radiograph. It should not be used to describe a positioning technique or projection.[3] Doctors usually attach the term *view* to whatever positioning technique was performed when naming the radiographic image; that is, the term *view* is used synonymously with *projection* and *position*.[4] For example, an anteroposterior projection is an anteroposterior view. However, one technical publication emphasizes that the term *view* means exactly the opposite of *projection*.[5] By this definition, the image produced by an anteroposterior projection should be called a posteroanterior *view*. Taken a step further, a view was named either by that part of the body closest to the film or by where the x-ray beam exits.[6]

The authors that distinguish between the terms *view* and *projection* by definition, however, fail to address the issue in practice. Figures illustrating positioning techniques in those texts are named as projections, but the radiographic images accompanying the technical descriptions are either named as a projection or not named at all! The term *view* is omitted intentionally. Another positioning textbook does not define how the term *view* is applied except that it is reserved for discussing the radiograph, not the technique.[3]

Discrepancies abound in the medical and technical literature regarding the names of positioning techniques and resultant images. A recent issue of *Clinics in Podiatric Medicine and Surgery* dedicated to radiology of the foot and ankle demonstrates this inconsistency. One article stresses routine use of the term *projection* for describing both technique and radiograph[7]; the projection is based on the body surface that the x-ray beam first enters. In contrast, another article consistently uses the term *view* when describing positioning techniques[8]; oblique positions are named by the surface nearest to the film, yet the dorsoplantar view is named by the direction of the x-ray beam.

This confusion appears to be rooted in the separation of a radiographic study into technical and diagnostic components. The technical component is three-dimensional and therefore appropriate terminology is needed to adequately describe the procedure. The radiograph, however, is only two-dimensional. It is not necessary to consider that the body part is being visualized from the film side, as suggested by Merrill. The radiograph looks the same no matter how the film is placed on the viewbox. In fact, anteroposterior and posteroanterior chest radiographs are customarily viewed as if the doctor were facing the patient (the patient's right is on the viewer's left, for example).[9] This practice has no regard for the patient's position relative to the film.

A final source of confusion pertains to usage of the term *lateral*. The term *lateral* can be defined two ways. (1) It can, generally speaking, refer to any side of the body; in this case, both sides of the foot are considered lateral. Lateral positions of the foot simply correspond to side positions of the body relative to the film. The term does not differentiate between true lateral and medial sides. Therefore *medial* refers to the center or midline of the foot or ankle.[10] (2) The second definition of *lateral* corresponds to true lateral, that is, that aspect of the foot farther from the body's midline, the latter being located between both extremities and separating them into right and left.[11] In this case, medial corresponds to that side of an extremity that is closer to the midline of the torso. In radiography, the designation "lateral position" is not specific and corresponds to the first definition. The modifier "lateromedial" or "mediolateral projection" must be added to specify the precise positioning technique. The second definition (true medial and lateral) is applied when describing projections.

The lateral foot and ankle positions were originally performed with the patient not bearing weight and with the true lateral aspect of the extremity positioned against the film. More specific terminology was not necessary to further identify the technique performed. The weight-bearing lateral foot and ankle techniques were developed later. The true medial aspect of the foot or ankle was positioned against the film, not the lateral. However, instead of naming it a lateral position/lateromedial projection, technicians named it by that aspect of the extremity closer to the x-ray tube (i.e., by the surface the x-ray beam enters first). The two techniques were differentiated as being either weight bearing or recumbent.[12]

## The Solution

One goal of this textbook is to standardize the terminology applied to positioning techniques and radiographic images of the foot and ankle. This can be easily accomplished without grossly changing the terminology or routines already being practiced. Definitions for the terms *projection, position, view,* and *positioning technique* are followed by specific applications.

**Position:** Pertains to that aspect of the body closest to the film. It is used to name the oblique and lateral (not the true lateral but a side) positioning techniques. A directional term *(projection)* and other adjectives *(weight bearing* or *non–weight bearing,* for example) should be used with the oblique and lateral positions to further define the positioning technique.

**Projection:** The direction that the x-ray beam travels through the body. This direction is described as being anteroposterior or posteroanterior, dorsoplantar or plantodorsal, or lateromedial or mediolateral. (The latter terms refer to true lateral and medial.) The projection is used in addition to a position term to further describe a particular oblique or lateral position. The term *projection* is used to describe a positioning technique; it does not refer to the radiographic image.

**View:** Pertains to the radiographic image only. The terminology used to describe the positioning technique will simply be applied to the image, but the word *view* will replace the term *position* or *projection.* For example, the technique for a dorsoplantar projection produces a dorsoplantar view, the technique for a lateral position (lateromedial projection) produces a lateral (or lateromedial) view, and the technique for a medial oblique position produces a medial oblique view. View is not the opposite of projection. Additional terms should be included when appropriate, such as *weight bearing or non–weight bearing.*

**Positioning Technique:** The actual method of performing the study, including the position of the patient, tubehead, and film and the projection of the x-ray beam.

## Application

As noted earlier, numerous positioning techniques are possible for imaging the foot and ankle. Each is discussed in detail in the following sections. The terminology will adhere to the definitions just noted. Some positioning techniques have been named after the authors who first described them. Their names are included with the description of the positioning technique.

Positioning techniques that produce images of the ankle and foot in the coronal and transverse planes, respectively, should be named by projections alone. Ankle techniques are anteroposterior projections, and foot techniques are typically dorsoplantar projections. The descriptor *weight-bearing* or *non–weight-bearing* should precede the name. The radiographic image has the same name except the word *view* replaces the term *projection*. An example of a positioning technique and corresponding view is the weight-bearing dorsoplantar projection and weight-bearing dorsoplantar view.

Descriptions of lateral positioning techniques, in contrast, require two designations, a position term accompanied by a projection term. The term describing the projection of the x-ray beam follows the position term. The designation *weight-bearing* or *non–weight-bearing* precedes the term *lateral position*; for example, "weight-bearing lateral position (lateromedial projection)".

The four lateral positioning techniques, including the weight-bearing mediolateral and lateromedial projections and the non–weight-bearing mediolateral and lateromedial projections, produce views that look similar to one another. The resultant images or views can all be named lateral views; the projection terms need not be included (especially if the full positioning technique has been previously described).

Oblique positioning techniques may or may not require additional position and projection terms. Non–weight-bearing oblique positioning techniques should include a term designating that aspect of the extremity closest to the film. An example is the non–weight-bearing medial oblique position. Weight-bearing oblique positions (which are **not** advocated for the reasons listed below in "Special Considerations") do not need the position term *plantar* added to the title. The term *weight bearing* implies that the plantar surface of the foot is closest to the film; including it would be redundant. However, a projection term is required to designate the direction of the x-ray beam through the extremity. The two weight-bearing oblique positioning techniques are either mediolateral or lateromedial oblique

projections. Radiographic images are named the same except the term *view* replaces the words *position* or *projection*. An example of an oblique positioning technique and corresponding view is the non–weight-bearing medial oblique position and the non–weight-bearing medial oblique view.

## Special Considerations

Weight-bearing oblique foot-positioning techniques with the tubehead angled at 45 degrees have been advocated by some doctors of podiatric medicine. One reason for this practice has been to standardize performance of the technique. Weight-bearing techniques alone, however, do not necessarily standardize the resultant view. It has been shown that foot positioning (supination and pronation) influences the radiographic positional relationships of the bones during weight bearing.[13] Another attempt to standardize positioning techniques is by positioning the extremity in its angle and base of gait.[14] This technique is used so that biomechanical measurements of the foot are standardized and reproducible.[15] Biomechanical measurements, however, are only performed on dorsoplantar and lateral radiographs, not on oblique views.

Magnification and distortion of the image results from weight-bearing oblique positioning techniques. If true magnification is desired, a magniposer can be used to increase the object-to-image distance (OID); the geometric distortion is much less than that obtained by the weight-bearing oblique study. Occasionally, distortion of the object may be desirable in an attempt to better visualize a particular pathology. If so, the distorted oblique projection should be performed adjunctively as a special technique. A non–weight-bearing oblique position, with the foot tilted 45 degrees and the tubehead directed perpendicular to the film, should be performed initially. Non–weight-bearing oblique foot positions can be accurately performed with a radiolucent foam wedge positioning aid. The foot should be positioned perpendicular to the leg as the sole of the foot rests against the wedge. The only other time that the distorted weight-bearing oblique positioning technique should be performed is if the patient cannot position his or her extremity properly for the non–weight-bearing oblique study. On a final note, the non–weight-bearing oblique requires a lesser exposure technique and, as an economical consideration, can be performed on half of an 8- × 10-inch or 10- × 12-inch film. The weight-bearing oblique may require the use of a separate sheet of film for each extremity.

Positioning techniques for imaging the foot and ankle should be relatively simple to perform by both technician and patient. The type of x-ray unit being used, however, may already impose limitations. Many techniques can be performed with lower extremity-specific x-ray units. Orthoposer-mounted units offer convenience (the source-to-image distance [SID] is fixed) and safety (the patient can hold on to an attached railing, and the weight of the tubehead holds the orthoposer unit steady); they are best for performing weight-bearing studies. However, it is difficult, if not impossible, to perform non–weight-bearing ankle studies with these particular units. Wall-mounted x-ray units with flexible arms, in contrast, can serve two purposes if mounted properly: non–weight-bearing studies can be performed with the patient lying on an examination chair or table; weight-bearing studies can be performed on an orthoposer platform placed adjacent to the chair or table. Greater technical expertise, however, is necessary to position the tubehead properly with flexible wall-mounted units. Extremity-positioning aids are useful for performing certain techniques, such as the weight-bearing sesamoid axial projection. (Chapter 2 describes the x-ray units and positioning aids available and lists manufacturers and distributors for obtaining these devices.)

## Overview of Positioning Techniques

The following is an outline of the positioning techniques that can be performed on the foot and ankle. They are categorized as foot-, toe-, sesamoid-, tarsal-, and ankle-positioning techniques. Each category is further subdivided into dorsoplantar (plantodorsal) or anteroposterior (posteroanterior) projections, oblique positions, and lateral positions, when applicable.

  I. Foot-Positioning Techniques
     A. Dorsoplantar projections
        1. Weight bearing
        2. Non–weight bearing
           a. Foot flat
           b. Forefoot angled 15 degrees
     B. Oblique positions
        1. Non–weight bearing
           a. Medial
           b. Lateral
        2. Weight bearing
           a. Lateromedial oblique projection
           b. Mediolateral oblique projection
     C. Lateral positions (may be performed weight bearing or non–weight bearing)
        1. Lateromedial projection
        2. Mediolateral projection
 II. Toe-Positioning Techniques
     A. Dorsoplantar projection (weight bearing or non–weight bearing)
     B. Oblique positions
        1. Non–weight bearing
           a. Medial
           b. Lateral
        2. Weight bearing
           a. Lateromedial oblique projection
           b. Mediolateral oblique projection
     C. Lateral positions (may be performed weight bearing or non–weight bearing)
        1. Lateromedial projection
        2. Mediolateral projection
III. Sesamoid-Positioning Techniques
     A. Posteroanterior sesamoid axial projections
        1. Weight-bearing axialposer
        2. Lewis method
     B. Anteroposterior sesamoid axial projection (Holly method)
     C. Lateromedial tangential projection (Causton method)
 IV. Tarsal-Positioning Techniques
     A. Dorsoplantar calcaneal axial projection
     B. Plantodorsal calcaneal axial projection
     C. Harris-Beath
     D. Broden
     E. Isherwood
     F. Anthonsen
  V. Ankle-Positioning Techniques (may be performed weight bearing or non–weight bearing)
     A. Anteroposterior projection
     B. Mortise position
     C. Oblique positions
        1. Internal (or medial) oblique
        2. External (or lateral) oblique
     D. Lateral positions
        1. Lateromedial projection
        2. Mediolateral projection

## Terminology

1. **Angle of gait:** The angle formed between the feet and line of progression while walking: approximately 10 to 15 degrees of abduction in the normal individual.
2. **Base of gait:** This is the distance between both medial malleoli while walking (approximately 2 inches).
3. **Midline of foot:** The imaginary line that enters the center of the heel and exits through the second digit, thereby dividing the foot into two halves.
4. **Central ray (CR):** The most direct beam of radiation from the tube.
5. **Dorsum (dorsal):** In reference to the top of the foot.
6. **Plantar:** Bottom (sole) of foot.
7. **Lateral** (two definitions):
   a. Away from the torso's midline (outer side of the extremity).
   b. Away from the midline of the extremity (inner or outer side of the extremity)
8. **Medial:** Inner side of the extremity (toward the torso's midline).
9. **Extension:** The process of straightening the joint.

10. **Flexion:** The process of bending the joint in an angle.
11. **Supine:** Lying face up.
12. **Prone:** Lying face down.
13. **Specific body position:** Describes the placement of the foot or ankle relative to the x-ray film/cassette. Non–weight-bearing oblique positions are named by that aspect of the extremity nearest the film/cassette.
14. **Positioning:** Manner in which the tubehead, film, patient, and central ray are placed to obtain a radiographic image of a particular body part.
15. **Projection:** The direction that the primary x-ray beam travels through the body part. Used to describe anteroposterior (dorsoplantar), lateral, and weight-bearing foot oblique positioning techniques. For example, the x-ray beam enters the dorsal aspect of the foot and exits the plantar aspect in the dorsoplantar projection.
16. **Tubehead angulation:** The number of degrees the tubehead is set from vertical (0 degrees.)
17. **View:** This term refers to the image in the radiograph. It is not a positioning term.[16]
18. **Oblique:** The condition when the plane of a body part is neither perpendicular nor parallel to the film.
19. **Axial:** The long axis of a structure or body part.
20. **Cassette:** Film holder.
21. **Orthoposer:** Platform used to perform weight-bearing studies.

## GENERAL CONSIDERATIONS

Most views of the foot and ankle can be obtained with either a weight-bearing or a non–weight-bearing positioning technique. The patient being considered for weight-bearing positioning techniques should be ambulatory, able to walk without assistance. If not, partial weight bearing or non–weight bearing may be preferable. The added weight of a lead apron or shield to a patient whose mobility is questionable poses a considerable risk for injury if an unsteady patient is positioned on an orthoposer for a weight-bearing study. Partial or non–weight bearing should be considered for the patient who is not surefooted or uses an ambulation assistance device (e.g., walker, cane, or crutches). Patients who have recently had a cast put on or who have undergone a surgical procedure may not be stable enough to allow full weight bearing. Non–weight-bearing positioning techniques are necessary for individuals who are confined to a wheelchair, have recently undergone an extensive surgical procedure, or have acute pain (secondary to recent trauma, for example).

Positioning techniques can be modified as needed. This is especially true for oblique positions if you are trying to view a specific anatomic landmark or location.

If a lesion marker is placed on the skin, only dorsoplantar and lateral positioning techniques should be performed. Marker position cannot be accurately assessed with oblique views. Furthermore, the tubehead must be positioned vertically (0 degrees) for the dorsoplantar projection. Any other tubehead angulation will alter the position of the marker relative to the internal foot structures.

## PREPARATION FOR THE RADIOGRAPHIC STUDY

Preparation of the radiography room expedites patient turnaround and minimizes the chance for mistakes. Several aspects of the study should be considered and performed before the patient is brought into the room. Initially, the desired views must be selected; positioning techniques are chosen that will result in the desired images. The radiographer can then gather all applicable items pertaining to the study: cassettes with film, positioning aids, and identification markers, for example. (Many of these items are discussed in Chapter 2.) Standard technical factors (mA, kVp, time, and SID) should be posted by each unit's control panel for all positioning techniques. Any modifications should be determined in advance. Tubehead and cassette placement, lead film blocker, identification markers, and control panel adjustments can be ready for the first positioning technique before the patient enters the radiography room.

Once the patient is in the radiography room, he or she must be given precise instructions as to what to do and what is expected for each of the positioning techniques. The patient must clearly understand these instructions so that the necessity for repeat studies is minimized. Image blurring caused by patient movement is probably the most common reason for repeating any particular study. Clear instructions must also be given to the parent or guardian who remains in the room and is helping to maintain an infant's or young child's position. Occasionally, a patient, particularly a trauma or geriatric patient, may express discomfort during positioning of the extremity. If it becomes unreasonable to perform a certain positioning technique, an alternative position or projection or even a non–weight-bearing technique should be considered.

A final check should be made by the radiographer to make sure that all technical parameters are correct: patient positioning, identification markers, and technical factors. This should be done for each positioning technique. Error regarding any of these parameters can result in having to repeat a study.

Lead aprons must be provided for and used by each patient who is being examined. This also applies to the infant or child patient. An apron and lead gloves must be

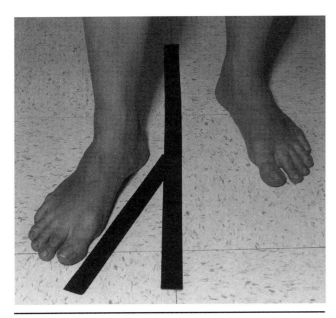

Figure 3-1    Angle of gait.

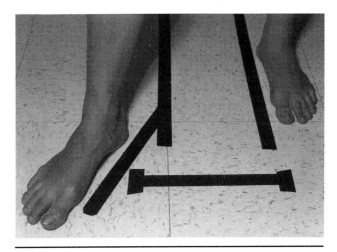

Figure 3-2    Base of gait.

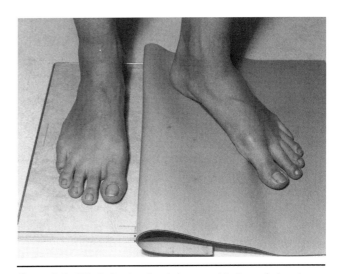

Figure 3-3    Weight-bearing dorsal plantar positioning technique in angle and base of gait. The patient's right foot is positioned on the right half of the film/cassette. The left foot is then positioned such that both feet are in angle and base of gait. This usually means that the opposite foot will partly be off the edge of the cassette. Ideally, another block of material of the same thickness of the cassette should be placed against the side of the cassette; this ensures patient comfort and full weight bearing without any compensation by the patient. This example demonstrates the use of a soft sheet of foam.

provided to any individual who remains in the room during the exposure to assist in positioning.

## ANGLE AND BASE OF GAIT POSITIONING

Weight-bearing dorsoplantar and lateral foot radiographs have been advocated for decades, as early as 1943.[17] The weight-bearing attitude is felt to create an anatomic image that is most feasible for assessing normal versus pathological biomechanical conditions under the stresses and strain of body weight.[18] Shortly after Sgarlato[19] described the kinesiologic and structural relationships of the angle of gait, Hlavac[20] demonstrated that foot position has a profound influence on the radiographic relationships and forms of osseous structures and angular biomechanical measurements. Weight-bearing foot radiography with the foot positioned in angle and base of gait is considered standard technique in podiatric practice for dorsoplantar and lateral foot radiographs and has since been advocated to the orthopedic community.[21]

The purpose of using angle and base of gait is to standardize the weight-bearing radiographic technique in order to visualize positional relationships of the foot bones in a midstance attitude.[22] The radiographer must first study the relationship of the foot to the line of progression in the patient's gait cycle. The degree of abduction or adduction of the foot from the midline (line of progression) is known as the angle of gait (Figure 3-1). The separation or distance between both heels during the gait cycle is referred to as the base of gait (Figure 3-2). Because both heels are not on the ground at the same time during gait (as they are in foot radiography), base of gait is an attempt to maintain a normal midstance relationship of the tibia to the ground.[22] The radiographer must then position the patient's foot relative to the x-ray film and central beam such that angle and base of gait is reproduced. When using an orthoposer, the x-ray film/cassette and tube are first positioned for the desired technique (dorsoplantar or lateral) and the patient's stance is adjusted to place the foot in proper position. Figures 3-3 and 3-4 show examples of dorsoplantar and lateral positioning techniques, respectively, in angle and base of gait.

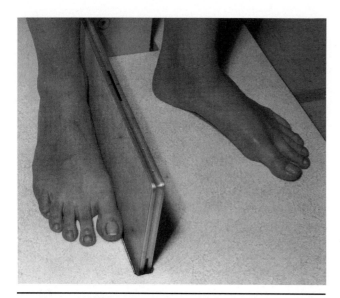

Figure 3-4  Weight-bearing lateral positioning technique in angle and base of gait. The patient's right foot is positioned against the film/cassette. The left foot is then positioned such that both feet are in angle and base of gait.

## ■ FOOT-POSITIONING TECHNIQUES

*Note:* Weight-bearing techniques can also be performed as partial weight bearing. The only difference in positioning is that the patient places most of the weight on the opposite foot while partially bearing weight on the foot being studied. If there is any question whether or not a patient can safely step onto or stand on the orthoposer, perform the study non–weight bearing, with the patient seated.

### Dorsoplantar Projections

1.  Weight-bearing dorsoplantar projection (Figure 3-5)

    Film placement: flat (horizontal) on orthoposer; long side of cassette parallel to long side of orthoposer.
    Tubehead angulation: 15 degrees from vertical directed posteriorly.
    Foot position: flat on cassette with foot's midline parallel to long side of cassette. The opposite foot is placed in angle and base of gait.
    Central ray direction: second metatarsocuneiform joint.
    Other considerations: It has been advocated that dorsoplantar projections be performed with the tubehead angled 5, 10, or even 20 degrees posteriorly, depending on metatarsal declination. On the average, metatarsal declination is 15 degrees relative to the plane of support. A 15-degree tubehead angulation should be performed initially for dorsoplantar projections; tubehead angulation at 5, 10, or 20 degrees should be performed only as an adjunctive

study, if needed. A standardized tubehead angulation eliminates another variable when interpreting the resultant view. If the tubehead is angled at different degrees for each patient, it will be difficult to appreciate the form and position of foot bones relative to normal expectations; in other words, is a bone's shape, size, or position viewed in the radiograph distorted by the non-standard tubehead angulation?

2.  Non–weight-bearing dorsoplantar projection

    Film placement: flat (horizontal) on radiographic table.
    Tubehead angulation: 15 degrees from vertical directed posteriorly.
    Foot position: flat on cassette with foot's midline parallel to long side of cassette. The knee must be flexed so that the foot fully purchases the cassette. A sandbag should be placed along the front edge of the cassette to prevent it from sliding.
    Central ray direction: second metatarsocuneiform joint.
    Other considerations:

    (a) To perform this technique with an orthoposer, the patient must be seated, facing the orthoposer. The long axis of the cassette is perpendicular to the long side of the orthoposer. The patient places the sole of the foot in contact with the cassette. The tubehead is directed posteriorly toward the second metatarsocuneiform joint at 15 degrees from vertical.
    (b) A variation of this technique angles the tubehead 0 degrees (vertical). The foot can either remain flat on the cassette, or a 15-degree radiolucent wedge can be placed beneath the forefoot so the metatarsals are parallel to the film.

### Oblique Positions

1.  Non–weight-bearing medial oblique position (Figure 3-6)

    Film placement: flat (horizontal) on radiographic table.
    Tubehead angulation: 0 degrees (vertical).
    Foot position: Patient lies supine and flexes knee. The sole of the foot is placed flat on the cassette. The knee should be flexed such that the lower leg is nearly perpendicular to the foot. The foot's midline should be parallel to the long side of the cassette. The knee is then turned inward so that the medial side of the foot is closer to the cassette and the sole forms a 45-degree angulation with the cassette. A 45-degree radiolucent positioning wedge can be placed under the sole of the foot to aid in positioning. (A variation of this technique positions the foot so that it is angulated 30 degrees.)
    Central ray direction: third metatarsocuneiform joint.

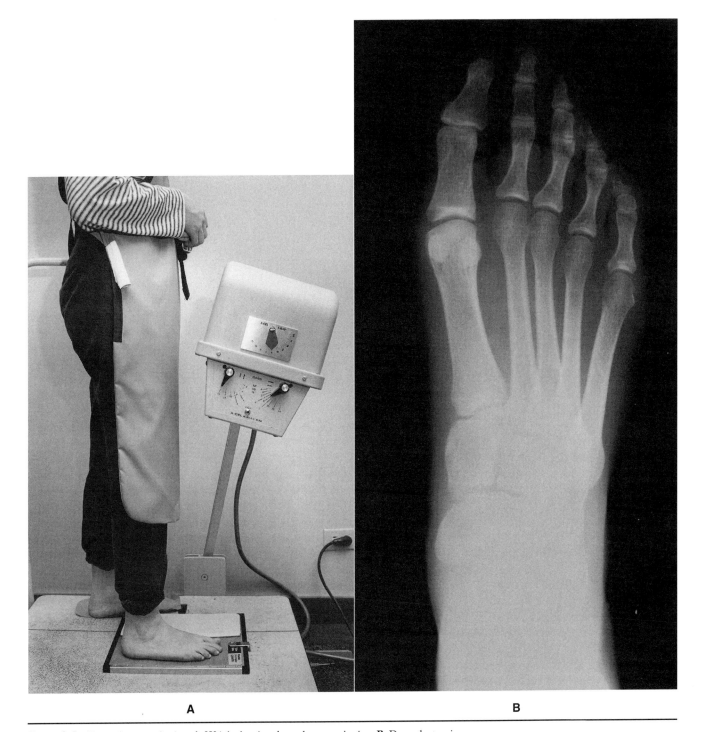

Figure 3-5    Dorsoplantar projection. **A,** Weight-bearing dorsoplantar projection. **B,** Dorsoplantar view.

Other considerations: To perform this technique with an orthoposer, the patient must be seated, facing the orthoposer. The long side of the cassette is perpendicular to the long side of the orthoposer. The tubehead, foot, and central ray are positioned or directed as just noted.

2.  Non–weight-bearing lateral oblique position (Figure 3-7)

Film placement: flat (horizontal) on radiographic table.
Tubehead angulation: 0 degrees (vertical).
Foot position: Patient lies supine and flexes knee. The sole of the foot is placed flat on the cassette. The knee

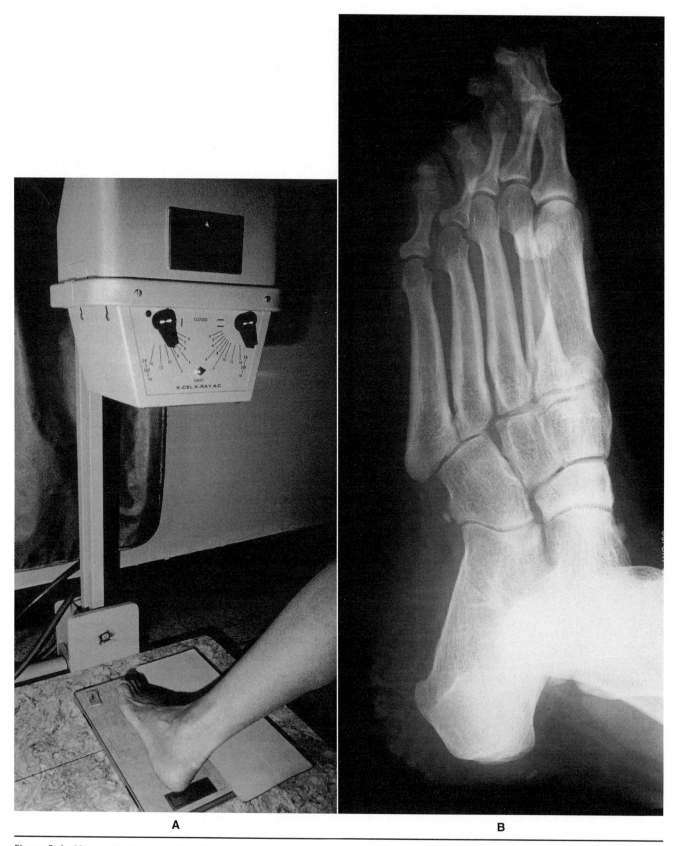

**A**

**B**

Figure 3-6    Non–weight-bearing medial oblique position. **A**, Non–weight-bearing medial oblique position. **B**, Non–weight-bearing medial oblique view.

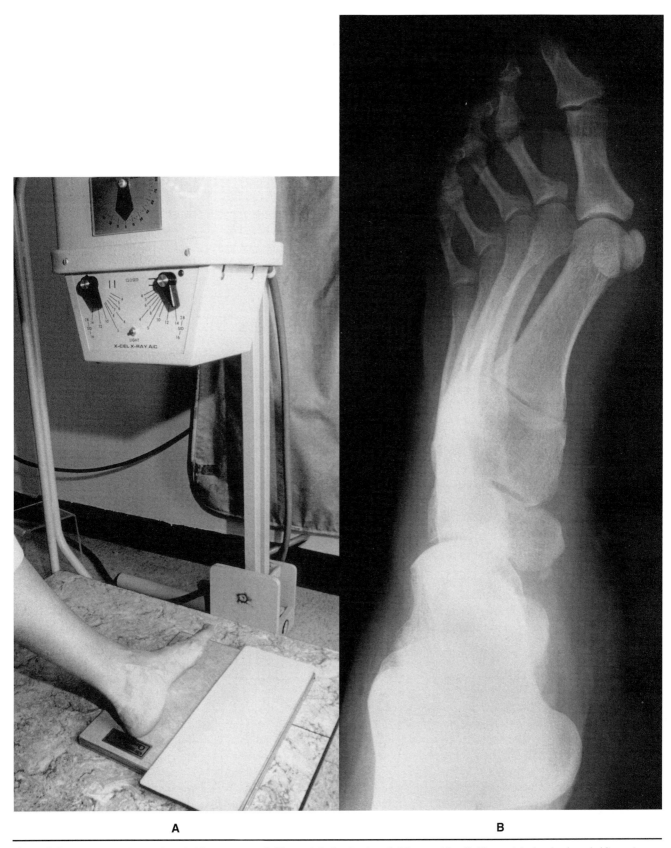

A                                                                          B

Figure 3-7    Non–weight-bearing lateral oblique position. **A,** Non–weight-bearing lateral oblique position. **B,** Non–weight-bearing lateral oblique view.

should be flexed such that the leg is nearly perpendicular to the foot. The foot's midline should be parallel to the long side of the cassette. The knee is then turned out so that the lateral side of the foot is closer to the cassette and the sole forms a 45-degree angulation with the cassette. A 45-degree radiolucent positioning wedge can be placed under the sole of the foot to aid in positioning. (A variation of this technique positions the foot so that it is angulated 30 degrees.)

Central ray direction: first metatarsocuneiform joint.

Other considerations: To perform this technique with an orthoposer, the patient must be seated, facing the orthoposer. The long axis of the cassette is perpendicular to the long side of the orthoposer. The tubehead, foot, and central ray are positioned or directed as noted earlier.

3. Weight-bearing lateromedial oblique projection

Film placement: flat (horizontal) on orthoposer; long axis of cassette parallel to front end of orthoposer.

Tubehead angulation: 45 degrees from vertical.

Foot position: Lateral aspect of foot faces the tubehead. The patient stands on the cassette so that the foot's midline is parallel to the long side of the cassette. The lateral aspect of the foot should be positioned along the long side of the cassette if dividing the film into halves for two views per film. The 45-degree angulation of the tubehead results in image distortion (unequal magnification), and the foot therefore takes up a larger portion of the film than it does with the non–weight-bearing oblique position.

Central ray direction: fourth metatarsocuboid joint.

4. Weight-bearing mediolateral oblique projection

Film placement: flat (horizontal) on orthoposer; long axis of cassette parallel to front end of orthoposer.

Tubehead angulation: 45 degrees from vertical.

Foot position: Medial aspect of foot faces the tubehead. The patient places the foot on the cassette so that its midline is parallel to the long side of the cassette. The medial aspect of the foot should be positioned along the long side of the cassette if dividing the film into halves for two views per film. The opposite foot must be positioned behind and to the side of the foot under study; the patient is instructed to hold onto a support rail to limit movement caused by imbalance and as a safety precaution. The 45-degree tubehead angulation results in image distortion, and the foot therefore takes up a larger portion of the film than it does with the non–weight-bearing oblique position.

Central ray direction: first metatarsocuneiform joint.

## Lateral Positions (Figure 3-8)

1. Weight-bearing lateromedial projection

Film placement: upright (vertical) in slot or well of orthoposer.

Tubehead angulation: 90 degrees from vertical.

Foot position: Patient stands on the orthoposer with the medial aspect of the forefoot positioned against the cassette and the midline of the foot parallel to the cassette. This may require that the heel be pulled away from the cassette a small distance. Also, the tubehead must be precisely positioned at 90 degrees. If not, the plantar aspect of the foot may be cut off the film by the orthoposer. Because it may be difficult to achieve an exact and accurate 90-degree tubehead angulation, have the patient stand on ¼- or ½-inch felt blocks. The opposite foot is placed in angle and base of gait and should also be placed on top of felt, if applicable.

Central ray direction: lateral cuneiform/cuboid.

2. Non–weight-bearing lateromedial projection

Film placement: flat (horizontal) on radiographic table.

Tubehead angulation: 0 degrees (vertical).

Foot position: For a right-foot study, the patient lies on the left body side and vice versa. The medial aspect of the foot is positioned against the cassette. The foot must be nearly perpendicular to the lower leg.

Central ray direction: lateral cuneiform/cuboid.

Other considerations: To perform this technique with an orthoposer, the patient must be seated, facing the orthoposer. The cassette stands vertical in the well of the orthoposer. The medial aspect of the forefoot is positioned against the cassette with the midline of the foot parallel to the cassette. The tubehead must be precisely positioned at 90 degrees. If not, the plantar aspect of the foot may be cut off the film by the orthoposer. Because it may be difficult to achieve an exact and accurate 90-degree tubehead angulation, place the foot on a ¼- or ½-inch felt block. The central ray is directed as already noted.

3. Non–weight-bearing mediolateral projection

Film placement: flat (horizontal) on radiographic table.

Tubehead angulation: 0 degrees (vertical).

Foot position: For a right-foot study, the patient lies on the right body side and for the left foot, on the left body side. The lateral aspect of the foot is positioned against the cassette. The foot should be nearly perpendicular to the lower leg and the sole of the foot should be perpendicular to the cassette.

Central ray direction: medial cuneiform.

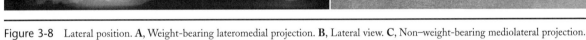

Figure 3-8    Lateral position. **A,** Weight-bearing lateromedial projection. **B,** Lateral view. **C,** Non–weight-bearing mediolateral projection.

Other considerations: To perform this technique with an orthoposer, the patient must be seated, facing the orthoposer. The cassette lies flat on the orthoposer. The lateral aspect of the foot is positioned against the cassette so that the sole of the foot is perpendicular to the cassette. The tubehead angulation and direction of the central ray are as noted earlier.

## TOE-POSITIONING TECHNIQUES

### Dorsoplantar Projections

1. Weight-bearing and non–weight-bearing dorsoplantar projections

These projections of the toes are performed in the same manner as the weight-bearing and non–weight-bearing dorsoplantar projections of the foot with the following exceptions:

The tubehead angulation is 0 degrees (vertical).

The central ray is directed toward the second digit proximal phalanx if viewing all digits or the digit in question if only one digit.

### Oblique Positions

Non–weight-bearing medial and lateral oblique positions and

Weight-bearing lateromedial and mediolateral oblique projections

The oblique positioning techniques of the toes are performed in the same manner as the oblique positions of the foot with the following exception: The central ray is directed toward the third digit proximal phalanx if viewing all digits or the digit in question if only one digit.

### Lateral Positions

The following descriptions pertain to standard film sizes (10 by 12 inches or 8 by 10 inches). However, an option is to use dental film.[23] The unexposed dental film is placed vertically behind the toe in question. Occasionally, nonstandard positioning of the foot (turned slightly inward or outward, for example) may enhance visibility of the toe in question in the radiograph.

1.  Weight-bearing lateromedial projection (Figure 3-9)

    Film placement: upright (vertical) in slot or well of orthoposer.
    Tubehead angulation: 90 degrees from vertical.
    Foot position: Patient stands on the orthoposer with the medial aspect of the hallux positioned against the cassette. Place a roll of gauze beneath the digit of concern to raise it above the remaining digits. (If there is a history of trauma, place the roll of gauze beneath the remaining toes to raise them above the digit under study.) An 8-foot length of tube gauze can also be used to isolate a digit. The toe is positioned at the midpoint of the tube gauze; the patient is instructed to pull the affected or adjacent digit(s) up or down (this depends on which toe is to be isolated and whether or not there are digital deformities) with the two ends of tube gauze.
    Central ray direction: toe in question.

2.  Non–weight-bearing lateromedial projection

    Film placement: flat (horizontal) on radiographic table.
    Tubehead angulation: 0 degrees (vertical).
    Foot position: For a right-foot study, the patient lies on the left body side and vice versa. The medial aspect of the hallux is positioned against the cassette. The affected toe can be further isolated with tube gauze as described for the weight-bearing lateromedial projection.
    Central ray direction: toe in question.
    Other considerations: To perform this technique with an orthoposer, the patient must be seated, facing the orthoposer. The cassette stands vertical in the well of the orthoposer. The medial aspect of the hallux is positioned against the cassette. The central ray is directed as noted earlier.

3.  Non–weight-bearing mediolateral projection

    Film placement: flat (horizontal) on radiographic table.
    Tubehead angulation: 0 degrees (vertical).
    Foot position: For a right-foot study, the patient lies on the right body side and for the left foot, on the left

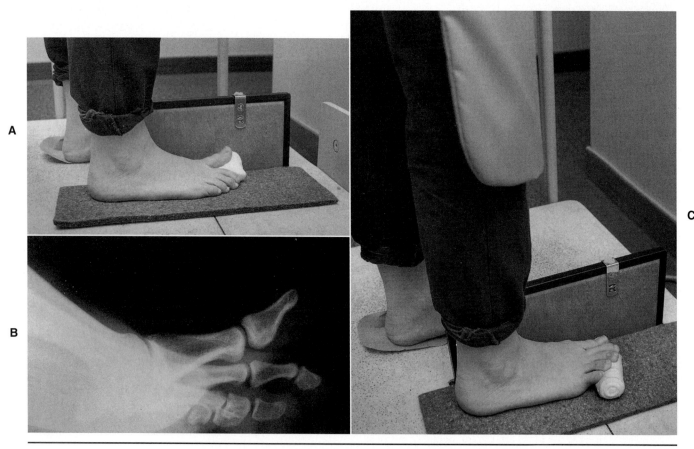

**A**
**B**
**C**

Figure 3-9    Lateral toe positions. **A,** Weight-bearing lateromedial projection of the hallux (hallux elevated). **B,** Lateral view of the hallux. **C,** Weight-bearing lateromedial projection of the hallux (lesser toes elevated).

body side. The lateral aspect of the fifth toe is positioned next to the cassette. The affected toe can be isolated with tube gauze as described for the weight-bearing lateromedial projection.

Central ray direction: toe in question.

Other considerations: To perform this technique with an orthoposer, the patient must be seated, facing the orthoposer. The cassette lies flat (horizontal) on the orthoposer. The lateral aspect of the foot is positioned against the cassette so that the sole of the foot is perpendicular to the cassette. The tubehead angulation and direction of the central ray are as noted earlier.

## ■ SESAMOID-POSITIONING TECHNIQUES

### Posteroanterior Sesamoid Axial Projections

*Note:* The lead apron should be reversed so that it is placed over the patient's back.

1.  Weight-bearing axialposer method[24,25] (Figure 3-10)

    Film placement: upright (vertical) in slot or well of orthoposer.
    Tubehead angulation: 90 degrees from vertical.

Foot position: The front of the axialposer positioning device is placed against the cassette so that the toes will be closest to the film and the heel farthest. The patient stands on the axialposer (heel and toes are elevated so that the metatarsophalangeal joints are the most inferiorly positioned anatomic structures). (The tubehead is behind the patient.)

Central ray direction: center of back of axialposer device.

Other considerations: If an axialposer is not available, the following variation can be performed: Film placement and tubehead angulation are as just described. A ¼-inch felt pad is placed under the ball of the foot. The digits (toes) are placed against the cassette, and dorsiflexion is maintained. The patient then elevates the heel. The central ray is aimed at the plantar surface of the metatarsal head, usually at the third metatarsal head surface. The lead apron is worn in reverse. If the patient has difficulty in maintaining the dorsiflexion of the digits against the cassette, a 3-inch roll of gauze can be placed beneath the toes to provide support.

2.  Lewis method[26] (Figure 3-11, *A*)

    Film placement: flat (horizontal) on radiographic table.
    Tubehead angulation: 0 degrees (vertical).

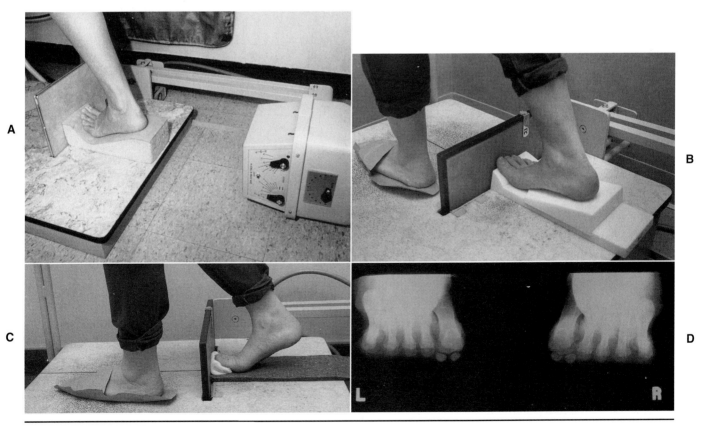

**Figure 3-10**  Weight-bearing sesamoid axial projections. **A,** Weight-bearing axialposer method (precut Styrofoam device). **B,** Weight-bearing axialposer method (adjustable axialposer device). **C,** Weight-bearing sesamoid axial projection without axialposer device. **D,** Weight-bearing sesamoid axial view.

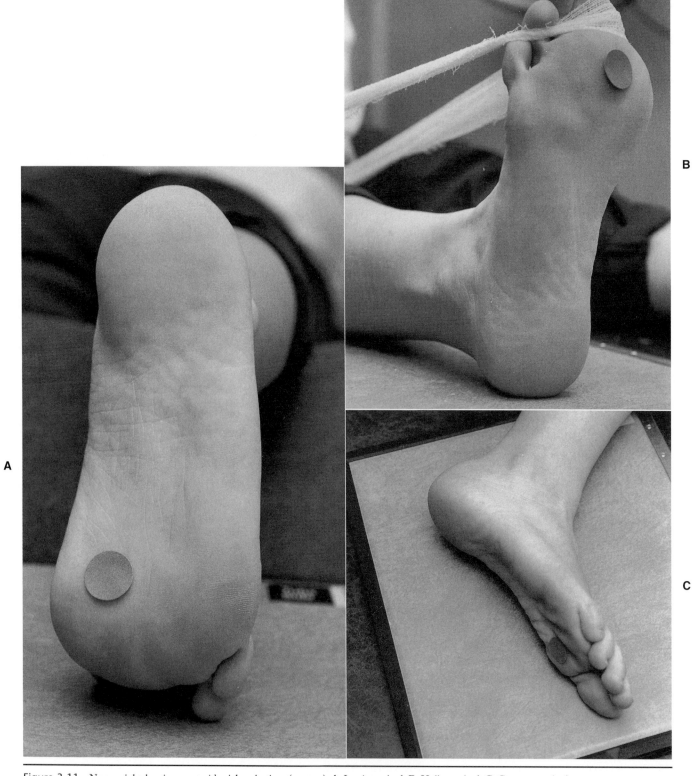

**Figure 3-11**   Non–weight-bearing sesamoid axial projections (see text). **A,** Lewis method. **B,** Holly method. **C,** Causton method.

Foot position: Patient lies prone on the radiographic table. The knee should rest on a foam cushion. The toes are forcibly dorsiflexed as they are positioned against the film.

Central ray direction: ball of foot.

## Anteroposterior Sesamoid Axial Projection (Holly Method[27]) (Figure 3-11, *B*)

Film placement: flat (horizontal) on radiographic table.

Tubehead angulation: 0 degrees (vertical).

Foot position: Patient lies supine on the radiographic table. The heel is placed against the film, and the foot is upright and slightly plantarflexed. The toes are forcibly dorsiflexed by the patient with a long strip of tube gauze placed around the toes.

Central ray direction: ball of foot.

## Lateromedial Tangential Projection (Causton Method[28]) (Figure 3-11, *C*)

Film placement: flat (horizontal) on radiographic table.

Tubehead angulation: 40 degrees from vertical directed posteriorly.

Foot position: Patient lies on the radiographic table on

unaffected body side with knees flexed. The medial aspect of the affected foot is placed against the film; the sole is perpendicular to the cassette.

Central ray direction: sesamoids.

## ■ TARSAL-POSITIONING TECHNIQUES

### Dorsoplantar Calcaneal Axial Projection (Figure 3-12, *A* and *B*)

*Note:* The lead apron should be reversed so that it is placed over the patient's back.

Film placement: flat (horizontal) on orthoposer.

Tubehead angulation: 25 degrees from vertical directed anteriorly.

Foot position: Patient stands on the cassette. (The tubehead is behind the patient.) The heel is placed so that its posterior aspect is about 1 to 1½ inches away from the edge of the cassette closest to the x-ray tube. The patient can be instructed to flex the knees slightly into a "ski jump" configuration so that the foot is dorsiflexed at the ankle joint.

Central ray direction: posterior aspect of foot between the Achilles tendon insertion and the ankle joint.

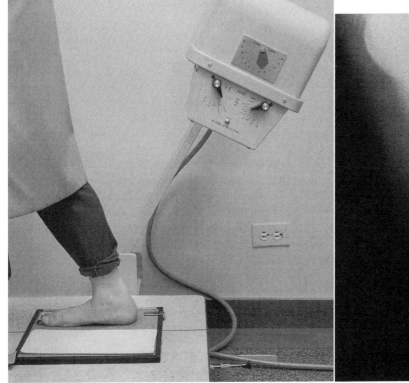

**A**

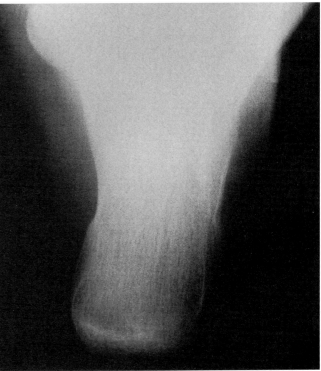

**B**

Figure 3-12, cont'd   Calcaneal axial projections. **A,** Dorsoplantar calcaneal axial projection.

*Continued*

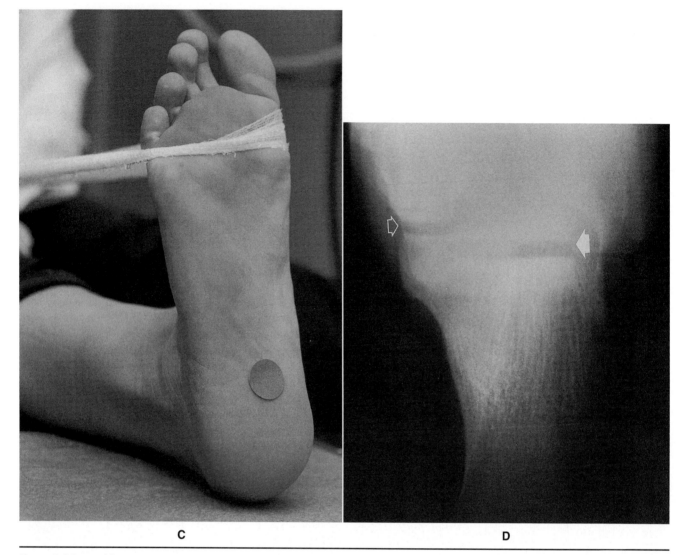

C

D

Figure 3-12, cont'd   Calcaneal axial projections. **C,** Plantodorsal calcaneal axial projection. **D,** Calcaneal axial (Harris-Beath) view (45 degrees).

Other considerations:

1. One variation of this positioning technique is known as the posterior tangential projection.[29] The film placement, foot position, and central ray position is the same as just described except that the patient stands erect (no additional dorsiflexion is needed at the ankle joint). The tubehead is positioned at 45 degrees from vertical and directed toward the midpoint between the inferior aspects of the malleoli. The resultant view shows the middle and posterior articular facets in addition to the calcaneal body.

2. Another variation is known as the calcaneal apophysis or superoinferior calcaneus projection.[30] It is used to assess the posterior calcaneal surface (Achilles tendon enthesis) in the adult and the apophysis in the child. Film placement and foot position is the same as described earlier except that the patient is instructed to

place both hands on the support rails and lean forward while the heels still purchase the cassette. The heels are parallel to each other on the film and the lower limbs are bent slightly forward. The tubehead angulation is 0 degrees (vertical). Some modification of tubehead angulation may be necessary to adequately visualize the Achilles tendon enthesis and to see different aspects of the apophysis. The central ray is directed toward the posterior aspect of the heel.

## Plantodorsal Calcaneal Axial Projection
(Figure 3-12, *C*)

Film placement: flat (horizontal) on radiographic table.

Tubehead angulation: 40 to 45 degrees from vertical directed posteriorly.

Foot position: Patient lies supine on the radiographic

table. The back (posterior aspect) of the heel is placed against the cassette, and the toes point upward. The lateral and plantar aspects of the foot should be perpendicular to the cassette. The patient then forcibly dorsiflexes the forefoot with a long strip of tube gauze placed around the ball of the foot and grasped by both hands at its ends.
Central ray direction: center of heel.

## Harris-Beath Calcaneal Axial Projection

*Note:* The lead apron should be reversed so that it is placed over the patient's back.

The resultant image is also known as the "coalition position"[5] (Figure 3-12, *D*). Lilienfeld[31] first described this for assessment of talocalcaneal coalition. It has been further described and used by Harris and Beath,[32] Coventry,[33] and Vaughan and Segal.[34] The positioning is similar to the dorsoplantar calcaneal axial projection except for the tube angulation.

Film placement: flat (horizontal) on orthoposer.
Tubehead angulation: depends on the angle that the posterior subtalar facet forms with the weight-bearing plantar surface. This can be measured on a standard weight-bearing lateral projection. The usual tube angle is at 40 degrees, but can vary anywhere from 35 to 45 degrees.
Foot position: Patient stands on the cassette. (The tubehead is behind the patient.) The heel is placed so that the posterior aspect of the heel is about 1 to 1½ inches away from the edge of the cassette closest to the x-ray tube. The patient is instructed to flex the knees slightly into a "ski jump" configuration.
Central ray direction: center of heel.

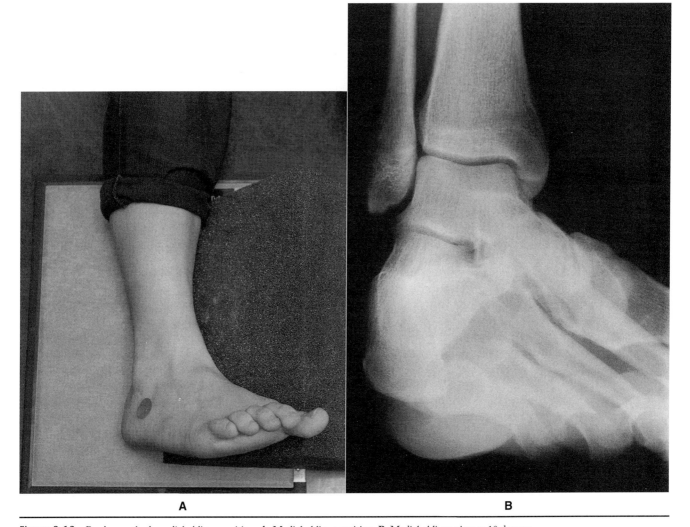

**A**                                                         **B**

Figure 3-13    Broden method: medial oblique position. **A,** Medial oblique position. **B,** Medial oblique view at 10 degrees.

*Continued*

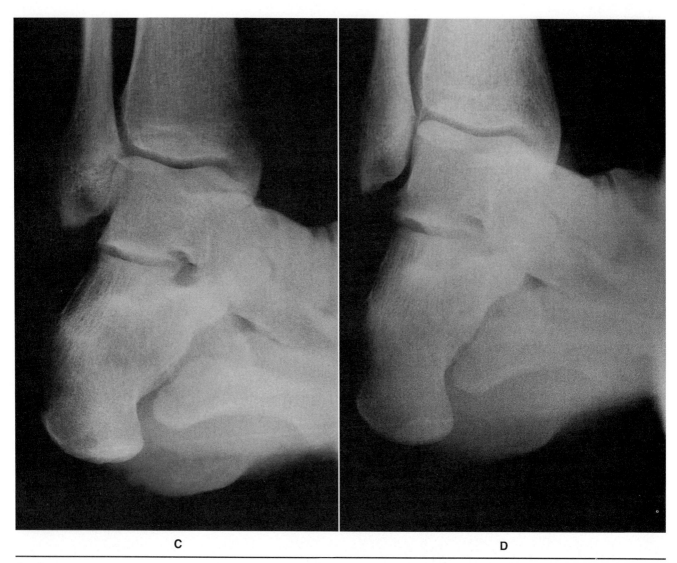

|        C        |        D        |

Figure 3-13, cont'd    Broden method: medial oblique position. **C,** Medial oblique view at 20 degrees. **D,** Medial oblique view at 30 degrees.

*Continued*

## Broden Method[35]

Multiple positioning techniques are performed to assess different aspects of the posterior subtalar joint:

1.  Medial oblique positions (Figure 3-13)

    Film placement: flat (horizontal) on radiographic table.
    Tubehead angulation: Four positioning techniques are performed at 10, 20, 30, and 40 degrees from vertical, directed posteriorly and cephalad.
    Foot position: Patient lies supine on the radiographic table. The back (posterior aspect) of the heel is placed against the cassette, and the toes point upward. (The posterior aspect of the heel is placed about 1 to 1½ inches away from the edge of the cassette closest to the x-ray tube.)

A 45-degree positioning wedge is placed along the medial aspect of the foot and ankle. The leg and foot are turned inward and rest on the wedge. The patient dorsiflexes the foot so that it is perpendicular to the lower leg. This can be maintained with a long strip of tube gauze placed around the ball of the foot and grasped by the patient with both hands at its ends.
    Central ray direction: between the fibular malleolus and fifth metatarsal base.

2.  Lateral oblique positions (Figure 3-14)

    Film placement: flat (horizontal) on radiographic table.
    Tubehead angulation: Two positioning techniques are performed at 15 and 18 degrees from vertical, directed posteriorly and cephalad.

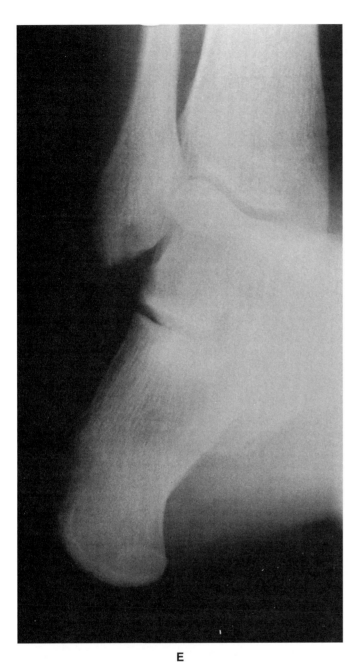

**Figure 3-13, cont'd**  Broden method: medial oblique position. **E,** Medial oblique view at 40 degrees.

Foot position: Patient lies supine on the radiographic table. The back (posterior aspect) of the heel is placed against the cassette, and the toes point upward. (The posterior aspect of the heel is placed about 1 to 1½ inches away from the edge of the cassette closest to the x-ray tube.) A 45-degree positioning wedge is placed along the lateral aspect of the foot and ankle. The leg and foot are turned outward and rest on the wedge. The patient dorsiflexes the foot so that it is perpendicular to the lower leg. This can be maintained with a long strip of tube gauze placed around the ball of the foot and grasped by the patient with both hands at its ends.

Central ray direction: between the tibial malleolus and navicular tuberosity.

## Isherwood Method[36,37] (Figure 3-15)

Three positioning techniques are performed to assess the anterior, middle, and posterior subtalar joints:

1. Medial oblique position (to assess the anterior articulation)

*Note:* This positioning technique is the same as the non–weight-bearing medial oblique foot position except for the central ray direction.

Film placement: flat (horizontal) on radiographic table.
Tubehead angulation: 0 degrees (vertical).
Foot position: Patient lies on the unaffected side and flexes knee. The knee of the affected extremity sits on the table and the medial side of the foot lies against the cassette; the foot is held perpendicular to the lower leg. A 45-degree positioning wedge is placed beside the sole of the foot; the knee is lifted off the table so that the medial side of the foot stays against the cassette and the sole of the foot rests against the wedge, forming a 45-degree angulation with the cassette.
Central ray direction: between the fibular malleolus and cuboid.

2. Medial oblique axial position (to assess the middle articulation)

Film placement: flat (horizontal) on radiographic table.
Tubehead angulation: 10 degrees from vertical directed posteriorly and superiorly.
Foot position: Patient sits supine on the radiographic table. The back (posterior aspect) of the heel is placed against the cassette and the toes point upward. The foot is held perpendicular to the lower leg. A 30-degree positioning wedge is placed beside the medial aspect of the foot. The knee is slightly flexed and the extremity turned internally so that the back of the heel remains against the cassette and the medial side of the foot and ankle rests against the wedge, forming a 30-degree angle with the cassette. A pillow or sandbag should be placed under the knee for support. The patient is instructed to dorsiflex and invert the foot. This can be maintained with a long strip of tube gauze placed around the ball of the foot and grasped by the patient with both hands at its ends.
Central ray direction: between the fibular malleolus and cuboid.

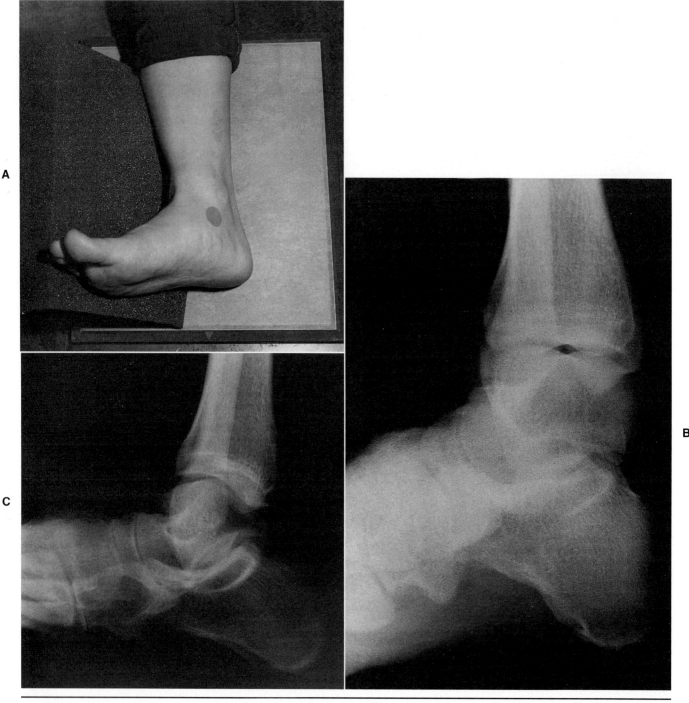

**Figure 3-14** Broden method: lateral oblique position. **A,** Lateral oblique position. **B,** Lateral oblique view at 15 degrees. **C,** Lateral oblique view at 18 degrees.

3. Lateral oblique axial position (to assess the posterior articulation)

Film placement: flat (horizontal) on radiographic table. Tubehead angulation: 10 degrees from vertical directed posteriorly and superiorly.

Foot position: Patient sits supine on the radiographic table. The back (posterior aspect) of the heel is placed against the cassette, and the toes point upward. The foot is held perpendicular to the lower leg. A 30-degree positioning wedge is placed beside the lateral aspect of the foot. The knee is slightly flexed and the extremity turned externally so that the back of the heel remains against the cassette and the lateral side of the foot and ankle rests against the wedge, forming a 30-degree angulation with the cassette. A pillow or sandbag should be placed under the knee for support. The patient is instructed to dorsiflex and evert the foot. This can be maintained with a long strip of tube gauze placed around the ball of the foot and grasped by the patient with both hands at its ends.

Central ray direction: between the tibial malleolus and navicular tuberosity.

## ANKLE-POSITIONING TECHNIQUES

### Anteroposterior Projections

1.  Weight-bearing anteroposterior projection (Figure 3-16)

    Film placement: upright (vertical) in slot of orthoposer; long axis of cassette perpendicular to orthoposer surface.

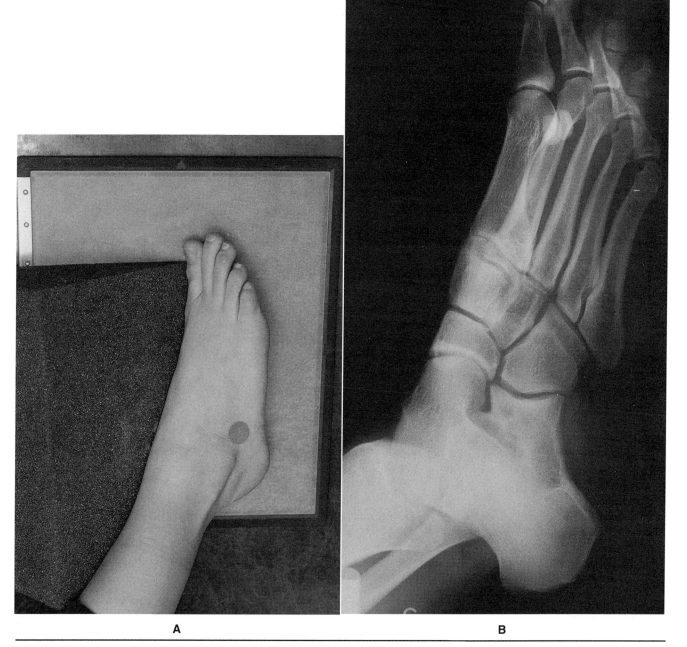

| A | B |

Figure 3-15    Isherwood method. **A**, Medial oblique position. **B**, Medial oblique view.

*Continued*

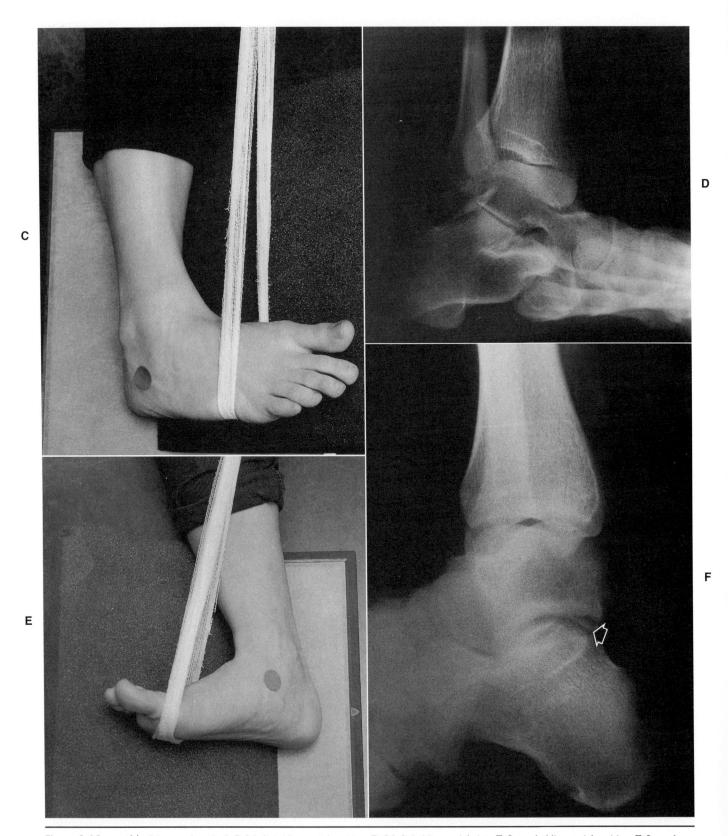

Figure 3-15, cont'd    Isherwood method. **C,** Medial oblique axial position. **D,** Medial oblique axial view. **E,** Lateral oblique axial position. **F,** Lateral oblique axial view.

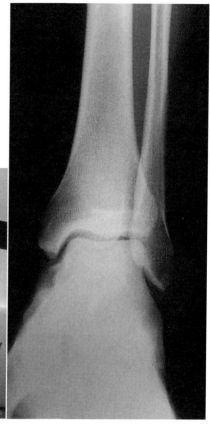

Figure 3-16    Anteroposterior projection. **A**, Weight-bearing anteroposterior projection. **B**, Anteroposterior view.

Tubehead angulation: 90 degrees from vertical.
Foot position: Back of heel is placed against the cassette.
    The foot's midline axis is perpendicular to the cassette.
Central ray direction: center of ankle joint.

2.    Non–weight-bearing anteroposterior projection

Film placement: flat (horizontal) on radiographic table.
Tubehead angulation: 0 degrees (vertical).
Foot position: Patient lies supine or sits on radiographic
    table. The back of the heel is placed against the cassette,
    and the toes point upward. The knee is nearly straight;
    a small pillow or sandbag can be placed under the knee
    for patient comfort. The foot's midline axis is perpen-
    dicular to the cassette. The foot should be held nearly
    perpendicular to the leg; a sandbag can be propped
    against the sole of the foot to aid in positioning.
Central ray direction: center of ankle joint.

## Mortise Position

1.    Weight-bearing mortise position (Figure 3-17)

Film placement: upright (vertical) in slot of orthoposer;
    long axis of cassette perpendicular to orthoposer surface.

Tubehead angulation: 90 degrees from vertical.
Foot position: Back of heel is placed against the cassette.
    The ankle joint axis (an imaginary line running
    through both malleoli) is aligned so that it lies parallel
    to the cassette. This is best achieved by placing an
    index finger on each malleolus and visualizing the axis
    through the ankle. A slight internal rotation of the
    extremity is required, anywhere from 5 to 15 degrees.
    After positioning the extremity, recheck the malleolar
    axis; excessive pronation causes exaggerated internal
    rotation of the talus and lower leg on weight bearing,
    resulting in an oblique view of the ankle.
Central ray direction: center of ankle joint.

2.    Non–weight-bearing mortise position

Film placement: flat (horizontal) on radiographic table.
Tubehead angulation: 0 degrees (vertical).
Foot position: Patient lies supine or sits on radiographic
    table. The back of the heel is placed against the cassette.
    The knee is nearly straight; a small pillow or sandbag
    can be placed under the knee for patient comfort. The
    ankle joint axis (an imaginary line running through
    both malleoli) is aligned so that it lies parallel to the

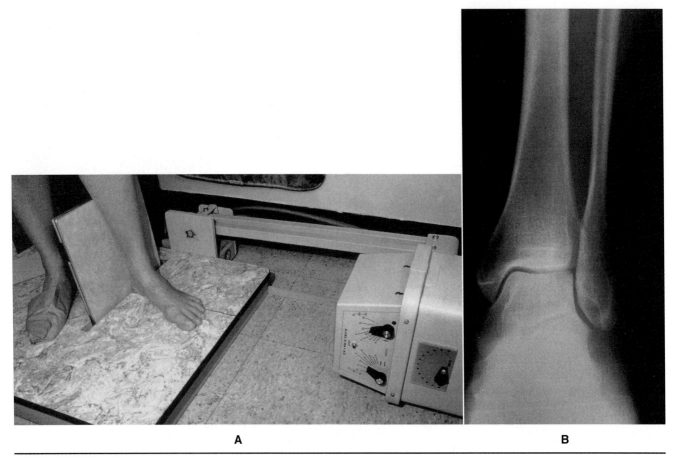

**Figure 3-17**    Mortise position. **A,** Weight-bearing mortise position. **B,** Mortise view.

cassette. Or rotate the limb until the medial and lateral malleoli are equidistant from the cassette.[38] This is best achieved by placing an index finger on each malleolus and visualizing the axis through the ankle. A slight internal rotation of the extremity is required, anywhere from 5 to 15 degrees. The foot should be held nearly perpendicular to the leg; a sandbag can be propped against the sole of the foot to aid in positioning.
Central ray direction: center of ankle joint.

## Oblique Positions

1. Weight-bearing medial (internal) oblique position (Figure 3-18)

   Film placement: upright (vertical) in slot of orthoposer; long axis of cassette is perpendicular to orthoposer surface.
   Tubehead angulation: 90 degrees from vertical.
   Foot position: Back of heel is placed against the cassette. The lower extremity (foot and leg) is internally rotated

45 degrees so that the medial surface of the extremity faces the cassette. A 45-degree positioning wedge can be used to assist in positioning.
Central ray direction: center of ankle.

2. Non–weight-bearing medial (internal) oblique position

   Film placement: flat (horizontal) on radiographic table.
   Tubehead angulation: 0 degrees (vertical).
   Foot position: Patient lies supine or sits on radiographic table. The back of the heel is placed against the cassette. The knee is nearly straight; a small pillow or sandbag can be placed under the knee for patient comfort. A 45-degree positioning wedge is placed along the medial aspect of the foot and ankle. The lower extremity (foot and leg) is internally rotated 45 degrees so that the medial surface rests against the wedge. The foot should be held nearly perpendicular to the leg; a sandbag can be propped against the sole of the foot to aid in positioning.
   Central ray direction: center of ankle.

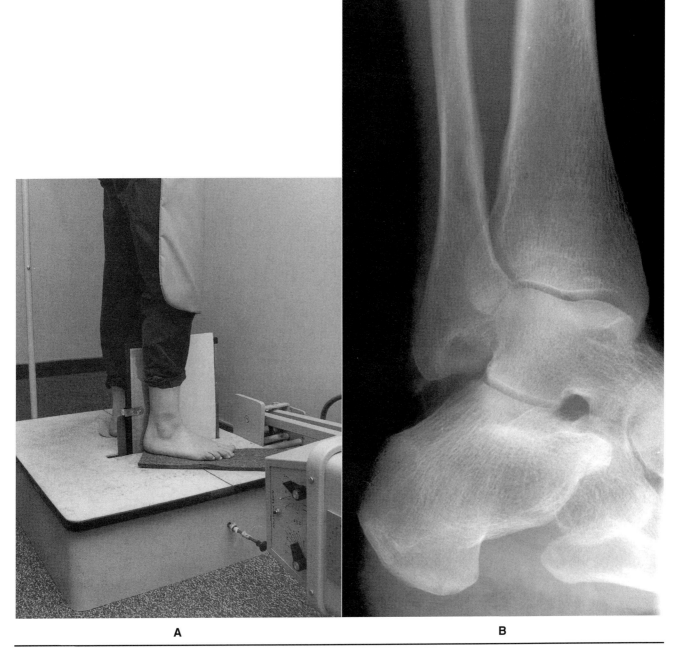

**A**                                              **B**

Figure 3-18    Internal oblique position. **A**, Weight-bearing internal oblique position. **B**, Internal oblique view.

3. Weight-bearing lateral (external) oblique position (Figure 3-19)

Film placement: upright (vertical) in slot of orthoposer; long axis of cassette is perpendicular to orthoposer surface.

Tubehead angulation: 90 degrees from vertical.

Foot position: Back of heel is placed against the cassette. The lower extremity (foot and leg) is externally rotated 45 degrees so that the lateral surface of the extremity faces the cassette. A 45-degree positioning wedge can be used to assist in positioning.

Central ray direction: center of ankle.

4. Non–weight-bearing lateral (external) oblique position

Film placement: flat (horizontal) on radiographic table.

Tubehead angulation: 0 degrees (vertical).

Foot position: Patient lies supine or sits on radiographic table. The back of the heel is placed against the

**Figure 3-19**    External oblique position. **A,** Weight-bearing external oblique position. **B,** External oblique view.

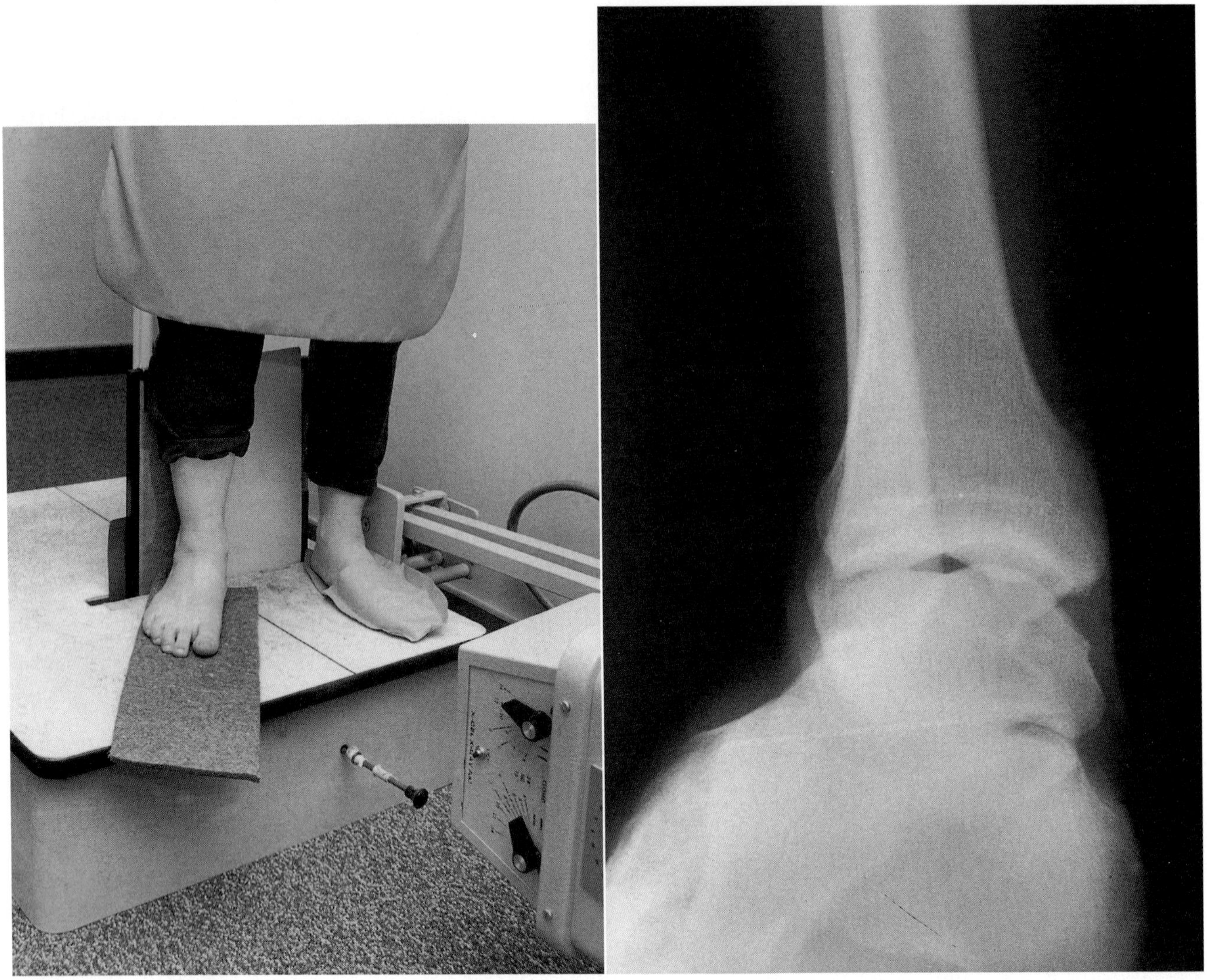

cassette. The knee is nearly straight; a small pillow or sandbag can be placed under the knee for patient comfort. A 45-degree positioning wedge is placed along the lateral aspect of the foot and ankle. The lower extremity (foot and leg) is externally rotated 45 degrees so that the lateral surface rests against the wedge. The foot should be held nearly perpendicular to the leg; a sandbag can be propped against the sole of the foot to aid in positioning.

Central ray direction: center of ankle.

## Lateral Positions (Figure 3-20)

1. Weight-bearing lateromedial projection

   Film placement: upright (vertical) in slot or well of orthoposer.

Tubehead angulation: 90 degrees from vertical.

Foot position: Patient stands on the orthoposer with the medial aspect of the ankle positioned against the cassette so that the ankle joint axis (an imaginary line running through both malleoli) is perpendicular to the cassette. This is best achieved by placing an index finger on each malleolus and visualizing the malleolar axis through the ankle. The heel may have to be pulled away from the cassette a small distance to achieve a perpendicular position. The foot should be nearly perpendicular to the lower leg.

Central ray direction: center of ankle.

2. Non–weight-bearing lateromedial projection

   Film placement: flat (horizontal) on radiographic table.
   Tubehead angulation: 0 degrees (vertical).

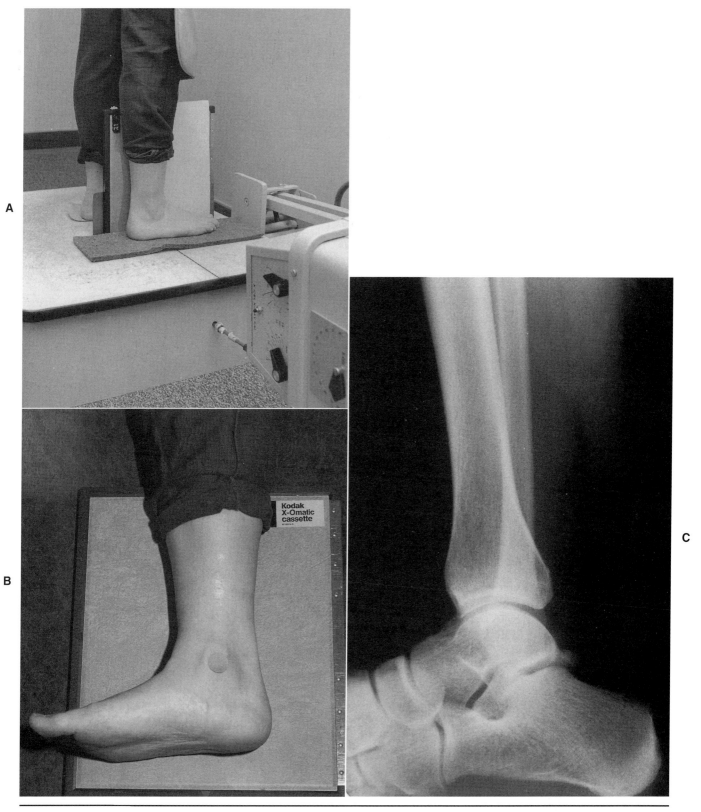

Figure 3-20    Lateral ankle positions. **A**, Weight-bearing lateromedial projection. **B**, Non–weight-bearing mediolateral projection. **C**, Lateral view.

Foot position: For a right-ankle study, the patient lies on the left body side and vice versa. The medial aspect of the ankle is positioned against the cassette. The foot should be held nearly perpendicular to the leg; a sandbag can be propped against the sole of the foot to aid in positioning.

Central ray direction: center of ankle.

Other considerations: To perform this technique with an orthoposer, the patient must be seated, facing the orthoposer. The cassette stands vertical in the well of the orthoposer. The medial aspect of the ankle is placed against the cassette so that the ankle joint axis lies perpendicular to the cassette. The tubehead is angled at 90 degrees (horizontal), and the central ray is directed at the center of the ankle.

3.  Non–weight-bearing mediolateral projection

Film placement: flat (horizontal) on radiographic table.
Tubehead angulation: 0 degrees (vertical).
Foot position: For a right-foot study, the patient lies on the right body side and for the left foot, on the left body side. The lateral aspect of the foot is positioned against the cassette. The foot should be nearly perpendicular to the lower leg; a sandbag can be propped against the sole of the foot to aid in positioning.

Central ray direction: center of ankle.

## References

1. Meschan I: *Roentgen signs in diagnostic imaging,* vol 2, ed 2, Philadelphia, 1985, WB Saunders.
2. Juhl JH: *Paul & Juhl's essentials of roentgen interpretation,* ed 4, Philadelphia, 1981, Harper & Row.
3. Bontrager KL, Anthony BT: *Textbook of radiographic positioning and related anatomy,* Denver, 1982, Multi-Media Publishing.
4. Merrill V: *Atlas of roentgenographic positions,* ed 3, St Louis, 1967, Mosby.
5. Ballinger PW: *Merrill's atlas of radiographic positions and radiologic procedures,* ed 5, St Louis, 1982, Mosby.
6. Weissman, SD: *Radiology of the foot,* ed 2, Baltimore, 1989, Williams & Wilkins.
7. Weissman, S: Standard radiographic techniques for the foot and ankle, *Clin Podiatr Med Surg* 5(4):767, 1988.
8. Kaschak TJ, Laine W: Surgical radiology, *Clin Podiatr Med Surg* 5(4):797, 1988.
9. Squire LF, Novelline RA: *Fundamentals of radiology,* ed 4, Cambridge, MA, 1988, Harvard University Press.
10. Greenfield GB, Cooper SJ: *A manual of radiographic positioning,* Philadelphia, 1973, Lippincott.
11. *Dorland's illustrated medical dictionary,* ed 27, Philadelphia, 1988, WB Saunders.
12. Gamble FO, Yale I: *Clinical foot roentgenology,* ed 2, Huntington, NY, 1975, Robert E Krieger Publishing.
13. Hlavac HF: Differences in x-ray findings with varied positioning of the foot, *J Am Podiatr Med Assoc* 57:465, 1967.
14. Sgarlato TE: The angle of gait, *J Am Podiatr Med Assoc* 55:645, 1965.
15. Ruch JA: Significance and use of radiographs in the angle and base of gait, *PAL Perspectives* 1(2):1, 1980.
16. Bontrager KL, Anthony BT: *Textbook of radiographic positioning and related anatomy,* Denver, 1982, Multi-Media Publishing.
17. Gamble FO: A special approach to foot radiography, *Radiography and Clinical Photography* 19(3):78, 1943.
18. Gamble FO: *Applied foot roentgenology,* Baltimore, 1957, Williams & Wilkins.
19. Sgarlato TE: The angle of gait, *J Am Podiatr Med Assoc* 55(9):645, 1965.
20. Hlavac HF: Differences in x-ray findings with varied positioning of the foot, *J Am Podiatr Med Assoc* 57(10):465, 1967.
21. Brand PW, Coleman WC: A standard for dorsal-plantar and lateral radiographic projections of the feet, *Orthopedics* 10(1):117, 1987.
22. Ruch JA: Significance and use of radiographs in the angle and base of gait, *PAL Perspectives* 1(2):1, 1980.
23. Blass BC, Imanuel HM, Marcus S: Technique for radiographic digital isolation, *J Am Podiatr Med Assoc* 64:870, 1974.
24. Downey MA, Dorothy WL: A radiographic technique to demonstrate the plantar aspect of the forefoot in stance, *J Am Podiatr Med Assoc* 59:140, 1969.
25. Fuson SM, Blau K, Beilman BA: A new sponge axial poser, *J Am Podiatr Med Assoc* 69:681, 1979.
26. Lewis RW: Non-routine views in roentgen examination of the extremities, *Surg Gynecol Obstet* 69:38, 1938.
27. Holly EW: Radiography of the tarsal sesamoid bones, *Med Radiogr Photogr* 31:73, 1955.
28. Causton J: Projection of sesamoid bones in the region of the first metatarsophalangeal joint, *Radiology* 9:39, 1943.
29. Kleiger B, Mankin HJ: A roentgenographic study of the development of the calcaneus by means of the posterior tangential view, *J Bone Joint Surg (Am)* 43:961, 1961.
30. Helal B, Wilson D: *The foot,* vol 1, New York, 1988, Churchill Livingstone.
31. Lilienfeld L: *Anordnung der normalisierten rontgenaufnahmen des menschlichen korpers,* ed 4, Berlin, 1927, Urban &

Schwarzenberg. Cited in Ballinger PW: *Merrill's atlas of radiographic positions and radiologic procedures,* ed 5, St Louis, 1982, Mosby.

32. Harris RI, Beath T: Etiology of peroneal spastic flatfoot, *J Bone Joint Surg (Br)* 30:624, 1948.

33. Coventry MB: Flatfoot with special consideration of tarsal coalition, *Minn Med* 33:1091-1097, 1950. Cited in Ballinger PW: *Merrill's atlas of radiographic positions and radiologic procedures,* ed 5, St Louis, 1982, Mosby.

34. Vaughn WH, Segal G: Tarsal coalition, with special reference to roentgenographic interpretation, *Radiology* 60:855-863, 1953. Cited in Ballinger PW: *Merrill's atlas of radiographic positions and radiologic procedures,* ed 5, St Louis, 1982, Mosby.

35. Broden B: Roentgen examination of the subtaloid joint in fractures of the calcaneus, *Acta Radiol* 31:85, 1949.

36. Isherwood I: A radiological approach to the subtalar joint, *J Bone Joint Surg (Br)* 43:566, 1961.

37. Pinsky MJ: The Isherwood views, *J Am Podiatr Med Assoc* 69:200, 1979.

38. Montagne J, Chevrot A, Galmiche JM: *Atlas of foot radiology,* New York, 1981, Masson Publishing.

## Suggested Readings

Anthonsen W: An oblique projection for roentgen examination of the talo-calcanean joint, particularly regarding intra-articular fracture of the calcaneus, *Acta Radiol* 24:306, 1943.

Baron RL, Strugielski C: X-ray positioning. Pt I: Weight bearing projections, *Podiatric Staff* (February):65, 1989.

Baron RL, Strugielski C: X-ray positioning. Pt II: Non–weight bearing and partial weight bearing projections, *Podiatric Staff* (March):41, 1989.

Baron RL, Knight BL, Strugielski C: X-ray positioning. Pt III: Specialty radiographs, *Podiatry Today* (September):25, 1989.

Brand PW, Coleman WC: A standard for dorsal-plantar and lateral radiographic projections of the feet, *Orthopedics* 10:117, 1987.

Cahoon JB: Radiography of the foot, *Radiogr Clin Photogr* 22:2, 1946.

Cobey JC: Posterior roentgenogram of the foot, *Clin Orthop* 118:202, 1976.

Dreeban S, Thomas PBM, Noble PC et al: A new method for radiography of weight bearing metatarsal heads, *Clin Orthop* 224:260, 1987.

Gabriel GR, Burger ES: Angular plates for fixed angle radiography, *J Am Podiatr Med Assoc* 57:1, 1967.

Goff CW: Weight bearing x-rays of the feet, *Am J Orthopedic Surg* 10(1):13, 1968.

Holly EW: Oblique anteroposterior projection for medial bones of foot, *Med Radiogr Photogr* 31:118, 1955.

Inchaustegui N: Modified lateral view of the distal foot and hand for the evaluation of phalanges, *Revista Interamericana de Radiologia* 6:61, 1981.

Keim HA, Ritchie GW: Weight bearing roentgenograms in the evaluation of foot deformities, *Clin Orthop* 70:133, 1970.

Kirby KA, Loendorf AJ, Gregorio R: Anterior axial projection of the foot, *J Am Podiatr Med Assoc* 78:159, 1988.

Samuelson KM, Harrison R, Freidman MAR: A roentgenographic technique to evaluate and document hindfoot position, *Foot Ankle Int* 1:286, 1985.

Warren AG: Radiographic examination of the feet, *Lepr Rev* 44:131, 1973.

# CHAPTER 4

# Exposure Techniques and Special Considerations

CASIMIR F. STRUGIELSKI

The radiologic examination is an important adjunct in determining the etiology(ies) of a patient's complaint. It becomes equally important that the finished radiograph(s) be of the highest quality, providing as much information as technically possible. Just as no two patients are alike, so will situations and technical factors that produce the image vary. The fundamental concept is that the finished radiograph should exhibit sufficient radiographic density, acceptable contrast, optimal detail, and minimal distortion (Figure 4-1).[1-4]

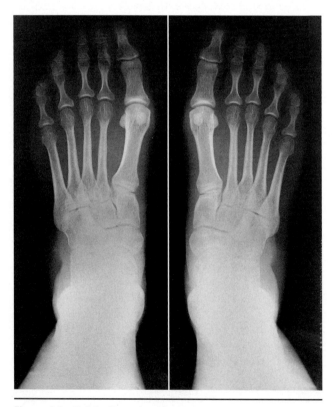

Figure 4-1   Pedal radiograph exhibiting an appropriate gray scale.

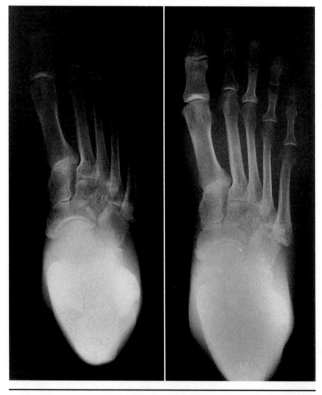

Figure 4-2   As time or mA changes, a corresponding change in density (law of reciprocity) occurs. Left image: $^{16}\!/_{60}$ s at 15mA and 60 kVp. Right image: $^{8}\!/_{60}$ s at 15mA and 60 kVp.

## ■ RADIOGRAPHIC DENSITY

The radiographic density should be such that the proper range of grays is present for the particular area of anatomic interest (see Figure 4-1).[2]

Milliampere–seconds (mAs) is the primary controlling factor for radiographic density. The mAs is a product of milliampere multiplied by the exposure time expressed in seconds (s).

$$mAs = mA \cdot s$$

**Example:** $\frac{8}{60}$ s $\times$ 15 mA = $\frac{120}{60}$ = 2 mAs
   A. $\frac{8}{60}$ s at 15 mA    28 in SID    60 kVp
   B. $\frac{4}{60}$ s at 30 mA    28 in SID    60kVp

Both sets of exposure factors yield the same mAs value; therefore, both (A and B) films should exhibit the same radiographic density. Also, it is important to remember that as mAs increases, both x-ray quantity and radiographic density increase proportionally. This is known as the law of reciprocity (Figure 4-2).[2,3,5]

**Examples:**
   A. $\frac{4}{60}$ s at 15 mA = 1 mAs
   B. $\frac{8}{60}$ s at 15 mA = 2 mAs
   C. $\frac{16}{60}$ s at 15 mA = 4 mAs

To cause a visible shift in radiographic density, a ±30% alteration is necessary to produce this effect (Figure 4-3). This is the minimum change required that will be perceived by the human eye. If adjustment in density is necessary, however, changes should be made by factors of 2 (either double or half).[2] A film that displays insufficient density and that was originally exposed using 2 mAs, for example, should be repeated at 4 mAs (Figure 4-4).

The radiograph in question should be outside the acceptable limits to justify a repeat exposure, either very light or very dark. Basically this means that the viewer is unable to adequately distinguish the necessary anatomic structures. The appropriate change would be to either double or half the mAs. Remember to change *either* mA *or* exposure time: Changing both will increase the mAs value above the half or double value required.

Other influencing factors for density are kilovoltage, distance, film/screen combination, and film processing, discussed as follows.

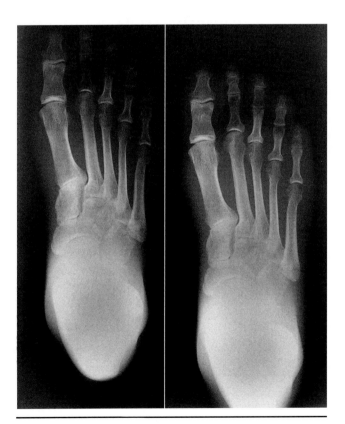

**Figure 4-3**   mAs technique of the left image is 30% greater than that of the right image.

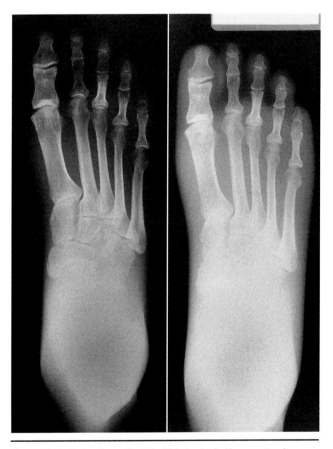

**Figure 4-4**   Rule of twos (half/double) 4 mAs (left) versus 2 mAs (right). (kVp and SID are unchanged).

## Kilovoltage

Kilovoltage alters both the quality (energy) of the x-ray beam and the quantity of x-ray photons produced. Increases in kilovoltage also increase kVp and therefore have a tremendous impact on the image presentation. The operator must know how kVp adjustments alter radiographic density. These changes are presented in Boxes 4-1 and 4-2 and in Figures 4-5 and 4-6.

## Distance

Changes in distance between the x-ray tube and film, also referred to as the source-to-image distance (SID) will alter the number of photons striking the film (quantity of radiation). This will affect the background density: If the tube is too far away from the film, an insufficient number of x-ray photons strike the film, producing a light film (decreased radiographic density) (Figure 4-7). Also, if the tube is too close to the film, a greater number of x-ray photons than are required strike the film, producing a very dark film (radiographic density) (Figure 4-8). This is known as the inverse square law.[1-6] This is expressed using the following formula:[1]

$$\frac{I_1}{I_2} = \frac{(D_2)^2}{(D_1)^2}$$

$I_1$ = Original intensity
$I_2$ = New intensity
$D_1{}^2$ = Original distance squared
$D_2{}^2$ = New distance squared

**Example:**
**Original technique:**
28 in SID

$$\frac{2}{X} \text{ mAs} = \frac{36^2}{28^2} \text{ in}$$

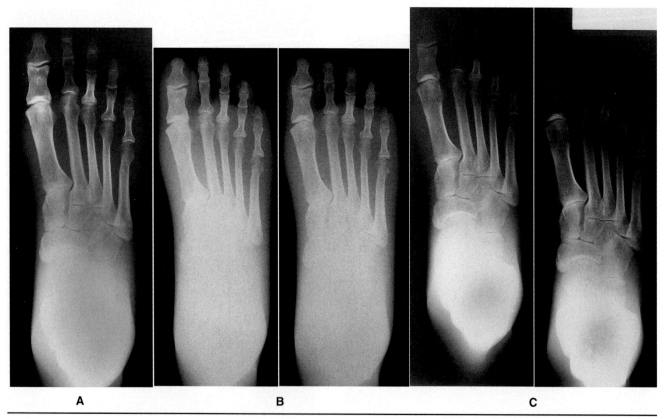

|  A  |  B  |  C  |

**Figure 4-5**   15% rule effect. **A**, Normal exposure factors. **B**, Left image: kVp decreased by 15%. Right image: exposure (mAs) decreased by half. Both images exhibit decreased radiographic density. **C**, Right image: exposure time increased by doubling. Both images exhibit increased radiographic density.

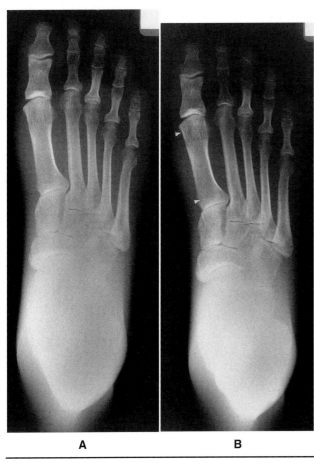

**Figure 4-6**    kVp changes. **A**, Normal kVp (60). **B**, kVp increased approximately 7% to 65 kVp. Note change in gray scale in the metatarsal and tarsal areas.

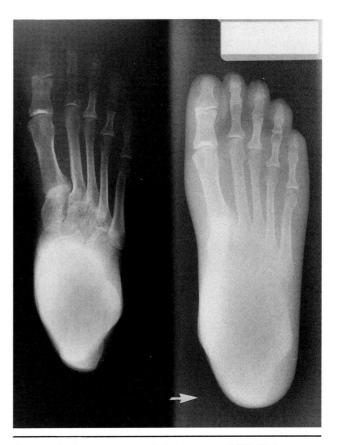

**Figure 4-7**    Inverse square law. Left image: normal SID. Right image: tube distance from film (SID). Note the diminished radiographic density.

2 mAs                      $\dfrac{2}{X}$ mAs $= \dfrac{1296}{784}$ in

**New technique:**
36 in SID                  1296 $X$ = 1568 mAs
                           $X$ = 1.2 mAs

Short method:

| | |
|---|---|
| **Divide new distance into old:** | 28 ÷ 36 = .77 |
| Square result: | 0.77 × 0.77 = 0.59 |
| Multiply this value times old mAs: | 0.59 × 2 mAs = 1.18 |
| | mAs ≅ 1.2 mAs |

To maintain the same density at different distances (SID), the following formula may be used:

$$\frac{mAs_1}{mAs_2} = \frac{(D_1)^2}{(D_2)^2}$$

Using the previous example:

**Old technique:**
28 in SID          $\dfrac{2\ mAs}{X} = \dfrac{28\ in^2}{36\ in^2}$

2 mAs              $\dfrac{2\ mAs}{X} = \dfrac{784\ in}{1296\ in}$

**New technique:**
36 in SID    784 in $X$ = 1296 in × 2 mAs
$X$ = mAs    784 in $X$ = 2,592 in
                        $X$ = 2592 ÷ 784
                        $X$ = 3.3 mAs

Short method:

| | |
|---|---|
| Divide new SID by old SID: | 36 ÷ 28 = 1.28 |
| Square result: | 1.28 × 1.28 = 1.64 |
| Multiply this value by the old mAs: | 1.64 × 2 mAs = 3.28 mAs |

This type of scenario will arise when using x-ray units with variable SID versus fixed SID. This is a common problem in portable/mobile radiography and intraoperative radiography.

## Film/Screen Combinations

The speed of the system can be expressed in numeric terms, developed by the manufacturers, referred to as relative speed (RS) value. This refers to the sensitivity or response that the intensifying crystals have to x-ray photons.

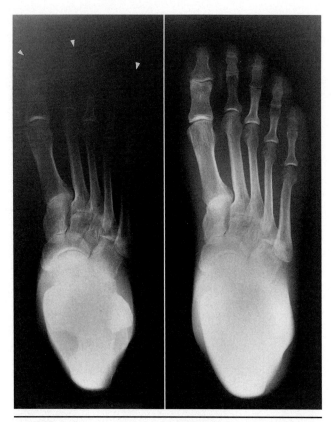

**Figure 4-8** Inverse square law. Left image: SID decreased by half (normal SID for right image). Note increased radiographic density and poor visualization of distal structures.

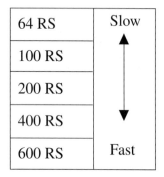

Previously, film/screen speed was divided into three groups as follows:

Slow (detail)          Double the average screen mAs
Average (medium, par)  Baseline
Fast                   Half average screen speed

The higher the number, the faster the film. This means less radiation is needed to produce an image; however, there is a compromise with reduction in image sharpness (detail).

With the availability of rare-earth phosphor crystals in imaging technology, the compromise between detail and speed has diminished. A balance between speed or photon

sensitivity and resolution (detail) has been accomplished. However, film/screen technology continues to advance toward even better improvements in phosphor response and better-recorded detail.[3]

Should it become necessary to use or change factors because you are employing different speed systems, the following formula can be used (Figure 4-9)[1,5]:

$$\frac{mAs_1}{mAs_2} = \frac{RS_2}{RS_1}$$

$mAs_1$ = Old mAs
$mAs_2$ = New mAs
$RS_1$ = Old relative speed
$RS_2$ = New relative speed

**Example 1**
2 mAs, 200 $RS_{old}$ (slow)
400 $RS_{new}$ (fast)

$$\frac{2\ mAs}{X} = \frac{400\ RS}{200\ RS}$$

400 RS $X$ = 400 RS
$X$ = 1 mAs or ½ old mAs

**Example 2**
2 mAs, 400 $RS_{old}$ (fast)
100 $RS_{new}$ (slow)

$$\frac{2\ mAs}{X} = \frac{100\ RS}{400\ RS}$$

100 $X$ = 800
$X$ = 8 mAs or 4 times old mAs

Short method for Example 2:

Old RS ÷ New RS
400 RS ÷ 100 RS = 4

Multiply this result by the old mAs value

4 × 2 mAs = 8 mAs

In addition to adjusting the speed of screens (2 screens per cassette) by altering size, thickness, and phosphor layer size, one can adjust the speed by employing single-screen cassettes (Figure 4-10). Adjustments are made by increasing the mAs (quantity of radiation) value by a factor of 2 (double):

**Original double-screen technique:**
2 mAs

**New single-screen technique:**
2 × (2 mAs)
4 mAs

A single screen may be employed to image the extremities. This system improves the sharpness of detail. However, when using a single-screen imaging cassette, the correct film type (single emulsion) must be used. Care must be taken when loading the film into the cassette. The film emulsion, generally the dull side, must face the single screen. This can be accomplished by making sure the notch of the film is placed in the correct position to have the film emulsion side face the screen surface (Figure 4-11).

## Effects of Film Processing

When proper temperature, replenishment rate, and sequence of film processing are maintained, then processing will not be an influencing factor concerning radiographic density. However, development temperature is a crucial

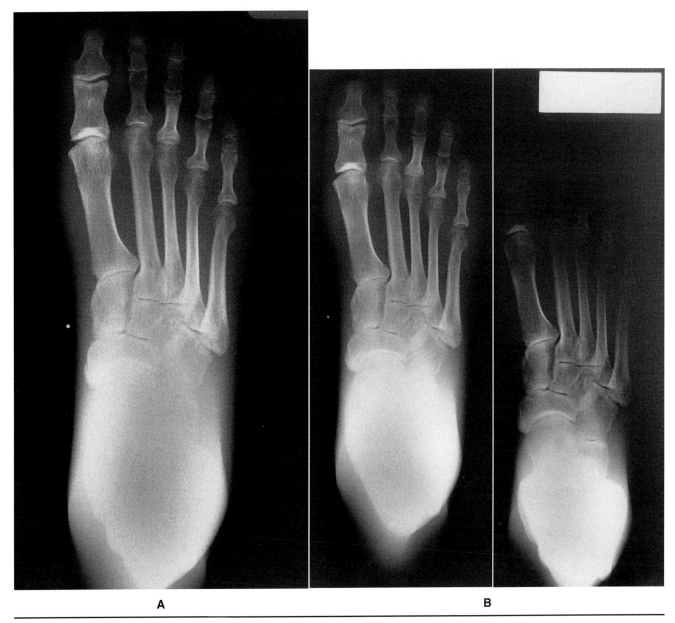

**Figure 4-9**   Screen speed. **A,** Slow speed (detail) system at standard technique. **B,** Medium speed system. The right image was produced using the same technical factors as in **A.** (Note the increased film density.) The left image was produced with corrected technical factors. In this example the time was decreased by half. This film closely resembles Figure 4-10.

factor. This temperature is that of the developer solution. For each specific type of film, a recommended temperature and time chart has been compiled by each manufacturer.

As the temperature increases, the time of immersion in the developer solution should decrease. If a film is immersed beyond this period of time, the radiographic density increases. Likewise, as solution temperature decreases, the immersion time should increase. When the film has not been in the developer for the required length of time, this film will exhibit decreased radiographic density.

Adequate replenishment rates must be maintained to have proper activity level of the processing chemicals. Improper replenishment, either too high or too low, will affect the radiographic density. To ensure proper activity of the processing solutions, new chemicals should be prepared every one to two months.

Automatic processors should be monitored for correct temperature levels, replenishment rates, proper roller transport function, proper water circulation, and sufficient dryer blower function. Some form of preventive maintenance

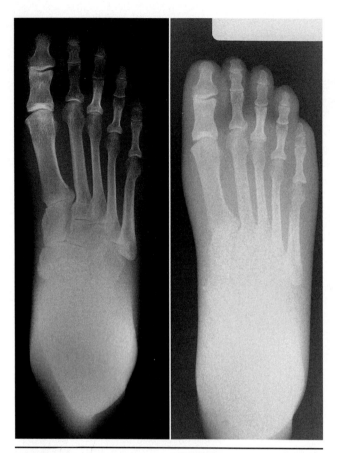

Figure 4-10    Single-screen system. The right image was produced with the same technical factors as that used for double-screen detail system (see Figure 4-9, A). The exposure time was increased 2½ times to produce the image seen on the left (compare to Figure 4-9, A).

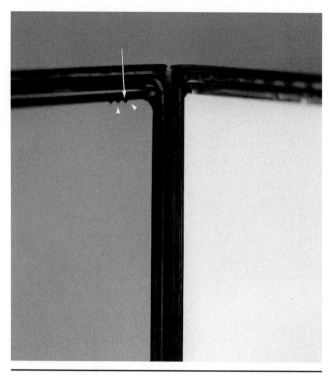

Figure 4-11    Single-screen system. Position of notches aid in proper placement of the film's emulsion side adjacent to the intensifying screen.

should be scheduled and performed at least monthly to provide proper film development quality.

## ■ CONTRAST

Contrast is primarily responsible for allowing the visibility of detail. Simply stated, contrast is the variation or difference in densities that allows one to discern between two adjacent densities within the image.[1-6] The two scales of contrast are differentiated in Box 4-3 and Figure 4-12.

Kilovoltage is the primary controlling factor in determining the type or scale of contrast produced. The scale of contrast is determined by area, tissue type, and pathologic condition.[1-6]

There are no hard-and-fast rules governing the scale or level of contrast. This area of concern becomes subjective with the individual(s) viewing the radiograph(s). As a rule, you must have sufficient kilovoltage to expose any body area. Therefore, you should adequately visualize any given anatomic region/area.

| BOX 4-3 | Contrast | |
|---|---|
| Short Scale | Long Scale |
| High contrast | Low contrast |
| Limited number of gray shades | Increased number of gray shades |
| Increased contrast | Decreased contrast |
| Lower level of kilovoltage | Higher level of kilovoltage |
| Limited areas of visibility (thinner structures) | Thicker areas more visible |

Generally speaking, the higher kVp levels will produce low contrast and low kVp will produce high contrast. To produce a visible or noticeable contrast change, the kVp should be changed by 4% to 12%, dependent on the kVp level (Box 4-4).[2]

When the desired contrast is not present on the finished radiograph, the kVp should be altered ±8% to 15%. The radiograph in question should be outside the acceptable limits to necessitate a repeat radiograph.

The ability to distinguish the contrast of different tissues may be hindered when the image has poor density. In those cases a contrast mask (Figure 4-13), may be useful in eliminating adjacent densities for better evaluation.[2]

The two remaining qualities, detail and distortion, deal with geometric integrity of the recorded image.

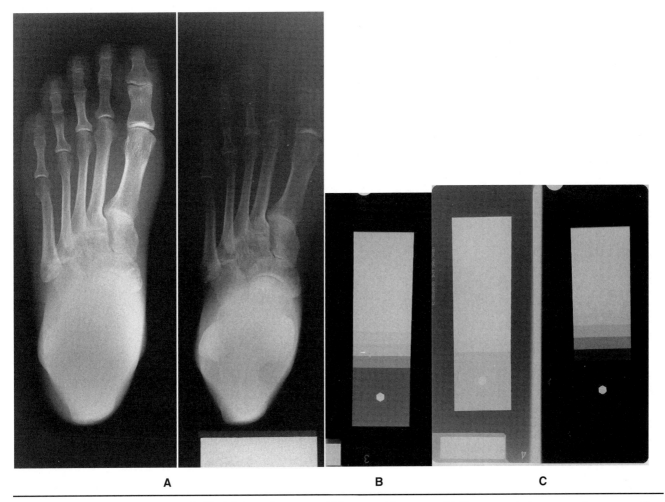

**Figure 4-12** **A,** Example of contrast scale: The left image demonstrates high contrast (short gray scale). Compare to the low contrast (long gray scale) image seen on the right. **B,** Aluminum step wedge: This image was produced by the same technical factors used to produce a dorsoplantar view of the foot (60 kVp). **C,** Aluminum step wedge: The left image was produced using 50 kVp. It demonstrates higher contrast (short gray scale, smaller number of steps). The right image was produced with 70 kVp and demonstrates lower contrast (long gray scale, larger number of steps).

---

**BOX 4-4**    **15% Rule**

To lengthen the scale of contrast, ↓ mAs by ½ and ↑ kVp 15%.
To shorten the scale of contrast, ↑ mAs by 2 and ↓ kVp 15%.

---

### ■ DETAIL

Detail (resolution, sharpness, definition) is the recorded accuracy of the structures imaged.[1-6] The image structures may appear either sharp/crisp or blurred/ill-defined depending on the degree of detail recorded. This property also involves how well two closely placed objects are perceived or seen as two distinct objects. This differentiation becomes crucial when dealing with minute structures.

Recorded detail may be influenced by geometry, material, film/screen contact, and motion.

### Geometry

*Focal-spot size:* Size of area electrons strike on target (anode); Larger focal-spot size will result in decreased detail.

*Object–image distance (OID):* The greater the distance the object is away from the film, the less detail or sharpness will be recorded (blurred image).

*Source–image distance:* Longer SID generally means the image will be much sharper.

### Material (Films/Screens)

Slower-speed systems mean sharper recorded image. This sharpness is caused by the crystal size and phosphor layer thickness.

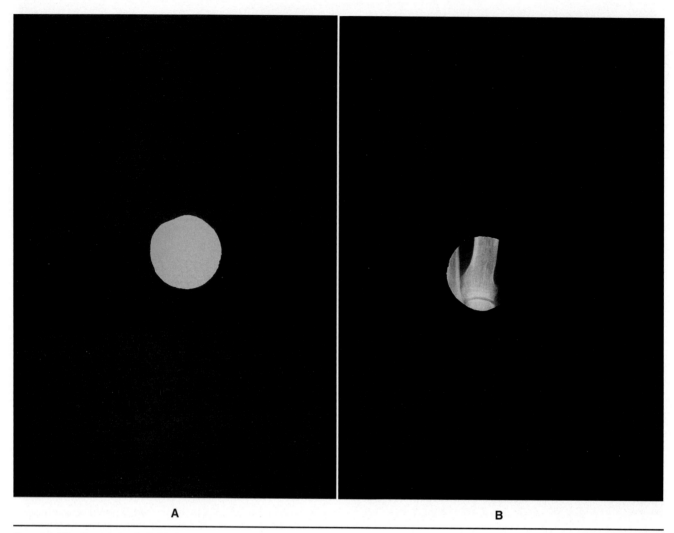

**A**                              **B**

Figure 4-13   Contrast mask. **A,** Mask made from black construction paper with 4.5-cm-diameter viewing area. **B,** Contrast mask placed on radiograph. At base of first metatarsal cuneiform joint left foot.

**Screens and Attributes**

Slow (detail)

- Small crystal size
- Thinner layer
- Greater detail

Fast

- Larger crystal size
- Thicker layer
- Less detail

## Film/Screen Contact

Uniform film/screen contact must be maintained throughout the entire film surface or localized area(s) of blurring may occur.[1-6] This problem with detail may manifest itself as specific area(s) of blurring regardless of proper instructions to patient, immobilization, and exposure factors. The key in identifying this type of problem is that the suspicious area of blurring appears in the same area(s) when the cassette is employed either on different patients or positions.

The operator can perform a test for this problem.[1,3,7] Place a fine wire screen (the type employed in windows or doors) on the cassette in question (make sure the screen is in contact with the entire cassette front). Then make an exposure using normal factors for average-size dorsoplantar foot projection. Develop this film normally. Now check the image for irregularities in sharpness and density. When this test is positive, replacement of the screen is indicated. To help in identifying this and other problems (artifacts), the screen should be numbered to better identify the problem cassette(s) (Figure 4-14).

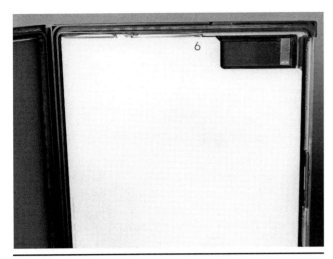

**Figure 4-14**   Cassette with ID number. Rub-on number 6 placed on intensifying screen to better identify problem cassette. The number will show up on exposed x-ray film.

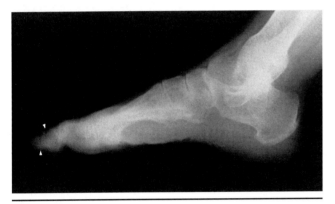

**Figure 4-15**   Motion blur. The patient's forefoot moved during the exposure, resulting in image blur, especially at the toes *(arrowheads)*. Note lack of sharpness of detail in the forefoot.

## Motion

Two types:

I.  Patient (Figure 4-15)
    Voluntary motion: under direct control of patient
    Involuntary motion: not under direct control of patient (neurologic disorder)
    Pediatric patients
II.  Equipment
    Vibration or drift of x-ray tube housing because locking devices have failed; suspected when multiple films exhibit blurring effect

Reduction of exposure time, immobilization of body part, or in some cases (pediatric) sedation may be indicated to limit motion blur. Periodic equipment inspections should be performed to check that the locking mechanisms are functioning properly.

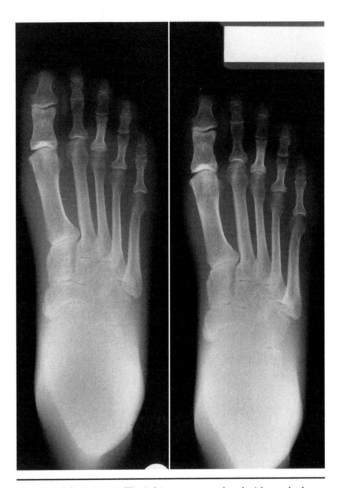

**Figure 4-16**   15% rule. The left image was produced with standard technical factors. The right image was produced by decreasing the exposure time by half and increasing the kVp by 15%. Note the density of both images are similar.

The 15% rule states that to decrease the exposure time by half and maintain the same density, you should increase kilovoltage by 15% (Figure 4-16).[2]

**Example:**

| Old Factors | New Factors |
|---|---|
| 15 mA | 15 mA |
| $^{16}\!/_{60}$ s | $^{8}\!/_{60}$ s |
| 28 in SID | 28 in SID |
| 60 kVp | New kVp = (60 kVp × 15%) + 60 kVp = 69 |

The two films should exhibit equal densities. This can be applied to pediatric or geriatric patients, or to individuals whom you determine may not hold still for the duration of the x-ray exposure.

## ■ DISTORTION

Distortion is the misrepresentation of size (magnification), shape, or positional relationships of recorded structures (Figure 4-17).[1-7]

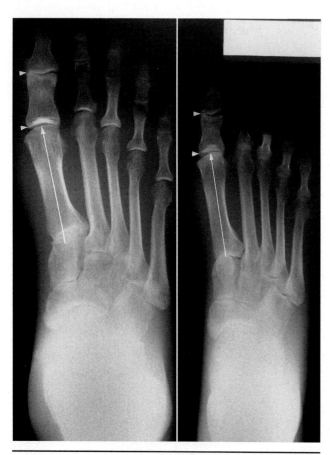

Figure 4-17   Magnification and distortion. The left image demonstrates magnification caused by an increased OFD. The right image demonstrates shape distortion caused by tube head angulation not perpendicular to the film. Note the second to fourth metatarsal heads and bases (the OFD is 0 inches).

**BOX 4-5**   **Indications of Magnification Use**

- Articular disorders
- Infections
- Fractures
- Foreign bodies
- Neoplasms (osseous involvement)
- Metabolic

inherent and unavoidable. Longer SID values decrease magnification. The most common SID range is 36 to 40 inches, which is employed in diagnostic radiology. For certain examinations (erect chest), 72 inches SID is used, to neutralize the effect of inherent magnification.

The SID of lower extremity specific x-ray units may be fixed at 22 to 28 inches. The image magnification that is produced should be negligible.

Shape distortion is the unequal magnification of the actual structures(s) involved.[1-7] Elongation projects the object so as to have the image appear longer. This occurs when either the tube or film is improperly aligned.[2] Foreshortening projects the object so as to have the image appear shorter than normal object length. This only happens when the part is improperly aligned.[2]

It is important to have the area of interest, the central ray or the x-ray beam, and film in proper alignment to avoid shape distortion, or positional changes. Ideally the tube should be perpendicular to the film and part.

Careful attention to part placement, film placement, and tube angulation (degree and direction) will help minimize distortion. One must be familiar with the various projections and positions, because of the different degrees of distortion that present themselves on the finished radiograph. Distortion is occasionally used to reduce superimposition or to enhance visualization of difficult areas (consider the Harris-Beath and Broden views).[7]

Shape distortion is usually accomplished by three means. The first is by manipulating the tube angle so that the central beam is not perpendicular to the film and/or body part (Figure 4-18). Greater distortions occur with greater tube angles. Compare non–weight-bearing obliques of the foot (0° tubehead angle) with the weight-bearing counterparts (45°) (Figure 4-19).

The second way distortion is created is by part rotation or angulation so that the plane of the body part is not parallel to the film (Figure 4-20). Finally, shape distortion occurs if the x-ray beam is not centered over the middle of the body part to be examined.

Each of the three methods distort the image in varying degrees. Attempts should be made to minimize distortion. However, distortion may be created on purpose, to assist in visualizing difficult areas or specific structures. Proper use of

Magnification (size) distortion (see Figure 4-17) is caused by increases in object–film distance (OFD).[7] The amount of magnification or magnification factor can be determined by dividing SID by source–object distance (SOD). Source–object distance is found by subtracting object–film distance (OFD) from SID.

**Example:**

6 in OFD    28 in SID    28 in – 6 in = 22 in SOD

$$\frac{28 \text{ in SID}}{22 \text{ in SOD}} = 1.27 \text{ Magnification Factor}$$

Translated, this means that the magnification will be 27%, or the image will be 127% of the object size. This applies to each structure that is in that same OFD plane. This magnification is uniform throughout the OFD plane.

Applied correctly, magnification can aid in diagnosis.[8] Some indications are listed in Box 4-5.

Even if the object (or foot) is placed against the film, the bones may be one or more centimeters away from the film. Therefore, some magnification of internal structures is

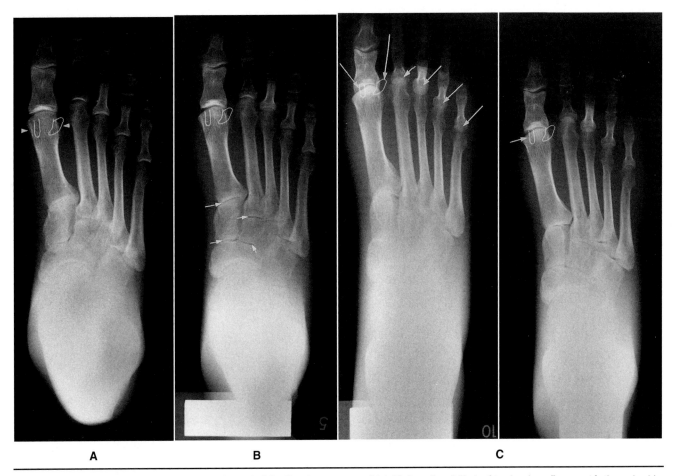

|  A  |  B  |  C  |

**Figure 4-18** **A,** Dorsoplantar foot view at 0° tube angle. Metallic wires represent tibial (U-shaped) and fibular (circular-shaped) sesamoids *(arrowheads)*. **B,** Tube angle 15°. Note: Sesamoid markers appear to move distally. The first metatarsal-cuneiform, second metatarsal-cuneiform, and medial and intermediate cuneiform-navicular joints are now visible. **C,** The tube angle for the right image was 30°. Note the distal sesamoid marker position and elongation of the metatarsals. The tube was angulated at 45° for the image on the left. Again, the sesamoids are seen more distal. Also note the loss of joint space at all metatarsophalangeal joints and in the midfoot.

the tube, part, or film angulation can be an adjunct to routine projection.

## ■ TECHNIQUE GUIDES

To achieve optimal radiographs, it is necessary to develop and employ a technique chart. This chart is required by many state licensing organizations. It must be posted near each piece of x-ray generating unit that the user owns. The guides must include the following:

1. Patient's size versus technique factors
2. Type and size of film/screen to be used
3. SID to be used

Recommend:

Room location

Unit type
Projection listing
Film placement
Tube angle used

The first consideration is the technique system, or exposure system. There are various types of exposure systems[1,2,4,9,10]; the two applied in podiatric radiology are fixed kilovoltage and variable kilovoltage systems.

### Fixed Kilovoltage

Using the fixed kilovoltage system, the kVp is held constant while the mAs is varied per the part thickness. An optimal kVp is used that produces appropriate contrast typically 60 kVp for the foot and ankle. Generally speaking, higher kVp settings are used, fixed kVp technique versus variable kVp techniques.

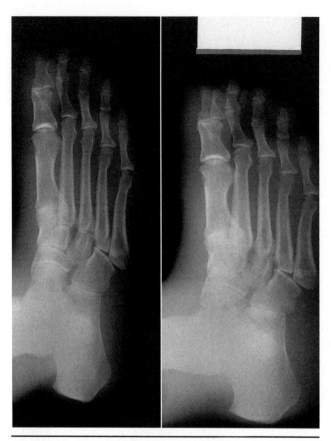

**Figure 4-19**  Distortion caused by tubehead position. There is unequal magnification of all bones in the weight-bearing medial oblique view *(right image)* compared to the non–weight-bearing oblique view *(left image)*.

**Advantages:**
>   Decreases patient dose
>   Uniform radiographic contrast
>   Lower x-ray tube heating
>   Lengthens exposure latitude
>   Extends tube life
>   Decreases exposure time

**Disadvantages:**
>   Lower contrast levels
>   Produces more scattered radiation
>   Small incremental changes not possible

## Variable Kilovoltage

Uses varied kVp, which depends on part thickness and use of one mAs value for that specific part regardless of size.

**Advantages:**
>   Small incremental changes possible
>   Higher contrast levels

**Disadvantages:**
>   Varying contrast levels
>   Varying radiation dose to patient.

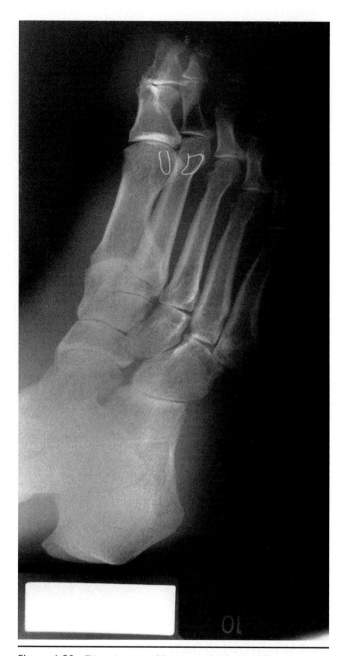

**Figure 4-20**  Distortion caused by nonparallel foot and film.

| BOX 4-6 | Average | | | | |
|---|---|---|---|---|---|
| **Adult Part Thickness** | | | | | |
| Foot: | AP | 6-8 cm | Ankle: | AP | 8-10 cm |
| | LAT | 7-9 cm | | LAT | 6-9 cm |

A typical variable-kVp chart is set up by measuring the thickness of the area in question and selecting the appropriate kilovoltage for the varying part thicknesses (Boxes 4-6 and 4-7).

| BOX 4-7 | Suggested kVp Range |
|---|---|
| Small extremities | 50-60 kVp |
| Medium extremities | 55-65 kVp |
| Large extremities | 60-70 kVp |

To determine the kilovoltage for a particular area, use one of the following:

$$(2 \text{ kVp} \times \text{cm part thickness}) + 40 \text{ kVp} = \text{New kVp}$$

$$(2 \text{ kVp} \times \text{cm part thickness}) + 50 \text{ kVp} = \text{New kVp}$$

**Example:**

Dorsoplantar thickness foot (dorsal navicular area to plantar aspect) = 8 cm
$(2 \text{ kVp} \times 8 \text{ cm}) + 40 \text{ kVp}$
$= 16 \text{ kVp} + 40 \text{ kVp}$
$= 56 \text{ kVp}$

It is important to remember no amount of mAs will compensate for insufficient kilovoltage.[9]

It is very important, regardless of the type of technique chart employed, that the part is measured properly. Proper use of a caliper device is important (Figure 4-21). To use the caliper device properly, the longer side should represent the central ray (CR). Now place the device so this longer side mimics the CR path through the desired anatomical area. Also, measure at the thickest part for that particular projection. (For example, dorsoplantar foot: Measure at base of second metatarsal, dorsally. For digital problems, measure at the metatarsal-phalangeal joints, proximally.) Make sure the two shorter arms are placed so that they remain parallel to each other when obtaining the proper centimeter measurement (Figure 4-22).

Also, to ensure that on the next visit for a serial x-ray study the quality is consistent, write down the factors employed on the back of the patient's x-ray folder.

## OTHER CONSIDERATIONS

The importance of maintaining optimum quality by monitoring various factors of the imaging process must be stressed. This means monitoring temperatures of the processing chemicals and replenishment rates of exhausted chemicals, checking the prime factors (mA, time, distance, kVp), measuring correctly, and making adequate preparations (positioning, instructions) in producing the radiograph(s).

Variation in technique will occur when examining the pediatric patient, geriatric patient, presentation of certain pathologies, use of magnification, and soft tissue radiography.

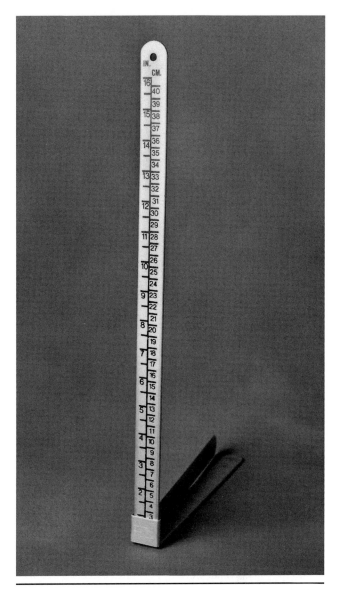

Figure 4-21    Caliper device. This device is used to measure anatomic regions for proper factor setting in conjunction with technique guide (right side in centimeters; left side in inches).

## Children

The pediatric patient may pose a problem for the operator. With the pediatric patient, the tissues have a greater percentage of water.[1,11] This causes more scattering of the remnant radiation. Use of lower kVp ranges may be useful in producing a diagnostic radiograph. Many facilities group the children into age groups (three or four) to the age of 12 while varying the mAs (Boxes 4-8 and 4-9).[1]

Children younger than 5 years of age may need a parent or guardian present in the room to assist in the examination process. This person must be provided with a lead apron and must wear it during the x-ray examination. Radiographic

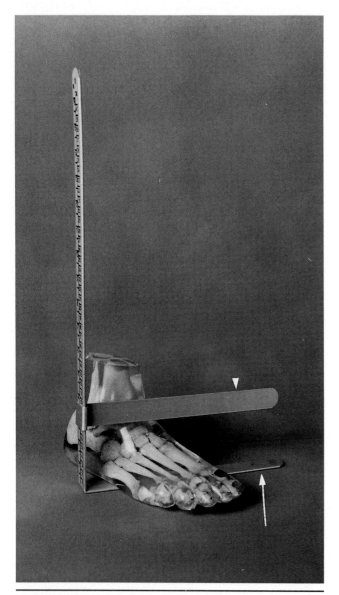

Figure 4-22   Proper method for measuring using caliper.

| BOX 4-8 | Pediatric kVp Technique |
|---------|---------------|
| Birth to 2.5 years | .3 × Adult mAs |
| 2.6 years to 6 years | .5 × Adult mAs |
| 7 years to 12 years | .75 × Adult mAs |

studies may be performed "simulated weight bearing" for those infants unable to stand (weight bearing). The parent holds the child under the arms to simulate weight bearing. The younger infant may have to be examined while supine. The key is using the quickest exposure time possible to eliminate motion artifacts. Proper instructions must be given to parents/guardians as to how to help hold the child.

| BOX 4-9 | Pediatric mAs Technique |
|---------|---------------|
| Birth to 1 year | .25 × Adult mAs |
| 1 year to 3 years | .5 × Adult mAs |
| 3 years to 7 years | .70 × Adult mAs |
| 7 years to 12 years | .9 × Adult mAs |

Some pediatric patients may vary in size because of their development.

Some points to remember:

1. Explain procedure to assistant (parent, guardian, and so on).
2. Explain procedure to those children who may understand.
3. Use patience and understanding.
4. Use reliable technical factors.
5. Check that restraining devices do not interfere with projection.

## Geriatrics

The geriatric patient may require alterations to the technical factors.[1]

The following must be considered:

1. Osteoporosis (common in Caucasian women)
2. Muscle tone (atrophy, disuse)
3. Difficulty in positioning

Secondary considerations include the following:

1. Decline in auditory senses
2. Decline in vision
3. Decrease in stability (use non–weight-bearing studies)
4. Decline in ability to remain still for study

Generally speaking the mAs can be decreased 25% to 30% for patients with poor muscle tone; kVp can be decreased 6% to 8% for patients with known or suspected osteoporosis.

Use the best combination of mA and time for the shortest exposure time possible, thereby minimizing exposure. Use clear, concise instructions for positioning. To decrease the chance of injury, assist the patient.

Some instances require immobilizing or holding the foot or ankle for required projections/positions. The person who is holding the patient should wear a lead apron and gloves. Before completing the radiographic study, check the first film of multiple-projection studies for quality.

## Pathological Considerations

Different pathologic conditions may warrant changes in technique. These changes are either increases ("additive" pathology) or decreases ("destructive" pathology) in mAs.[1,2] The additive pathologies are those that increase either the volume or density of the soft tissues or osseous structures. This warrants an increase in the amount of radiation to properly penetrate the area and expose the film. The destructive pathologies are those that decrease either volume or density of the soft tissues or osseous structures. Because of this effect, the amount of radiation must be decreased to adequately expose the film. Box 4-10 lists pathologies that may be encountered in the foot and ankle.

The changes should be in either mAs or kVp. The minimum change in mAs is 30%. Likewise, the change in kVp should be 5% to 8%. These changes provide for a visible alteration in the image contrast/density. There is no set value for each change. The change in technique will depend on the patient's condition (Figure 4-23).

| BOX 4-10 | Skeletal System |
|---|---|
| Additive | Destructive |
| Paget's disease | Active osteomyelitis |
| Acromegaly | Gout |
| Osteopetrosis | Osteoporosis |
| | Carcinoma |

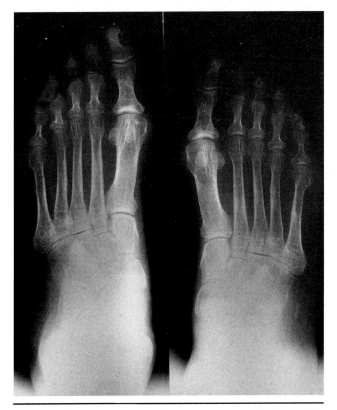

Figure 4-23    Geriatric patient with known osteoporosis. Radiograph is exposed with decreased factors to compensate for stated condition.

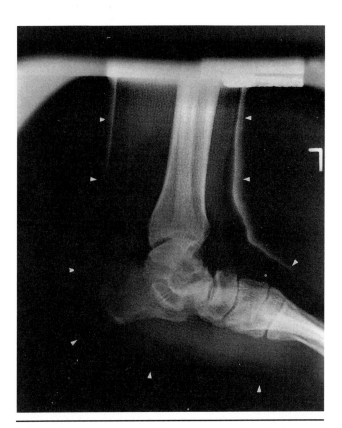

Figure 4-24    Cast radiography. Note the increased tissue density caused by the fiberglass cast outline.

## Cast Radiography

It may be necessary to make x-ray studies of patients who have casts because of postoperative procedures, have trauma, or have other indications for immobilization (Figure 4-24). The cast may either be wet or dry. A wet cast tends to be more radiopaque than a dry cast. A general guideline is presented in Box 4-11. Measure the contralateral part to determine normal mAs value, consult the technique chart, and make the appropriate adjustment increases.

## Magnification

Magnification is a useful adjunct in diagnosing various conditions. This technique is achieved via two methods,

| BOX 4-11 | Cast Radiography |
|---|---|
| Plaster* | Fiberglass* |
| Wet: 3 × Normal mAs or + 15 kVp | Wet: 2 × mAs or + 10 kVp |
| Dry: 2 × Normal mAs or + 10 kVp | Dry: 1½ × mAs |

Based on normal cast thickness
*Thickness of cast is important. Some areas may have greater amounts than surrounding areas(s).

optical and radiographic. A thorough discussion can be found in numerous articles and texts (also see Chapter 16 for more information).[2-4,7-9,12-15]

These two methods can be modified for use with lower-extremity–specific x-ray units.

*Optical:* Use fine (detail) screens. Normal SID. Use 10× hand-held loupe to selectively magnify desired areas of the radiograph.
*Radiographic:* Use fine (detail) screens.
Normal SID
Varying OFD

It is important to remember that large OFDs produce greater magnification and also produce greater decreases in sharpness.

When deciding on the type of magnification to use (either optical or radiographic), consider the following:

* *Type of imaging system resolution:* This is the ability to record detail. This ability may decrease (less detail/sharpness) when increasing the OFD to achieve larger magnification factors. In general, slower-speed systems tend to have better resolution. Faster speed systems tend to have decreased resolution.

| BOX 4-12 | Comparison of Various Magnifications at Varying SIDs | |
|---|---|---|
| **21 in SID** | | **40 in SID** |
| 2 in OFD = 1.10 MF | | 2 in OFD = 1.05 MF |
| 4 in OFD = 1.23 MF | | 4 in OFD = 1.11 MF |
| 6 in OFD = 1.40 MF | | 6 in OFD = 1.14 MF |
| 8 in OFD = 1.61 MF | | 8 in OFD = 1.24 MF |
| 10 in OFD = 2.00 MF | | 10 in OFD = 1.33 MF |
| | | 20 in OFD = 2.00 MF |
| **28 in SID** | | **36 in SID** |
| 2 in OFD = 1.07 MF | | 2 in OFD = 1.05 MF |
| 4 in OFD = 1.16 MF | | 4 in OFD = 1.12 MF |
| 6 in OFD = 1.27 MF | | 6 in OFD = 1.20 MF |
| 8 in OFD = 1.40 MF | | 8 in OFD = 1.27 MF |
| 10 in OFD = 1.55 MF | | 10 in OFD = 1.37 MF |
| 14 in OFD = 2.00 MF | | 18 in OFD = 2.00 MF |

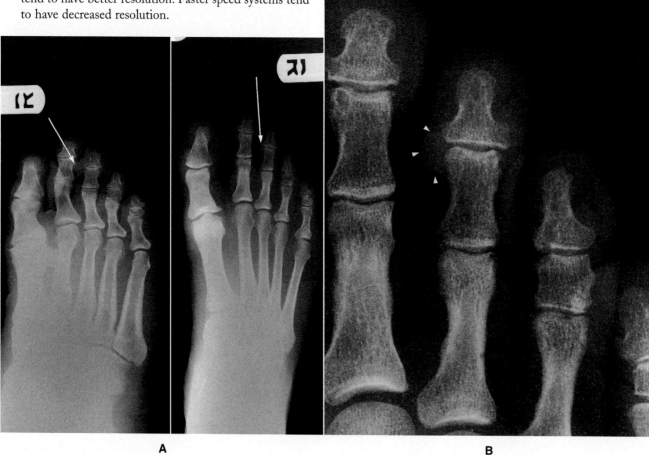

**A**　　　　　　　　　**B**

Figure 4-25　Soft tissue radiography. **A,** Small soft tissue mass medial aspect third digit distal interphalangeal joint (DIPJ), right foot. (Note that bone appears white.) **B,** Closeup of third digit right foot. Note soft tissue mass outline (DIPJ). Medial side change in soft tissue density.

- *Magnification factor (MF):* This choice will depend on how well the image system will be able to record detail (sharpness) at varying OFDs. Higher MFs may increase the visibility of difficult or minute anatomic detail area(s).
- Longer OFD = High MF
- Shorter OFD = Low MF

This choice also depends on the SIDs employed for routine radiologic studies (Box 4-12).

To determine the magnification factor, the SID is divided by the SOD (distance from tube to object).[16] The SOD can be determined by subtracting the OFD from the SID.

**Example:**

28 in SID
4 in OFD

SOD = SID − OFD
SOD = 28 in − 4 in
SOD = 24 in

$$MF = \frac{SID}{SOD}$$

Using the preceding values:

$$MF = \frac{28 \text{ in}}{24 \text{ in}}$$

$$MF = 1.16$$

Using this technique increases the radiation dose to the tissue because of the object being in closer proximity to the x-ray tube. Because the magnified images are not sharp, this procedure should be used in selective instances rather than as a routine type of procedure.[8]

## Soft Tissue

In certain clinical presentations, it may be desirable to enhance the soft tissue densities.[16,17] This may be accomplished by having a film that exhibits high contrast. To achieve this high contrast, decrease the kVp used for the examination. This can be done by decreasing kVp by 15% and doubling the mAs value. Another method is by decreasing the kVp by appropriate percentage (see Box 4-2, Figure 4-25). It is important to remember that with the decrease in kVp a resultant increase in bone density will be seen (Figure 4-26).

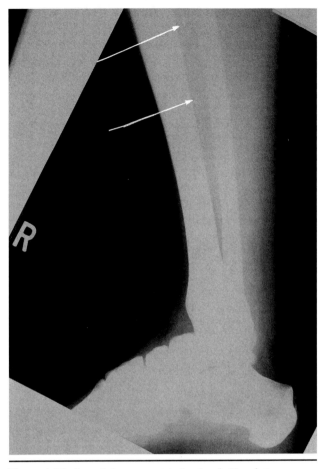

Figure 4-26    Lateral view non–weight bearing. Ankle soft tissue radiograph; note the metallic vascular clips.

Some of the clinical applications of the preceding techniques may be soft tissue masses, articular disorders, Achilles tendon pathology, and some embedded foreign bodies (e.g., metal, glass, wood chips, plastics).

Soft tissue technique must be used in selective cases. Because of the lower kVp used, the area receives greater radiation to the tissues. When properly exposed, soft tissue radiographs serve as adjuncts to conventional diagnostic plain films.

## References

1. DeVos DC: *Basic principles of radiographic exposure,* Philadelphia, 1990, Lea & Febiger.
2. Carlton RR, Adler AM: *Principles of radiographic imaging, an art and a science,* Albany, NY, 1992, Delmar.
3. Bushong SC: *Radiologic science for technologists: Physics, biology and protection,* ed 3, St Louis, 1984, Mosby.
4. Malott JC, Fodor J: *The art and science of medical radiography,* St Louis, 1993, Mosby.
5. Sprawls P: *Physical principles of medical imaging,* Rockville, MD, 1987, Aspen.
6. Curry TC, Dowdey JE, Murry RC: *Christensen's physics of diagnostic radiology,* ed 4, Philadelphia, 1990, Lea & Febiger.

7. Health Sciences Market Division: Kodak Publication NO-M1-18, *The fundamentals of radiography,* ed 12, Rochester, NY, Eastman Kodak.

8. Genant HK, Resneck D: Magnification radiography. In Resnick D, editor: *Bone and joint imaging,* Philadelphia, 1989, WB Saunders.

9. Eastman T: *Radiographic fundamentals and technique guide,* St Louis, 1979, Mosby.

10. Cullinan JE, Cullinan A: *Illustrated guide to x-ray technics,* ed 2, Philadelphia, 1980, JB Lippincott.

11. Heinlein CW: Radiographic technique for infants and children, *Radiol Technol* 38:25, 1966.

12. Genant HK, Doi K: High-resolution skeletal radiography: image quality and clinical applications, *Curr Probl Diagn Radiol* 7:3, 1978.

13. Weiss A: A technique for demonstrating fine detail in bones of the hands, *Clin Radiol* 23:185, 1972.

14. Genant HK, Doi K, Mall JC: Optical versus radiographic magnification for fine-detail skeletal radiography, *Invest Radiol* 10:160, 1975.

15. Sundaram M: The clinical value of direct magnification radiography in orthopedics, *Skel Rad* 3:85, 1978.

16. Fischer E: Low kilovolt radiography. In Resnick D, editor: *Bone and joint imaging,* Philadelphia, 1989, WB Saunders.

17. Ngo C, Yaghmai I: The value of immersion hand radiography in soft tissue changes of musculoskeletal disorders, *Skel Rad* 17:259, 1988.

18. Kath K: *Pocket reference to radiographic exposure techniques,* St. Louis, 1993, Mosby.

# Troubleshooting: Poor Film/Image Quality Checklist

## ■ VISIBILITY OF STRUCTURES

1. Film too light (lack of radiographic density)
   Causes:
       Short exposure time
       Low mA
       SID too long (x-ray tube further than normal)
       kVp too low
       Inadequate developer solution:
           Temperature too low
           Time of development too short
2. Film too dark (excessive radiographic density)
   Causes:
       Long exposure time
       High mA
       SID too short (x-ray tube closer than normal)
       kVp too high
       Inappropriate developer solution:
           Temperature too high
           Time of development too long
3. Image appears gray (film fog)
   Causes:
       kVp too high (produces excessive scatter radiation)
       Abnormal chemistry (developer: temperature and date)
       Light leaks (portions of image may be obscured)
       Cassette(s): poor foam seals
       Darkroom: door, film bin, and film box leaks or cracks
4. Image appears light (bones are white, soft tissue highlighted) and the background radiographic density is adequate.
   Causes:
       Low kVp: insufficient kVp to penetrate desired area.
           Remeasure area (+kVp 8%-15%)
       Exposure factors too low
           Remeasure patient at correct area
5. Image appears dark (soft tissue dark, bones appear various grays) and the background radiographic density is adequate.
       High kVp: overpenetration of area(s) to visualize
           Remeasure area (−kVp 8%-15%)
       Exposure factors too excessive
           Remeasure patient, consult chart
       Processing tanks
           *Manual:* Are tanks securely covered?
           *Automatic:* Is cover completely on?
       Opened door/turned on light too early; before signal (audible) given by processor

## ■ GEOMETRY OF IMAGE

1. Image blurred
   Causes:
       Patient motion
       Poor film/screen contact
       Faulty locking mechanism
2. Shape of object altered
   Causes:
       Greater tube angulation than normally employed (elongation)
       Object position changed from normal (foreshortening)
       Object rotated
       Object angulated
       Film not in normal position
3. Position of object altered
   Causes:
       Check tube position—central ray location
       Check tube angulation
       Check part placement

# Formulas for Exposure Calculation

1. Milliamperage-Time (equal densities between old exposure and new exposure) To find exposure time when changing milliamperage or to find new milliamperage when changing exposure time:

$$\frac{mA_{old}}{mA_{new}} = \frac{Time_{new}}{Time_{old}}$$

   High mA = Short exposure time
   Low mA = Long exposure time

2. Inverse Square Law
   To determine amount of radiation (intensity) reaching the film at a new distance

$$\frac{Intensity_{old}}{Intensity_{new}} = \frac{[Distance\ (SID)_{new}]^2}{[Distance\ (SID)_{old}]^2}$$

3. Milliamperage-Seconds
   To find mAs value for given exposure factors

$$mA \times Exposure\ time\ (s) = mAs$$

4. Time-Distance (to maintain equal densities)
   To find exposure time when changing distance (SID)

$$\frac{Time_{old}}{Time_{new}} = \frac{(Distance_{new})^2}{(Distance_{old})^2}$$

5. Milliamperage-Distance (to maintain equal densities)
   To find mA when changing distance (SID)

$$\frac{mA_{old}}{mA_{new}} = \frac{(Distance_{new})^2}{(Distance_{old})^2}$$

6. Milliampere-Seconds (mAs) Distance (maintain equal densities)
   To find mAs value when changing distance (SID)

$$\frac{mAs_{old}}{mAs_{new}} = \frac{(Distance_{new})^2}{(Distance_{old})^2}$$

7. Fifteen Percent Rule (to reduce exposure time and maintain equal densities)
   Decrease exposure time by half (50%), increase original kVp by 15%

8. Speed of Intensifying Screen/mAs Value
   When changing speed of system when relative speed (RS) is known for old and new screens.

$$\frac{mAs_{old}}{mAs_{new}} = \frac{Relative\ speed_{new}}{Relative\ speed_{old}}$$

**Short Method**

   Old RS ÷ New RS = New RS factor

   New RS factor × Old mAs value = New mAs value

**Board System Speed Change (nonnumeric method):**
   When numeric value for relative speed is not known; general guideline (some minor adjustments may be necessary).
   Slow (detail) to medium = Decrease slow mAs by ½
   Medium (par speed) to fast = Decrease medium speed mAs by ½
   Slow to fast = Decrease slow mAs by ¼
   Fast to medium = Multiply fast mAs value by 2
   Medium to slow = Multiply medium mAs value by 2
   Fast to slow = Multiply fast mAs value by 4

9. Change Contrast Scale
   High contrast needed: ↑ original mAs by 2 and ↓ original kVp 15%
   Low contrast needed: ↓ original mAs by ½ and ↑ original kVp 15%

10. Determine Magnification Factor (MF)
    Source–image distance (SID) ÷ Source–object distance (SOD) = MF

11. Determine kVp for a Particular Area (double part thickness)

    2 kVp × cm measurement + 35 kVp

    2 kVp × cm measurement + 40 kVp

    2 kVp × cm measurement + 50 kVp

12. Cast

| Plaster | Fiberglass |
|---|---|
| Wet: 3× normal mAs or +15 kVp | Wet: 2× normal mAs or +10 |
| Dry: 2× normal mAs or +10 kVp | Dry: 1½ normal mAs |

13. Tube Angulation Increase[18]

| From 0 degrees to: | Percentage Increase (add to original mAs value) |
|---|---|
| 5 degrees | No change |
| 10 degrees | 25% increase |
| 15 degrees | 40% increase |
| 20 degrees | 60% increase |
| 25 degrees | 120% increase |
| 30 degrees | 175% increase |
| 35 degrees | 175% increase |

14. Collimation[18]

Decrease field size by half, increase mAs value by 50%.

15. kVp-Distance Formula[18]

$$\text{New kVp} = \frac{D_2 \times kVp_1}{D_1}$$

$D_1$ = Old distance

$D_2$ = New distance

$kVp_1$ = Old kilovoltage

# CHAPTER 5

# Film Quality

DAVID E. WILLIAMSON

## ■ THE HISTORY OF X-RAY FILM

Silver halide photographic imaging had been fairly well perfected by the late 1800s when Wilhelm Conrad Roentgen was working with his phosphors. From the announcement of Louis-Jacques-Mandé Daguerre's imaging discovery in 1839 to the late 1890s, photo imaging had evolved significantly. The daguerreotype was beautiful and stunningly sharp but terribly slow and frightfully fragile. The daguerreotype also was a singular image—that is, it could not be used to create multiple copies. Early attempts at coating paper with light-sensitive emulsions from which multiple prints could be made were headed in the right direction, but were not successful because image quality was not good. Other media were tried, resulting in the common tintypes, ambrotypes, and glass plates. Around the 1870s glass plates coated with collodion began to be used by most serious photographers. The images of the western United States made by Timothy O'Sullivan and Alexander Gardiner gave testimony to the remarkable sharpness and reality-capturing capability this art and science had achieved. Within another decade, George Eastman had perfected production of dry plates, and as 1900 approached, flexible roll film was about to be invented.

The glass plate was the state of the art in photography in Roentgen's time. Roentgen knew that if you could see something, you could probably capture it through photographic means. Dry glass plates were available from a variety of sources. Roentgen obtained his recording medium from Adox, a Frankfurt-based photographic firm. After recording images produced by the vacuum tubes on plates provided by Adox, Roentgen wrote to Dr. Carl Schleussner, the owner of Adox, commending him on the superb quality of the glass plates he had obtained for experimentation. Being a scientist, Roentgen correctly named the rays he discovered as x rays, as x stood for the unknown in mathematics.

Using photographic plates to record x-ray images excited George Eastman, who was looking for every avenue he could possibly find to propel his young company into the leadership role in photo imaging. Eastman was prompt to size up the opportunity that this branch of imaging offered and established a separate department to focus on this area. Of course, dry glass plates were the medium used. Almost simultaneous with the discovery of x rays, scientists began to look for ways to intensify the x-ray image. They recognized almost immediately that direct x-ray exposure was a horribly slow imaging system. They knew that certain phosphors gave off light when excited by x-radiation. It was actually from the fluorescence of a barium platinocyanide screen that Roentgen visualized the first x-ray shadows. The light given off by substances when excited is known as actinic light. Cardboard was coated with phosphors such as calcium tungstate, and the intensifying screen was born. Using an Edison screen, the first radiograph using an intensifying screen and a glass plate is credited to Dr. Michael Pupin at Columbia University in February 1896, just three months after Roentgen's disclosure. Thomas A. Edison had started work within weeks of Roentgen's announcement and began to produce fluorescent intensifying screens that amplified the direct x-ray exposure and matched the spectral sensitivity of the glass photographic plate. The result was the screen-and-film system that persists today, even though the phosphors have changed and the image-recording medium has progressed from glass to cellulose nitrate to cellulose acetate and finally polyester.

Photographic substances must be kept dark to be protected against unwanted exposure so that when they are exposed to record the desired information, that is the only exposure they get. This necessity gave birth to the x-ray cassette, which in essence is a light-tight film holder into which the film (glass plate, and so on) is inserted in the dark. This cassette may contain two, one, or no intensifying screens, depending on the use. There were even screen books that held as many as 15 pairs of screens; between each pair a film was inserted, and the whole "block" was put into a special light-tight holder. Cassettes have been made of wood, metal, and plastic. The basic requirements for a good cassette are that it remain light-tight, provide intimate contact of the film and the screens, allow transmission of x-radiation (not attenuate too much), and be of a durable material to withstand use.

Radiography without intensifying screens requires increases in dosage up to as much as 95%. Many x-ray pioneers, not aware of the hazards, were reckless when it came to radiation safety, and judicious use of exposure when it came to the patient was not a consideration. Some persisted in radiographing extremities with direct x ray only (no intensifying screens); this method disappeared as film/screen systems increased in sharpness and awareness of radiation hazards grew. Cardboard film holders used for extremity use are probably now found only in the archives or kept for historic purposes.

Until World War I, glass was used as the support for x-ray plates. It was the shortage of optical-quality glass plates caused by the war that prompted American photographic manufacturers to speed up their research on flexible base, the result of which was x-ray film on cellulose nitrate base. Cellulose nitrate was hazardous to store; it was extremely flammable, actually incendiary. Almost as soon as cellulose nitrate was being delivered, work was in progress to make a suitable substitute, which was cellulose acetate, which gave way to cellulose triacetate and finally polyester-based film that is known today by trade names such as Estar and Cronex.

Advances in the emulsion or image-capturing medium have progressed similarly to the base. Although all photographic film is naturally blue sensitive, within the past three decades green-sensitive film has emerged. Without compromising trade secrets, a grossly simplified but adequate description is that an x-ray film is made green sensitive by additional sensitization and adding dyes that do not filter out green light. Of course, the screens have to emit green actinic light, and to do so they must be made of different compounds. The screen progression is commented on shortly. The latest advances in film technology involve such words as *tabular* and *rapid access*. Tabular films were introduced in the amateur photographic market about twenty years ago. They produce sharper images achieved by the physical construction of the emulsion. This was translated into x-ray film, where sharpness and detail are much-sought-after attributes. The terms *rapid access* and *short cycle time* refer to the time it takes to process a film. Today a film can be processed from dry latent image status to a finished readable image in as short a time as 45 seconds. Digital imaging is knocking at the door; as yet there is no image-capturing medium that has as great an amplification nor as sharp an imaging resolution or is as cost effective as the silver halide wet-processed film, but it is coming.

Earlier I mentioned that Roentgen was working with phosphors when he discovered x rays. It was actually the desire to understand the phosphors that led to the discovery of x rays. Within months of Roentgen's discovery, scientists like Edison had already isolated chemical compounds that were capable of producing actinic light when exposed to x-radiation. Nearly fifty such compounds were identified quickly, most of which were either too slow to be pursued or cost too much to make. The result was that for close to eighty years, the stalwart phosphor used was calcium tungstate. This is the material that went into the screens known as par speed.

Not all screens were used to expose film. For direct in-line visualization of a barium swallow, for example, a radiologist might have used an iodide- or barium-based phosphor imbedded in glass, which would have been placed in front of the patient, with the x-ray tube being positioned behind the patient. The doctor could move the fluoroscopic screen, as it was called, around in front of the patient to see the internal organs. Needless to say, the dosages to both patient and doctor were tremendous. Today fluoroscopy is performed with image intensifiers and monitors. Although the physician may still be in the room with the patient, the dosage to both is minimized by using much faster systems, collimation, and protective shielding.

Understanding the difference between phosphorescence and fluorescence is important. The latter is useful in radiography because it produces light only when excited by x rays. Phosphorescent substances will have an afterglow, which would not be suitable for x-ray screens.

## ■ THE HISTORY OF INTENSIFYING SCREENS

About 99% of the exposure on x-ray film comes from the light emitted by the intensifying screen. X rays are horribly inefficient in producing density. Because x-radiation is absorbed by tissue (and accumulated), any method to reduce dosage and yet provide usable images is desirable. The intensifying screen is primarily responsible for making x-ray imaging a relatively safe medical diagnostic tool. Intensifying screens are unique in that they fluoresce when exposed to x-radiation.

In 1850 a Frenchman, Antoine-Henri Becquerel, first studied and measured the phenomenon of fluorescence. He demonstrated that a large number of solids had the ability to absorb energy of one wavelength and through transformation could emit energies of longer wavelength. Most dramatic of his discoveries was that short ultraviolet wavelength radiation could be absorbed by most fluorescent substances and be transformed into wavelengths that were visible to the eye. Shortly thereafter, in 1852, Sir George Stokes of Cambridge, England, applied Becquerel's principles by painting a piece of paper with a finely pulverized mixture of barium platinocyanide. He then exposed this paper to ultraviolet radiation and observed that the paper glowed with visible light. Although quite crude, this could be labeled the first demonstration of a fluorescent screen. Sir William Crookes and Eugen Goldstein extended the fluorescence phenomenon into areas of the unknown through the excitation of known fluorescent materials in cathode ray tubes. Another pioneer, Philip Lenard, was able to produce luminescence of fluorescent materials outside a Crookes tube. There was a lot of interest in the physics world in this area of converting one wavelength to another. In 1895, while Wilhelm Roentgen was investigating the excitation of a Crookes tube he discovered a radiation that had the ability to penetrate black paper and other opaque substances. Actually, he was using a fluorescent screen for the first time as a fluoroscopic screen. The news of his discovery of the unknown rays, or *x rays* as he named them, spread rapidly. So did the use of this flimsy, unstable, and expensive fluorescent screen.

In February 1896, Professor Michael S. Pupin placed a fluorescent screen on a photographic plate and put a patient's hand on top of the screen. With an x-ray exposure of a few seconds he obtained a roentgenogram of much greater contrast than had been seen up to that time. Thomas Edison had provided Pupin that screen. Edison had been working on improving the incandescent lamp and discovered that calcium tungstate crystals had the ability to increase the intensity severalfold over barium platinocyanide. The screen of calcium tungstate was crude and the quality was poor, if judged by modern standards, but the research did demonstrate that the intensifying screen had practical applications in the medical field. Indeed, if the fluorescent screen had not been used to enhance the x-ray image, the use of radiation in medical diagnoses would have been sidetracked significantly.

In March 1896 while continuing to work on improvements connected with the incandescent lamp, Edison conceived of the fluoroscope. His invention consisted of a piece of cardboard on which he affixed calcium tungstate crystals by means of a matrix of collodion. Collodion had been used successfully for sticking photographic emulsions to glass for approximately fifty years, so it was natural to use this concept to make a fluoroscopic device. The fluorescent screen was inserted into a truncated pyramidal box. The other end of the box was narrower and shaped to fit closely over the forehead and eyes. It was lined with black feathers to prevent external light from interfering with the acuity of the eye while the observer watched the shadows on the screen at the other end. This device was highly successful

and before long was being mass produced under Edison's direction at a firm in Orange, New Jersey, known as Aylsworth and Jackson. A major drawback of these screens was the phosphorescent lag and rapid deterioration. In addition, the surface, being quite rough, picked up dirt readily, which reduced usability. These difficulties, however, were accepted, because there were no substitutes, and Edison's screens remained the standard for almost fourteen years.

In the period between 1896 and 1912 an exhaustive search was conducted for more efficient, longer-lasting, and cheaper screens. English and German firms entered into the production of screens, with trials at overcoming the shortcomings of the American screens. Most efforts were fruitless. One German screen even had a binder that dissolved when moistened, which certainly prevented it from being cleansed with soap and water. In 1912, Dr. Herbert Threkeld-Edwards succeeded in making a hardened emulsion of calcium tungstate. This durable screen was also faster and cut down on radiation. The Snook Company in Philadelphia produced a screen that had less lag and produced sharper images. The research for this screen was headed by Carl V. S. Patterson. In 1914, Patterson left the Snook Company to return to his home in Towanda, Pennsylvania. Rumor has it that his attention was focused on producing a lagless screen because he had a broken bone set improperly as a result of the use of a screen that was unsharp and with considerable lag. (Patterson walked with a limp his entire life as a result of the improperly set broken bone.) Patterson was successful in developing a screen that did not deteriorate with use or age. This screen, the Patterson Standard Fluoroscopic Screen, created a new standard for medical fluoroscopic use. He created a company known as the Patterson Company and headed up the research, having hired Frederick W. Reuter to head up manufacturing. By 1918, the Patterson Company was experimenting with the idea of having two screens instead of one to increase the fluorescence. Eastman Kodak was trying the same idea only with film. Kodak was coating both sides of film with light-sensitive emulsion. The combination of Patterson's screens and Kodak's "duplitized" film created the format that is still used today in medical radiography, primarily because of the dosage reduction.

Patterson did not rest on their laurels, however; by 1921 they were producing screens that were "waterproof" or at least could be washed and had a tough-enough surface to resist abrasive wear. These screens touted a nonalcoholic protective surface and could be cleansed with alcohol, a common solvent in most medical facilities.

By 1922, Kodak decided to enter into the manufacture of screens. Kodak researchers coated their fluorescent emulsions onto a cellulose backing, similar to that used with their flexible films; however, this backing proved unsuccessful, and they reverted to the use of cardboard such as the Patterson Screen was coated on. (Not until Du Pont perfected Mylar was a flexible, dimensionally stable plastic back used as the basis for screens.)

Throughout the 1920s and well into the 1930s, Patterson continued to dominate both the fluoroscopic and medical screen business, even though viable competition arose in the form of such companies as Buck, in St. Louis, Missouri. This period could be characterized as one when various phosphors were used in attempts to decrease the early deficiencies of lag, unsharpness, and durability. Different phosphors were found more effective for fluoroscopy and film recording. One such fluoro screen was made in 1933 by two English inventors, Leonard Levy and Donald W. West. Their screen used zinc cadmium sulfide and was particularly sensitive to soft radiation and could be used at lower voltages. In those days it was common to directly capture the x ray–transmitted image through the body by means of a fluorescent screen. The Patterson Company imported this phosphor and incorporated it in the Patterson B Fluoroscopic Screen, which dominated this application until the introduction of image intensifers.

By the mid 1930s the availability of higher-powered equipment permitted the introduction of lower-speed, finer-grained screens. Patterson, again the leader, introduced the Detail Screen, which was advertised as producing the finest definition possible, almost as good as with a nonscreen technique, but with the higher contrast provided by screens. In 1935, Patterson began marketing an improved combination called the Par-Speed. The phosphor of choice was calcium tungstate, still the standard of the industry.

In 1937, General Electric made a device that would photograph the fluoroscopic screen. Because the screens in use at the time emitted green light and the film used to photograph was basically blue sensitive, there was a mismatch. Paterson was again consulted, to produce a screen that would match the film's sensitivity. The outcome was the Patterson Type D Photo Roentgen blue fluorescing screen. This was the beginning of the image-intensifying work and the capturing of the fluoroscopic image with film rather than by the eye.

Patterson was purchased by Du Pont in the early 1940s. Du Pont had been in the medical x-ray film manufacturing business since 1931, and could use the addition of a sister business that was a market leader. Du Pont scientists were challenged to make faster, more durable, and sharper screens. In 1948 they succeeded in making a new screen, based on zinc cadmium sulfide, that was 40% faster than the earlier Patterson model. They also made a new fast screen called Hi-Speed, which was only slightly less sharp than Par-Speed, but because of its motion-stopping capability, was able to produce an overall more uniform sharpness

image. This line of screens was also the first to be coated on a plastic support of Mylar. This essentially removed the problems of moisture delamination. Additional breakthroughs included the production of uniform-thickness screens that could be used as front or back screens, interchangeably. Prior to this most screens had a specific screen orientation of thin front and thick back.

The U.S. Radium Corporation entered the field of screen manufacturing in the 1940s, marketing three types of screens, intensifying, fluoroscopic, and photofluorographic screens. Eastman Kodak, in an endeavor to correct poor contact problems, tried to market a special cassette with an air bag designed to create a pneumatic cushion and provide superior contact. It failed because of leakage. Du Pont watched the air bag results with interest, and even tried to market separate air bags, but abandoned this approach in favor of felt backing, which, although not providing as good a contact as a properly installed air bag, was more reliable. In 1952, Kodak dropped its intensifying screen promotion. It re-entered the market in the early 1970s with revolutionary screens and a plastic cassette.

Artifacts generated by screens are among the worst offenders in the x-ray department because unless the offending screen is located and taken out of use, the artifact persists in interrupting accurate diagnoses. Locating the artifact is often not possible with the naked eye and white light inspection. An ultraviolet "black light" often displays the artifact-causing area, but not always. To assist in locating faulty cassettes, Du Pont began a distinctive serial numbering system on all "Patterson" screens beginning in 1954. This numbering system helped the user maintain a record throughout the useful life of each screen, and because the number was recorded on each film that exposed, there was a positive method of determining the screen that had the artifact.

Radiologists, becoming more and more aware of the hazards of radiation, both to the patient and the technologist, demanded faster and faster systems. To answer this challenge, the Du Pont Patterson's "Lightning Special" screen proved especially useful in portables, spot filming, operating room, and angiographic studies. This screen used barium lead sulfate, a departure from the old stand-by, calcium tungstate.

Simultaneous with Kodak's departure from the screen business in 1952, other screen manufacturers took advantage of the void and entered the arena. Names such as Intensi, Buck X-Ograph, Siemens, Kruppa, Dr. Streck, Della Volpe, Phillips, Levy-West, Ilford, Aver, Kalicon, and Massiot emerged. Screens began to be manufactured in every major industrial country. The major exchange however was between the United States and European countries. Japan manufactured for its own market until the mid 1960s, when it began to have a presence in the United States. By 1990 the leading screen manufacturers were Du Pont (Sterling), Kodak, Siemens, Toshiba, Kyokko, Agfa, and 3M, not necessarily in that order. Today's screen manufacturer needs to have "clean rooms" and employ high-technology practices to produce the tight tolerances required in this field.

Throughout the 1950s and 1960s, the standards continued to be calcium tungstate and barium lead sulfate phosphors. As radiology progressed and became more sophisticated and demanding, faster and sharper systems were designed. The emergence of rare-earth phosphors in the early 1970s ushered in a new era in imaging. Today an x-ray department has a plethora of screens emitting in the blue, green, and even ultraviolet spectra, matched to films of the same wavelengths providing a wide range of standardized speed systems from 50 to 1600 arithmetic and resolutions exceeding 15 line pairs per millimeter—beyond the naked eye's capability to see! Although challenged by the electronics, silver halide films and the intensifying screen system combination is predicted to survive well into the twenty-first century.

## ■ OBJECT OF RADIOGRAPHY

The purpose of producing a radiographic image is to provide the greatest amount of usable information for a diagnostician. In photography, art and science are often combined to create social statements or illusions, in medical radiography there is no tolerance for anything other than the closest to reality that one can achieve. Consistency and most faithful recording of anatomical structures with optimum detail are primary goals. Anything less is unacceptable for both the physician's and the patient's interests.

Quality can be described as a level of excellence. There are many adjectives used to clarify it. In medical imaging, one must think of matching the physician's trained eye with the optimum image capturing characteristics of the film. When the image can be visualized to allow the most concise and informative interpretation, one can say the highest level of radiographic quality has been attained. Many factors contribute to or detract from the end product quality. The following discusses many of those factors.

When a film is labelled "high quality," it usually has low fog, appropriate contrast to display small differences in density for the type of examination, and sufficient speed to overcome unsharpness caused by motion, and all this embodied in an emulsion that has grain structure fine enough not to impair the definition of the part being radiographed. This is no small task.

In medical radiography, many different products have been designed to offer a vast array of speed levels and contrasts as specified by the body part being radiographed. Certainly, imaging uniform soft tissue such as the breast

requires considerably different treatment, both in exposure and choice of film and even processing, from the choices, say, for a lateral lumbar spine or calcaneus. In general the inherent speed of a film depends on the grain size, grain structure, sensitization, choice of developer, and time and temperature the film is processed. It naturally follows that the larger the grain, the faster the speed of the film and the less the exposure. Combinations of different-size grains are used to create the desired characteristic curves. It would be wrong to oversimplify or make light of the methodology or technology that goes into the design and manufacture of a film. What is intended here is to offer general concepts that are used in assessing radiographic quality and the factors that the clinician can control and measure.

## ■ STRUCTURE AND MANUFACTURE OF X-RAY FILM

The process really begins with the manufacture of polyester film base (Figure 5-1). Molten polymer is sent through a vacuum reservoir and a barometric column, passing through a metering pump and extruded through a hopper to a casting wheel, which gives the polyester its surface. The polyester is at that point a thick band of flattened molten mass. It goes through a cooling bath, and then into a dryer, where it stiffens up. Then it is stretched longitudinally and laterally to a preset width. After reaching the proper width and thickness, it is given a memory by heat setting and cooling and then wound up on a master roll, to be coated later with emulsion.

Polyester base is manufactured by combining ethylene glycol with dimethyl terephthalate. This combination produces polyethylene terephthalate chains known to most under the brand names Cronar, Mylar, and Dacron.

Photographic film manufacture requires many complicated operations and extensive quality control tests at every step to ensure a product with high quality and uniform characteristics. There are basically five steps in the production of x-ray film (Figure 5-2):

1. Prepping the emulsion, which involves coagulation and washing the emulsion
2. Coating the actual emulsion on film
3. Drying
4. Finishing
5. Packaging

The typical film structure is composed of base covered with a subcoat onto which the emulsion is then coated. This is topped with an overcoat. If the film is intended for general radiographic use, it is probably coated on both sides exactly the same or "duplitized" (this doubles the speed of the film). If the film is intended to record images where dosage is not

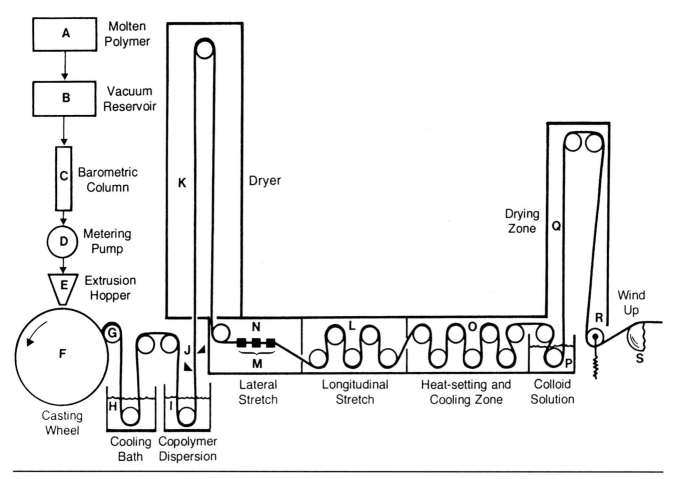

**Figure 5-1**    Manufacture of polyester film base. (Courtesy DuPont Photo Products, Wilmington, DE)

a factor, it is then coated on one side with a photosensitive emulsion. The other side is coated with an antihalation layer to prevent light scattering through the base, which would degrade the image sharpness.

The layers of an x-ray film (Figure 5-3) and their functions are as follows:

*Overcoat:* A protective layer that aids in scratch protection both before and after processing

*Emulsion:* The light-sensitive layer, made up of silver halide suspension in a high-grade gelatin support

*Subcoat:* A very thin coating that ensures adherence of the emulsion to the base support

*Base support:* The material that forms the structural support onto which the other sensitive and protective layers are coated

*Backing:* Another gelatin layer, sometimes used to prevent curl, inhibit light piping, and improve image quality or to act as a filter to make the film insensitive to certain wavelengths

## ▪ IMAGE FORMATION

The formation of a radiographic image is one of straight photographic exposure and development. The science is the same for radiographers and photographers. There are major differences in the equipment used and the subjects imaged, but the image formation and processing is identical. Simply put, it is black-and-white photographic imaging. The difference is that instead of using a camera and reflected light to capture the image, intensifying screens in a cassette give off actinic light when excited by x-radiation, and that light exposes the film. Understanding the concepts of the photographic theory are prerequisite to the physician and clinician if they are to be able to control the outcome and thereby achieve the desired degree of excellence, or quality.

A good starting point for understanding what happens to a film when it is exposed and processed into a visible image requires a short discussion of sensitometry. Although often avoided because it is not an exciting subject, it is

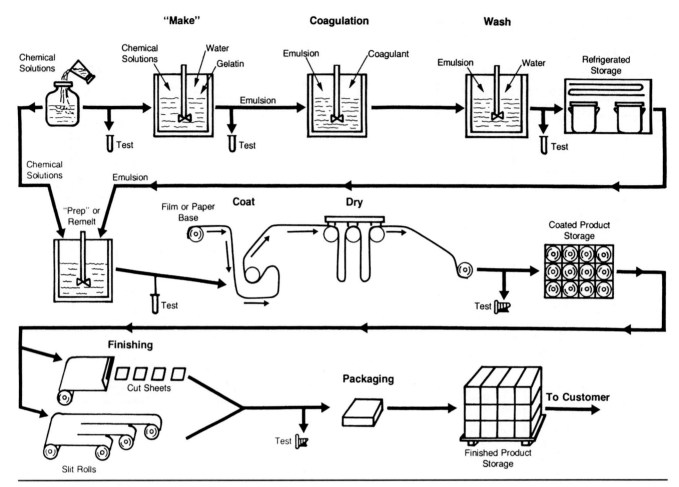

**Figure 5-2**    Manufacture of photographic film and paper. (Courtesy DuPont Photo Products, Wilmington, DE)

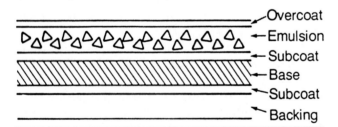

**Figure 5-3**    X-ray film cross section.

simply the study of a film's response to exposure and processing, factors that must be understood in order to achieve high-quality images.

## Sensitometry

In the early days of photography, those who made exposures and processed images did so by trial and error. Just shortly before the discovery of x rays, two British photographers, Hurter and Driffield, described the relationship between exposure and density. Prior to their work, predicting a specific photographic result was limited by the uncertainties of the process. Their work explained the mystery of exposure and development and aided the rapid expansion of photography and radiography. Once these factors were clarified and simplified, one could predict the technical factors required both in exposure and processing to achieve a desired image. This kind of thing is taken for granted today. Those who have tried to make an image without knowing the speed of a film or activity level of the chemistry understand the dilemma that Hurter and Driffield solved. The graphic basis of sensitometry—the H&D curve—has remained the single most important tool for scientists and manufacturers in measuring the photographic system. Although this tool is of extreme importance to the physicists, chemists, and engineers who are making films, those who expose or view the finished product will probably benefit more from having a practical overview of the subject. In short, knowing the relationships between exposure and density is much more important to the practitioner than dwelling on the science of the system.

Density and adequate differences in density, or contrast, are considered the most important properties of a radiograph. Proper densities and adequate contrast are required to give visibility to the structural detail of a subject.

Radiographic density is defined as the amount of blackening, which is the result of a deposit of metallic silver remaining on a film after exposure and processing. A useful method of measuring the amount of that blackening is to shine a light through the film. The more the blackening, the more light is absorbed and the less is transmitted. Densities are read by a specialized light meter called a densitometer, and the results are measured in logarithms. Logarithms are used because they provide the mathematical shorthand to reduce large numbers to little ones. For example, the log of 10 is 1, the log of 100 is 2, and the log of 1000 is 3. Applied to sensitometry, density is defined as the common logarithm of the ratio of the amount of light striking one side of the film, compared to the amount of light coming out of the other side. When 10 units of light are shined at a film and only one unit comes out the other side, the film is said to have a density of 1; there is a 10:1 ratio. When the ratio is 100:1, the density is 2, and when the ratio is 1000:1 the density is 3, and so on.

To produce an H&D curve, the film is first exposed to a calibrated step wedge that has a series of equal-increment step changes. The film is processed, and each step of density is read and plotted on special graph paper.

Figure 5-4 is a characteristic curve of an x-ray film exposed with intensifying screens and processed in x-ray chemistry. The portion of the curve designated as the "toe" demonstrates the response of the emulsion to relatively small amounts of radiant energy. With an increase in exposure, the density builds slowly until the "straight line" portion of the film is achieved. Along this straight line portion the density increases uniformly with the logarithm of the exposure until the shoulder of the curve is reached. In the shoulder region additional exposure results in smaller increases in density to a point where additional exposure does not produce any greater density. In fact, if sufficient exposure is given, the density will actually decrease.

The dictionary definition of the verb *contrast* is "to stand out," "to exhibit noticeable difference when compared side by side." Radiographically, contrast is the difference in two or more densities. As a radiograph is viewed on an illuminator, the difference in brightness of the various parts of the image is called radiographic contrast. This is the product of two distinct factors:

1. *Film contrast:* Inherent in the film and influenced by development
2. *Subject contrast:* Result of varied x-ray absorption by the patient

Although radiographic contrast can be altered by changing one or both of these factors, it is good practice to standardize

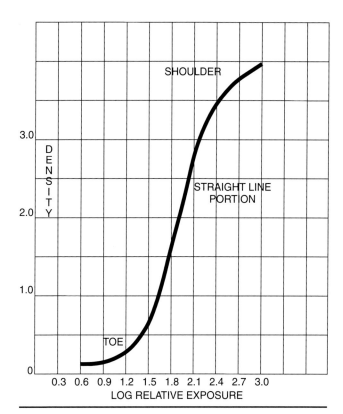

**Figure 5-4**   Characteristic curve of x-ray film.

the film and processing procedure and control radiographic contrast by altering the quality of the radiation by adjusting the kilovoltage. Sensitometrically, the term *contrast* refers to the slope or steepness of the characteristic curve of the film; *contrast* is a generic term. There are different contrasts depending on where they are "read" on the characteristic curve, as follows.

*Gradient* is the contrast of the film at a given density. When a straight line is drawn tangent to the characteristic curve at a particular density, this line forms a slope that is the gradient (or contrast) at this density (Figure 5-5).

*Average gradient* is found most often in radiography because it is more useful to have a single number to indicate the effective contrast of a film. This number, known as the average gradient, is determined by drawing a straight line between two selected densities on the characteristic curve. The two densities used for this measurement are those most often at the thresholds of where the information in the radiograph falls—from 0.25 to 2.00 (Figure 5-6).

Another term used to describe density is *gamma*: the slope of the straight line portion of the characteristic curve. This term is seldom used in radiography, because the curves of radiographic films have relatively short straight line portions. It is, however, used commonly to describe films used in a camera. Also, this portion of the curve may not coincide with the density range that is most useful in

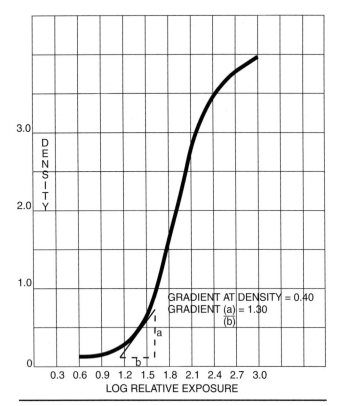

Figure 5-5  Calculation of gradient.

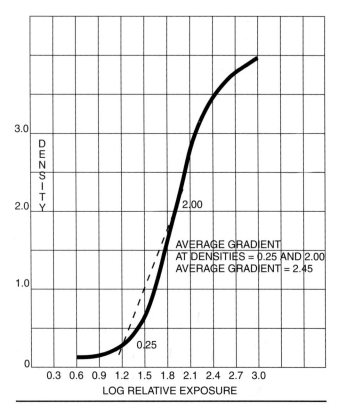

Figure 5-6  Determination of average gradient.

radiology. If gamma is a reference, it is best to determine exactly which of the "contrasts" is being referred to.

Exposure is defined as intensity multiplied by time. This can be expressed in either absolute exposure units (ergs per square cm of x-radiation) or in relative units. Relative exposure is much more convenient and equally useful to us. In radiography, we refer to exposure in terms of milliampere-seconds (mAs). In general, when the mAs is doubled the exposure is doubled, kVp remaining constant.

In plotting a characteristic curve, we most often plot density against the log of relative exposure. If the kilovoltage remains constant, the ratios of the exposures reaching the film through two different regions of the subject are always the same, regardless of the values of the milliamperage, time, or what the focal film distance might be. On a logarithmic scale, any two exposures whose ratio is constant will always be separated by the same distance on the exposure scale, regardless of the absolute values. For example, two exposures, one of which is twice the other, will always be separated by 0.3 on the logarithmic scale (the logarithm of 2 is 0.3).

It has been determined that the contrast of a film is indicated by the *shape* of the characteristic curve. Speed is indicated by the location of the curve along the exposure axis. The faster a film is, the more it will lie toward the left of the graph. The faster it is, the less relative exposure it will

take to reach the speed point density. The separation of two films plotted on the same graph may be measured at the speed point to determine the speed difference (Figure 5-7).

The convenience of using relative exposures also applies to speed. The speed of one film can be expressed on a relative basis to another when one is made the standard of comparison. The reference film can be assigned any arbitrary speed value, such as 100. If another film only requires half as much exposure to reach the same density as the reference film, then the faster film will have a relative speed of 200.

A density of 1.0 above base plus fog has been designated by the American Standards Association as the density for computing film speeds. This density was chosen because it represents the average of the useful density range (0.25 to 2.00). However, a density of 0.25 above base plus fog appears to be the approximate density most often viewed in the diagnostic region of a typical radiograph. For practical purposes, relative speeds are often calculated at this lower density.

In the dictionary, *latitude* is defined as "freedom from narrow limits." Radiographically, we think of latitude in terms of the freedom of exposure ranges and processing times and temperatures.

Of the variable factors, we think of film exposure being controlled by varying the time of exposure, the milliamper-

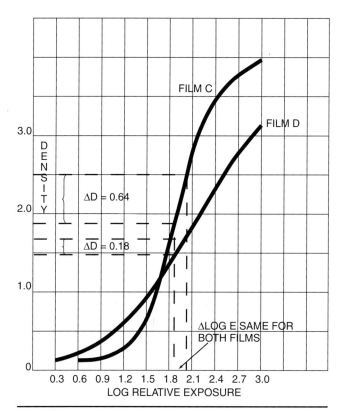

**Figure 5-7** Differences of film contrast and speed results in changes of curve shape and position, respectively.

age, or the kilovoltage. Exposure latitude is simply a measure of the magnitude of error that is permitted in each of these factors while still yielding a usable radiograph. When a film is said to have wide latitude, it has the ability to accept large changes in exposure without producing excessive density changes.

The tolerable variations in processing solutions, developer temperature, and time of development are known as developing latitude. Materials that permit variations in development without significant influence on density, contrast, or fog are considered to possess good processing latitude.

## Film Processing/Development

**Overview.**  When light strikes the emulsion, an invisible image is formed. This image is referred to as the latent image. Going from latent to visible requires a process known as development. There are two kinds of development, chemical and physical. Chemical development involves chemical reduction of silver halide crystals into metallic silver by a solution containing reducing agents, which offer electrons to the ionic silver salt to produce metallic silver. In physical development, silver salts are actually deposited where the latent image was captured from a solution that has

a great deal of silver in it. In today's production of a radiograph, mostly chemical development is used. There may be some physical development because of silver being present in the developer from previously developed films; however, physical development is no longer of practical value. Chemical development is more economical, less sensitive to temperature changes, less temperamental overall, and therefore easier to control.

The reduction to metallic silver is done in total darkness or under safelight conditions. While in contact with the developer, prior to contact with the fixer, the image is unstable and if exposed to light will be obliterated by formation of a uniform dense blackness or maximum density. Ideally, during development, only the crystals of silver halide that were exposed to light will be converted to metallic silver. Normally the unexposed silver halide crystals are dissolved into solution in the fixing bath. Following development and fixation, the film must be washed to remove the hypo-fixing agent and other chemicals remaining in the emulsion after the fixing, leaving a layer of clear, clean gelatin holding the inert metallic silver particles that make up the image. Following the wash cycle, the film is then dried and ready for viewing.

The image visualized in a black-and-white negative or x-ray film is composed of minute particles of metallic silver. The more the silver, the greater the density. X-ray film is a typical (black and white) negative emulsion that has emulsion coated on both sides (or "duplitized"—a Kodak invention), to increase system speed. X-ray film is normally sensitized to blue and ultraviolet light, sometimes extended sensitization to green light as well, but thus far not made sensitive to all light (panchromatic). The spectral sensitivity of the film must match the actinic output of the intensifying screen. A side benefit of the blue or blue-green spectral sensitivity is that x-ray film can be handled in illumination called safelight, usually some form of deep orange or red to which the x-ray film is insensitive.

**Chemicals.**  Processing chemistry is marketed already mixed, ready to use or in concentrates that must be mixed on site, either by hand or in an automated chemical mixer/blender apparatus. If the chemistry is delivered premixed, it may be mixed properly or may be a source of problems. If mixed on site in the replenisher tank, there is a prescribed method. Deviations can and more than likely will result in disaster.

The user's choices when purchasing chemistry are as follows:

1. Buy concentrate and mix on site in replenisher tanks.
2. Buy dealer premixed solutions and have periodic delivery.
3. Buy concentrate and use a chemical mixer.

There are tradeoffs with each choice:

| Choice | Good News | Bad News |
| --- | --- | --- |
| 1 | Consistent quality | Probably highest cost |
| | | User must store and provide labor to mix |
| 2 | No hassle for user | If stale, chemicals lose potency |
| | | No assurance of quality |
| 3 | Easiest on-site mixing | Quality can be degraded |
| | | Malfunctions can cause oxidation and precipitation |

The tests to make sure the developer and fixers are mixed properly are pH, specific gravity, bromide ion concentration, amount of hydroquinone, and clearing time.

Usually, developers come in two- or three-part concentrates, fixers usually come in two-part concentrates. The concentrates are marked A, B, and C and must be mixed in that order. The key is to put in a prescribed amount of water, followed by Part A, and then B, and so on. If there is insufficient water, or the water is too high a temperature or not stirred enough, or if the parts are installed out of order, precipitation may occur and render the chemical useless. It is important that chemical mixtures be stirred to ensure total mixing, as insufficient stirring will cause layering or separation of the chemicals by their weight. Excessive stirring of the developer, such as beating the solution, is not recommended, either, as it can fold air into the developer, which promotes aerial oxidation. Chemistry may also come in a mixture of powders and liquids, the only difference being the amount of time it takes to mix the solutions from a powder to a clear liquid.

Weak-looking images can be the direct result of improper dilution of developer and fixer. Sensitometric and physical results can be altered dramatically. Overdilution decreases the activity of the solution; underdilution may cause either increase or decrease in the activity level. Developer overdilution produces films of slower speed and lower contrast. With fixer, either overdilution or underdilution will result in increased clearing time, often compounded by drying problems. Dilution is most accurately measured by using a hydrometer, which measures how much solid there is in solution (specific gravity) and by a pH test to measure hydrogen ion concentration (acidic or basic levels). Suppliers who mix chemistry are quite familiar with these tests, but very few hospitals or clinics would ever check their solutions this way. Even if the hospital staff mix their own chemistry from concentrates or powders, they probably don't do analytical checks.

Dilution problems occur frequently, but they can be easily avoided. All that is required is to follow the mixing instructions provided, making sure to measure the water accurately. A quick and simple approach to use when mixing solutions is to know the volume of the tank used for mixing. Some have gallonage markings on the side; many have

nothing. Knowing the number of gallons per inch of solution, it is easy to add precise amounts to a partially filled replenisher tank. The formulas for figuring out the number of gallons for different shaped containers are pretty straightforward:

For rectangular tanks:

$$\text{Gallonage} = \frac{\text{Height} \leftrightarrow \text{Length} \leftrightarrow \text{Width (in inches)}}{231}$$

For cylindrical tanks:

$$\text{Gallonage} = \frac{3.14 \leftrightarrow \text{Radius}^2 \leftrightarrow \text{Height (in inches)}}{231}$$

With either tank, the number of gallons merely has to be divided by the height to get the number of gallons per inch. The gallons/inch could be marked on the side of the tank. Then measure up from the fluid level to the desired number of gallons and fill to that point.

**Charging a processor.**    Assuming the chemicals have been mixed properly, they now must be put into the processor. If the processor is being charged initially, from a dry state, it is important to know how much is required for the developer tank, because you must add a solution to the developer called a starter. The manual will tell the volume of the tank; if it doesn't, then use the rectangular formula just given, less the displacement of the rack, to determine the usable volume of the developer tank. The addition of starter brings the developer to a state of equilibrium, where the activity will remain constant by the process of regeneration. As films are processed, they carry some developer out of the processor into the fixer tank. At the same time, some of the developing agents are consumed, leaving residual gelatin and salts from the film in the developing solution. This is where the replenishment process achieves the equilibrium state. Just enough new chemistry is introduced to offset what is depleted or carried out of the developer tank. The reason for using the starter is to approximate that equilibrium state from the first film in a recharged processor. If the starter is left out, there will probably be an increase in activity, which translates into increased density and contrast and usually into wasted films and unnecessary exposure for patients.

It doesn't matter whether the developer or the fixer is put in first, as long as care is taken not to splash fixer into the developer tank. It is safer to put the fixer in first so any accidental fixer that spills into the developer tank can be flushed out with water, reducing the chance for contamination.

The wash tank must be full, and the flow must be set properly. The dryer must be up to the prescribed temperature, and the processor is ready to accept films.

**Stages of processing and chemical components.**
The developer is the only creative chemical. All the other

chemistries in the process do no more than halt some action or remove something. Developers are generally composed of two reducing agents, one for automatic processing that creates quick soft tones (phenidone), and the other that produces rich blacks and therefore contrast (hydroquinone). An alkali or accelerator must be present. These are buffered by a restrainer and are held in check by a preservative; all are dissolved in the medium of water. What goes on in the development action? First, phenidone donates electrons to the exposed silver bromide crystal to change it into black metallic silver. Phenidone works fast and provides development of lower densities and some degree of contrast. It is adversely affected by excess accumulations of bromide in the solution, as discussed later.

Hydroquinone also donates electrons to amplify the image; it is a reducing agent that starts slowly but when combined with phenidone becomes more active. Hydroquinone provides high contrast and rich maximum densities. It is temperature sensitive, however; if cold, it loses activity. In addition, too low a pH reduces its activity, which results in lower contrast and density.

The alkalis or accelerators are usually carbonates or hydroxides. They provide pH levels 9 to 11, which swell the emulsion and promote the release of electrons from the developing agents. Generally, although not always, the higher the pH, the higher the contrast and speed.

The restrainer, usually a potassium or sodium bromide, holds back the reducing agent from attacking the unexposed silver bromide crystals. There are also antifoggants present to maintain low fog levels. Antifoggants such as benzotriazole depress the production of unwanted density. Depending on the choice of the metal combined with the bromide, the color of the image may be altered. Sodium tends to produce slightly less blue-black images than do the potassiums. Bromide is the important ingredient, because it acts as a conditioner, maintaining a constancy. Recall the addition of the starter? Well, in essence, it is the addition of this bromide.

The preservative is usually a sodium or potassium sulfite. The sulfite leads to sulfination of early oxidation products of development, stopping their interference in the development process. Further, sulfites also have a minor solvent action on the silver halides.

The final ingredient is water, which must be relatively clear of metal ions such as iron or copper, because these accelerate oxidation and result in fogs. Hard water (with too much calcium, bicarbonate) can react with the sodium carbonate and sodium sulfite and form insoluble calcium. This forms so-called lime deposits on the side of the tanks and rollers. Finally, de-ionized or distilled water should not be used, because it would allow excessive swelling of the emulsion as well as be too expensive.

Earlier, I mentioned that time and temperature were important. Assuming a given chemical activity, controlling time and temperature in the developing process is the only way to ensure accurate and consistent sensitometric results. Time and temperature control in the other areas of the image production are not as crucial as in the developing stage.

As with developers, radiographic fixing baths are generally water vehicle solutions in which a variety of chemicals are dissolved to react principally on unexposed silver bromide crystals and provide permanence to the image. The basic ingredients in fixers are the buffering agent, fixing solvent, preservative, and hardener.

The buffering agent is usually an acid. Acetic acid and metabisulfites are common. Acids neutralize the developer and create the right environment for the other chemicals to work properly. The best working strength is around 4.5 pH. Below a pH of 4 the fixer will be unstable and might result in decomposition of sulfur. At too high a pH, the hardeners lose their effectiveness.

Actual fixing agents are usually sodium or ammonium thiosulfate. These are commonly referred to as hypo. Thiosulfate, a silver solvent, dissolves the unexposed silver bromide salts making them easier to wash out. (If films are left in fixer for extended periods, such as overnight, the image may be totally dissolved!)

The preservative prevents deposition of sulfur in the solution. It reacts with sulfur to reform sodium thiosulfate, and thus is self-regenerating. Anther preservative is sodium acetate, which when coupled with acetic acid forms a very good buffering medium, keeping the pH high as needed when hardeners are used in the fixing bath. Boric acid used to be a common ingredient used to prevent aluminum from combining with hydroxide, which can scavenge gelatin, which redeposits a sludge on the film surface. Borates are now banned in citrus-growing states because they are absorbed into such fruit.

Hardeners such as chrom alum, aluminum sulfate, and aluminum chloride have the effect of tanning or hardening the film surface to give permanence to the visible image.

Replenishment of both the developer and fixer, if done on the basis of usage as well as maintenance of pH levels, and bromide (in the developer) fosters a state of equilibrium that may continue until a long period of inactivity or contamination occurs. It is not uncommon for processors to be used several months without problems, merely with the addition of replenisher and minor cleaning of the crossovers between the tanks.

Once fixation is complete, the film will be ready for washing and drying. If the fixation portion of the process is incomplete, the films do not dry properly, come out of the dryer tacky, and have an opalescent appearance. This commonly leads to an early archival breakdown, with a brown staining known as dichroic stain, which is the result of residual developer. If the film is cleared or fixed sufficiently but not washed thoroughly, it may also suffer from a darkening of the image known as hypo retention. There are rules imposed by law that state how long the film should last unchanged. These rules are not uniform, but the minimum storage time is generally seven years. The current standard for residual thiosulfate retention is 40 micrograms per square inch. At this level or lower, the image is not impaired during its normal storage life.

Recycling and closed-loop systems are being promoted because of economic and ecological issues. Fixer can be reconstituted relatively easily; recycling of developer is not as simple. If recycling is done, the archival property of the films must be checked carefully.

Washing and drying are the final two steps. The purposes are obvious, to get rid of the chemicals involved in fixing and make the film suitable for prolonged storage. In general, present-day processors are called "cold water," because they do not require tempered water. In practice, the wash water is roughly no greater than 10° Fahrenheit less than the fixer, which in turn is between the developer and wash.

Common temperatures used in automatic processors are as follows: developer 92° to 95° F, fixer 85° to 90° F, wash 70° to 75° F, and dryer 120° to 140° F.

Drying requires clean, warm air passing evenly over both surfaces of the film equally. The swollen wet film reduces to about 20% of its wet thickness, the density increases, and the silver metal image becomes more reflective.

**Manual chemistry versus machine chemistry.** All processing is a function of time, temperature, and chemical activity. There are differences between manual and machine developing in terms of all three factors. With proper procedures and care, the results should be identical. The differences are listed in Table 5-1.

For users who wants to mix their own x-ray chemistry, it usually comes packaged to make 2 × 5 gallons. It is usually composed of three parts, A, B, and C. One merely has to add about 14 quarts of water to make 5 gallons of working solution for machine use.

These developers can also be used as a manual developer merely by omitting the addition of part C and making up for that volume with water. At 68° F, with agitation for 5 seconds every minute, the recommended times of immersion are usually 3 minutes minimum and a maximum of 5 minutes development. Recommended replenishment is at the rate of 1 gallon of developer for every 100 sheets of 14- × 17-inch film (or equivalent) processed. The simplest method to do this is to drain each film from the corner as it is extracted from the developer, and after 100 sheets, remove 1 gallon of the working solution and replace with fresh developer replenisher.

Fixers come packaged to make the same volume as developer. Fixers usually have two parts, A and B, to which adding about 15 quarts of water will make 5 gallons of working solution for machine use. Fixers can be used as manual solutions merely by omitting the addition of part B and making up that volume with water.

Fixer immersion time recommended is a minimum of two times the clearing time. Clearing time varies depending on the condition of the fixer. Clearing time is measured by immersing a strip of green film into the fixer and measuring the time it takes to clear. With fresh fixer, medical screen film should clear in no more than 10 seconds. For this condition, the fixing time should be no less than 20 seconds. As the fixer becomes used, the clearing time will increase, and so should the total time in the fixer, according to the formula just given. If the clearing time is longer than 1 minute, the fixer is too weak and should be replaced. Replenishment of 2 gallons per 100 sheets of 14 × 17 inch (or equivalent), done the same way as with the developer will maintain the fixer indefinitely.

With the advent of machine processing, a whole host of darkroom cleanliness problems disappeared, unfortunately to be replaced with a new set of handling problems that occur only in machine processing. Table 5-2 presents a few problems that one may encounter in manual processing.

| TABLE 5-1 | Differences Between Manual and Machine Developing | |
| --- | --- | --- |
| Factor | Manual | Machine |
| Developer component | No hardener required | Has hardener |
| Developer temperature | 68°-75° F | 85°-95° F |
| Developer immersion time | 1.5-5 min | 20-35 s |
| Fixer component | No hardener required | Has hardener |
| Fixation time | 1-3 min | 20-35 s |
| Fixer temperature | 68°-75° F | 5° F lower than developer temperature |
| Wash time and temperature | 5-20 min if running water at 68°-80° F | 20-35 s at temperature equal to or 5° F lower than fixer |
| After treatment | Photo-Flo solution will minimize water marks | None |
| Drying | 10-30 min at room temperature or heated air box (100°-120° F) | 20-25 s at 120°-140° F |

| TABLE 5-2 | Manual Processing Problems | |
|---|---|---|
| Problem | Symptoms | Cure |
| Finger marks | Light or dark finger marks on films | Make sure hands are not contaminated by fixer or developer and that they are dry. |
| Kill marks | Clear areas on films | Make sure no air bubbles remain on films and that films are not touching during development process. |
| Chemicals on screens | Stains on screens, resulting in light areas on films | Care when handling films wet with developer or fixer. Also separate wet and dry areas in darkroom. |

Most problems that one encounters in manual processing can be overcome by observing good practices, common sense, and cleanliness.

## AUTOMATED PROCESSING

In today's x-ray department, mere automation of processing does not immunize against processing problems. In fact, when the automatic processor came into use in the late 1950s it ushered in a whole new set of artifact-producing problems involving transport, such as film jams, abrasions, cocked films, pressure marks, gelatin pick-off, and overlapped films. This does not suggest that automatic processors are problem producers, but for every problem that was eliminated with the discontinuation of the manual mode, a new one emerged in the processor.

Radiographic processing is performed with an automatic processor to achieve consistent quality. Because the processing system is a chemical process that has specific conditions of time and temperature based on a given chemical activity, using an automatic processor with set temperatures and immersion times ensured more consistent results than could have been achieved manually unless extreme care were exercised.

A basic key to maintaining uniform sensitometry is to keep the developer activity level as close to constant as possible.

Film quality can change dramatically in a very short period. For example, if a high-use processor is not replenished (because of a kinked line or empty replenisher tank), the dropoff in gradient and background can happen in a matter of minutes. Conversely, if a low-use processor is running continuously without replenisher to compensate for aerial oxidation and evaporation, the resulting sensitometry can be extremely erratic.

A delicate balance is needed with regard to the bromide content of a developer solution. Most other chemistries have starters that add the bromide at the initial startup to bring it to the equilibrium state that will produce uniform sensitometry. As films are processed, bromide builds up in the developer. Because bromide is a restrainer, the more bromide, the more the development will be suppressed. To offset bromide buildup in the developer, the solution is replenished. This is the only way to keep bromide at the desired level. Overreplenishment with most chemistries may cause rises in activity levels, upsetting the equilibrium state.

Over a decade ago, Du Pont introduced a developer with a revolutionary approach to solving this problem. The developer, HSD (High Stability Developer) has bromide in the replenisher, and therefore it is almost impossible to overreplenish the developer. Whether in high- or low-use processors, that delicate state of equilibrium can be maintained.

For years, Du Pont was the only manufacturer able to make claims for and actually produce high stability. Other chemistries had to be dumped and recharged much more frequently. With newer, more sophisticated replenisher systems being incorporated in the new processors, such as area replenishment, longer stability is becoming more achievable.

## QUALITY CONTROL

Processing quality control is merely a procedure of monitoring to see if there is consistency. To achieve consistency, first one must be aware of those things that can be controlled and what they do; then one can make the necessary modifications. Like anything mechanical, processing quality control requires cleaning and maintenance, making necessary adjustments to tolerances, and replacing worn parts. The manufacturer usually provides a checklist and procedure to do this. Whether contracted out or done internally, it must be done. There are no shortcuts for maintaining quality processing conditions. To skimp on preventive maintenance will only result in massive headaches at times when one can least afford to have them.

When the processor is known to be in proper working order and a film and chemistry combination have been chosen, a processor quality control can be implemented.

The first ingredient in setting up a processor quality control program is to have a source for uniformly exposed

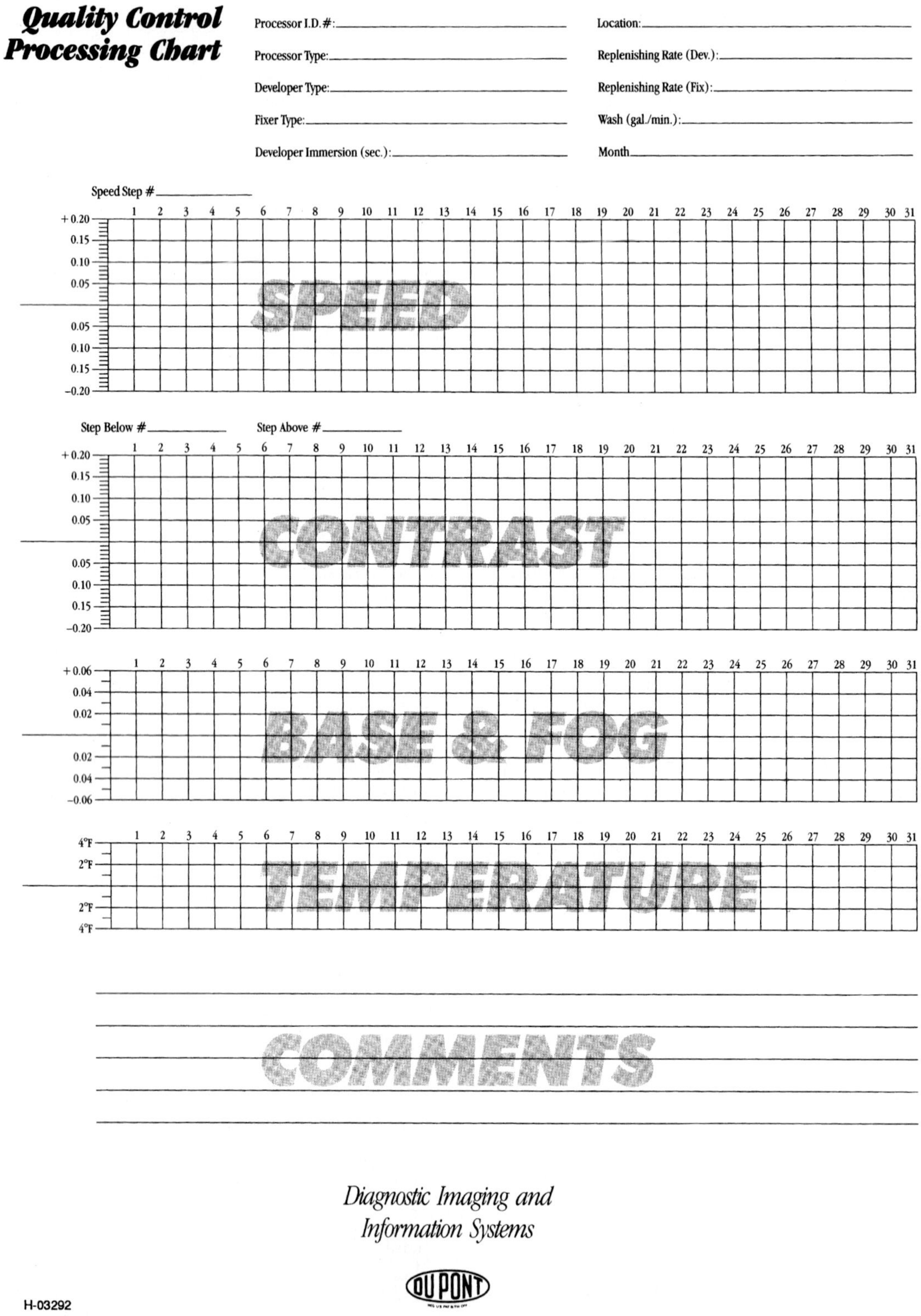

*Quality Control*
*Processing Chart*

Processor I.D.#:_____     Location:_____

Processor Type:_____     Replenishing Rate (Dev.):_____

Developer Type:_____     Replenishing Rate (Fix):_____

Fixer Type:_____     Wash (gal./min.):_____

Developer Immersion (sec.):_____     Month_____

Speed Step #_____

|  | 1 | 2 | 3 | 4 | 5 | 6 | 7 | 8 | 9 | 10 | 11 | 12 | 13 | 14 | 15 | 16 | 17 | 18 | 19 | 20 | 21 | 22 | 23 | 24 | 25 | 26 | 27 | 28 | 29 | 30 | 31 |
|---|---|---|---|---|---|---|---|---|---|---|---|---|---|---|---|---|---|---|---|---|---|---|---|---|---|---|---|---|---|---|---|

+0.20 / 0.15 / 0.10 / 0.05 / 0.05 / 0.10 / 0.15 / −0.20

SPEED

Step Below #_____     Step Above #_____

+0.20 / 0.15 / 0.10 / 0.05 / 0.05 / 0.10 / 0.15 / −0.20

CONTRAST

+0.06 / 0.04 / 0.02 / 0.02 / 0.04 / −0.06

BASE & FOG

4°F / 2°F / 2°F / 4°F

TEMPERATURE

_____
_____
_____
_____

COMMENTS

*Diagnostic Imaging and*
*Information Systems*

H-03292

Figure 5-8   Quality control processing chart. (Courtesy DuPont Photo Products, Wilmington, DE)

sensitometric strips to use in monitoring the processor. Although a step wedge could be used to make exposures with an x-ray tube, it is better to use a sensitometer to make exposures with because it removes the variables that may be introduced by x rays. It is the processor that is to be under control; the care and maintenance of the x-ray system is a topic for another discussion.

Technicians recommend using a separate box of film for monitoring. Using this film, an exposure is made with the sensitometer, processed, and set aside as the master control film. With a densitometer, read the speed step (closest to density of 1) and plot on a form (see Figure 5-8). Second, select two steps, measure the difference, and calculate a contrast value (Figure 5-9). In addition, plot base plus fog and temperature readings.

On a regular basis—some recommend several times per day, but no less than daily—expose another sheet of film sensitometrically and compare with the master control film. If the films do not match but are within acceptable limits, make note of this by recording the density shift. If convenient, check the specifications such as temperature and replenishment. Usually, acceptable limits are ±15%. If films do not match or are beyond the acceptable limits, a second film may be exposed to verify the validity of the test. Then a complete check of the processing condition should be made to identify which of the variables is out of limits. There may be more than one. Depending on how severely out of limits a variable is, development of patient films may have to be suspended until the situation is corrected. Once located, the offending variable should be readjusted or corrected and recorded. Another film should be processed to verify acceptable processing conditions have been achieved.

Periodically, no less often than weekly, all records should be reviewed and updated, and trends noted. Any time a major repair is made to the processor, or after major cleanings and chemical recharging, test films should be run.

An automatic processor is capable of consistently producing high-quality radiographs. Knowledge of the basics and adherence to a quality control regimen will ensure that this quality level is achieved.

Proper mixing of chemistry is important. It's cookbook style—quite straightforward. If the right amounts are mixed as prescribed, uniform, repeatable results are achieved. High-quality results require photo-grade ingredients in the right proportions, mixed according to directions. Deviations or attempted shortcuts will sabotage the goals.

Radiographic films today have reached a such a high standard of quality and uniformity that it is safe to say that in most cases, defects are caused by faulty storage, handling, and or processing. Faulty exposure techniques and positioning are not being addressed here; those were covered in previous chapters. Actual defects are almost limitless. However, two basic classes of defects exist, physical and photographic. Physical defects include marks on the film, blemishes caused by transport, rough handling, scratches, kinks, and any direct physical damage to the emulsion surface. Usually a routine examination or audit of what the film was subjected to and how it was handled can reveal the cause of most physical defects. An example of severe handling is the kink mark. Kink marks prior to exposure can be either light or dark, depending on the severity. After exposure the kink mark can only be dark (see Figure 5-10). Photographic defects may be more difficult to determine, because they are usually caused by the presence or absence of chemicals or a physical or chemical reaction in or on the film emulsion. Such defects are manifested by deposits on the film, stains, and fog. Samples of films with deposits or stains can be analyzed to find the chemical cause creating the artifact.

## ◼ DARKROOM

The darkroom is a vital link in the production of images. It is the funnel through which all light-sensitive silver halide film receptors must pass. More film artifacts are caused in the darkroom than anywhere else in the imaging chain, and the darkroom is often the last area to be designed and installed in the radiology department. This makes about as much sense as it would to design the kitchen for a cafeteria last, cramming it into a limited available space after all other construction was finalized! This neglect in the planning stages causes long-term headaches, because placement of equipment is often not conducive to making the work flow easy and productive. Another problem that can become increasingly difficult to overcome is the cleanliness issue. A crammed, ill-designed darkroom is difficult if not impossible to keep clean, and cleanliness is paramount in producing artifact-free films.

### Special Considerations

Different problems are encountered when dealing with an existing darkroom and when dealing with one in the design stage. There are common concerns as well, of course. First considerations should be cleanliness and of course light tightness. Dust, dirt, contaminants, and stray light cause most artifacts. If these can be minimized, the overall quality of the finished radiograph is enormously improved. To adapt an existing darkroom, make sure that it is upgraded to provide adequate ventilation and that the equipment and work areas are placed so wet areas are safely separated from storage and work surfaces where raw films will be handled. Dirt and dust are the two most insidious artifact-causing problems and are the most difficult to overcome. For example, a suspended ceiling may serve as a shelf for construction dust, which will be a constant source of filtering dust. If the

## *How to Measure Processing Variations with a CRONEX® Sensitometer*

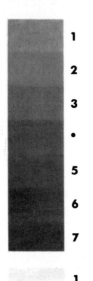

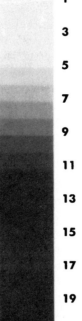

### *The 7-Step Wedge to Monitor Speed Visually*

Processor control by visual comparison is practical with the seven step wedge. The test film is placed next to the standard on the viewbox. The standard represents optimal results achieved at the onset of the quality control program, utilizing the CRONEX® Sensitometer. If the test film exactly matches the standard, the variation is zero. When matching densities requires displacement of the test film standard by one step, the variation from standard is equivalent to 15%. A one step offset from the standard is acceptable. When the test film must be displaced by two steps, the processing variation is equivalent to 30%. A two step variation indicates the need for corrective action. "A Guide to Common Processing Problems", is available from your DuPont Technical Representative, to assist you in processor troubleshooting. Results are not plotted on the daily monitoring chart on the other side.

### *Using the 21-Step Wedge*

#### SPEED

- Determine the step number within a density range of 1.00-1.30 on the 21-step wedge, that step becomes the Speed Step.
- Enter the step number and density reading on the chart on the other side. This step should be used for all future readings.
- Measure and plot the density of the Speed Step daily.
- Variations greater than ± 0.15 indicate the need for corrective action.

#### CONTRAST

- Determine the density of the steps *above* and *below* the Speed Step.
- Subtract these densities for a contrast reading. The same two steps should be used for all future contrast readings.
- Calculate and plot this density difference daily.
- Variations greater than ± 0.15 indicate the need for corrective action.

#### BASE + FOG

- Read an area of the film that has received no exposure.
- Enter reading in the space provided on the chart.
- Measure and plot Base + Fog *daily.*

#### TEMPERATURE

- With a calibrated thermometer, measure developer temperature and enter the reading on the chart. (Always measure at the same location in the tank).
- Measure and plot developer temperature *daily.*
- Variations greater than ± 2°F (1.1°C) indicate the need for corrective action.

Figure 5-9   Processing chart variables.

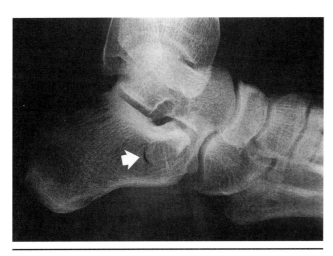

Figure 5-10   Kink mark—severe enough to cause sensitization.

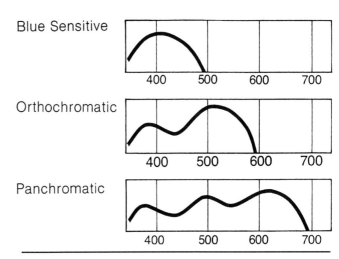

Figure 5-11   Film spectral response.

ceiling debris is constantly unsettled by the opening and closing of the darkroom door or from the exhaust of the processor, dirt will cascade into the darkroom for years. Modern shrink-wrap plastic sheeting may be used to minimize this kind of artifact-causing condition. Artifacts caused by dust and dirt on a screen and/or on a film when it is exposed can be examined with a magnifying glass. Usually these artifacts have somewhat amorphous edges. Artifacts can be by eruptions, gouges, and scratches; emulsion may be torn from the film, and the edges will be very sharp. If the artifact appears only on one side of the film, it usually has a physical source. Artifacts that are on both sides of the film are mostly photographic.

Light tightness is a must and goes hand in hand with good construction. Normally, there are no windows in a darkroom; if there are, they should be able to be totally light tight. As far as the ventilation is concerned, there should be a method of removing dead air from the darkroom. Ideally there should be a slight negative air pressure around the darkroom, which will draw air out of it. If the reverse is true, any lint, airborne dirt, or fumes will be drawn in. If there is space to install a revolving darkroom door, doing so is highly recommended. Not only do such doors ensure the integrity of the dark, but they also allow for continuous access to the darkroom without interrupting work. Basically, such a door is designed as two cylinders, one inside the other; the outer cylinder is constructed of two arcs with openings to both the light and dark sides of the opening. The inner sleeve has a single opening and revolves, allowing for entry without disturbing internal activities.

Light switches should be placed with protective covers so they are not inadvertently switched on. Fluorescent tape (that which emits a faint green glow) is often used to designate switch locations. If such a tape is used, it must first be checked out to determine its emission, to avoid fogging the film in use.

## Safelights

Although early darkrooms were painted black because that was thought safer, any color can be used as long as the safelights are correct. In choosing safelights, it is necessary to match safelight filtration to the spectral sensitivity of the films to be used (Figure 5-11) so that accidental fogging does not occur. Even then, the best practice is to use the inverse square law to place safelights as far away from the work surfaces as possible and to use a bulb of the lowest wattage possible to provide enough illumination for the darkroom worker to know where things are and yet have time to handle films safely. Exposed films are much more sensitive to fogging than are raw films prior to exposure. A good rule of thumb for safelights: use Wratten 6B for blue films, Kodak GBX2 for either blue or green rare-earth films, and no safelights for panchromatic films. Until a few years ago x-ray film was sensitive only to blue and ultraviolet light, matching the color emitted by calcium tungstate intensifying screens, which were the standard from the discovery of x rays until the advent of green rare-earth screens more than two decades ago. Deep orange or reddish filters such as Kodak Wratten 6B or DuPont 55X filters were "safe" for the blue-sensitive films, because their sensitivity did not extend into the red end of the spectrum. Green-emitting rare-earth screens required green-sensitive film, and to prevent the safelights from fogging these green-sensitive films, safelight filters were required that passed wavelengths above the sensitivity of the film. The answer was GBX2.

A 7.5-watt bulb at a distance of no less than 4 feet from a work surface provides adequate illumination.

## VIEWING EQUIPMENT

Probably the last consideration in designing or maintaining an x-ray department is the viewing equipment. Even though viewboxes are probably one of the least expensive and most important pieces of equipment, they are nevertheless neglected. Uniform brightness and color are achieved by using the same color temperature bulbs and making sure the plastic screens are clean and free from color changes. Hot lights, at one time commonplace in viewing areas, have diminished in popularity as automated exposure devices with phototiming have reduced the incidence of overexposed films.

## STORAGE

Film should be stored in humidity and temperatures that are comfortable for humans. A relative humidity of 40% to 60% and a constant 70° F temperature are ideal for storage. The fog of x-ray film will rise gradually, because of cosmic radiation, but should be well within limits during the two years or so that the producer dates the film forward from date of manufacture. Film responds to any stimulus it gets; if it is handled roughly or subjected to stress, pressure, humidity, or radiation, it will record the damage.

## TROUBLESHOOTING

The result of major manufacturer quality controls and production protocols makes consistent artifact-free imaging products available for all consumers. Users can be assured of uniform quality if they use prescribed products and follow directions. Problems of incompatibility arise when shortcuts are attempted or mixing of products that were not intended to be mixed takes place. Today's imaging products are quite sophisticated, were designed as systems, and function best when used that way. That said, if problems occur, there is a protocol for determining the cause. Solving problems that occur with imaging products requires a full knowledge of the total system, from image formation to processing and all the handling in between. Usually by process of elimination, the source(s) of the problem can be found. Asking what the problem is and what it is not can quickly eliminate tangential investigations, which, although informative, may not find causes of the problem. An example is a scratch on a piece of film that is in an arc shape versus one that is perfectly straight. It is safe to say that the arc scratch originated in handling in the darkroom, because in manufacturing and in the roller processor, the film travels in straight lines. It is in the handling that short, curved motions occur that would cause an arc scratch. The question of when the scratch took place, either before exposure, after exposure and before processing, or after processing can often be determined through careful examination of unprocessed films and simulating or recreating the handling procedure. This requires close examination and note keeping on what the problem is and what it is not. There is an answer for the problem, and with careful examination and all the facts, it can be solved. All too often the symptom is treated rather than the cause. When this happens, the problem is bound to surface again. Often it is useful to work backward through the path the product took to find the source of the problem. If the film went through an automatic processor, start at the dryer end and work backward from the dryer, to the wash, to the fixer, to the developer. Common causes of unsatisfactory radiographs are listed in Box 5-1.

## ARTIFACTS

Artifacts are basically unwanted information that has been recorded on the film. Artifacts can be lumped into two major categories, physical and sensitometric. They often can be "read" around, but when they are more than an annoyance, they can and often do result in poor diagnoses. Discussed next are some common artifacts, their causes and possible sources, and hints on how to avoid them.

### Static

Static is elusive and insidious. It often obliterates valuable information. All static is caused by a discharge of electricity. It is actually the light from a spark of electricity that exposes the film. If the electrical charge is slight, the result is smudge static; if it is severe, the result is tree static (Figure 5-12). Note that in the center of the tree static there is an amorphous area that is the smudge referred to. Static is less a problem when the relative humidity is 40% to 60%. It often occurs when the atmosphere is extremely dry, such as in temperate zones during the winter when the heat is on. If static snaps from your hand to a doorknob, you will be sure to see it on your films. To minimize static, humidifiers are often used to replace the moisture. Care should also be taken when cleaning screens. If screens are rubbed too vigorously, static could result. Often screen cleaners contain an antistatic solution. If mild soap and water are used in place of a screen cleaner, use a gentle motion to clean the screens.

### Fog

Fog is unwanted density that fills in the toe density, reducing the contrast of the fine detail in that area. Fog can be caused by radiation, white light (Figure 5-13), overexposure to safelights, age of film, and chemical reaction. Although it is

| BOX 5-1 | Common Causes of Unsatisfactory Radiographs |

**LOW DENSITY**

1. **Underexposure**
    A. Wrong exposure factors
        1. Too low kilovoltage
        2. Too low milliamperage
        3. Too short exposure
        4. Too great focal-film distance
    B. Meters out of calibration
    C. Timer out of calibration
    D Inaccurate settings of meters or timer
    E. Drop in incoming line voltage
        1. Elevators, welders, furnaces, blowers, etc., on same circuit
        2. Insufficient size of power line or transformers
    F. Photocell timer out of adjustment
    G. Incorrect centering of patient to photocell
    H. Central ray of x-ray tube not directed on film
        1. X-ray tube rotated in casing
    I. Distance out of grid radius
    J. Bucky timer inaccurate
    K. One of more valve tubes burned out (full wave rectifying machines)

II. **Underdevelopment**
    A. Improper development
        1. Time too short
        2. Temperature too low (hydroquinone inactive below 55° F or 13° C)
        3. Combination of both 1 and 2
        4. Inaccurate thermometer
    B. Exhausted developer
        1. Chemical activity used up
        2. Activity destroyed by contamination
    C. Dilluted developer
        1. Melted ice from cooling attempt
        2. Melted ice from cooling attempt
        3. Water overflowed from wash tank
        4. Insufficient chemical mixed originally because tank actually was larger than rating
        5. Improper additions
    D. Incorrectly mixed developer
        1. Exact capacity of tank unknown
        2. Mixing ingredients in wrong sequence
        3. Omission of ingredients
        4. Unbalanced formula composition
        5. Overdose of sodium bicarbonate as retarder in concentrated developer during hot weather

**HIGH DENSITY**

1. **Overexposure**
    A. Wrong exposure factors
        1. Too high kilovoltage
        2. Too high milliamperage
        3. Too long exposure
        4. Too short focal-film distance
    B. Meters out of calibration
    C. Timer out of calibration

    D. Inaccurate setting of meters or timer
    E. Surge in incoming line voltage
    F. Photocell timer out of adjustment
    G. Incorrect centering of patient to photocell

II. **Improper development**
    A. Time too long
    B. Temperature too high
    C. Combination of both A and B
    D. Inaccurate thermometer
    E. Insufficient dilution of concentrated developer
    F. Omission of bromide when mixing

III. **Fog—see section on "fog"**
    A. Light struck
    B. Radiation
    C. Chemical
    D. Film deterioration

**LOW CONTRAST**

I. **Overpenetration from too high kilovoltage**
    A. Overmeasurement of part to be examined
    B. Incorrect estimate of material or tissue density
    C. Meters out of calibration
    D. Meters inaccurately set
    E. Surge in incoming line voltage
    F. Undermeasurement of focal-film distance

II. **Scattered radiation**
    A. Failure to use Bucky diaphragm
    B. Failure to use stationary grid
    C. Failure to use cutout diaphragm
    D. Failure to use suitable cones
    E. Failure to use lead backing cassette

III. **Too short exposure**
    A. Timer out of calibration
    B. Timer inaccurately set
    c. Overload relay kicked out

IV. **Improper development**

**HIGH CONTRAST**

I. **Underpenetration from too low kilovoltage**
    A. Undermeasurement of part to be examined
    B. In parts of varying thickness, setting of kilovoltage for thinner sections
    C. Meters out of calibration
    D. Meters inaccurately set
    E. Drop in incoming time voltage
        1. Elevators, welders, furnaces, etc., on same line
        2. Insufficient size of power line or transformer
    F. Overmeasurement of focal-film distance

II. **Too long exposure**
    A. Timer out of calibration
    B. Timer inaccurately set

III. **Improper development**

*Continued*

## BOX 5-1    Common Causes of Unsatisfactory Radiographs—cont'd

**FOG**

**I. Unsafe light**
   A. Light leaks into processing room
      1. Leaks through doors, windows, etc.
      2. Poorly designed labyrinth entrance
         a. Bright light at outer entrance
         b. Reflection from white uniforms of persons passing through
      3. Sparking of motors
         a. Ventilating fans
         b. Dryer fans
         c. Mixers—barium
      4. Light leaks in film-carrying box
   B. Safelights
      1. Bulb too bright
      2. Improper filter
         a. Not dense enough
         b. Cracked
         c. Bleached
         d. Shrunken
   C. Turning on light before fixation is complete
   D. Luminous clock and watch faces
   E. Lighting matches in darkroom
   F. Where film is carried from machine to darkroom in containers, container may leak light

**II. Radiation**
   A. Insufficient protection
      1. During delivery or transportation in laboratory or shop
      2. Film storage bin
      3. Loaded cassette racks—steel back should face toward source of radiation
      4. Not enough protected for loading darkroom
   B. Improper storage
      1. Radium
      2. Isotopes
      3. X-ray machines

**III. Chemical**
   A. Prolonged development
   B. Developer contaminated
      1. Foreign matter of any kind (metals, etc.)

**IV. Deterioration of film**
   A. Age (Use oldest film first)
   B. Storage conditions
      1. Too high temperatures
         a. Hot room
         b. Cool room but near radiator or hot pipe
      2. Too high humidity
         a. Damp room
         b. Moist air
      3. Ammonia or other fumes present in darkroom or other working area
   C. Delivery conditions
      1. Moisture precipitation when cold box of film is opened in hot, humid room

2. Fresh boxes should be stored overnight at room temperature before opening

**V. Excessive pressure on emulsions of unprocessed film**
   A. During storage
   B. Durig manipulation in darkroom

**VI. Loaded cassettes stored near heat, sunlight, or radiation**

**STAINS ON RADIOGRAPHS**

**I. Yellow**
   A. Exhausted, oxidized developer
      1. Old
      2. Covers left off
      3. Scum on developer surface
         a. Oil from pipelines
         b. Impure water used when mixing
         c. Dust
   B. Prolonged development
   C. Insufficient rinsing
   D. Exhausted fixing bath

**II. Dichroic**
   A. Old, exhausted developer
      1. Colloidal metallic silver
   B. Nearly exhausted fixer
   C. Developer containing small amounts of fixer or scum
   D. Films partially fixed in weak fixer, exposed to light and refixed
   E. Prolonged intermediate rinse in contaminated rinse water

**III. Green tinted**
   A. Prolonged immersion in chrome alum fixing bath
   B. Insufficient washing

**DEPOSITS ON RADIOGRAPHS**

**I. Metallic**
   A. Oxidized products from developer
   B. Silver salts reacting with hydrogen sulfide in air to form silver sulfide
   C. Improper solder used in repair of hangers
   D. Silver loaded fixer

**II. White or crystalline**
   A. Milky fixer
      1. Acid portion added too fast while mixing
      2. Acid portion added when too hot
      3. Excessive acidity
      4. Glacial acetic acid mistaken for 28%
      5. Developer splashed into fixer
      6. Insufficient rinsing
   B. Prolonged washing

**III. Grit**
   A. Dirty water
   B. Dirt in dryer

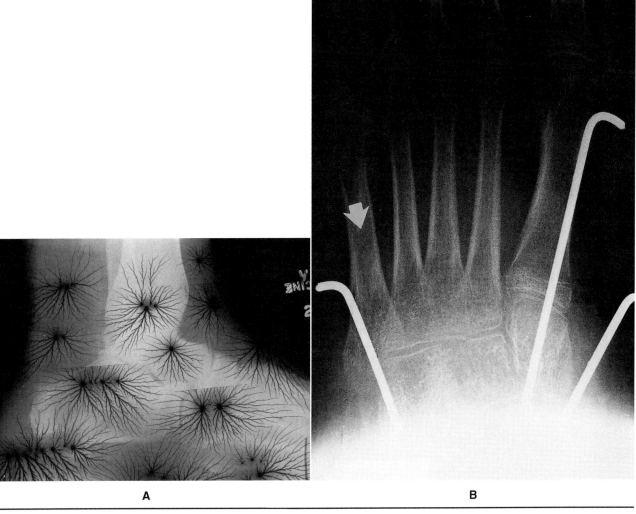

**Figure 5-12**  Static artifact. **A**, Tree static. **B**, Smudge static.

difficult to determine the exact cause of fog after the fact, some general guidelines may help reduce it. Keep cassettes out of the exposure room. Keep them as far away from radiation as possible. Radiation fog creates an overall gray appearance, and because it is penetrating, will record objects between the source and the film. If too high a kilovoltage level is used for the part being radiographed, then the secondary and scattered radiation will be recorded as fog. White light fog results in much greater densities and is not as uniform unless the entire film is exposed to the beam of light. Safelight fog is usually caused by too high a level of illumination, too short a distance between the safelight and the film, an improper filter for the film being used and too long a time of exposure to the safelight. Often these causes are combined. By process of elimination, this kind of fog can often be minimized. Note that after an initial exposure to radiation and to the light from the screens, films are more

sensitive to subsequent exposure to safelight. In the photographic world this is known as latensification. It is best to keep exposed films from too much safelight exposure as possible. Often, merely the placement of the safelight over the feed tray of the processor or over the hand tank is enough to cause safelight fogging. Relocating the safelight will eliminate the problem.

When fresh, film has a base plus fog range from 0.15 to 0.20 normally. As the film ages, it increases in fog. Once the fog reaches 0.25 and higher in density, information is being lost. Usually if film is stored at constant temperatures with relative humidity of 40% to 60% it will remain at the lower fog level throughout the period prior to expiration date. If it is stored longer, or exposed to high heat levels and high humidity, the fog will rise to objectionable levels.

Old chemistry or too high a temperature can result in chemical fogging. If the lead blocker position, which is

**Figure 5-13** Edge fog. Film bin or storage box exposed to white light along film edge. Normally not seen on a radiograph because maximum exposure is given to edge of film.

usually clear and bright, is fogged, the source may be chemical.

## Stain (Figure 5-14)

Chemical drops on the film prior to development or on the intensifying screen prior to exposure can result in unwanted artifact. Fixer stain is a frequent culprit. Keep intensifying screens at a distance from all chemicals; inspect them regularly, and clean or replace as needed.

## Scratches

As mentioned earlier, rough handling of processed film and during processing will result in unwanted artifacts. Figure 5-15 demonstrates some examples.

## Technical Error

Errors in positioning or technique frequently require repeat films. Examples include inadequate exposure (Figure 5-16, *A*) and double exposure (Figure 5-16, *B*).

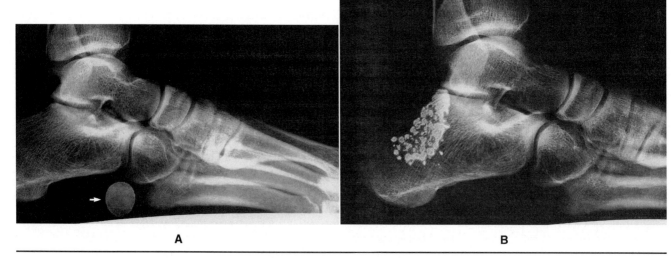

| A | B |

**Figure 5-14** Stain. **A**, Drop of fixer came in contact with film prior to development. **B**, Fixer stain on screen.

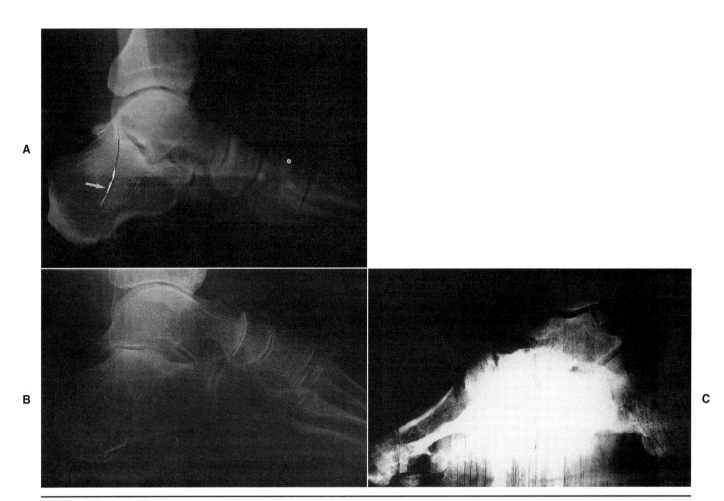

**Figure 5-15**   Scratches. **A**, Deep gouge from rough handling during processing (arrow). Also note stain artifacts. **B**, Scratches caused during automatic processing. **C**, Scratches caused by film being in contact with rough surface, probably in developer, with another film.

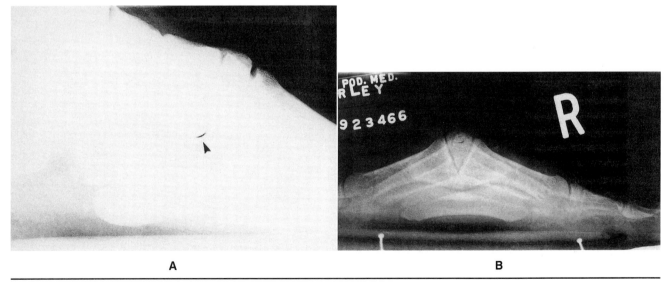

**Figure 5-16**   Technical error. **A**, Underexposure. Also note kink mark (arrow). **B**, Double exposure.

## Suggested Readings

Chamberlain WE, Henny GC: *Medical physics*, St Louis, 1944, Mosby.

Fuchs AW: *The science of radiology*, Springfield, Ill., 1933, Charles C Thomas.

John DHO: *Radiographic processing in medicine & industry*, New York, 1967, Focal Press.

McKinney WEJ: *Radiographic processing & quality control*, Philadelphia, 1988, Lippincott.

Mees CEK, James TH: *The theory of photographic process*, ed 3, New York, 1966, Macmillan.

Miller TH, Brummitt W: *This is photography*, New York, 1945, Garden City Publishing.

Patterson CVS: *Roentgenography: Fluoroscopic and intensifying screens, medical physics*, vol 2, St Louis, 1950, Mosby.

*Patterson intensifying screens*, Wilmington, Del., 1950, E. I. Du Pont de Nemours & Co.

Sprawls Jr. P: *The physical principles of diagnostic radiology*, Baltimore, 1977, University Park Press.

# SECTION 2

# Radiographic Anatomy

# CHAPTER 6

# Principles of Radiographic Interpretation

ROBERT A. CHRISTMAN

Radiographic interpretation is an art form. Effective film evaluation requires selecting appropriate views for the radiographic study (Chapter 11), use of the proper viewing tools, a consistent means for placing the film(s) on a viewbox, understanding basic concepts of image formation, and using a systematic approach for image assessment (Chapter 12). This chapter focuses on the fundamentals of plain film evaluation and image formation.

## ■ VIEWING TOOLS

The minimum requirements for an x-ray viewing room include a viewbox, magnifying glass, and spotlight.

### Viewbox

A viewbox should be used whose size is consistent with the size of film being viewed. For example, if 10- × 12-inch films are used, then the viewbox size should be 10 × 12 inches or multiples thereof. If the lit viewing area is larger than the film, extraneous light escapes around the sides of the film and the user perceives less useful visual information from the radiograph. The radiograph appears more dense (blacker) if extraneous light surrounds the film.[1] To illustrate, place a high-contrast dorsoplantar foot radiograph on a fully lit viewbox that accommodates two or more films. Notice how parts of the image that are relatively darker, such as the toes, are barely visible. Then turn off or cover all remaining viewbox lights except for that being used to view the radiograph. Finally, take the x-ray folder and cover up the entire foot except for the toes. Notice how the toes become more visible with each step. Therefore, not only should the size of the viewbox correspond to the film size, but each single film-viewing area should have its own on/off power switch and there should be reflectors that divide and separate each 10- × 12-inch viewing area so there is no crossover illumination.

Overhead lighting can also impair the viewer's ability to interpret radiographs by producing glare and surface reflections. Therefore, all other light sources should be turned off or subdued when viewing films.

Cool white or daylight fluorescent lightbulbs are used as the viewbox light source. Cool white bulbs are preferable; daylight bulbs are "bluer" and do not appear to provide as much light through the illuminator surface and film. If the viewbox uses more than one lightbulb, be sure to use the same type of bulb in all fixtures. Colored (green) fluorescent bulbs are also available; one manufacturer claims they are less straining to the eyes. This is fine if you don't mind looking at a green radiograph! (Personally, I favor the black and white/shades of gray variety.)

A white, transparent illuminator surface diffuses light of uniform brightness for viewing the radiograph. This surface must be kept clean and free of scratches. Dirt or other foreign matter on the illuminator surface will appear as artifact or may mimic pathology in the radiograph.

### Magnifying Glass

Every viewing area should have an accessible magnifying glass. Glasses come in many shapes, sizes, and powers. Invest in a precision-cut piece of glass. Inexpensive, bargain-brand magnifiers tend to distort the image because they are improperly manufactured. A small hand-held magnifying glass suffices.

### Spotlight

A spotlight generally uses an incandescent bulb for its light source. The bulb wattage is typically 60 or 75 watts. The device can be purchased with or without a pedal or dial for variable adjustment of light intensity.

When viewing a film over a spotlight, be extremely careful not to damage the film. The proper method for viewing the film with this light source is to slowly but constantly move and/or rotate the film. A film will warp if it is held over the high-intensity light source too long. (Consider the following analogy: If your hand is held still over a lit match, the skin will burn. However, continually moving your hand in a circular motion over the flame will prevent the skin from burning.) The emulsion may eventually crack in the damaged area, ruining the image. Another way of knowing if the film is burning is to continually hold a finger against the film near the area being highlighted. If your finger feels intense heat, then you know the film is being damaged. Burning x-ray film also emits an unpleasant smell. This damage, by the way, is permanent and cannot be reversed.

## ■ FILM PLACEMENT

How should radiographs be placed on the viewbox? The conventional method entails placing the film so that the patient is facing the viewer. For example, the patient's left ankle is seen on the viewer's right. And, by this method, the dorsoplantar foot view would be placed so that the toes are at the bottom, rearfoot at the top. Most people do not view foot films in this manner, however. The film is commonly placed on the viewing surface (and reproduced in textbooks or journals) so that the patient's right foot is on the viewer's right and the toes are at the top. Although the foot may appear more visually acceptable in this position, it does not simulate the patient's foot as it would be examined clinically for correlation to the radiograph. Whatever method is employed, the important factor is consistency; that is, place the film consistently in the same position (however that may be) each time it is evaluated. Keep in mind that the radiograph is two-dimensional and does not have depth. Regardless of which side of the film faces the viewer, the image will not be altered.

Oblique views of the foot are best viewed in the same fashion that a dorsoplantar view is placed on the viewbox. There are three reasons for this: first, this viewing position simulates a dorsoplantar presentation except the foot is either inverted or everted. Second, if you are viewing a bilateral oblique study with both feet on the same film, it is much easier to compare symmetry between the feet. And, lastly, the film placed in this position fits best on a viewbox sized for 10- × 12-inch films.

Lateral views of the foot are certainly best analyzed with the sole of the foot positioned horizontally. Bilateral lateral foot views on the same film should in addition be analyzed with the feet vertical, to compare for symmetry.

Ankle views should be placed on the viewbox by conventional means as already noted; that is, as if the patient were facing you. The patient's left extremity is on the viewer's right, and vice versa.

## ■ BASIC CONCEPTS OF IMAGE FORMATION

The radiographic image is a two-dimensional representation of a three-dimensional body part. This is not a concept that can be grasped easily. Individuals vary in their ability to apply spatial relationships to radiography. To some it comes easily; others need to develop an appreciation for it.

An understanding of certain fundamental principles is necessary before attempting to interpret radiographs. They are as follows: First, any substance has a characteristic radiographic appearance that depends on its thickness, form, and atomic number; and, second, the image is a summation of anatomic shadows.

Let's first discuss how the radiographic image is formed. The useful x-ray beam comes into contact with the body part (in this case, the foot). These x rays either travel through the foot and exit or are absorbed by it. Those that exit the foot come into contact with the x-ray film and screen (if used). The x rays' photons (and light photons emitted from a screen) convert to atomic silver the silver halide crystals that are embedded in the film emulsion. This image is known as the latent image. Processing converts the latent image into the radiographic image.

The x-ray beam is composed of individual x-ray photons with varying degrees of energy. Higher-energy x-ray photons have shorter wavelengths. They are able to penetrate matter more readily than lower-energy photons. Therefore, higher-energy photons stand a greater chance of reaching the film; the foot absorbs the lower energy photons.

X rays interact with matter in different ways (see Chapter 1). X rays may be scattered in different directions (classic scatter and Compton effect), or they can be absorbed by an atom (photoelectric effect). Scattered x rays can fog the film and are of no diagnostic value. Whether an x-ray photon is absorbed or not depends on two factors: the energy of the photon (as already discussed) and the atomic number of the substance. The difference between those x rays absorbed by the foot and those that penetrate it is known as differential absorption. Objects with greater atomic numbers absorb x rays more readily than do those with lower atomic numbers. Therefore, the element lead, with an atomic number of 82, absorbs more x-ray photons than bone, made of calcium, which has an atomic number of 20.

Another factor to consider is the thickness of the material. The thicker any particular substance is, all other factors remaining unchanged, the more x rays it absorbs. This process is known as attenuation.

The term *radiopaque* applies to those substances that absorb x rays; representative areas appear white on the exposed x-ray film. The term *radiolucent* refers to substances that x rays penetrate more readily; representative areas appear dark or black on the film.[2] When dealing with shades of gray, as in radiography, radiodensities are discussed in relative terms. Bone is radiopaque relative to muscle, but radiolucent compared to a heavy metal such as lead. How does all this relate to formation of the radiographic image? Because radiopaque objects absorb more x-ray photons than those that are radiolucent, fewer x rays reach the film. Therefore, fewer silver halide crystals are ionized, and a radiopaque object appears whiter. Figure 6-1 lists matter found in the foot and their relative radiodensities.

A thicker foot appears more radiodense than a thinner foot, assuming all other factors, such as radiographic technique, remain the same when exposing the two feet. Also, areas containing fluid (edema, for example) add density to that part of the image.

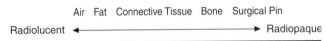

Figure 6-1   Relative radiodensities of matter seen in the foot.

Next we need to consider the form of the object being viewed radiographically. Interpreting radiographs requires imagination and logical analysis. This is especially true if the object in question is not parallel to the x-ray film or has a complex form. (You are encouraged to read the introductory chapters of *Fundamentals of Radiography*, by Lucy Frank Squire.[3] He presents an excellent discourse on this subject matter.)

If a solid, flat object such as a quarter lies parallel to the x-ray film, and the x-ray beam is perpendicular to the object and film, the shape of the quarter will be recognized true to form. However, if this same object is "obliqued" or turned vertically, its circular shape will not be distinguished (Figure 6-2).

Let's consider complex objects. As an exercise, close your eyes and try to imagine what an egg would look like. Next imagine a conch shell with and without spines. Check your imaginative pictures with Figures 6-3 and 6-4. An x-ray image is not a picture per se, but a collection of shadows. Think of these shadows being laid on one another layer by layer. The egg, for example, is not a homogeneous density. The outer shell is made of calcium; the inner fluids and pocket of air are less radiodense. The resultant image is a summation of the inner substances superimposed on the outer shell, which is viewed, roughly speaking, as a flat sheet.

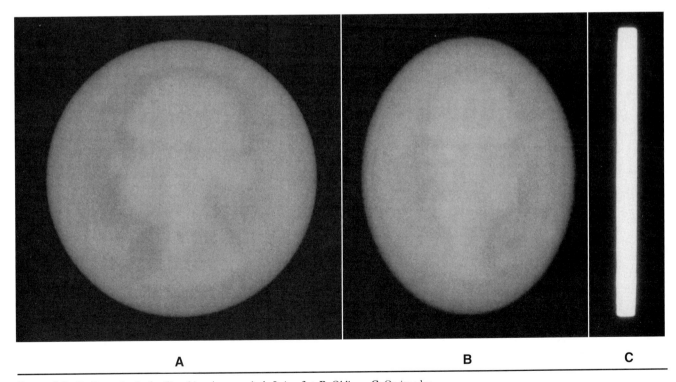

**A**                                      **B**                    **C**

Figure 6-2   Radiograph of a familiar object (a quarter). **A,** Lying flat. **B,** Oblique. **C,** On its edge.

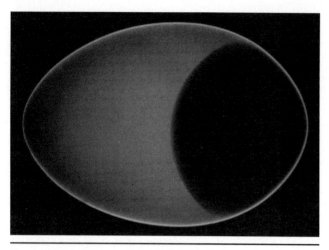

Figure 6-3    Radiograph of an infertile emu egg.

Note the radiopaque periphery or margin of the egg. As a rule, a curved object will appear radiopaque if it is perpendicular to the film and parallel to the x-ray beam. It will appear relatively radiolucent if parallel to the film and perpendicular to the x-ray beam, as in the center of the egg. Did you imagine the conch shell to appear the way it does in Figure 6-4? The shell is physically the same density throughout, yet many shadows of differing densities are appreciated radiographically. Apply the concept just described regarding the curved object and its position relative to the film and x-ray beam to the conch shell.

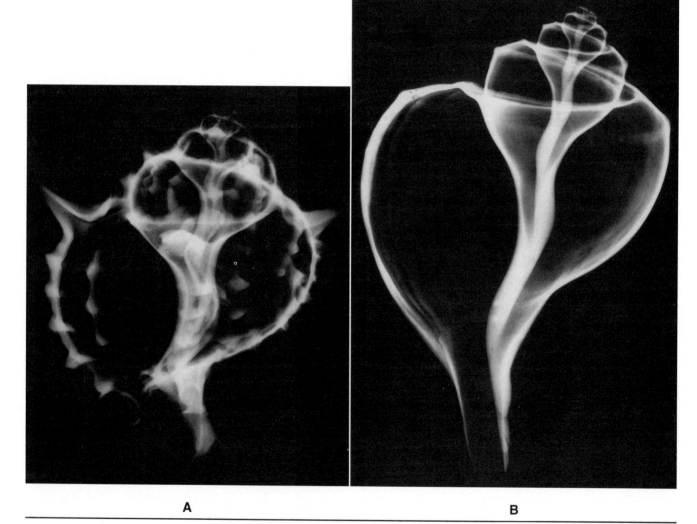

A                                    B

Figure 6-4    Radiograph of a conch shell. **A,** With spines. **B,** Without spines.

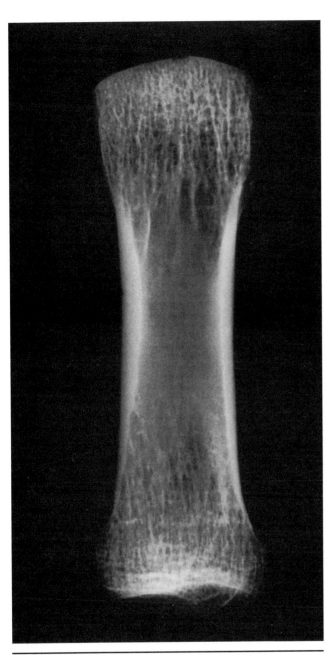

Tubular objects are commonly encountered in a foot radiograph. The characteristic image of a tubular object, such as the metatarsal, is shown in Figure 6-5. The periphery of the metatarsal is radiopaque. This is because the curved margin of the shaft is perpendicular to the film and parallel to the x-ray beam. The center consists of a less dense material, the bone marrow; cortical bone is superimposed on the marrow but is nearly parallel to the film and perpendicular to the x-ray beam. Therefore the center of the tube appears relatively lucent.

An object with complex form can look different in many ways simply because of the way it is positioned relative to the x-ray film and beam (Figure 6-6).

Interpreting foot radiographs is particularly challenging because multiple bones are superimposed on one another, especially in the tarsal region. You will eventually become familiar with the radiographic appearance of each bone. Always think in layers: Shadows are layers of objects superimposed on one another. The boundary of an object generally appears as a well-defined shadow on the radiograph. Separate each shadow mentally, subtracting everything else. This concept is extremely important and is emphasized again in the following chapter dealing with normal radiographic anatomy.

**Figure 6-5**  Radiograph of a common tubular object found in the foot: The first metatarsal bone.

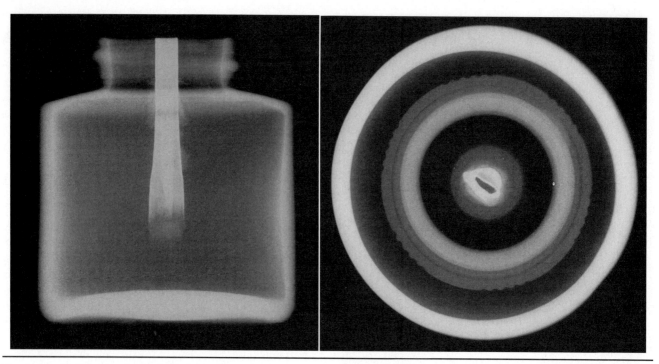

Figure 6-6    Radiographs of an ink bottle and applicator in two views perpendicular to one another.

Finally, think in terms of three dimensions. To mentally formulate a three-dimensional picture, two views that are perpendicular to one another are necessary. The most common examples are anteroposterior (dorsoplantar) and lateral views of the part in question. This is best illustrated by the fracture in Figure 6-7.

In summary, interpreting a radiograph is an exercise of imagination and reasoning. The formation of the image depends on the object's atomic numbers and thicknesses. The image is a summation of shadows superimposed on one another. So think in layers when viewing a radiograph. An object can be recognized by its form. However, a familiar object may look quite unfamiliar if it is positioned differently relative to the film and x-ray beam. Finally, think in terms of three dimensions, always correlating the two-dimensional radiographic shadows to the three-dimensional object.

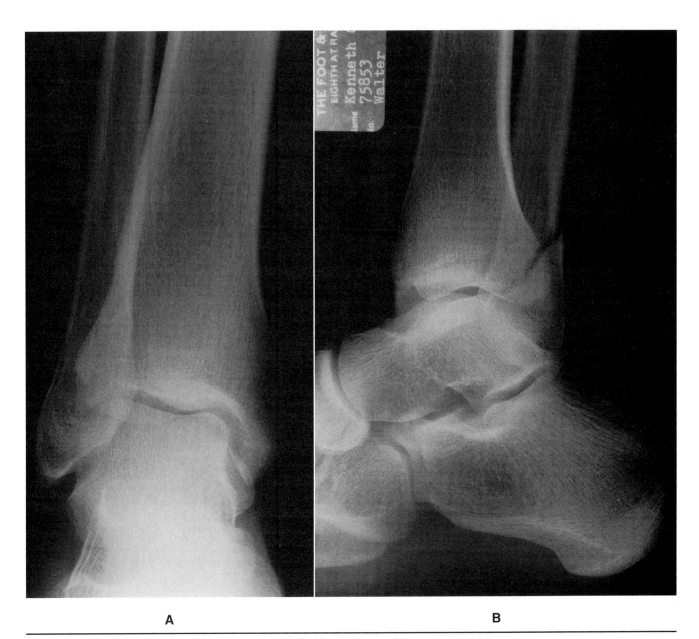

**A**                                                                **B**

Figure 6-7   Views of a distal fibular fracture. **A**, Anteroposterior. **B**, Lateral. Because the fracture is displaced only in the sagittal plane, it is nearly imperceptible in the anteroposterior view but fairly obvious in the lateral view.

## References

1. Fuchs AW: *Principles of radiographic exposure and processing*, ed 2, Springfield, Ill., 1958, Charles C Thomas.
2. *Dorland's illustrated medical dictionary*, ed 27, Philadelphia, 1988, Saunders.
3. Squire LF, Novelline RA: *Fundamentals of radiography*, ed 4, Cambridge, Mass., 1988, Harvard University Press.

# CHAPTER 7

# The Normal Foot and Ankle

ROBERT A. CHRISTMAN

Over the years I have observed that the most common pitfall when interpreting foot and ankle radiographs is mistaking normal anatomic shadows for pathology. To truly appreciate abnormalities of position, form, density, and architecture, the interpreter must have a working knowledge and appreciation of normal radiographic anatomy. In the foot and ankle, this requires correlation of normal three-dimensional osteology (the bone specimen) to two-dimensional radiographic anatomy (the film). The reader is therefore encouraged to compare the images to a foot skeleton.

The following collection of illustrations, tracings of "rectus" foot images, and their respective radiographs should be used as a general reference guide. Slight variations in the appearance of each bone occur depending on the position of the foot relative to the film. For example, a pronated or supinated foot affects the overall appearance of the entire foot as well as each individual bone. Therefore it is important to concentrate on the correlation of gross anatomy to the radiograph, not to memorize the appearance of each bone per se.

Sarrafian's *Anatomy of the Foot and Ankle*[1] was used as the reference for the terminology in the labels. Occasionally, however, I used the best generic term to label a radiographic "shadow" that Sarrafian had not specifically identified. The label key (Box 7-1) is located at the end of the chapter.

I have spent years studying foot and ankle bone specimens (normal three-dimensional osteology) and correlating them to two-dimensional radiographs.[2-6] The original manuscript for this chapter was written to serve as the complete reference guide to radiographic anatomy of the foot and ankle. However, because of its large size and numerous images, it has been replaced with this overview. The original completed manuscript will be submitted to and (I hope!) made available in the medical literature soon.

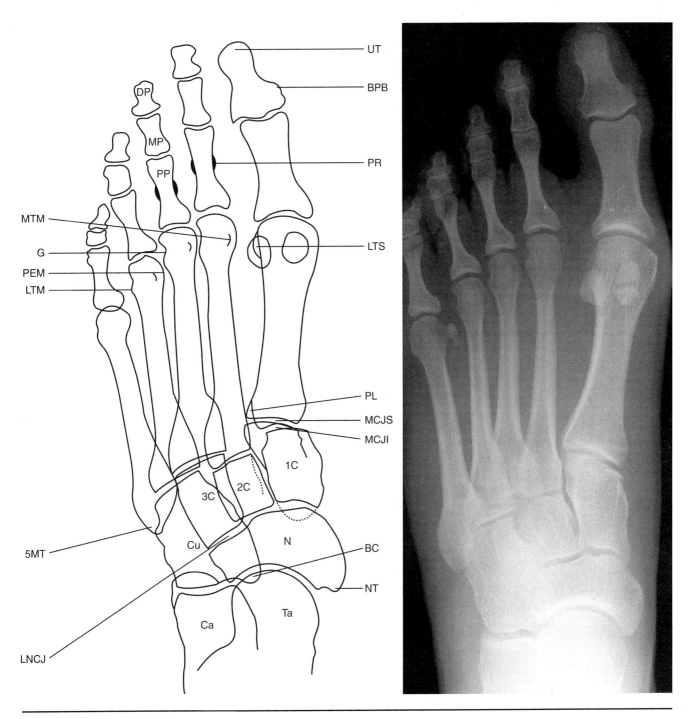

Figure 7-1    Dorsoplantar (DP) foot view.

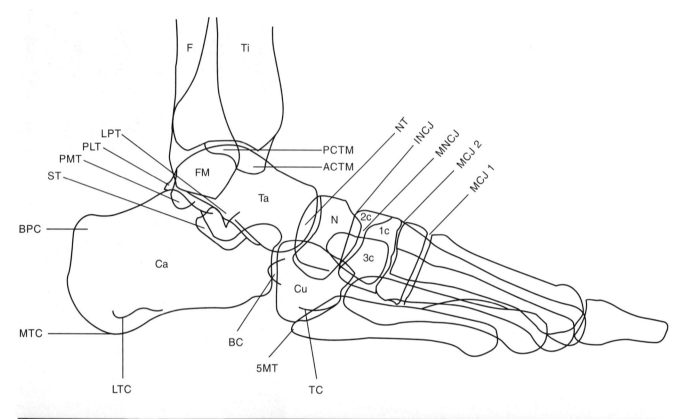

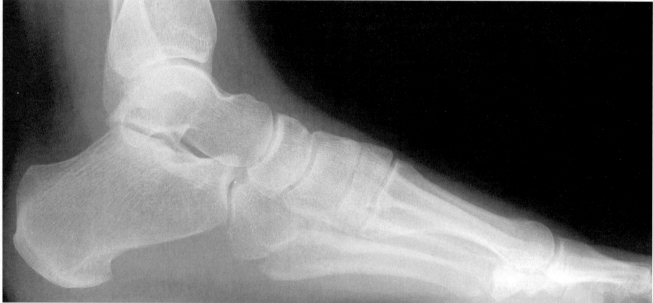

Figure 7-2   Lateral foot view.

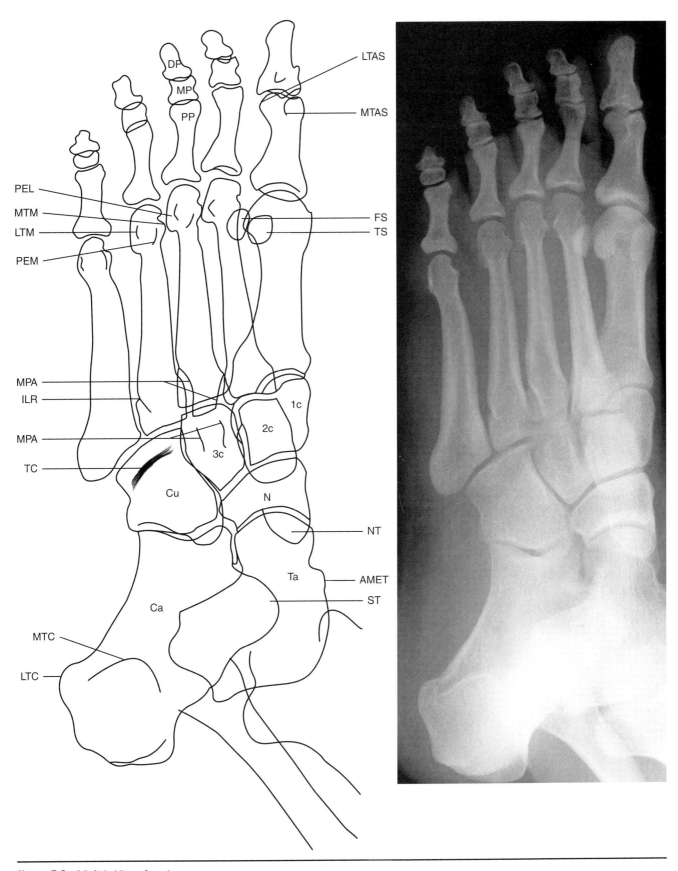

Figure 7-3    Medial oblique foot view.

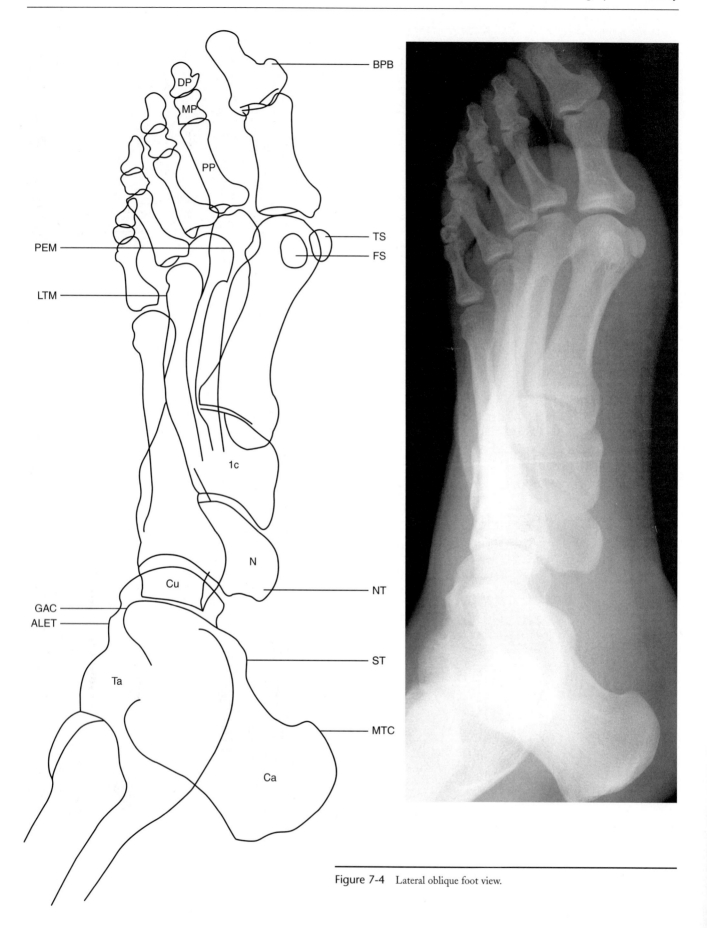

Figure 7-4  Lateral oblique foot view.

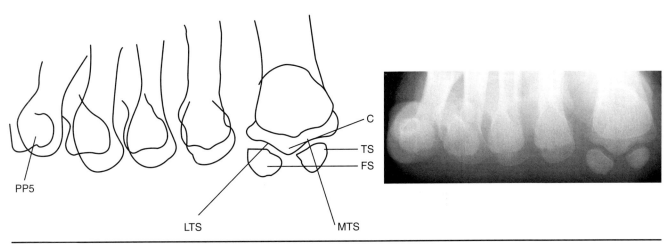

Figure 7-5    Sesamoid axial view.

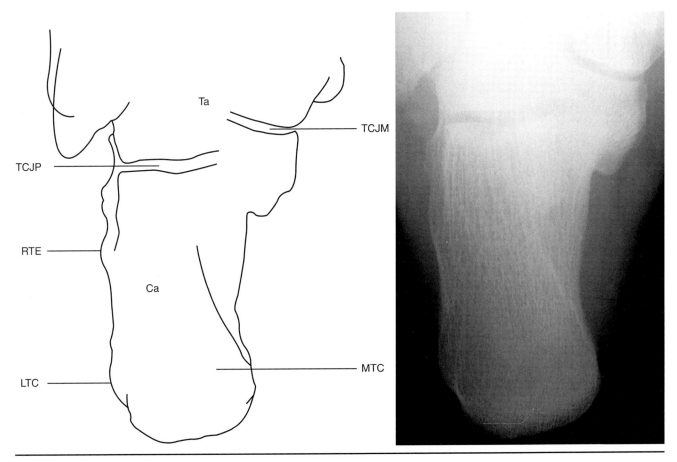

Figure 7-6    Calcaneal axial view.

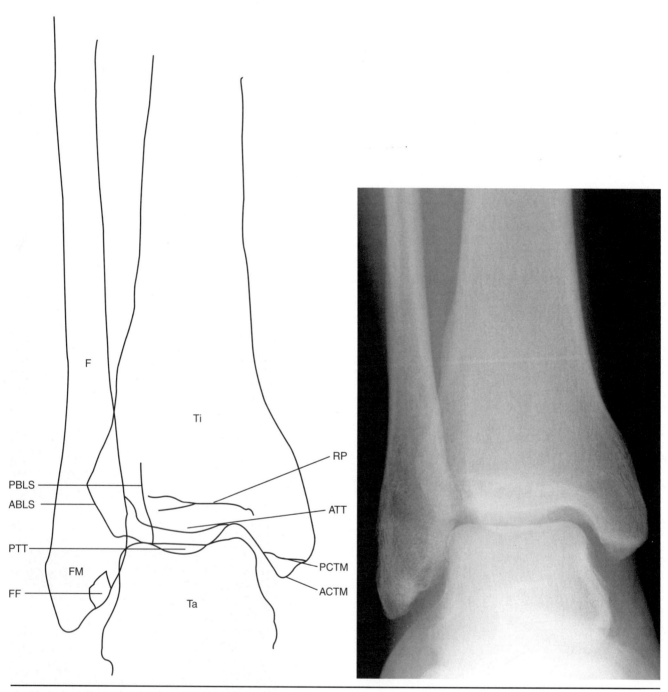

Figure 7-7   Anteroposterior (AP) ankle view.

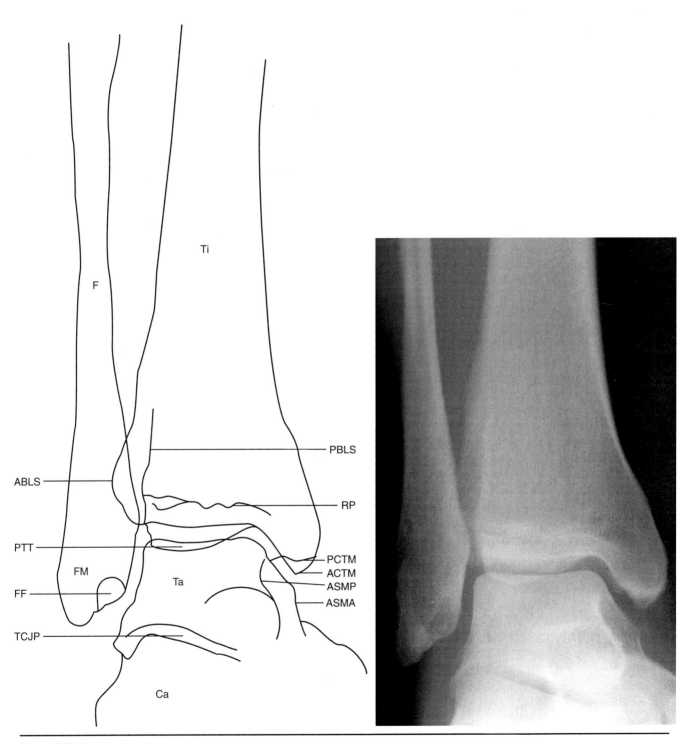

Figure 7-8    Mortise ankle view.

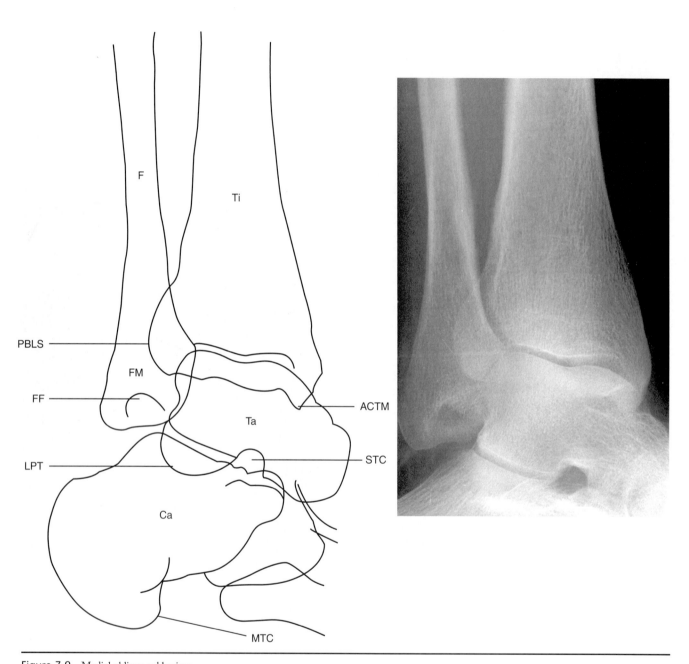

Figure 7-9  Medial oblique ankle view.

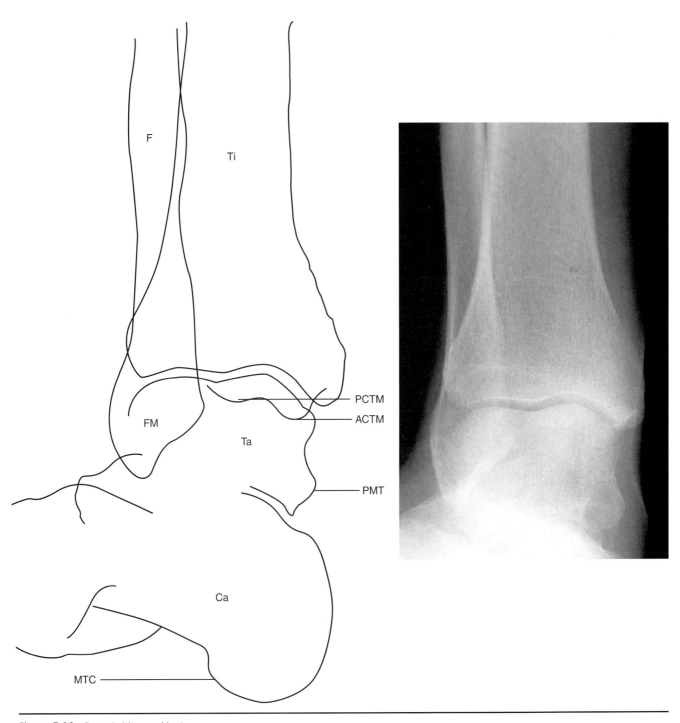

Figure 7-10    Lateral oblique ankle view.

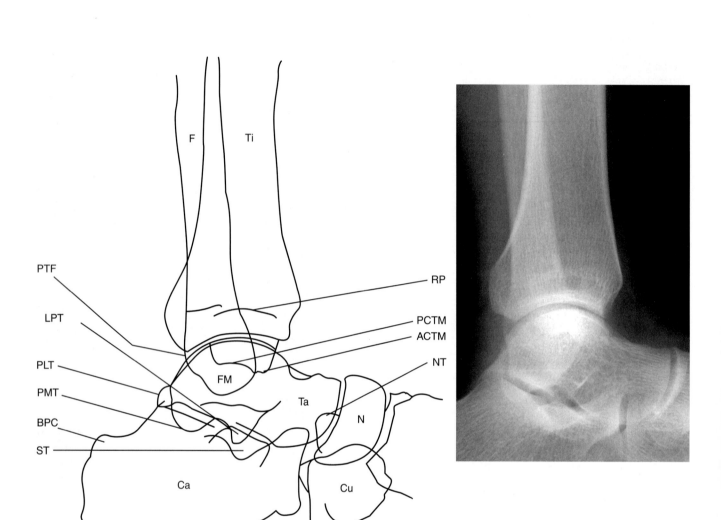

Figure 7-11   Lateral ankle view.

## BOX 7-1  Label Key

| | | | |
|---|---|---|---|
| 1C | First cuneiform (medial cuneiform) | MCJI | Inferior aspect of first metatarsocuneiform joint |
| 2C | Second cuneiform (intermediate cuneiform) | MCJS | Superior aspect of first metatarsocuneiform joint |
| 3C | Third cuneiform (lateral cuneiform) | MNCJ | Medial naviculocuneiform joint |
| 5MT | Tuberosity of fifth-metatarsal base | MP | Middle phalanx |
| ABLS | Anterior border of distal tibial lateral surface | MPA | Medial and lateral margins of plantar apex of bone |
| ACTM | Anterior colliculus (of tibial malleolus) | MTAS | Medial trochlear articular surface (hallux proximal phalanx) |
| ALET | Anterolateral extension of trochlear surface (talus) | MTC | Medial tuberosity (medial tubercle) |
| AMET | Anteromedial extension of trochlear surface (talus) | MTM | Medial tubercle (for metatarsophalangeal ligaments) |
| ASMA | Articular surface for medial malleolus, anterior margin | MTS | Medial trochlear surface (first met) |
| | | N | Navicular |
| ASMP | Articular surface for medial malleolus, posterior margin | NT | Tuberosity of navicular |
| | | PBLS | Posterior border of distal tibial lateral surface |
| ATC | Anterior tuberosity (anterior tubercle) | PCTM | Posterior colliculus (of tibial malleolus) |
| ATT | Anterior tibial tubercle | PEL | Proximal extension of metatarsal head articular surface, laterally |
| BC | Beak of cuboid | | |
| BPB | Bony projection, distal phalanx base (varies in size) | PEM | Proximal extension of metatarsal head articular surface, medially |
| BPC | Bursal projection, posterior calcaneus | | |
| C | Crista (crest of metatarsal head) | PL | Tubercle for insertion of peroneus longus tendon |
| Ca | Calcaneus | PLT | Posterolateral tubercle (talus) (trigonal process) |
| Cu | Cuboid | PMT | Posteromedial tubercle (talus) |
| DP | Distal phalanx | PP | Proximal phalanx |
| F | Fibula | PR | Phalangeal ridge |
| FF | Fibular (digital) fossa | PTF | Posterior tubercle (fibula) |
| FM | Fibular malleolus | PTT | Posterior tibial tubercle |
| FS | Fibular sesamoid | RP | Remnant of physis |
| G | Groove separating tubercle and articular surface | RTE | Retrotrochlear eminence |
| GAC | Great apophysis (anterior process of calcaneus) | ST | Sustentaculum tali |
| INCJ | Intermediate naviculocuneiform joint | STC | Sinus tarsi/tarsal canal |
| ILR | Interosseous ligament rugosity | Ta | Talus |
| LNCJ | Lateral naviculocuneiform joint | TC | Tuberosity of cuboid |
| LPT | Lateral process (talus) | TCJA | Talocalcaneal joint, anterior |
| LTAS | Lateral trochlear articular surface (hallux proximal phalanx) | TCJM | Talocalcaneal joint, middle |
| | | TCJP | Talocalcaneal joint, posterior |
| LTC | Lateral tuberosity (lateral tubercle) | Ti | Tibia |
| LTM | Lateral tubercle (for metatarsophalangeal ligaments) | TS | Tibial sesamoid |
| LTS | Lateral trochlear surface (first metatarsal) | UT | Ungual tuberosity (tuft of distal phalanx) |
| MCJ1 | First metatarsocuneiform joint | | |
| MCJ2 | Second metatarsocuneiform joint | | |

## References

1. Sarrafian SK: *Anatomy of the foot and ankle: descriptive, topographic, functional,* ed 2, Philadelphia, 1993, Lippincott.
2. Christman RA: Radiographic anatomy of the calcaneus. I. Inferior surface, *J Am Podiatr Med Assoc* 77(10):549-553, 1987.
3. Christman RA: Radiographic anatomy of the calcaneus. II. Posterior surface, *J Am Podiatr Med Assoc* 77(11):581-585, 1987.
4. Christman RA: Radiographic anatomy of the calcaneus. III. Superior surface, *J Am Podiatr Med Assoc* 77(12):633-637, 1987.
5. Christman RA: Radiographic anatomy of the calcaneus. IV. Lateral and medial surfaces. *J Am Podiatr Med Assoc* 78(1):11-14, 1988.
6. Christman RA, Ly P: Radiographic anatomy of the first metatarsal, *J Am Podiatr Med Assoc* 80(4):177-203, 1990.

# CHAPTER 8

# Normal Variants and Anomalies

ROBERT A. CHRISTMAN

Thirty bones compose the foot and ankle complex. (This number includes the distal tibia and fibula and the two sesamoids at the first metatarsophalangeal joint.) The previous chapter described the expected radiographic appearance of each bone in the many views available. However, variations in their appearance are not uncommon. Variations typically are incidental findings and asymptomatic, although symptomatology or pathology may occur secondary to a skeletal variation. More common examples of the latter include the accessory navicular and tarsal coalition.

Several words are frequently used when referring to variations of the skeleton. Their definitions are as follows (from *Dorland's Illustrated Medical Dictionary*[1]):

**Accessory:** supplementary to another similar and generally important thing.
**Anomaly:** marked deviation from the normal standard, especially as a result of congenital defects.
**Os:** bone; a general term that is qualified by the appropriate adjective to designate a specific type of bony structure or a specific segment of the skeleton.
**Ossicle:** a small bone.
**Partite:** having parts or divisions.
**Sesamoid:** a small, nodular bone embedded in a tendon or joint capsule.
**Supernumerary:** in excess of the regular or normal number.
**Synostosis:** the osseous union of bones that are normally distinct.
**Variant:** something that differs in some characteristic from the class to which it belongs, as a variant of a disease, trait, and so forth.

The terms *partite, supernumerary,* and *accessory bone* in the following discourse are differentiated thus: *Partite* can pertain to either a normally existing bone or an accessory bone that is subdivided, *supernumerary* pertains to

anomalous duplication of a normally existing bone, and *accessory bone* refers to those ossicles (not anomalous duplication) that are found in addition to the normally existing bones. Also note that although all sesamoid bones are ossicles, not all ossicles are sesamoid bones.

Variations can be expressed in several ways (Box 8-1). Examples of variations involving normally existing bones include variants of number, position, form (shape and size), density, and architecture. Accessory ossicles, in addition to the existing 30 bones, are not uncommon.

Variants of number include partite bones, supernumerary bones, and absence of bones. Bipartite sesamoids, for example, are common. Although rare, bipartite medial cuneiform and navicular bones may be encountered. Supernumerary bones include duplication of phalanges, metatarsals, and tarsal bones.

The axis of each bone has a characteristic position relative to the axes of adjacent bones. In the two-dimensional radiograph, this position can vary considerably among patients and depends heavily on foot type and the degree of pronation or supination during weight-bearing stance in angle and base of gait.[2] Variations of position can predispose for future pathology.

Most variations of existing bones are variants of form. Variants of form concern the girth, length, and contour of a bone. Synostosis/coalition is also a variation of form. Other

---

**BOX 8-1** **Expression of Variants in the Foot**

Variations Involving Normally Existing Bones
    Variants of number
    Variants of position
    Variants of form
    Variants of density
    Variants of architecture
Accessory ossicles

variants of form can be attributed to the position of the foot or ankle bones relative to each other and/or the film. For example, the navicular bone frequently appears rectangular in a pes cavus foot but wedge shaped in a pes planus foot. Varying forms may also be encountered in weight-bearing studies secondary to pronation and supination (internal and external leg rotation, respectively). (Angle and base of gait positioning provide a means for minimizing the technical variation that may occur.) Positional changes are predictable, however, and the experienced interpreter can recognize these alterations and correlate them to normal radiographic anatomy.

Variants of density can mimic abnormal or pathologic processes. More commonly, this appears as a relative radiolucency or decreased density. Occasionally, focal areas of increased density are seen.

Each bone has its own characteristic shadows. These shadows represent cortex, trabeculae, and superimposed osseous landmarks in the adult skeleton and constitute the architecture of the bone. The outer margin of the bone is its external architecture, and the remainder its internal architecture. Most architectural variants relate to the appearance of cortical bone and trabeculae. Variation of an osseous landmark's superimposed shadow may correlate to variant size, shape, or position of that landmark.

Variations of the existing 30 bones aren't the only variants one may encounter. Numerous accessory bones are commonly found in the foot and ankle. One may be an isolated finding, or, not uncommonly, multiple ossicles can occur throughout both extremities.

Appreciation of the summation of shadows concept and normal radiographic anatomy (Chapters 6 and 7, respectively) are the first steps of film interpretation. The interpreter must then become familiar with the numerous variations of normal. Many of these variants appear unilaterally and can mimic fractures or other pathology. Bilateral studies, therefore, are not always useful for their differentiation and can be misleading. Furthermore, even if they are bilateral, they may be asymmetric in appearance. The purpose of this chapter is to present the gamut of radiologic variants that one may encounter in the adult foot and ankle.

## VARIANTS OF NUMBER

### Partite Sesamoids at the First Metatarsophalangeal Joint

It is common to see partite tibial and fibular sesamoids; they are typically bipartite (Figure 8-1). Partitioning may involve one or both sesamoids and be unilateral or bilateral. Furthermore, if only the tibial sesamoid is partite in one foot, only the fibular sesamoid may be partite in the opposite

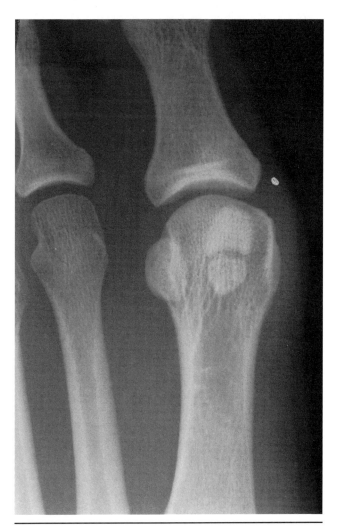

Figure 8-1    Bipartite tibial sesamoid.

foot. The presentations (partitioning, shape, size, and number) are extremely variable and follow no specific rule. For example, a bipartition may divide the sesamoid into equal or unequal halves; it typically is either transverse or oblique. The bipartition is rarely longitudinal.

An interesting variation is the presence of a third sesamoid at the first metatarsophalangeal joint. This extra sesamoid is located between the tibial and fibular sesamoids. It is best seen with the sesamoid axial view.

It is difficult to differentiate a fractured sesamoid from a partite sesamoid in most instances, especially in the dorsoplantar view. The presence of jagged edges alone is not a useful distinguishing feature, because both the bipartite and the fractured sesamoid can appear to have jagged edges. A partite sesamoid that is complicated by degenerative joint disease has spurs that give the appearance of a jagged edge, similar to that of a fracture. Furthermore, the coarse trabeculations that are normally found in the first-metatarsal

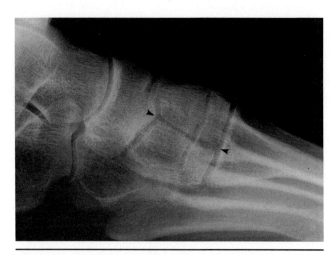

Figure 8-2　Bipartite medial cuneiform.

distal metaphysis are superimposed on the sesamoids. These shadows can exaggerate the perception of a jagged fracture line. Nor can fracture be determined by the amount of separation between the two segments. It is not uncommon to see apparent "distraction" in the asymptomatic, untraumatized bipartition. Fracture is best differentiated from variant bipartition with the sesamoid isolated, that is, with no superimposition on the metatarsal head (this can only be accomplished with the sesamoid axial and lateral oblique or modified non–weight-bearing lateral—or Causton—views). Certainly correlation with clinical history is important in these instances.

The sesamoids are initially evaluated with the dorsoplantar and sesamoid axial views. The lateral oblique view is invaluable for assessing tibial sesamoid pathology. The tibial and fibular sesamoids are superimposed on the first and second metatarsals, respectively, in the medial oblique view; this view generally does not provide any additional information apart from the dorsoplantar, lateral oblique, and axial views. The standard lateral view is useless for imaging the sesamoids; they are superimposed on each other in addition to other metatarsal and phalangeal bones.

## Bipartite Medial Cuneiform

In rare instances, the medial cuneiform presents as two entities in the adult skeleton, a variant known as the bipartite medial cuneiform. The partition classically divides the bone into upper and lower halves. It is best seen in the lateral view (Figure 8-2). A rare variation of the complete bipartition divides the bone into a small posterosuperior segment and a large anteroinferior one.

The classic bipartition, when present, is not readily identified by casual glance. It is fully superimposed on the remaining cuneiform bones and easily mistaken for other bone shadows. However, the transverse joint space identified

in the center of the medial cuneiform is its characteristic radiologic feature. This joint space typically is complete from anterior to posterior.

A variation may be encountered where the bipartition is incomplete. The medial cuneiform may be incompletely divided into two segments at its anterior and/or posterior margins but is "fused" centrally. Indentations are seen along the articular surfaces.

I have seen more than 25 patients with bipartite medial cuneiform; in those having bilateral foot studies, all were bilateral, although a few were incompletely bipartite unilaterally. In more than half of these patients, arch pain was associated with this entity. In one case the bipartite joint showed symptomatology suggesting synovitis or arthritis; symptoms were relieved initially with orthotics and, after recurrence of symptoms one year later, with an intra-articular cortisone injection.

## Bipartite Navicular

The bipartite navicular is a rare entity. The division separates the bone into a smaller superolateral segment and a larger inferior and medial segment (Figure 8-3). It may be found either bilaterally or unilaterally. The smaller bipartite segment appears closely associated with the intermediate cuneiform. The bipartition is best seen in the lateral view as a transverse linear lucency. Another, oblique, linear lucency may also be seen; however, after closer viewing and correlation with a normal gross anatomic specimen, this latter entity appears to represent the articulation between the lateral cuneiform and the larger navicular segment. The navicular is deformed in the dorsoplantar view; it is wedge shaped (apex laterally, base medially). Of interest, it appears that the third cuneiform has a variant form posteriorly that may even partially articulate with the talus. Variations of this entity have been seen. For example, the smaller segment may be positioned inferolaterally, or even dorsomedially.

The bipartite navicular may mimic a fracture if the partition is osteoarthritic, which is not infrequent; the adjacent margins are sclerotic; the segments are deformed; and the smaller superolateral segment is displaced and subluxed superiorly. Differentiation is usually based on the patient's age (the appearance of osteoarthritis increases with increasing age) and a thorough history (bipartite navicular is not associated with a history of trauma). Its presence bilaterally also weighs in favor of bipartition.

## Supernumerary Bones

Anomalous duplication of a bone is rare (Figure 8-4). The phalanges are most frequently affected. Metatarsal duplication is usually incomplete or dwarfed unless accompanied by tarsal duplication.

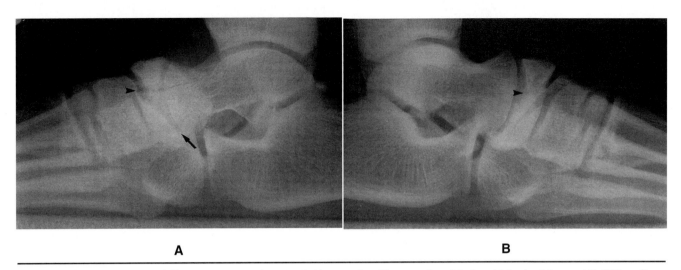

**Figure 8-3** Bipartite navicular. **A,** Transverse partition *(arrowhead).* Also note the odd presentation of the lateral joint *(straight arrow).* **B,** Oblique, linear lucency correlates to third naviculocuneiform joint; transverse partition is not clearly seen *(arrowhead),* probably because its position is not tangent to the x-ray beam. (Same patient as **A,** opposite foot.)

## Absence of Normally Existing Bones

On rare occasion one or several normally existing bones may be absent (Figure 8-5). The absence of a single bone may not be obvious clinically and is identified incidentally with radiographs; primary examples include absence of the tibial or fibular sesamoid and absence of a lesser-toe middle phalanx. Absence of a sesamoid and aphalangia may be either bilateral or unilateral. Neither is associated with symptomatology. In contrast, anomalous absence of multiple bones can present with gross deformity. A classic example is the so-called claw or lobster foot.

## ▮ VARIANTS OF POSITION

Each bone has a characteristic position in the foot and ankle. This is best assessed in the dorsoplantar and lateral views with the foot bearing weight in its angle and base of gait (described in Chapter 3). The axis of any particular bone lies at a particular position relative to other bones. All three anatomic planes should be considered when evaluating position. Unfortunately, with two-dimensional radiographs it is difficult to fully appreciate position in all planes. The frontal-plane position of a bone cannot be directly evaluated; assessment requires logical analysis and reasoning while looking at both the dorsoplantar (transverse plane) and lateral (sagittal plane) views.

Position variants predispose the patient to future symptomatology and pathology. Normal and abnormal position of foot bones, including foot structure, and their relationships to biomechanics, are discussed in Section 4 (Chapters 13, 14, and 15) of this text. A word of caution:

Altered positioning of the foot or leg relative to the x-ray film may profoundly affect the form and positional relationships of bones in the radiograph.

## Forefoot

The following variants of position occur in the forefoot and are seen in the dorsoplantar view: mild hallux abductus and, rarely, hallux adductus, interphalangeus abductus, adducto-varus lesser toes, reverse splaying of the second and third toes, abduction or adduction of the lesser-toe distal phalanx (secondary to variant form of its middle phalanx), juxta-position of lesser metatarsal heads, variation of the metatarsal length parabola, and sesamoid position variation relative to the first-metatarsal axis. Lateral view positional variants include digital contractures. Occasionally, in the sesamoid axial view, the inferior aspects of the second-, third-, and fourth-metatarsal heads may not be at the same level.

## Midfoot

Midfoot position variants include lateral splaying of the fifth metatarsal, metatarsus primus adductus, lesser-meta-tarsal adduction, and medial splaying of the medial cunei-form relative to the intermediate cuneiform (dorsoplantar view) (Figure 8-6). Lateral view variants include increased or decreased first-metatarsal declination and "subluxated" first metatarsocuneiform joint.

## Tarsus and Ankle

The following variations of position may be encountered in the tarsus and ankle: talar adduction and abduction (the

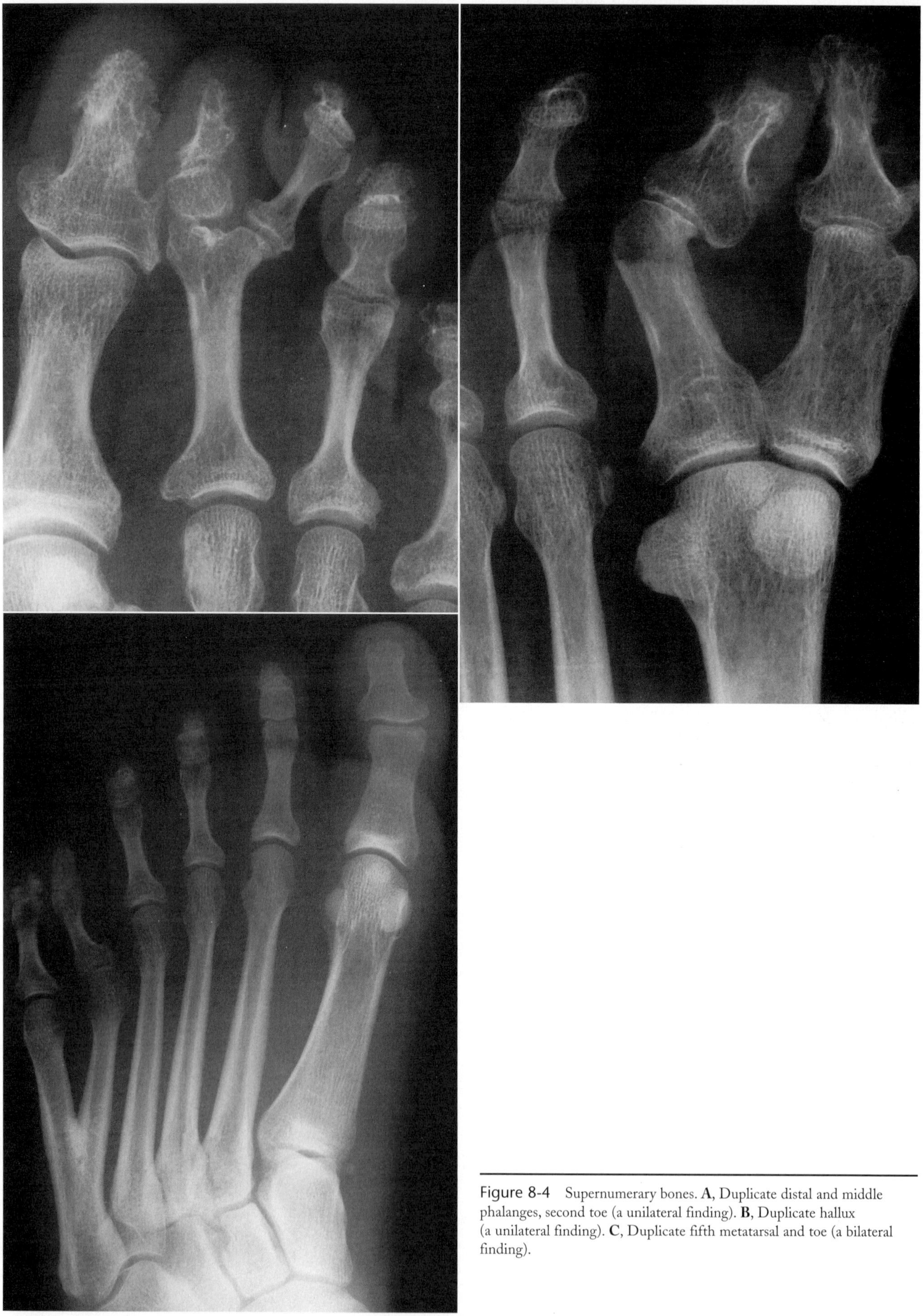

Figure 8-4 Supernumerary bones. **A,** Duplicate distal and middle phalanges, second toe (a unilateral finding). **B,** Duplicate hallux (a unilateral finding). **C,** Duplicate fifth metatarsal and toe (a bilateral finding).

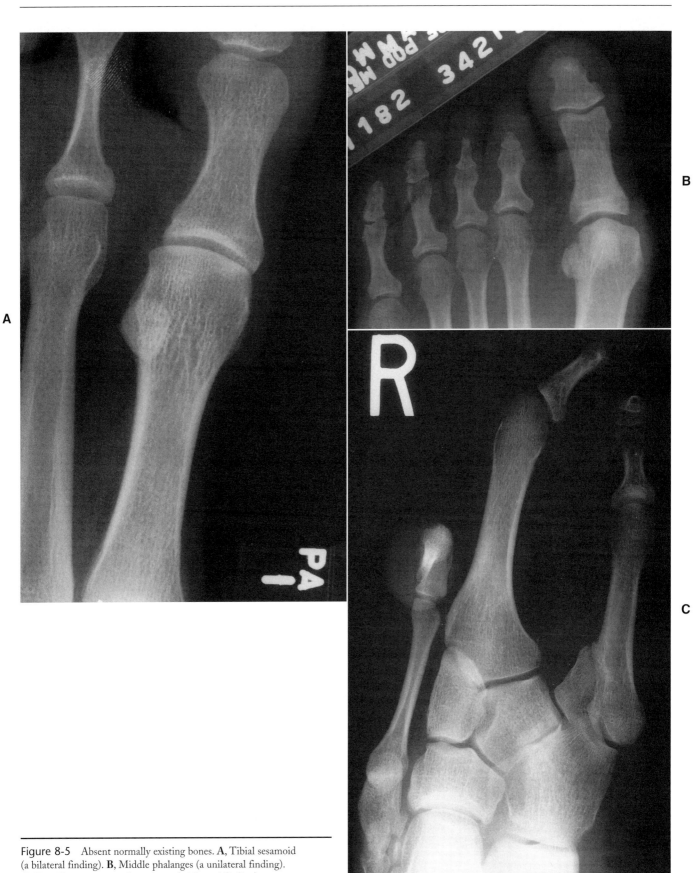

Figure 8-5    Absent normally existing bones. **A,** Tibial sesamoid
(a bilateral finding). **B,** Middle phalanges (a unilateral finding).
**C,** Cuneiforms, metatarsals, and toes (a bilateral finding).

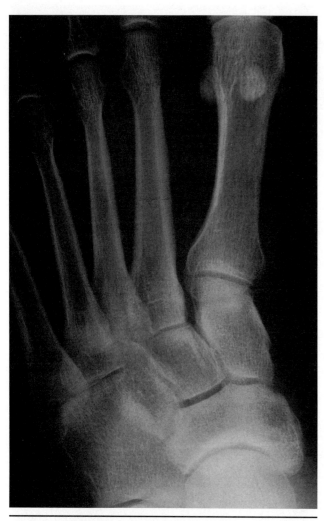

Figure 8-6    Midfoot variants of position: Medial splaying of medial cuneiform relative to intermediate cuneiform.

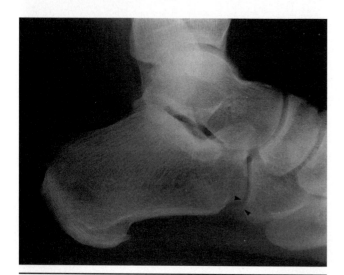

Figure 8-7    Tarsus positional variants: "Subluxated" calcaneocuboid joint.

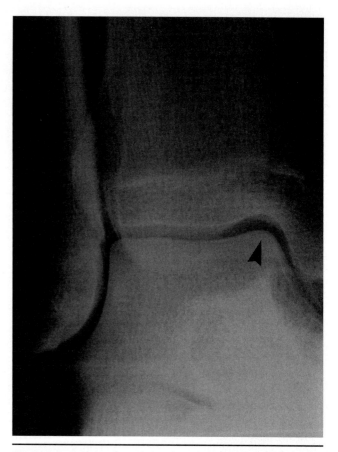

Figure 8-8    Tarsus/ankle positional variants: "Gapping" at superomedial corner of ankle joint.

former creates a gap between the anterior calcaneus and talar head), calcaneal adduction, and cuboid abduction (dorsoplantar view); increased or decreased calcaneal inclination and talar declination, naviculocuneiform fault, "subluxated" calcaneocuboid joint (Figure 8-7), and malleolar position (lateral view); and gapping at the superomedial corner of the ankle joint (Figure 8-8) and talar tilt (anteroposterior ankle view).

### ▇ VARIANTS OF FORM

### Distal Phalanx

Variations of the ungual tuberosity may be encountered in the dorsoplantar view (Figure 8-9). Its entire outer margin may be irregular or spiculated, simulating the reaction associated with inflammatory processes (chronic nail infection or psoriatic arthritis, for example). Another variation is absence of the medial or lateral margin; absence

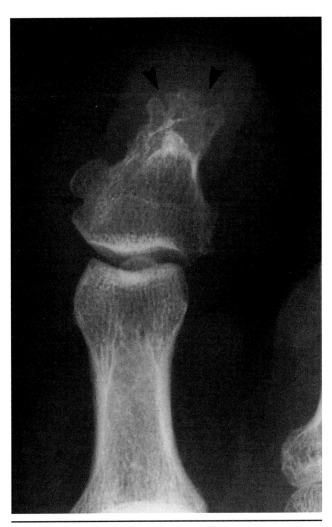

**Figure 8-9**   Varying presentations of the ungual tuberosity: Multiple distal indentations (hallux).

of both margins simulates the whittling of bone associated with forefoot neuropathic arthropathy. Occasionally the entire ungual tuberosity may be absent or appear atrophic. In a lesser toe, for example, the distal phalanx may appear triangular.

Spur formation is occasionally seen along the postero-inferior, medial, and lateral margins of the ungual tuberosity. It can be seen in the dorsoplantar and lateral views. The lateral interosseous ligaments insert along these margins.[3,4] A spur may be seen in the lateral view. This "mechanical" subungual spur may be related to hallux limitus.[5]

Occasionally variation of the length or girth of a distal phalanx is encountered (Figure 8-10). The phalanx may be increased or decreased in length or girth. Increased girth can many times be attributed to the flexor tuberosity that may be enlarged or hypertrophied. This is best identified in the isolated hallux lateral view. A wavy contour that mimics a periosteal reaction is infrequently seen along the shaft's medial and lateral margins. "Whiskering" may also be seen as a normal variation that is suggestive of psoriatic arthritis.

Variations of the hallucal distal phalanx base may also be encountered. The size of the basal inferomedial tubercle, for example, varies considerably, ranging from absent to quite enlarged radiographically (Figure 8-11). A recent investigation of this bony excrescence proposes that it probably represents a reaction of normal bone to repeated forces occurring during gait.[6] The lateral interosseous ligaments that run between the base and ungual tuberosity originate from the inferomedial and inferolateral basal tubercles. It infrequently calcifies, and spur formation may be noted at the entheses.

Occasionally variation of the lesser-toe distal phalanx base is seen. The base commonly flares medially and laterally in the dorsoplantar view. Often it appears quite pronounced relative to the narrow shaft. In rare instances the lateral aspect of the hallux distal phalanx base appears absent.

## Middle Phalanx

The shape of the lesser-toe middle phalanx may be either square or rectangular. The margins of a rectangular middle phalanx may either appear flat or indented (concave). The head of a middle phalanx occasionally is angulated laterally relative to its shaft, resulting in angulation of its respective distal phalanx (Figure 8-12).

## Proximal Phalanx

The proximal phalanx is a short, tubular bone. Variations in its length and girth are frequently encountered. For example, the phalanx may be shorter in length and wider in girth. This variant more frequently affects the lesser toes (Figure 8-13), although it also can involve the hallux. In contrast, a decreased diaphyseal girth may be seen. One example is the spool-shaped proximal phalanx.[7] The medullary canal may even appear obliterated in exaggerated cases.

Occasionally a proximal phalanx head is enlarged. This finding primarily involves the fifth digit and usually accompanies the clinical presence of an adductovarus contracture with a heloma durum overlying the hypertrophied head. A small exostosis may be seen along the head's superolateral aspect. A remnant of the phalangeal cleft may be identified in a similar location. Rarely, the hallux proximal phalanx head is enlarged.

A wavy contour and associated increased girth is commonly encountered along the medial and lateral margins of the diaphysis (Figure 8-14). This corresponds to the diaphyseal ridge in a lesser toe. Its size varies

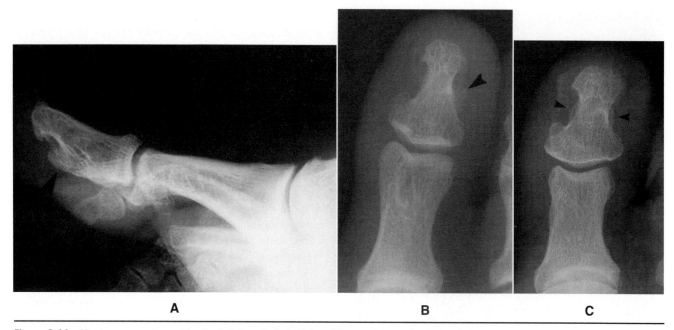

**A**                                    **B**                        **C**

Figure 8-10    Varying presentations of the distal phalanx shaft. **A,** Enlarged flexor tuberosity (lateral view). **B,** Enlarged flexor tuberosity (dorsoplantar view, a bilateral finding). **C,** Wavy medial and lateral margins mimicking periosteal reaction (a bilateral finding).

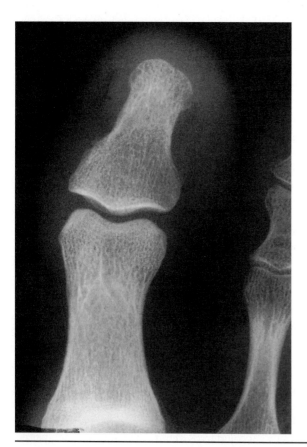

Figure 8-11    Varying presentations of the distal phalanx base: Absent tubercles (a bilateral finding).

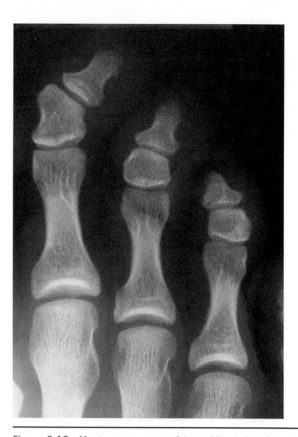

Figure 8-12    Varying presentation of the middle phalanx. Lateral aspect of second-toe middle phalanx is significantly shorter than the medial aspect, resulting in angulation of the distal phalanx laterally. Note also the square middle phalanges of the third and fourth toes.

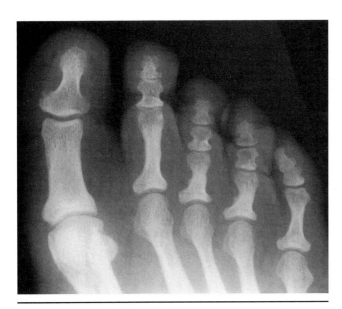

**Figure 8-13** Short proximal phalanx third and fourth toes, a bilateral finding.

considerably, and it may or may not be seen on all lesser-digit proximal phalanges of the same patient. The wing of the extensor hood apparatus and the fibrous flexor sheath insert along the diaphyseal ridge. Rotation of the digit obscures its visualization. A different type of cortical thickening and irregular contour is infrequently seen along the medial and lateral margins of the hallux proximal phalangeal distal diametaphysis.

## Sesamoids

The size of a sesamoid bone is fairly constant, although infrequently an enlarged or atrophic sesamoid may be encountered. They typically have smooth and regular margins. Occasionally, however, small protuberances resembling spurs may be seen along their posterolateral margins in the absence of any degenerative process or enthesopathy elsewhere. Rarely, a sesamoid may be much smaller in size than normally expected and when compared to its mate (Figure 8-15). Coalition of the two sesamoids has recently been reported.[8]

## Metatarsals

Metatarsals have a characteristic length pattern in the dorsoplantar view. Typically, the anterior end of the second metatarsal is most distal, followed by the first and third metatarsals (the anterior ends of both bones are nearly at the same position distally). The anterior end of the fourth metatarsal is more proximal relative to the third metatarsal, and the fifth is most proximal. Many variations are encountered regarding the lengths of each metatarsal relative to one another, some appearing longer, others shorter than the normal pattern described earlier (Figure 8-16). The short fourth metatarsal is typically anomalous.

The first-metatarsal head can have varying presentations (Figure 8-17). The shape of the distal articular surface may be round, demonstrate a central ridge, or be flat. Usually it is round. The medial and superior aspects of the first-metatarsal head vary in size and can be quite enlarged and hypertrophied. An enlarged tubercle may be seen medially at the diametaphyseal margin. The lateral tubercle is infrequently seen along the superior aspect of the first-metatarsal neck in the lateral view.

Regarding the lesser metatarsals (Figure 8-18), a head may (rarely) be flat distally with associated increased girth. The tubercles along the superomedial and superolateral aspects of their heads can be hypertrophied and prominent as seen in the medial oblique and dorsoplantar views, respectively. The neck's girth is consequently increased laterally when the superolateral tubercle is enlarged, simulating an old, healed fracture. The anatomic groove located between each tubercle and the anterior articular surface may be exaggerated in radiographic appearance. The posteroinferior articular extensions of the lesser-metatarsal heads may be pronounced in size. This finding, although superimposed, is identified in the dorsoplantar view. A lesser-metatarsal head may bow or angulate medially relative to the shaft, which is typically symmetric and bilateral.

Variations of the girth, contour, and form of a metatarsal shaft are encountered (Figure 8-19). The girth, for example, may be increased or decreased. Infrequently, a metatarsal shaft is overtubulated (overconstricted) and appears extremely narrow. Anatomic variations have been described that would correspond to this radiographic presentation.[9] Increased girth of a metatarsal shaft may be secondary to Wolff's law (increased stresses result in bone formation and remodeling). An example is the enlarged second-metatarsal shaft associated with a short first metatarsal (also known as the Morton's foot[10]). Occasionally the cortex along the inferolateral aspect of the first-metatarsal shaft proximally appears thickened. This site correlates anatomically to the insertion of the peroneus longus tendon. Lateral bowing of a metatarsal, especially the fifth, will be also seen. Increased girth of the fifth-metatarsal midshaft medially may accompany this finding and is symmetric bilaterally.

Along the margins of the metatarsal bases variations may be seen that could be mistaken for pathology (Figure 8-20). The medial and lateral aspects of the lesser-metatarsal bases normally are irregular; this finding is exaggerated by a deep

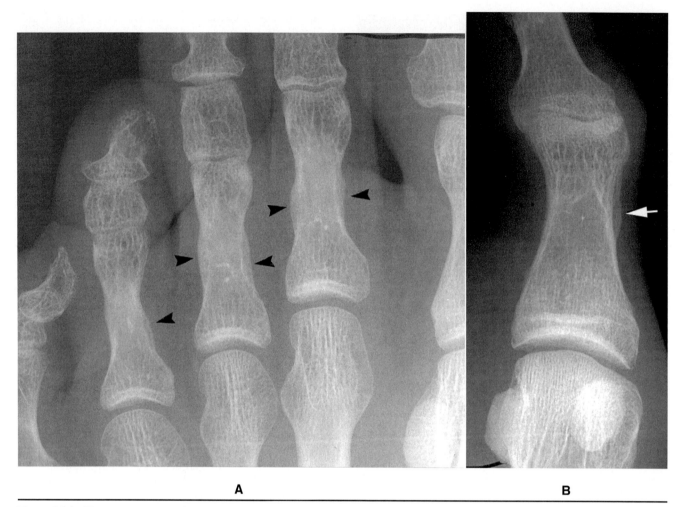

**A**                                                               **B**

Figure 8-14   Varying presentations of the proximal phalanx shaft. **A**, Phalangeal ridge (second, third, and fourth toes). **B**, Increased girth along the anterior aspect of the medial shaft (hallux) simulating a periosteal reaction. Present bilaterally.

groove located along the inferior and anterior aspects of the articular facet for the adjacent metatarsal. It is especially evident along the lateral aspects of the second-, third-, and fourth-metatarsal bases. An articulation is occasionally seen between the bases of the first and second metatarsals; the articulations between the lesser-metatarsal bases are rarely seen. A tubercle may be found, along the first-metatarsal base medially, that provides insertion for the tibialis anterior tendon. Another tubercle might be seen superiorly. The size of the fifth-metatarsal tuberosity is variable. It may appear absent, elongated posteriorly, or project laterally.

Variant articular surface shapes can also be encountered. The cuneiform articular surface of the first-metatarsal base may be flat or even concave. Occasionally the lateral cuneiform articular surface of the third metatarsal is also

concave, but in most cases it cannot be clearly identified, because adjacent structures are superimposed.

## Cuneiforms, Cuboid, and Navicular

Variability regarding the shape or form of the medial cuneiform is primarily positional in nature, but its form along the medial surface can vary. (The complete and incomplete bipartite medial cuneiform are discussed with variants of number.) One specific variant finding not related to position is a tubercle along the medial surface seen in the dorsoplantar view (Figure 8-21). The size and position of this tubercle varies, from small to large, and its position is inferomedial and is typically situated closer to the first-metatarsal articular surface, although it can also appear more

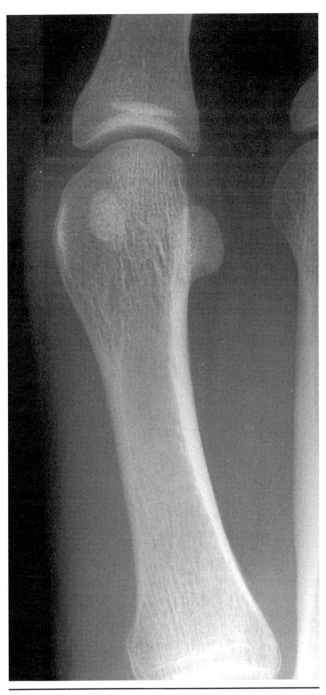

Figure 8-15  Varying presentations of the sesamoids: Smaller tibial sesamoid (bilateral).

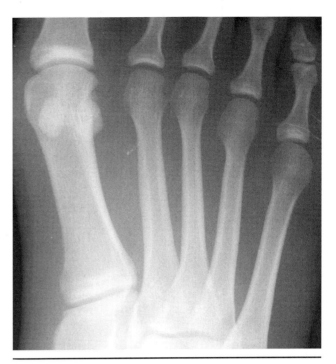

Figure 8-16  Variations of metatarsal length: Short second metatarsal.

posteriorly. It probably provides a gliding surface for the tibialis anterior tendon.

Superimposition of the midfoot bones is normally seen in the dorsoplantar view. This could lead to the misdiagnosis of a cubocuneiform coalition. Although trabeculations appear continuous between the two bones, the superimposed

shadows of the margins of this bone can still be identified. This latter finding would not be seen if the apparent continuity were a true coalition.

The cuboid has few variations to note (Figure 8-22). Its combined articular surface for the fourth and fifth metatarsals is typically flat or nearly flat; infrequently it has a prominent triangular ridge centrally separating the two articular surfaces, best seen in the medial oblique view. The anteromedial corner of the cuboid frequently juts medially toward the cuneiform, simulating an osteophyte or spur.

Most variants of the navicular's form are identified medially in the dorsoplantar or lateral oblique views. The navicular occasionally appears wedge shaped (its lateral half is narrow relative to the larger medial half in the dorsoplantar view), although it more frequently is somewhat rectangular. The tuberosity may be large, small, or absent in some individuals. When the tuberosity is elongated, it appears to wrap around the talar head. The elongated tuberosity may be related to a fused accessory navicular ossification center (see discussion of the accessory navicular later in this chapter). A large tubercle is infrequently seen along the navicular's medial surface anterior to the tuberosity (Figure 8-23). In yet other patients, the tuberosity may have an anomalous location medially; it classically is

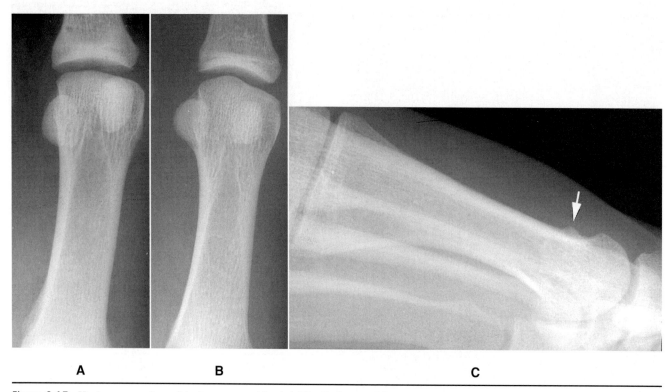

**Figure 8-17**  Varying presentations of the first-metatarsal head. **A,** Flat. **B,** Combined flat/ridge. **C,** Prominent lateral tubercle.

situated posteromedially. The medial margin of the navicular-medial cuneiform articular surface may be pronounced and extend away from the navicular anteriorly. A similar spurlike extension may be seen in the lateral view projecting anteriorly along the intermediate cuneiform articular surface. Variant form of the navicular simulating a bipartite navicular may be associated with a pronounced superoanterior margin. An unusual variant seen in the lateral view simulates an osteochondral lesion of the talar articular surface and typically is bilaterally symmetric. This latter finding may represent an incomplete bipartition (the bipartite navicular is discussed with variants of number). Finally, a tubercle may be seen in the medial oblique view for the cuboid articular surface.

## Talus

The talus is best seen in the lateral view. Its form is fairly consistent; however, occasionally it varies. The neck, for example, may be short or elongated. Less frequently, the body may appear flattened and the head/neck enlarged. Rarely, the head is flattened.

Spurs are frequently seen along the superior aspect of the talar head or neck. Anatomically, a small ridge is normally present along the superior surface at the junction of the talar head and neck that parallels the navicular articular surface. The talonavicular and talotibial joint capsules and ligaments insert here.[11] This ridge may be enlarged as a variation of normal. Occasionally an exostosis or hypertrophy is seen along the dorsum of the talar neck at the location of this ridge (Figure 8-24). Another spur is frequently identified on the talar head that is continuous with the navicular articular surface. This osteophyte is a feature of talonavicular joint osteoarthritis and is found in association with limited range of tarsal joint motion. However, its formation may be related to a prior injury.

The talar posterolateral process is continuous with the tibial articular surface of the talar dome and presents as a small protuberance. The process may be elongated and extend posteriorly. This is known as the trigonal process and probably represents a fused accessory ossification center (Figure 8-25) (see discussion of os trigonum later in this chapter).

The talar dome normally has a semicircular outline. If the ankle joint axis is not positioned perpendicular to the x-ray film, however, the medial and lateral shoulders of the dome are not aligned and give the appearance of a flattened talar dome (Figure 8-26). This appearance usually is positional in nature and is seen with a supinated/cavus foot in the weight-bearing lateral view.

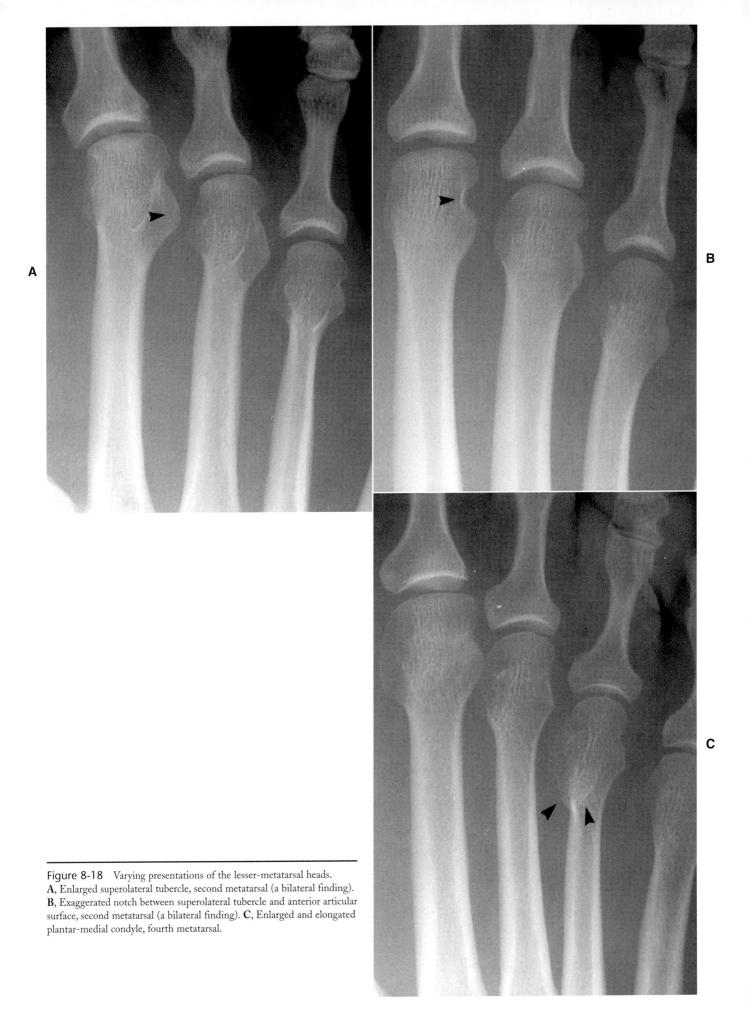

Figure 8-18   Varying presentations of the lesser-metatarsal heads.
**A,** Enlarged superolateral tubercle, second metatarsal (a bilateral finding).
**B,** Exaggerated notch between superolateral tubercle and anterior articular surface, second metatarsal (a bilateral finding). **C,** Enlarged and elongated plantar-medial condyle, fourth metatarsal.

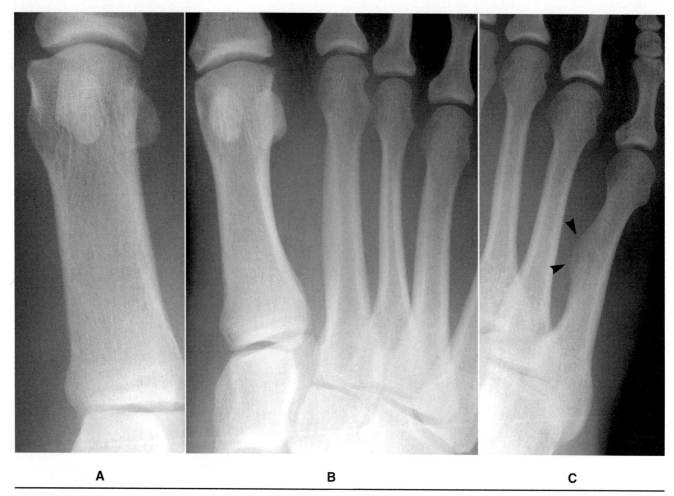

**Figure 8-19**    Metatarsal variants of form. **A,** Increased girth (first metatarsal). **B,** Decreased girth third metatarsal, increased girth second metatarsal. **C,** Fifth-metatarsal bowing with cortical thickening.

## Calcaneus

The form of the calcaneus is fairly constant. However, on occasion the overall shape appears somewhat rectangular and/or expanded, with distortion of its normal distinctive curves and lines. For example, the calcaneal length may appear elongated or foreshortened, the latter being the result of an enlarged posterior segment (Figure 8-27). Localized hypertrophy of the bursal projection (the posterosuperior aspect of the calcaneus) may or may not be associated with a clinical symptomatology. The superior or inferior surface rarely is flat (Figure 8-28). The anterior process may be enlarged and extend superiorly in the lateral view in the presence or absence of a calcaneonavicular coalition (Figure 8-29).

A projection of bone is rarely seen along the medial aspect of the calcaneus in the ankle anteroposterior view.

This variation articulates with an extension from the talar medial process and has been called the "assimilated os sustentaculum tali" because of its location. Anatomically, it is found along the posterior aspect of the sustentaculum tali. It may be identified as a bony palpable protuberance clinically and has been associated with symptomatology.[12] This probably represents an extra-articular talocalcaneal coalition (see discussion of synostosis and coalition later in this chapter).

The tubercles and tuberosities are occasionally enlarged and prominent (Figure 8-30). An enlarged peroneal tubercle or retrotrochlear eminence is infrequently seen along the lateral calcaneal body in the dorsoplantar and calcaneal axial views.[13] The anterior and lateral tuberosities may also be enlarged. The former is seen in the lateral view, the latter in the medial oblique and calcaneal axial views. The lateral tuberosity is rarely isolated in the lateral view.

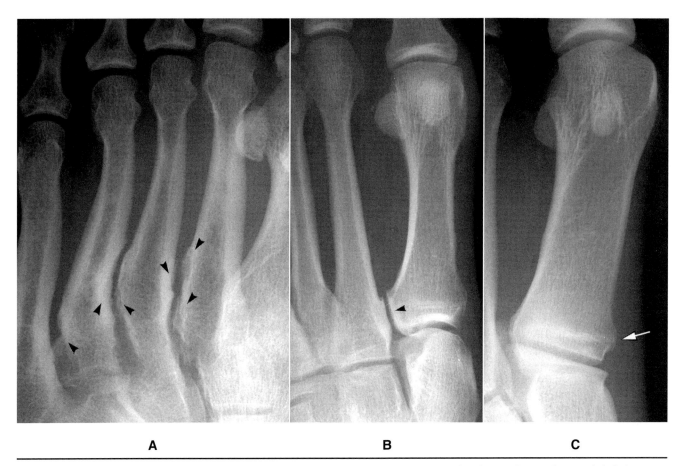

**Figure 8-20**   Varying presentations of the metatarsal base. **A**, Exaggerated, irregular intermetatarsal surfaces between bases and proximal shafts (a bilateral finding). **B**, Articulation between first- and second-metatarsal bases (a bilateral finding). **C**, Tubercle for tibialis anterior tendon insertion (a bilateral finding).

Anatomically, the middle and anterior articular surfaces for the talar head may be continuous or separate. Radiographically, the two surfaces generally appear continuous (this is only appreciated with the medial oblique view). It is unusual to see a separate articular surface for the anterior subtalar joint (Figure 8-31). The superior surface of the sustentaculum tali typically is flat in the lateral view; rarely, it appears curved. Also, the posterior aspect of the sustentaculum should not be continuous or articulate with the posteromedial talar process in the lateral view. Continuity is indicative of osseous coalition, articulation, or fibrocartilaginous union (see discussion of tarsal coalitions later in this section).

## Distal Tibia and Fibula

Form variants of the distal tibia or fibula are infrequent (Figure 8-32). For example, the tibial and fibular malleoli are occasionally elongated. An extended tibial malleolus

anterior colliculus may be related to ossification of the deltoid ligament at its enthesis. Elongation of the fibular malleolus may be accompanied by a hooklike extension at its inferior tip. Another variant of form is the presence of an enlarged tubercle or spur. It may be seen along the medial aspect of the tibial malleolus or the posterior aspect of either the tibial or fibular malleolus.

## Synostosis/Coalition

Union between two bones may be osseous, cartilaginous, or fibrous. Several terms have been used to describe these enigmas. The term *synostosis,* defined earlier, pertains to osseous union between two normally distinct bones. The term *coalition* is used more loosely and can pertain to osseous, cartilaginous, or fibrous union. The term *coalition* is frequently applied to anomalous union of tarsal bones. The term *ankylosis* refers to consolidation of a joint because of disease, injury, or surgical procedure. (For example, fibrous

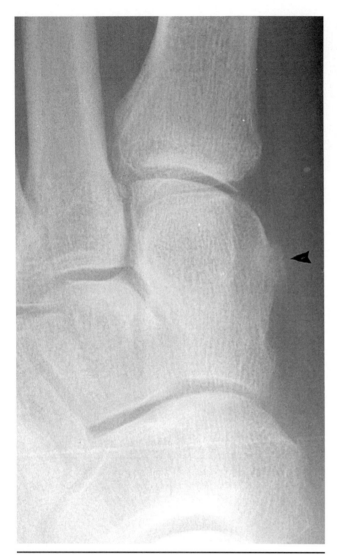

**Figure 8-21**    Tubercle along the medial surface of the medial cuneiform.

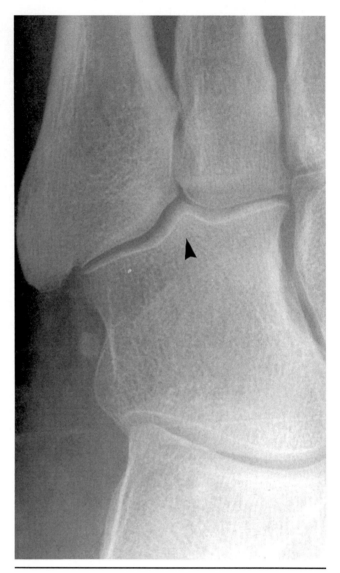

**Figure 8-22**    Cuboid variant of form: Ridge separating fourth- and fifth-metatarsal articulating surfaces.

or bony ankylosis may be seen as an end-stage presentation of inflammatory joint disease.) And *fusion* is defined as the operative formation of an ankylosis.[1]

Synostosis of a lesser-toe distal interphalangeal joint is the most common synostosis seen in the foot and typically is an incidental finding. Partial synostosis or bridging may be incidentally seen between metatarsal bones or at metatarsocuneiform joints. Tarsal coalitions, in contrast, are frequently associated with clinical symptomatology. This most likely is a result of faulty biomechanics and of limited range of motion between the affected bones.

Superimposition of two adjacent bones may mimic a synostosis. This can easily be distinguished by visually tracing the outer margin of each bone. If their outlines can be identified, there is no synostosis. It is not recommended to use continuity of the trabeculae in determining whether or not a synostosis exists. This finding is often misleading when bones are superimposed on one another.

*Interphalangeal joint synostosis* (Figure 8-33). Synostosis of the lesser-toe distal interphalangeal joint is frequently encountered in the foot. The fifth toe is most commonly affected. In decreasing order of frequency, distal interphalangeal joint synostoses of the fourth, third, and second digit occasionally are seen. Generally they are found bilaterally. A lesser

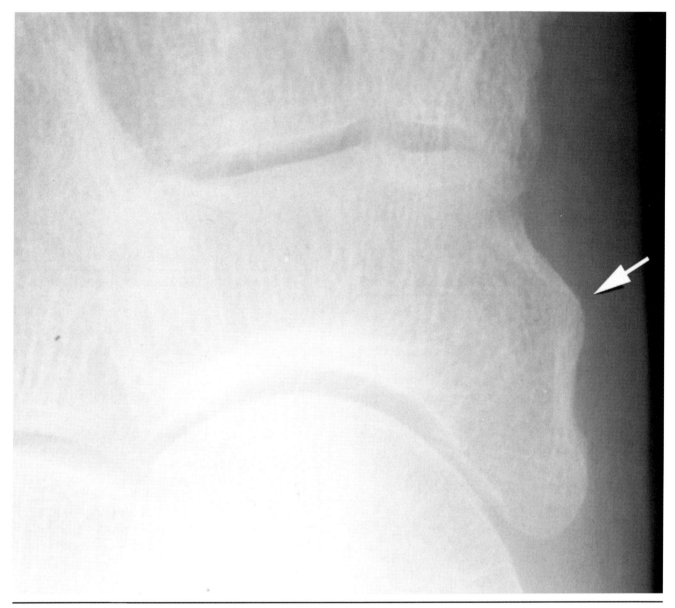

**Figure 8-23**    Navicular variants of form: Tubercle along medial surface anterior to the tuberosity.

digit that is clinically contracted (hammer toe or mallet toe, for example) radiographically appears as if it lacks a joint space, and simulates a synostosis. However, if the margins of the distal and middle phalanges are visually traced, the base and head of these bones, respectively, can be identified. They are superimposed on each other and collectively have an increased density relative to the remainder of each bone. The radiodensity of a synostosis is homogeneous and continuous with the middle and distal phalanges. No outline for the base or head can be visualized. Proximal interphalangeal joint synostosis is rarely seen.

*Intermetatarsal coalition.* Partial coalition between two metatarsals (rare) may or may not be entirely osseous and is frequently associated with other anomalies.

*Metatarsocuneiform coalition.* It is extremely rare to see synostosis between metatarsal and tarsal bones. They may be partial or complete.

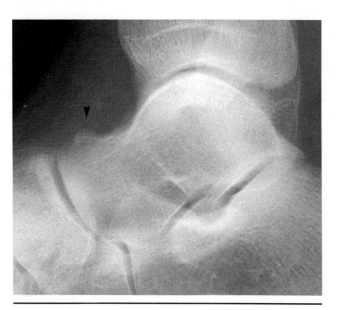

**Figure 8-24** "Exostosis" along talar head/neck superiorly: Slightly enlarged ridge.

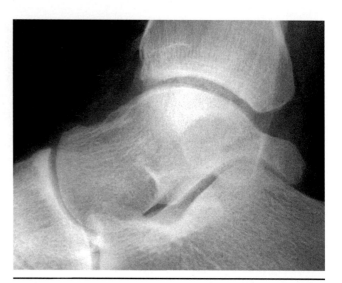

**Figure 8-25** Variants of talar posterolateral process: Prominent trigonal process.

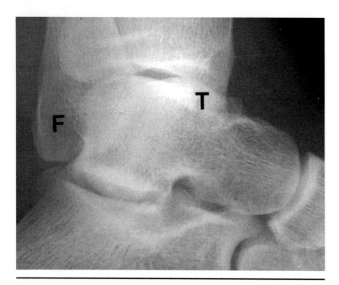

**Figure 8-26** The appearance of this "flattened" talar dome is purely positional in nature. Note that the fibular malleolus (F) is posterior in position relative to the tibial malleolus (T). Normally they should be superimposed.

*Tarsal coalition.* Synostosis may be seen between any two tarsal bones, but the most commonly encountered coalitions are calcaneonavicular and talocalcaneal. Talonavicular, calcaneocuboid, intercuneiform, naviculocuneiform, cubonavicular, and cubocuneiform coalitions are rarely identified (Figure 8-34).

The presence of a calcaneonavicular coalition (also known as calcaneonavicular bar) is not uncommon (Figure 8-35). It is best viewed in the medial oblique view, but calcaneonavicular coalition can also be recognized in the lateral view alone as an extension or elongation of the anterior calcaneal process superiorly. This finding has been referred to as the "anteater nose."[14] The appearance of the calcaneonavicular coalition in the medial oblique view varies, depending on the type of union. The superomedial aspect of the anterior calcaneal beak and inferolateral aspect of the navicular are continuous as one bony structure if there is osseous coalition. However, the fibrous or cartilaginous calcaneonavicular coalition is more frequently encountered. In this case, the two bones are in close apposition and appear to articulate with one another. The margin of each bone may be quite irregular and sclerotic, resembling degenerative arthritis. In contrast, the two bones may be found in close anatomic relationship to one another, yet no obvious articulation or marginal sclerosis is identified. Although this latter presentation represents a variant form, it is questionable whether or not it truly represents calcaneonavicular coalition. It has also been suggested that the os calcaneus secundarius, found at the same site, is related to the formation of the calcaneonavicular coalition.[15]

Identification of a calcaneonavicular coalition is best visualized if the foot is obliqued approximately 45 degrees relative to the x-ray film (the medial oblique view). If less than 45 degrees is attained, there is superimposition of the anterior calcaneus and navicular, mimicking a calcaneo-

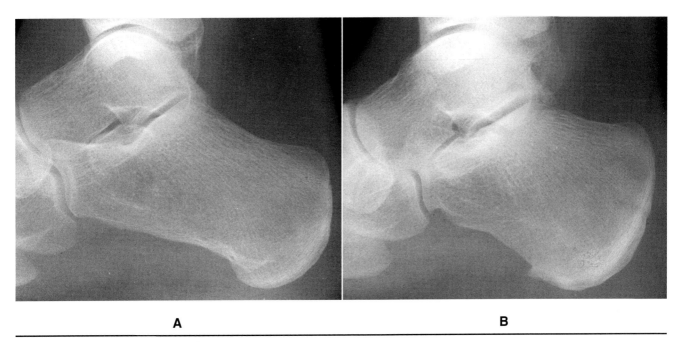

**Figure 8-27**   Variation of calcaneal form/length. **A,** Elongated with normal contours. **B,** Short with enlarged posterior segment.

navicular coalition. Proper foot position can be determined by examining the relationship of the cuboid and third cuneiform bones in the radiograph. If the two bones are separate and distinct (such that the cuboid is wholly isolated), the oblique position was performed properly. If not, a distinct space is not seen between the two bones. The latter case should also not be misinterpreted as coalition.

The talocalcaneal coalition receives the most attention in the literature of all the tarsal coalitions. Coalition of the middle talocalcaneal joint region is the most frequently encountered of the three possible talocalcaneal coalitions, anterior, middle, and posterior. Anatomically, the middle talocalcaneal coalition is either extra-articular (located between the posterior aspect of the sustentaculum tali and the talar body) and/or intra-articular.[16] It may either be complete, nearly complete, incomplete, or rudimentary.[17] Varying radiographic findings therefore can be attributed to variant presentations. In addition, the presence of an os sustentaculum tali has, like the os calcaneus secundarius, been suggested to contribute to the formation of coalition.[18]

Radiographically, the complete middle talocalcaneal coalition is best appreciated in the axial (Harris-Beath) view[19] (Figure 8-36). The joint space is obliterated if osseous coalition is present; gross joint space narrowing and subchondral sclerosis are seen if fibrocartilaginous. In the latter case, the middle subtalar joint appears obliquely oriented (at approximately 45 degrees). An os sustentaculum tali may rarely be identified in association with middle talocalcaneal coalition.

Although it is not obvious in the lateral foot view, specific radiographic findings may be identified, leading to its diagnosis (Figure 8-37). Normally the talar lateral process is triangular. When middle talocalcaneal coalition is present, this landmark frequently appears rounded or even flattened inferiorly. Also, the shadows of the sustentaculum tali and the talar posteromedial process are normally separate and distinct. In contrast, if middle talocalcaneal coalition is present, the inferior margins of these structures are continuous with one another. This finding has recently been coined the "C sign."[20] Less frequently one may see an osteoarthritic articulation between these two anatomic landmarks. A spur or "beak" along the superior aspect of the talar neck (at the ridge[10]) has also been associated with talocalcaneal coalition. But this latter finding is not a reliable indicator of coalition, because it can be seen when coalition is not present.

Anterior and posterior talocalcaneal coalition is rare. The anterior talocalcaneal coalition is identified in the medial oblique view. As already noted with the calcaneonavicular coalition, however, anterior talocalcaneal coalition is mimicked by superimposition of the two bones if the foot

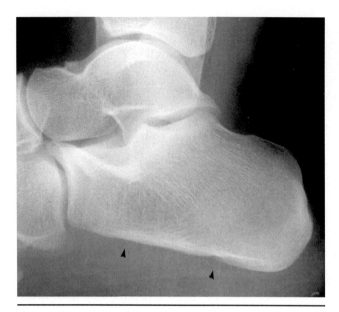

Figure 8-28    Flattened inferior calcaneal surface.

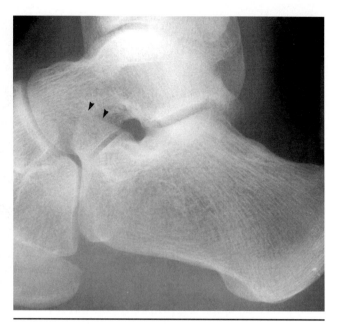

Figure 8-29    Variation of the anterior process: Enlarged and projecting superiorly, simulating an "anteater" calcaneus.

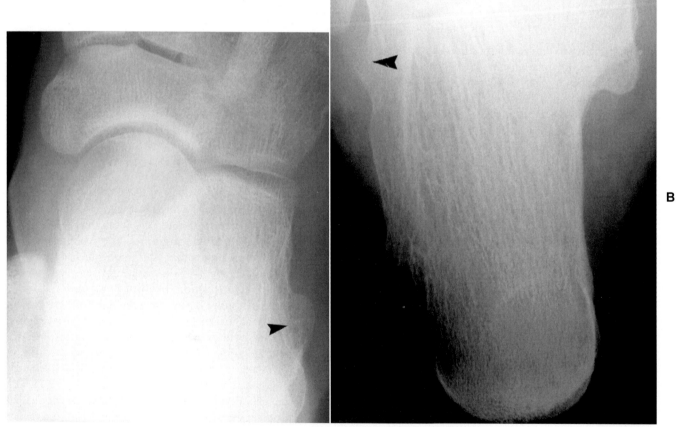

Figure 8-30    Variant calcaneal tubercles and tuberosities. **A**, Enlarged and prominent peroneal tubercle, dorsoplantar view. **B**, Large peroneal tubercle, axial view (different patient from **A**).

*Continued*

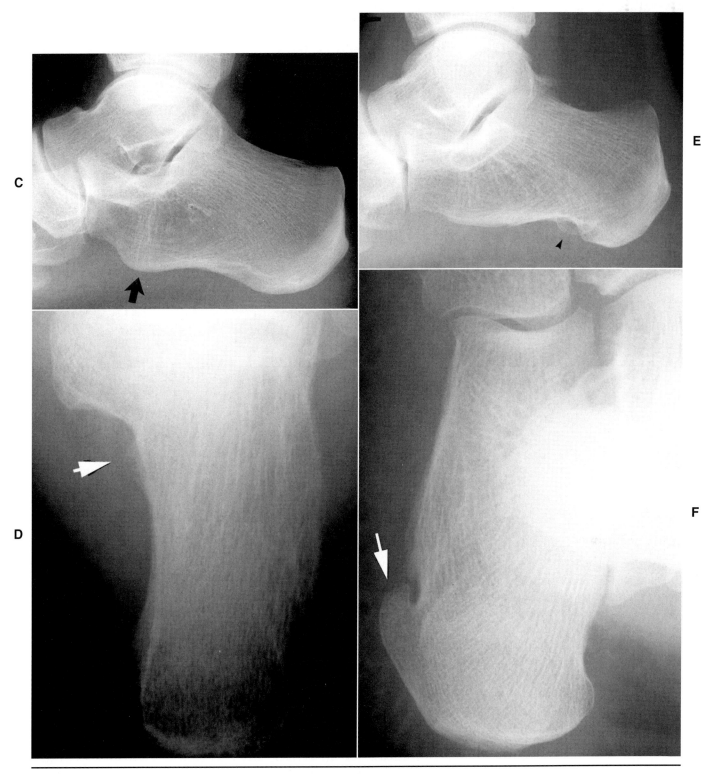

Figure 8-30, cont'd    Variant calcaneal tubercles and tuberosities. **C**, Large anterior tuberosity (lateral view). **D**, Medially prominent anterior tuberosity (axial view). **E**, Smaller, but still prominent lateral tuberosity seen in lateral view. **F**, Incomplete (probably developmental) hook-shaped lateral tuberosity and resultant foramina.

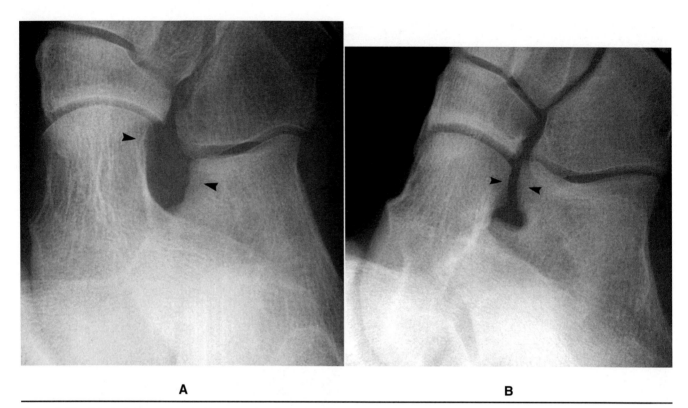

**A**                                                                     **B**

**Figure 8-31**    Subtalar joint variation. **A,** Absent anterior subtalar joint. **B,** Separate facet for anterior subtalar joint.

is not positioned properly. The posterior talocalcaneal coalition can only be seen in the axial view.

## ■ VARIANTS OF DENSITY

### Radiolucencies

At several anatomic locations, varying degrees of radiolucency may be encountered. They are found in the absence of any clinical symptomatology, appear bilaterally in most instances, and are variations of normal radiographic anatomy. For example, a central radiolucency may be seen in the hallux proximal phalanx diaphysis that mimics a geographic, solitary lytic lesion. Another example of a variant radiolucency is found in the medial aspect of the navicular in the dorsoplantar view, adjacent to the tuberosity. It typically is bilateral and symmetric. A larger area of radiolucency is occasionally encountered in the body of the calcaneus in the lateral view. The arrangement of trabeculae in this area is such that three patterns of stress trabeculae surround an oval or triangular central radiolucency, often referred to as the neutral triangle. Occasionally the margins of this radiolucency are well defined, simulating a geographic lytic lesion.

Other sites where variant radiolucencies are encountered include the metatarsal heads and the distal fibula. The medial aspect of the fifth-metatarsal head is commonly radiolucent. It simulates inflammatory joint disease, especially early rheumatoid arthritis. However, the subchondral bone plate is well defined and continuous when viewed over a spotlight. A similar radiolucency may be seen in the medial aspect of the remaining lesser-metatarsal heads. An oval geographic lucency is infrequently encountered in the lateral aspect of the second-metatarsal head. The well-defined radiolucency occasionally detected in the distal fibula relates to the superimposition of soft tissue shadows. It could easily be misinterpreted as a tumor or tumorlike lesion.

Small, well-defined, and round "punched out" radiolucencies are occasionally seen (Figure 8-38). It is not uncommon to see a tiny, round lucency in the distal metaphysis of the lesser-toe proximal phalanx. It is central in location. A similar finding may be encountered in the calcaneal body, in the "neutral triangle." Another round radiolucency is infrequently found adjacent to the calcaneal lateral tuberosity in the medial oblique view. This has been referred to in the literature as a nutrient foramen,[21] although it could also represent a developmental defect or incomplete ossification of the apophyseal growth center.

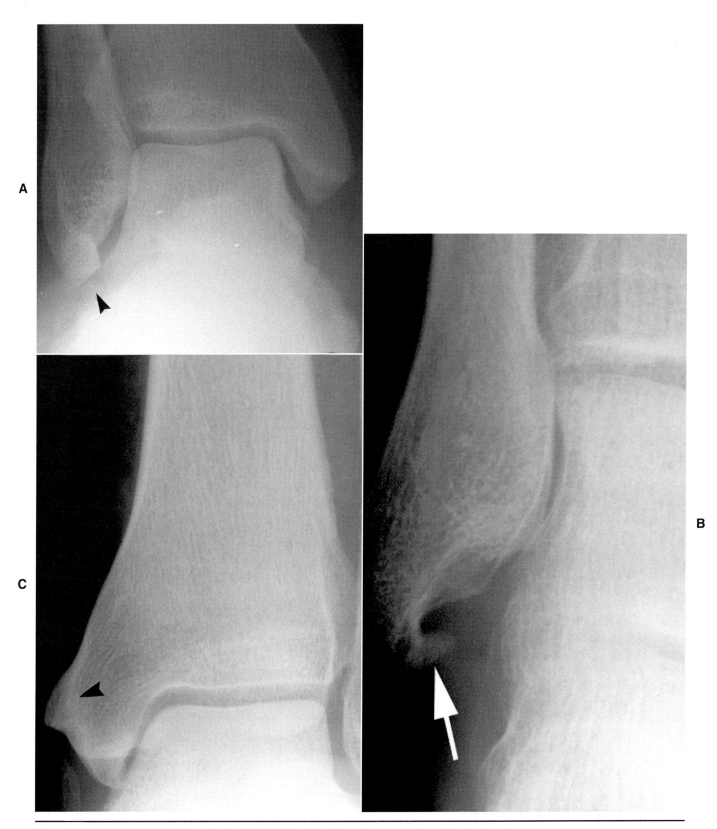

Figure 8-32    Distal tibial and fibular variants of form. **A,** Elongated fibular malleolus. **B,** Hooked fibular malleolus (a bilateral finding). **C,** Exostosis along medial aspect of tibial malleolus, a bilateral and symmetrical finding.

*Continued*

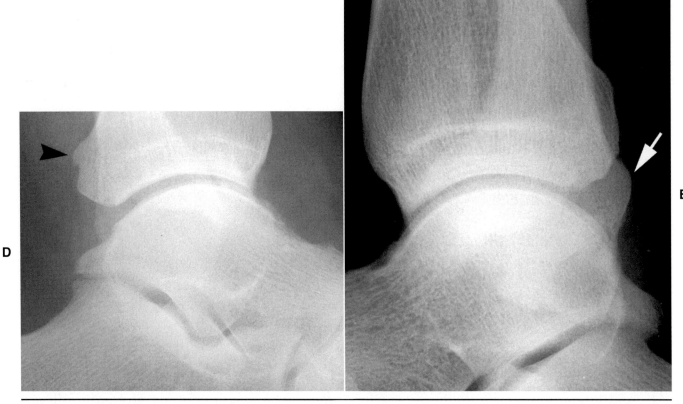

**Figure 8-32, cont'd** Distal tibial and fibular variants of form. **D,** Small exostosis along posterior surface of distal tibia, found bilaterally. **E,** Bony hypertrophy along the posterior aspect of the fibula, a bilateral finding.

## Increased Densities

A common variant of increased density appears as a solitary, geographic increased (cortical) density found in cancellous bone (Figure 8-39). This tumorlike lesion might be found in any foot bone and has been referred to as a bone island (also known as enostosis and endosteoma). Bone islands are incidental findings and are not associated with clinical symptomatology. A sesamoid, especially an accessory sesamoid, may appear homogeneously sclerotic. Its superimposition on the metatarsal head in the dorsoplantar view resembles a bone island.

Some increased radiodensities correspond to osteologic landmarks. For example, a curvilinear sclerosis may be seen in the hallux distal phalanx base in the dorsoplantar view that corresponds to the flexor tuberosity. Another sclerotic density is commonly seen in the body of the calcaneus in the lateral view, superior to the medial tuberosity. This curvilinear density corresponds to the lateral tuberosity; its position and outline varies among patients.

Occasionally the lower third of the posterior calcaneus is sclerotic relative to the body. This sclerosis extends from the Achilles tendon enthesis to the medial tuberosity inferiorly.

It appears to represent accentuation of the stress trabeculae along the posteroinferior calcaneus.

A severely contracted digit may be positioned such that a phalanx's shaft is parallel to the central x-ray beam in the dorsoplantar view. The resultant image appears as an intense, radiodense circle, corresponding to the diaphyseal cortex. This has been coined the "gun barrel" sign because it mimics the appearance seen when looking down the barrel of a gun.

Superimposed soft tissue structures may present an interesting finding. An infrequent finding is the appearance of a well-defined increased density in the anteroposterior ankle view that runs vertically through the center of the ankle joint. Its width spans at least half the width of the talar dome and widens superiorly. This shadow corresponds to the superimposed Achilles tendon (Figure 8-40).

## ■ VARIANTS OF ARCHITECTURE

### Cortical Bone

The cortex normally is radiopaque and homogeneous in density. Both the subperiosteal and endosteal surfaces should be smooth, continuous, and well defined. It is not uncommon, however, to see variations in the appearance of the cortex (Figure 8-41). Uniform increased or decreased thickness of the entire cortex is more directly related to increased or decreased girth (that is, form). In contrast, the contour of the lesser metatarsal's external margin may be irregular or wavy (but nonuniform) along its subperiosteal surface that can involve one or multiple bones. This finding is predominantly located along the proximal half diaphysis and is an incidental finding. The external margin of the cortex may also appear irregular at an enthesis. Increased girth along the endosteal surface of the cortex, usually localized, is encountered less frequently. This form of apposition is solid, homogeneous in density, and of the same radiodensity as the cortex proper. It may involve only one metatarsal, or several, unilaterally or bilaterally. It predominantly is seen in the second, third, or fourth metatarsal.

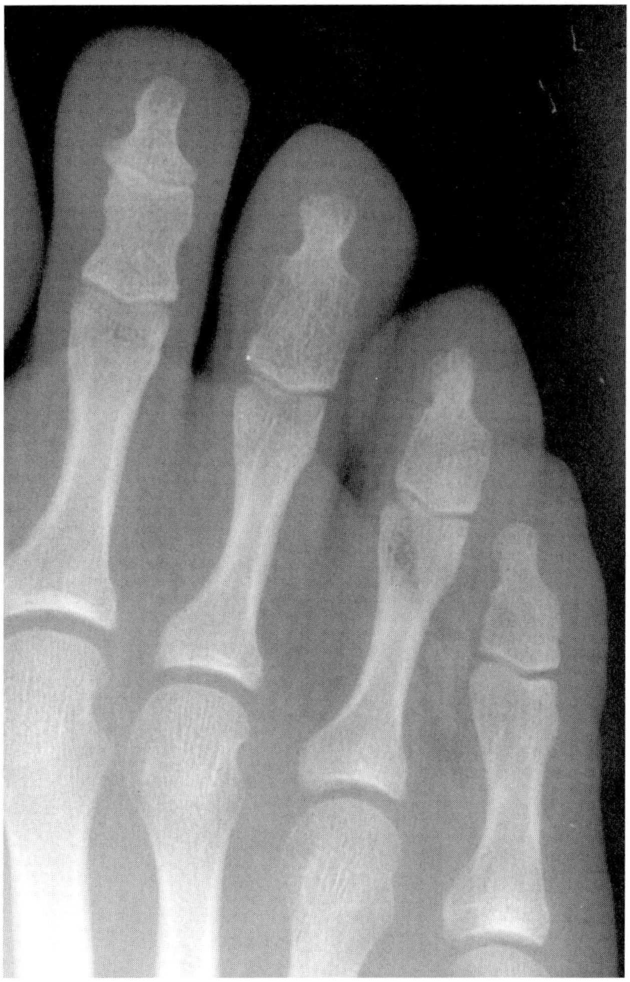

The cortex may appear to split apart or separate into longitudinal layers near the base of a lesser metatarsal, mimicking intracortical tunneling. This frequently occurs at

Figure 8-33    Interphalangeal joint synostosis: Third-, fourth-, and fifth-toe distal interphalangeal joints.

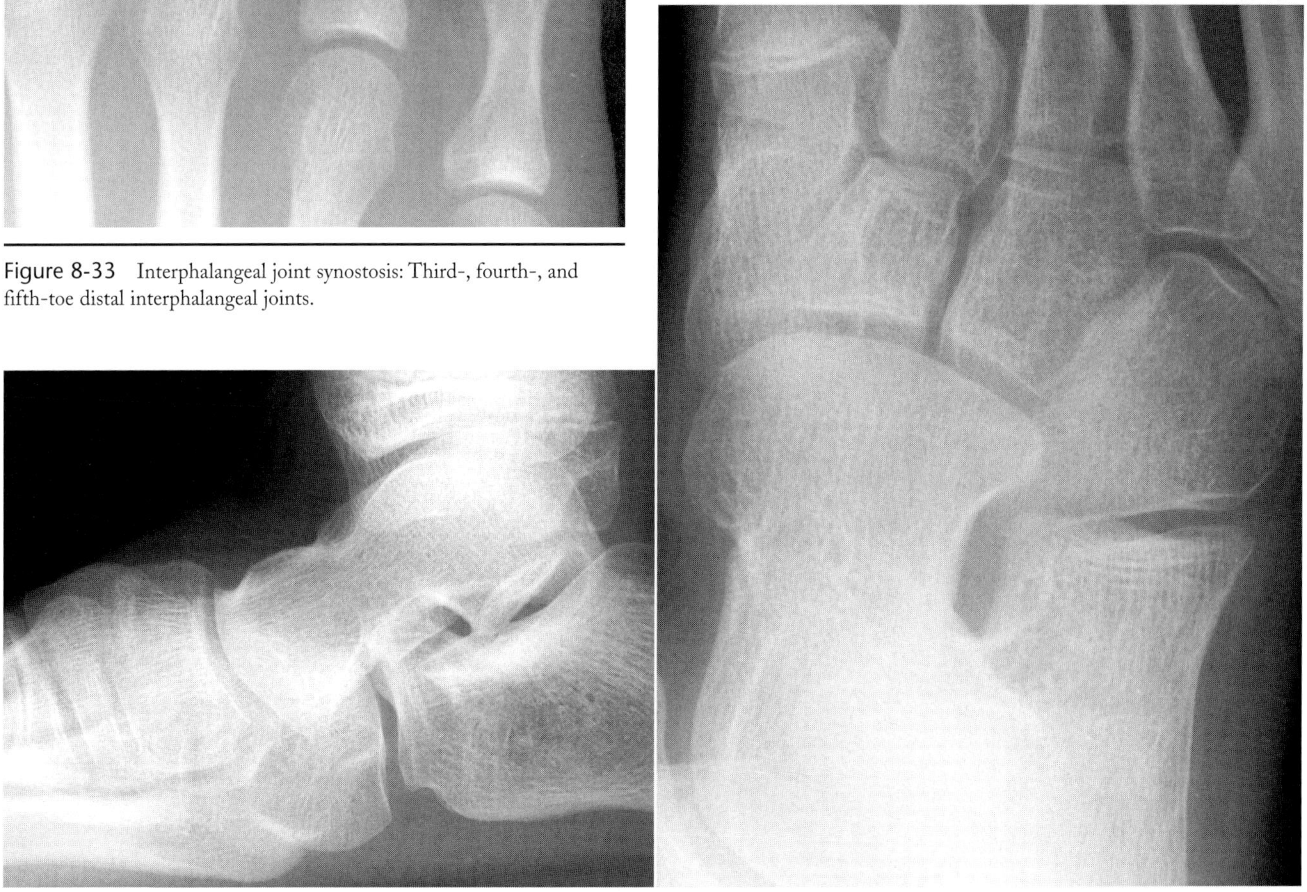

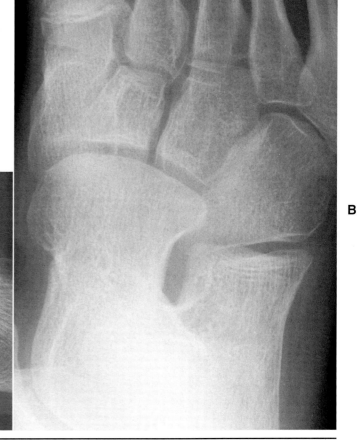

Figure 8-34    Rare intertarsal coalitions. **A,** Talonavicular coalition, lateral view. **B,** Talonavicular coalition, medial oblique view (same patient as **A**).

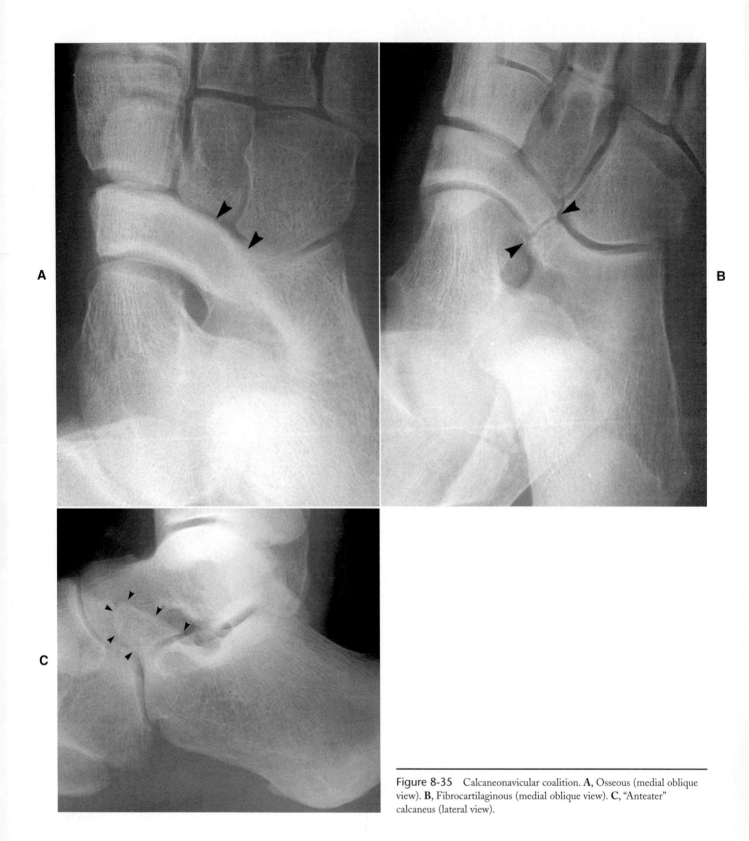

**Figure 8-35** Calcaneonavicular coalition. **A,** Osseous (medial oblique view). **B,** Fibrocartilaginous (medial oblique view). **C,** "Anteater" calcaneus (lateral view).

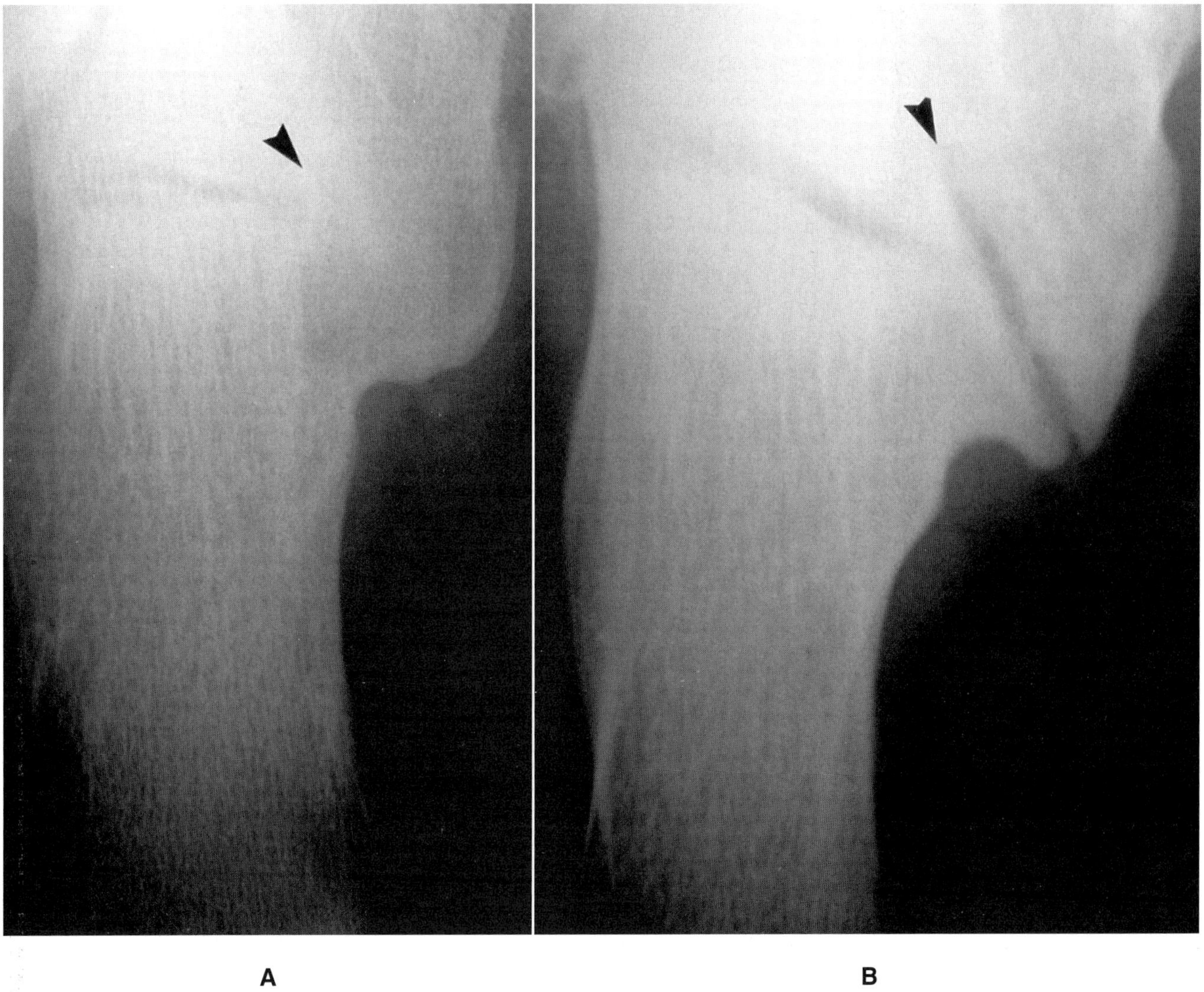

Figure 8-36   Middle talocalcaneal coalition, calcaneal axial view. **A,** Osseous (obliquely oriented). **B,** Fibrocartilaginous (obliquely oriented).

the diametaphyseal junction and is seen in the medial oblique view.

## Cancellous Bone

The trabecular pattern in the distal metaphysis of the first-metatarsal head is commonly coarse in appearance. These thickened trabeculae are normal and (if a solitary finding) do not represent osteopenia. The superimposition of these trabeculations on the sesamoids can simulate a fracture of the latter. A rare finding is a mosaic-like pattern of trabeculations, a generalized finding that is especially noticeable in the first metatarsal. A similar pattern may be localized to the proximal phalangeal heads.

Transversely oriented trabeculae are occasionally encountered in the medullary portion of tubular bones. These may be related to bone bars (reinforcement lines) in older patients but are not uncommon in younger adults.

## ◾ ACCESSORY OSSICLES

Numerous accessory ossicles are present in the foot. Although their anatomic locations are fairly consistent, the morphology of these ossicles can be quite complex and diverse. It is not uncommon to find them unilaterally. When present bilaterally, their size, shape, or number are frequently asymmetric. These presentations certainly can confound

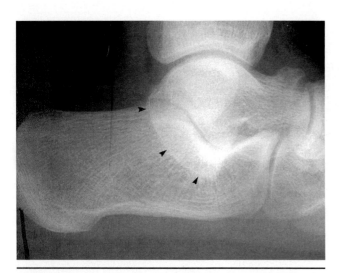

Figure 8-37    Middle talocalcaneal coalition, lateral view: "C sign" (continuity between sustentaculum and talar posteromedial process) and talar head exostosis.

interpretation of radiographs, especially when they are found in areas associated with clinical symptomatology. It is, therefore, of extreme importance that the interpreter be able to recognize the typical and atypical presentations of these enigmas.

## Os Interphalangeus

The os interphalangeus (Figure 8-42) is classically found along the inferior aspect of the hallux interphalangeal joint. It is rare to see this ossicle at the interphalangeal joints of the lesser toes. The position of the os interphalangeus is either central or eccentric; central is more common. These ossicles are round or oval. The centrally located os interphalangeus is considered a sesamoid bone because of its location in the plantar capsule and attachment to the flexor tendon.[16] (McCarthy and associates[22] have identified its location as in the joint capsule and the flexor hallucis capsularis interphalangeus.) The position of the eccentric os interphalangeus probably is intracapsular. Rarely, an ossicle may be encountered along the superior aspect of an interphalangeal joint.

The eccentric os interphalangeus appears to have a different genesis from that of the centrally located sesamoid. During development the basal epiphysis of the distal phalanx occasionally has multiple ossification centers. A segment of this ossification center may remain separate into adulthood and persist as the eccentric os interphalangeus. A defect in the adjacent phalangeal base is frequently observed that corresponds to the size and shape of the unfused ossification center in this case. Rarely, the ossicle is adjacent to a defect along the proximal phalanx head. The eccentric

os interphalangeus may also be the sequela of an old, unhealed fracture (that is, nonunion). However, the majority of these patients do not recall any history of trauma, and many times the radiographic finding is bilateral in presentation.

The os interphalangeus can be identified in either the dorsoplantar or isolated lateral view of the hallux. Its transverse-plane position is best determined with the dorsoplantar view. It is superimposed on the proximal phalanx head and appears as a fairly well-defined oval of increased density. Os interphalangeus can be clearly identified with the lateral view if the hallux is isolated from the lesser digits. The lateral or medial eccentric os interphalangeus can be isolated with the medial oblique or lateral oblique view, respectively. The central os interphalangeus is rarely bipartite.

## Accessory Sesamoids

A pair of sesamoid bones is consistently found at the first metatarsophalangeal joint. This occurs almost without exception. In addition, sesamoid bones may also be found along the inferior aspects of the lesser metatarsophalangeal joints, although not commonly (Figure 8-43). These latter ossicles are known as accessory sesamoids. They may be seen at any of the lesser metatarsophalangeal joints in varying combinations. For example, accessory sesamoids may appear at one, two, three, or all four lesser metatarsophalangeal joints. Furthermore, accessory sesamoids may exist as a single entity or occur in pairs. They appear circular or oval in shape and vary in size. Rarely, they are bipartite.

Accessory sesamoids are best isolated in the sesamoid axial view, seen along the inferomedial aspect of the metatarsophalangeal joint when solitary. The single sesamoid is superimposed on the medial aspect of the metatarsal head in the dorsoplantar view. The medial positioning of these sesamoids may be related to the normally inverted position of the lesser metatarsals relative to the x-ray film.

## Os Intermetatarseum

The os intermetatarseum (Figure 8-44) is situated superiorly between the first- and second-metatarsal bases. It is best seen in the dorsoplantar view. It can occasionally be seen in the lateral view superiorly, although it typically is superimposed on the first-metatarsal base. This ossicle may be round, oval, kidney-shaped, or linear, or may even resemble a rudimentary metatarsal. Its size also varies. The os intermetatarseum may articulate with the medial cuneiform or be attached to the first-metatarsal base. Calcification of the perforating branch between the dorsal and plantar metatarsal arteries may simulate an os intermetatarseum. An os intermetatarseum is rarely

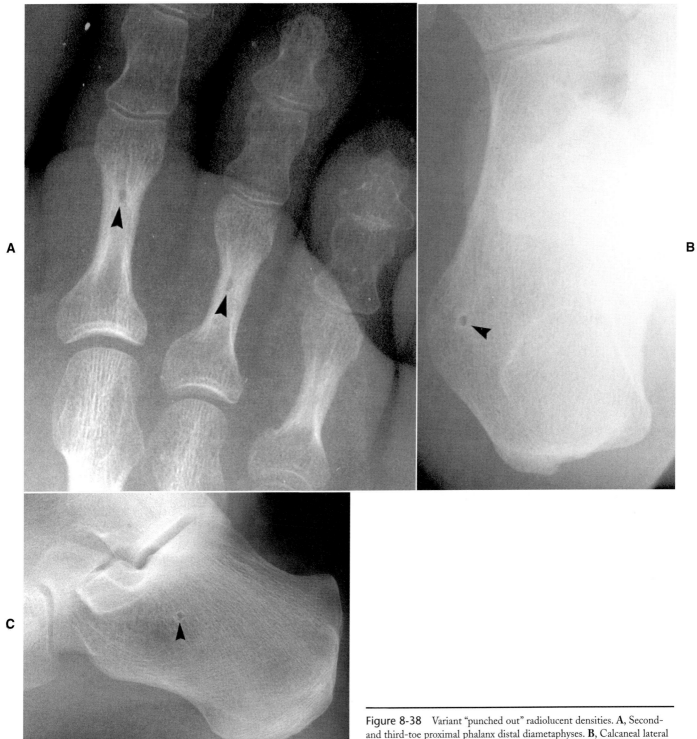

Figure 8-38    Variant "punched out" radiolucent densities. **A,** Second- and third-toe proximal phalanx distal diametaphyses. **B,** Calcaneal lateral tuberosity, small. **C,** Calcaneal body, central location.

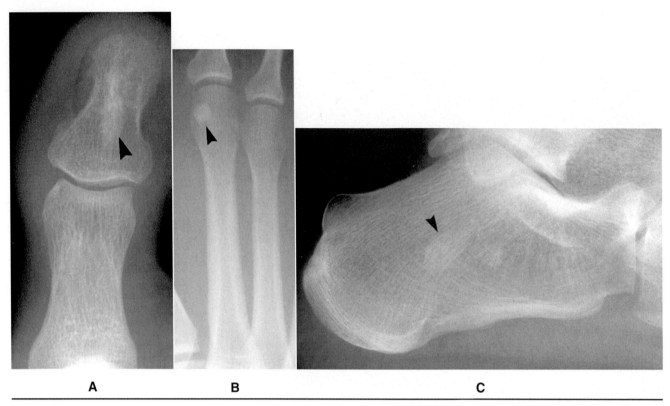

**Figure 8-39**    Variant increased densities in cancellous bone: Bone island. **A**, Hallux distal phalanx. **B**, Second-metatarsal head. **C**, Central calcaneus.

encountered at the second lesser metatarsocuneiform joint (also known as the os cuneometatarsale II dorsale). The os intermetatarseum is infrequently the cause of foot symptomatology.[23]

A sesamoid has been reported in the extensor hallucis brevis tendon at the level of the first metatarsocuneiform joint.[24] The lateral radiograph of this lesion looks similar to that of the os intermetatarseum, although the location of the former is slightly more superior.

### Tibialis Anterior Tendon Sesamoid

A sesamoid may infrequently be found in the tibialis anterior tendon near its insertion onto the first-metatarsal base (Figure 8-45). It is located adjacent to either the first metatarsocuneiform joint or the medial cuneiform[25] and is best seen in the dorsoplantar and, if located adjacent to the insertion site, lateral oblique views. This sesamoid may be either round, oval, or linear in shape. It may also be bipartite.

### Os Paracuneiforme (Os Cuneonaviculare Mediale)

An ossicle found adjacent to the medial aspect of the naviculocuneiform joint is known as the os paracuneiforme (Figure 8-46). It is rarely observed.

### Os Cuboid

Zimmer observed an ossicle between the anterior aspects of the cuboid and lateral cuneiform, adjacent to the fourth-metatarsal base (Figure 8-47).[26] He questioningly names it "os cuboid?" in the figure caption, for lack of a better term. This rare entity appears to provide an articular surface for the fourth-metatarsal base medially.

### Os Vesalianum

An accessory ossicle located at the posterior tip of the fifth-metatarsal tuberosity is known as the os vesalianum (Figure 8-48). The presence of this ossicle is quite rare, and its size and shape may vary considerably. It typically presents as a small, rounded calcific density. It is best seen in the medial oblique view. Ossification of the peroneus brevis tendon and old, unhealed (nonunion) fracture of the tuberosity may look similar to the os vesalianum. This ossicle is not the same entity as the persistent fifth-metatarsal apophysis (see next section).

### Persistent Fifth-Metatarsal Apophysis

The fifth-metatarsal tuberosity apophyseal ossification center may remain unfused into adulthood (Figure 8-49).

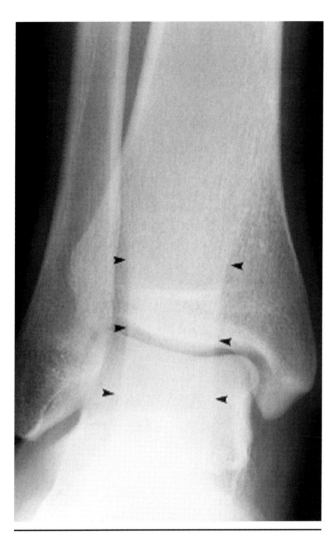

Figure 8-40    Achilles tendon shadow superimposed on distal tibia and talus in anteroposterior ankle view.

This is known as a persistent apophysis. It is large in size and appears to articulate with the metatarsal base. The persistent fifth-metatarsal apophysis is occasionally referred to as the os vesalianum, albeit incorrectly.[27] It is clearly identified with the medial oblique view and is frequently bilateral and symmetrical.

## Os Peroneum

The os peroneum is a sesamoid bone found in the peroneus longus tendon (Figure 8-50). It varies not only in size, but also in number: It commonly is partite. The os peroneum is classically situated beside the cuboid bone just proximal to where the tendon runs along the peroneal sulcus, but its position varies considerably. It is best isolated in the medial oblique view. The os peroneum generally is superimposed on the cuboid in the lateral and dorsoplantar views. However, it can be clearly identified in the lateral view if its position anatomically is more distal in the tendon; at this location it articulates with the anterior aspect of the cuboid's inferior tuberosity. This sesamoid may infrequently be found at a more proximal location, adjacent to the calcaneocuboid joint or anterior calcaneus. This latter entity may easily be misinterpreted as an avulsion fracture. Location of the os peroneum adjacent to the calcaneus as opposed to the cuboid may be variation[28] or may indicate a ruptured peroneal tendon with posterior sesamoid displacement.[29]

## Os Infranaviculare

An ossicle uncommonly found along the superior aspect of the naviculocuneiform joint is the os infranaviculare (Figure 8-51). It is best identified in the lateral view. This ossicle is seen infrequently along the superomedial aspect of the naviculocuneiform joint in the medial oblique view.

## Os Supranaviculare

The os supranaviculare is found along the superior aspect of the talonavicular joint (Figure 8-52). It is much more common than the os infranaviculare. Like the os infranaviculare, the os supranaviculare is typically found along the superior aspect of its respective joint, and infrequently superomedially. This ossicle has a multitude of configurations. It may appear as an entirely separate ossicle, as a continuation of the articular subchondral bone, or even as an attachment to the navicular. As with many of the accessory ossicles, it may be impossible to differentiate the os supranaviculare from an old, nonunion fracture.

## Os Supratalare

The accessory ossicle located along the superior surface of the talar head is known as the os supratalare (Figure 8-53). It typically is located over the ridge along the talar head/neck but may be seen distally over the head. It easily can simulate an old, ununited avulsion fracture and is only identified in the lateral view. Calcification of the talonavicular ligament may occasionally appear in the same location and mimic the appearance of an os supratalare.

## Accessory Navicular (Os Tibiale Externum)

An ossicle of varying size, shape, and position may be found adjacent to the navicular tuberosity (Figure 8-54). It is best identified in the lateral oblique view. The terms *accessory navicular* and *os tibiale externum* have been used interchangeably to identify this ossicle. However, some discre-

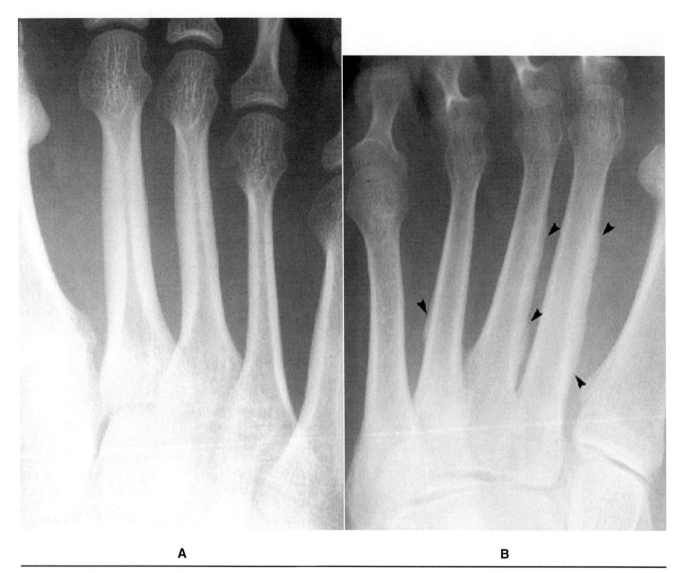

**A**

**B**

Figure 8-41    Variant architecture: Cortical bone. **A,** Cortical thickening, periosteal and endosteal, second and third metatarsals. **B,** Cortical thickening, periosteal, second, third, and fourth metatarsals.

pancy appears in the literature as to the definition and identification of this entity.

The ossicle that is found adjacent to the navicular tuberosity may either represent a sesamoid in the posterior tibial tendon or an accessory ossification center for the navicular tuberosity. The sesamoid characteristically is round, small, and located at a distance from the navicular tuberosity. The accessory ossification center, in contrast, is larger, oval or semicircular, and in close apposition to the tuberosity. Cartilage or fibrocartilage may attach it,[30] or it may articulate with the tuberosity, containing true synovial tissue.[31] Occasionally the accessory ossification center is fused to the tuberosity. This latter instance has been referred to as a "wraparound" navicular, cornuate or cornuted

navicular, gorilloid navicular, and the Kidner foot type. With so many varied presentations, one can see why the use of terminology for this ossicle has been confused!

Three distinct types of ossicles may be identified adjacent to the navicular tuberosity. Lawson[30] has classified them as follows:

*Accessory navicular type I:* sesamoid in the tendon
*Accessory navicular type II:* articulating accessory ossification center
*Accessory navicular type III:* fused accessory ossification center

This classification system best distinguishes between the varying forms of this enigma. The term *os tibiale externum*

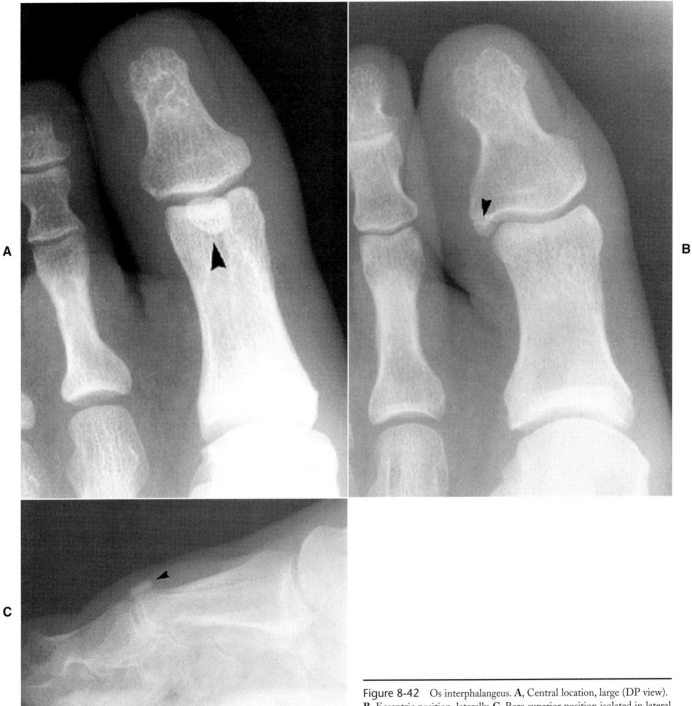

Figure 8-42   Os interphalangeus. **A,** Central location, large (DP view). **B,** Eccentric position, laterally. **C,** Rare superior position isolated in lateral view.

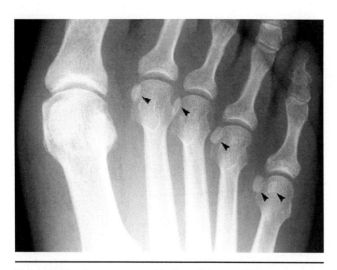

Figure 8-43　Accessory sesamoids: Second through fifth metatarsophalangeal joints.

should be used cautiously and applied only to the sesamoid entity (accessory navicular type I).

The accessory navicular type I may be partite. The partition could be either transverse or longitudinal. The articulation between the accessory navicular type II and navicular may be quite irregular and sclerotic. These findings most likely represent degenerative joint disease and can simulate the appearance of a hypertrophic nonunion fracture. Bone scintigraphy has been advocated for distinguishing between symptomatic and asymptomatic accessory navicular.[32]

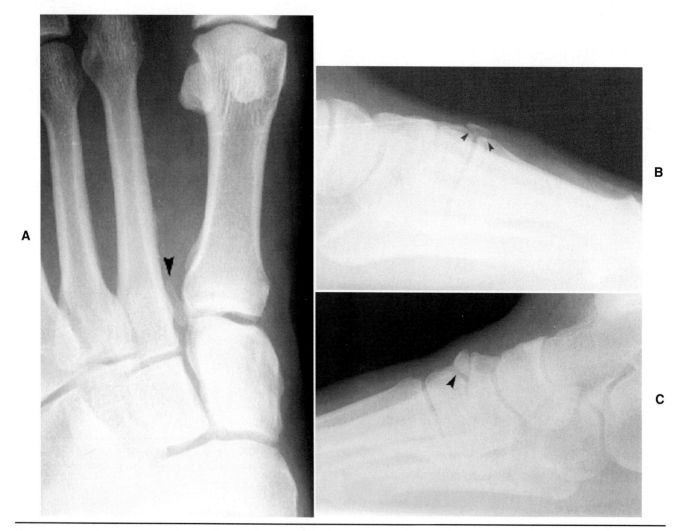

Figure 8-44　Os intermetatarseum. **A,** Long, linear. **B,** Large, triangular shape isolated in lateral view. **C,** Rare position at second metatarsocuneiform joint.

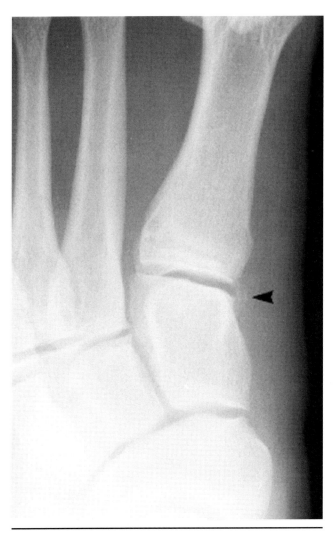

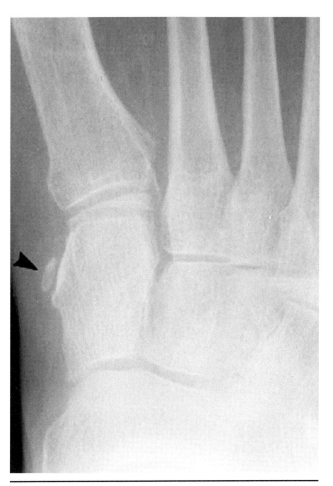

Figure 8-46    Os paracuneiforme?

Figure 8-45    Tibialis anterior tendon sesamoid: Adjacent to medial surface of medial cuneiform.

## Os Calcaneus Secundarius

The os calcaneus secundarius is best seen in the medial oblique view, adjacent to and in close apposition to the calcaneal anterior process along its superomedial surface (Figure 8-55). The ossicle is occasionally located centrally between the anterior calcaneus, talar head, cuboid, and navicular, especially when larger in size. It is not clearly seen in the lateral view because it is superimposed on the calcaneus and talus. The os calcaneus secundarius can be mistaken for a fracture of the anterior calcaneal process.

## Os Sustentaculum Tali

This rare ossicle, also known as the os sustentaculi, has been identified anatomically along the posterior aspect of the sustentaculum tali (Figure 8-56). It is best visualized with the axial view, although it is vaguely identified in the lateral view. Another rare condition that simulates this ossicle is known as the assimilated os sustentaculum tali.[12] Talocalcaneal coalition has been attributed to fusion of the os sustentaculum tali with the talus and calcaneus.[18,19] In support of this, Figure 8-56 demonstrates one case that reveals a large os sustentaculum tali in the one foot, a middle subtalar coalition in the opposite.

## Os Trochleare Calcanei

Rarely, an ossicle is found along the lateral aspect of the peroneal tubercle (or trochlea), between the peroneal tendons (Figure 8-57). It also has been referred to as the os calcaneus accessorius.[33] It is seen in the dorsoplantar or calcaneal axial views along the lateral surface of the anterior calcaneus, adjacent to the peroneal tubercle.

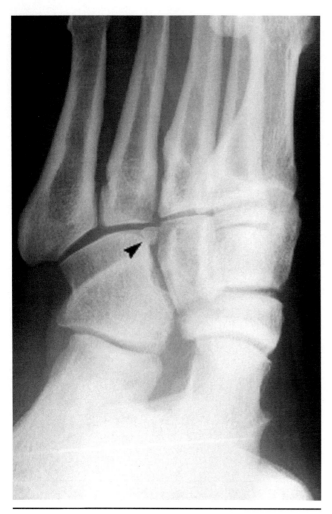

Figure 8-47   Os cuboid.

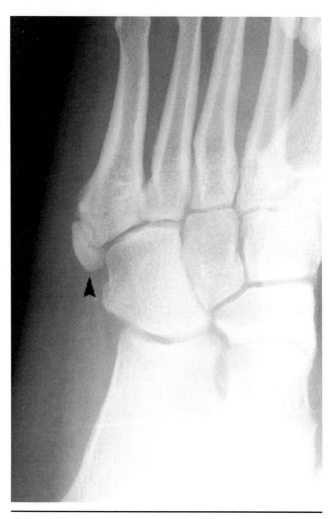

Figure 8-49   Persistent fifth-metatarsal apophysis.

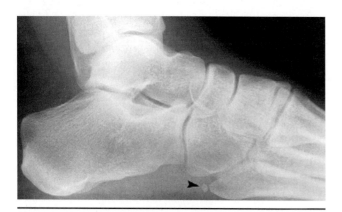

Figure 8-48   Os vesalianum (lateral view).

## Os Subcalcis

Another rare ossicle may be seen along the inferior aspect of the calcaneal tuberosity. This probably represents an unfused ossification center for the calcaneal apophysis. When it is located beneath the medial tuberosity, it is seen in the lateral view. However, when closely associated with the lateral tuberosity, it is clearly identified with the medial oblique view (see example in Chapter 9). Some reports describe instances of the os subcalcis in a more posteroinferior location. It is debatable whether or not this represents the same entity as the former.

## Os Aponeurosis Plantaris

An ossicle or ossicles located in the soft tissues of the plantar fascia has been referred to as the os aponeurosis plantare

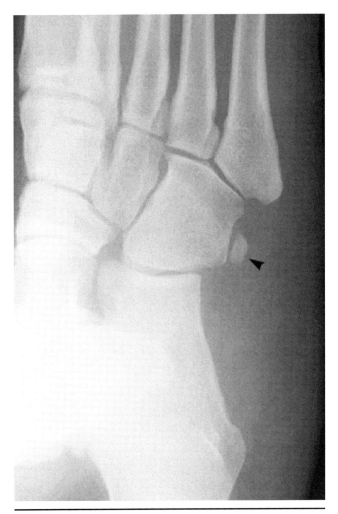

Figure 8-50    Os peroneum: Typical size and location adjacent to cuboid.

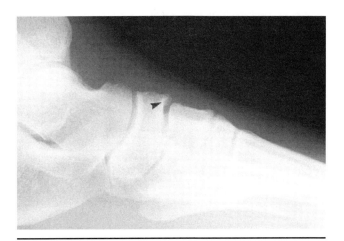

Figure 8-51    Os infranaviculare.

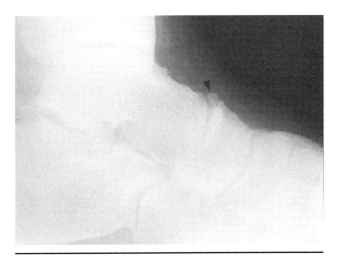

Figure 8-52    Os supranaviculare.

(Figure 8-58).[33] This entity may or may not be related to trauma (myositis ossificans).

## Os Trigonum

An accessory ossification center can be found along the posterior aspect of the talar posterolateral process (Figure 8-59). When fused to the talus, it is known as the trigonal (Stieda's) process. If it remains unfused and separate, it is known as the os trigonum. In either case, its inferior surface typically articulates with the calcaneus. The os trigonum may have a fibrous, fibrocartilaginous, or cartilaginous attachment to the talus.[16] A joint space may be identified between it and the posterior talus. Occasionally it may exhibit findings suggesting osteoarthritis. The size of this ossicle ranges from small to large. It is best seen in

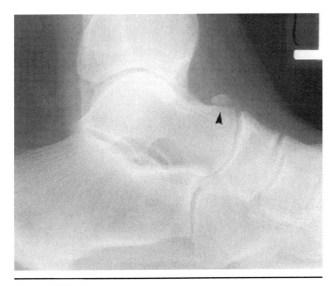

Figure 8-53    Os supratalare.

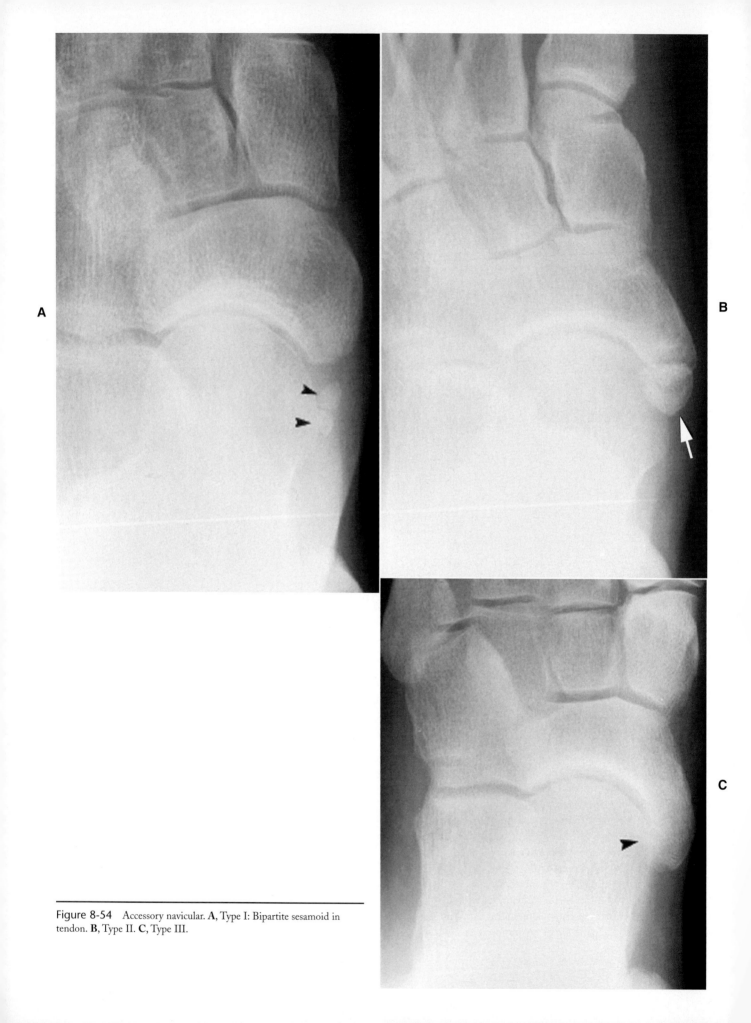

Figure 8-54   Accessory navicular. **A**, Type I: Bipartite sesamoid in tendon. **B**, Type II. **C**, Type III.

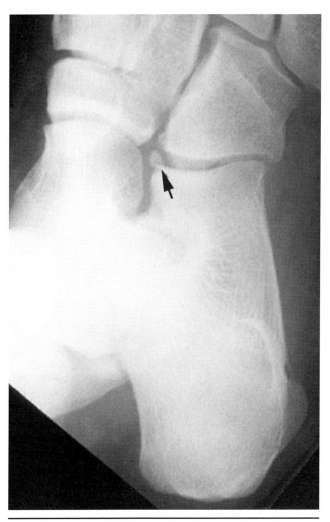

Figure 8-55   Os calcaneus secundarius.

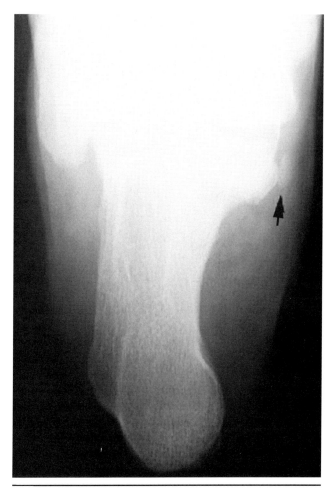

Figure 8-56   Os sustentaculum tali.

the lateral view but is infrequently viewed in the medial oblique view.

Bone scintigraphy may be a valuable diagnostic study for differentiation between symptomatic and asymptomatic os trigonum.[30] Focal intense uptake suggests degenerative disease and/or unhealed fracture.

## Os Supracalcaneum

The os supracalcaneum is an extremely rare ossicle (Figure 8-60). It is found along the superior surface of the posterior calcaneus. It can be mistaken for the os trigonum; however, the os supracalcaneum is not in direct apposition to the posterior talar process. The os supracalcaneum, when present, is large and not easily missed in the lateral view. Occasionally it is also found with an os trigonum just anterior to it.

## Os Talotibiale

An accessory ossicle infrequently seen along the anterior aspect of the ankle joint in the lateral view (Figure 8-61) is the os talotibiale. It is found in close apposition to the most anterior and inferior aspect of the tibia. It can easily be mistaken as a loose osseous body. However, the latter entity is usually associated with other degenerative findings. Rarely, an ossicle may present along the posterior aspect of the ankle joint. This unnamed ossicle, like the os talotibiale, is closely apposed to the tibia.

## Os Subtibiale

The os subtibiale is an ossicle found just inferior to the tibial malleolus (Figure 8-62). It varies considerably in size and shape, and can be mistaken for the following conditions: unfused malleolar accessory ossification center, loose osseous body, acute or nonunion avulsion fracture, and deltoid ligament ossification. It is directly apposed to the posterior

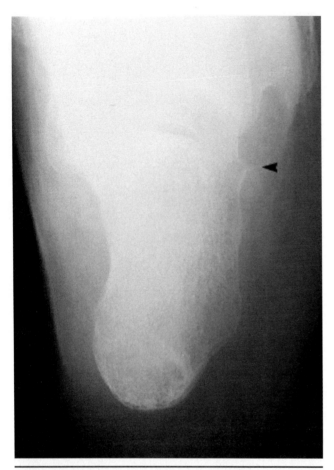

Figure 8-57   Os trochleare calcanei.

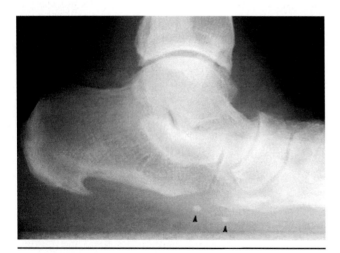

Figure 8-58   Os aponeurosis plantaris.

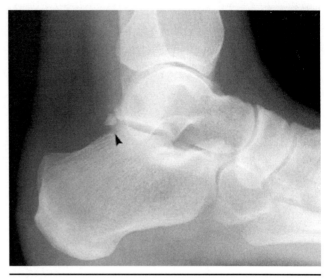

Figure 8-59   Os trigonum.

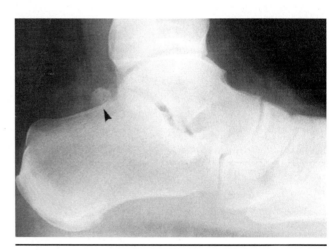

Figure 8-60   Os supracalcaneum.

colliculus of the tibial malleolus.[34] In contrast, malleolar avulsion fractures involve the anterior colliculus. This relationship is best appreciated in the lateral view. The os subtibiale and avulsion fracture may be impossible to differentiate from the anteroposterior and mortise ankle views alone.

## Os Subfibulare

An accessory ossicle found beneath the fibular malleolus is known as the os subfibulare (Figure 8-63). This can easily be misinterpreted as an avulsion fracture. Avulsion fractures of

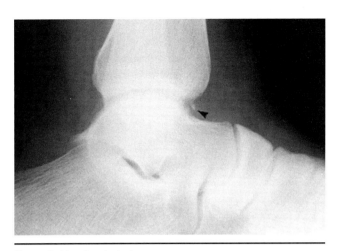

Figure 8-61    Os talotibiale.

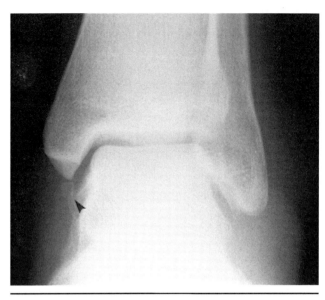

Figure 8-62    Os subtibiale.

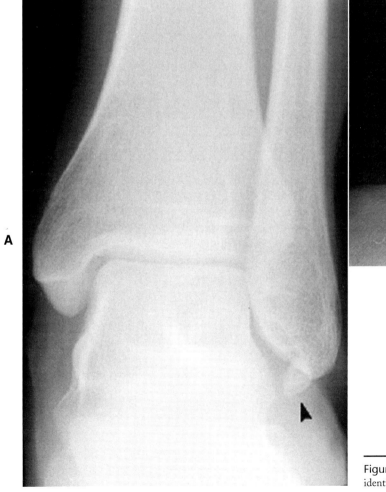

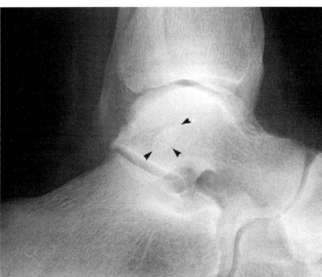

Figure 8-63    Os subfibulare. **A**, Anteroposterior view. **B**, Lateral view, identified along the anteroinferior margin of the fibular malleolus.

the fibular malleolus are usually ill defined and irregular. However, old, nonunion avulsion fractures may be identical in appearance to the accessory ossicle. The os subfibulare is seen in both the AP and mortise ankle views. It is not readily visible in the lateral view but can appear as a fairly well-defined increased density superimposed on the talus.

A large accessory ossification center for the fibular malleolus may be encountered in the same location as the os subfibulare. It has been shown to be directly related to ankle joint instability because of insertion of the calcaneofibular and/or anterior talocalcaneal ligaments and abnormal movement between the accessory ossification center and distal fibula.[35]

## References

1. *Dorland's illustrated medical dictionary*, ed 27, Philadelphia, 1988, Saunders.

2. Hlavac HF: Differences in x-ray findings with varied positioning of the foot, *J Am Podiatr Assoc* 57(10):465, 1967.

3. Winter WG, Iwerson LJ, Johnson ED: Lateral supporting ligament of the distal phalanx, *Foot Ankle* 9(6):310, 1989.

4. Shrewsbury M, Johnson RK: The fascia of the distal phalanx, *J Bone Joint Surg (Am)* 57A(6):784, 1975.

5. Lemont H, Christman RA: Subungual exostosis and nail disease and radiologic aspects. In Scher RK, Daniel CR: *Nails: Therapy, diagnosis, and surgery*, pp 250-257, Philadelphia, 1990, Saunders.

6. Lee M, Hodler J, Haghighi P et al: Bone excrescence at the medial base of the distal phalanx of the first toe: normal variant, reactive change, or neoplasia? *Skeletal Radiol* 21:161, 1992.

7. Sutro CJ, Sutro WH: Spool-shaped proximal pedal phalanges, *Bull Hosp Jt Dis* 46:122, 1986.

8. Saxby T, Vandemark RM, Hall RL: Coalition of the hallux sesamoids: a case report, *Foot Ankle* 13(6):355, 1992.

9. Bhargava KN, Malaviya G: Variations in the second metatarsal bone of man, *Indian J Med Sci* 15:100, 1961.

10. Morton DJ: Metatarsus atavicus, *J Bone Joint Surg* 9:531, 1927.

11. Resnick D: Talar ridges, osteophytes, and beaks: a radiologic commentary, *Radiology* 151:329, 1984.

12. Bloom RA, Libson E, Lax E et al: The assimilated os sustentaculi, *Skeletal Radiol* 15:455, 1986.

13. Ruiz JR, Christman RA, Hillstrom HJ: Anatomical considerations of the peroneal tubercle, *J Am Podiatr Med Assoc* 83(10):563, 1993.

14. Oestreich AE, Mize WA, Crawford AH et al: The "anteater nose": a direct sign of calcaneonavicular coalition on the lateral radiograph, *J Pediatr Orthopaed* 7:709, 1987.

15. Pfitzner W: Beiträge zur Kenntniss des menschlichen Extremitätenskelets. VII. Die Variationen im Aufbau des Fusskelets. In Schwalbe G: *Morphologischen Arbeiten*, vol 6, Jena, 1896, Fischer. (Cited in Webster FS, Roberts WM: Tarsal anomalies and peroneal spastic flatfoot, *JAMA* 146:1099, 1951.)

16. Sarrafian SK: *Anatomy of the foot and ankle*, Philadelphia, 1983, Lippincott.

17. Harris RI: Follow-up notes on articles previously published in the journal, *J Bone Joint Surg (Am)* 47A(8):1657, 1965.

18. Webster FS, Roberts WM: Tarsal anomalies and peroneal spastic flatfoot, *JAMA* 146:1099, 1951.

19. Harris RI, Beath T: Etiology of peroneal spastic flatfoot, *J Bone Joint Surg (Br)* 30B:624, 1948.

20. Lateur LM, Van Hoe LR, Van Ghillewe KV et al: Subtalar coalition: diagnosis with the C sign on lateral ankle radiographs of the ankle, *Radiology* 193:847, 1994.

21. Magilner AD: Normal roentgen variant: calcaneal nutrient canal, *Radiology* 136:10, 1980.

22. McCarthy DJ, Reed T, Abell N: The hallucal interphalangeal sesamoid, *J Am Podiatr Med Assoc* 76(6):311, 1986.

23. Reichmeister JP: The painful os intermetatarseum: a brief review and case reports, *Clin Orthop* 153:201, 1980.

24. Johnston FE, Lee RH: Anomalous accessory sesamoids associated with saddle deformity, *Curr Podiatr Med* (Jan-Feb):13, 1991.

25. Haliburton RA, Butt EG, Barber JR: The tibialis anterior sesamoid, *Can J Surg* 4:480, 1961.

26. Schmidt H, Freyschmidt J: *Kohler/Zimmer borderlands of normal and early pathologic findings in skeletal radiography*, ed 4, New York, 1993, Thieme Medical Publishers.

27. Shands AR: The accessory bones of the foot, *South Med Surg* (May):326, 1931.

28. Bloom RA: The infracalcaneal os peroneum, *Acta Anatomica* 140:34, 1991.

29. Thompson FM, Patterson AH: Rupture of the peroneus longus tendon. Report of three cases, *J Bone Joint Surg (Am)* 71A:293, 1989.

30. Lawson JP: Symptomatic radiographic variants in extremities, *Radiology* 157:625, 1985.

31. Lemont H, Travisano VL, Lyman J: Accessory navicular. Appearance of a synovial joint, *J Am Podiatr Assoc* 71(8):423, 1981.

32. Grogan DP, Gasser SI, Ogden JA: The painful accessory navicular: a clinical and histopathological study, *Foot Ankle* 10:164, 1989.

33. Trolle D: *Accessory bones of the human foot*, Copenhagen, Einar Munksgaard, 1948.

34. Coral A: The radiology of skeletal elements in the subtibial region: incidence and significance, *Skeletal Radiol* 16:298, 1987.

35. Karlsson J, Lansinger O: Separate centre of ossification of the lateral malleolus with instability of the ankle joint, *Arch Orthop Trauma Surg* 109:291, 1990.

## Suggested Readings

### General References on Variants

Bierman MI: The supernumerary pedal bones, *AJR* 9:404, 1922.

Birkner R: *Normal radiologic patterns and variances of the human skeleton*, Baltimore, 1978, Urban & Schwarzenberg.

Bizarro AH: On sesamoid and supernumerary bones of the limbs, *J Anat* 55:256, 1921.

Burman MS, Lapidus PW: The functional disturbances caused by the inconstant bones and sesamoids of the foot, *Arch Surg* 22:936, 1931.

Dwight T: *Variations of the bones of the hands and feet*, Philadelphia, 1907, Lippincott.

Geist ES: Supernumerary bones of the foot—a roentgen study of one hundred normal individuals, *Am Orthopedic Surg* 12:403, 1914.

Hark FW: Congenital anomalies of the tarsal bones, *Clin Orthop* 16:21, 1960.

Helal B: The accessory ossicles and sesamoids. In Helal B, Wilson D: *The foot*, vol 1, p 567, New York, 1988, Churchill-Livingstone.

Holland CT: On rarer ossifications seen during x-ray examinations, *J Anat* 55:235, 1921.

Kleinberg S: Supernumerary bones of the foot, *Ann Surg* 65:499, 1917.

O'Rahilly R: A survey of carpal and tarsal anomalies, *J Bone Joint Surg (Am)* 35A:626, 1953.

Pirie AH: Extra bones in the wrist and ankle found by roentgen rays, *AJR* 8:572, 1921.

### Partite Sesamoids

Dobas DC, Silvers MD: The frequency of partite sesamoids of the first metatarsophalangeal joint, *J Am Podiatr Assoc* 67(12):880, 1977.

Feldman F, Pochaczevsky R, Hecht H: The case of the wandering sesamoid and other sesamoid afflictions, *Radiology* 96:275, 1970.

Frankel JP, Harrington J: Symptomatic bipartite sesamoids, *JFS* 29(4):318, 1990.

Golding C: The sesamoids of the hallux, *J Bone Joint Surg (Br)* 42B(4):840, 1960.

Hubay CA: Sesamoid bones of the hands and feet, *AJR* 61(4):493, 1949.

Inge GAL, Ferguson AB: Surgery of the sesamoid bones of the great toe, *Arch Surg* 27:466, 1933.

Leonard MH: The sesamoids of the great toe: the pedal polemic, *Clin Orthop* 16:295, 1960.

Scranton PE, Rutkowski R: Anatomic variations in the first ray. II. Disorders of the sesamoids, *Clin Orthop* 151:256, 1980.

Walling AK, Ogden JA: Case report 666, *Skeletal Radiol* 20:233, 1991.

Weil LS, Hill M: Bipartite tibial sesamoid and hallux abducto valgus deformity: a previously unreported correlation, *JFS* 31(2):104, 1992.

### Bipartite Medial Cuneiform

Barclay M: A case of duplication of the internal cuneiform bone of the foot (cuneiforme bipartitum), *J Anat* 67: 175, 1932.

Dellacorte MP, Lin PJ, Grisafi PJ: Bilateral bipartite medial cuneiform, *J Am Podiatr Med Assoc* 82:475, 1992.

### Bipartite Navicular

de Fine Licht E: On bipartite os naviculare pedis, *Acta Radiol*, Stockholm 22:377, 1941.

Waugh W: Structural deformities of the outer third of the adult tarsal navicular, *Proceedings of the Royal Society of Medicine* 49:965-967, 1956.

Wiley JJ, Brown DE: The bipartite tarsal scaphoid, *J Bone Joint Surg (Br)* 63B:583, 1981.

### Supernumerary Bones

Acker I: Residuum of a supernumerary phalanx 30 years after surgery, *J Am Podiatr Assoc* 56:124, 1966.

Cole M: Three uncommon anomalies, *J Am Podiatr Assoc* 60:400, 1970.

Gold AG, Katz M, Comerford JS: Distal accessory phalanx of the foot, *J Am Podiatr Med Assoc* 80(6):323, 1990.

Rao BR: Supernumerary toe arising from the medial cuneiform, *J Bone Joint Surg (Am)* 61A:306, 1979.

Wishnie PA, London E, Porat S: Complete duplication of an accessory first ray, *JFS* 29(5):471, 1990.

### Absence of Bone

Carroll BW, Greenberg DC, Simpson RR: The two-phalanged fifth toe: development, occurrence and relation to heloma durum, *J Am Podiatr Assoc* 68(9):641, 1978.

Zinsmeister BJ, Edelman, R: Congenital absence of the tibial sesamoid: a report of two cases, *JFS* 24(4):266, 1985.

### Variants of Form

Berenter JS, Goldman FD: Surgical approach for enlarged

peroneal tubercles, *J Am Podiatr Med Assoc* 79(9):451, 1989.

Bisceglia CF, Sirota AD, Dull DD: An unusual case of hypertrophied peroneal tubercles, *J Am Podiatr Assoc* 73(9):481, 1983.

Scranton PE: Pathologic anatomic variations in the sesamoids, *Foot Ankle* 1(6):321, 1981.

Techner LM, DeCarlo RL: Peroneal tubercle osteochondroma, *JFS* 31(3):234, 1992.

*Synostosis/Coalition*

Agostinelli JR: Tarsal coalition and its relation to peroneal spastic flatfoot, *J Am Podiatr Med Assoc* 76(2):76, 1986.

Bonk JH, Tozzi MA: Congenital talonavicular synostosis, *J Am Podiatr Med Assoc* 79(4):186, 1989.

Bullitt JB: Variations of the bones of the foot. Fusion of the talus and navicular, bilateral and congenital, *AJR* 20:548, 1928.

Carson CW, Ginsburg WW, Cohen MD et al: Tarsal coalition: an unusual cause of foot pain: clinical spectrum and treatment in 129 patients, *Semin Arthritis Rheum* 20(6):367, 1991.

Cavallaro DC, Hadden HR: An unusual case of tarsal coalition, *J Am Podiatr Assoc* 68(2):71, 1978.

Cohen AH, Laugner TE, Pupp GR: Calcaneonavicular bar resection, *J Am Podiatr Med Assoc* 83(1):10, 1993.

Downey MS: Tarsal coalitions: a surgical classification, *J Am Podiatr Med Assoc* 81(4):187, 1991.

Frost RA, Fagan JP: Bilateral talonavicular and calcaneocuboid joint coalition, *J Am Podiatr Med Assoc* 85(6):339, 1995.

Green MR, Yanklowitz B: Asymptomatic naviculocuneiform synostosis with a ganglion cyst, *JFS* 31(3):272, 1992.

Hart DJ, Hart TJ: Iatrogenic metatarsal coalition: a postoperative complication of adjacent v-osteotomy, *JFS* 24(3):205, 1985.

Jack EA: Bone anomalies of the tarsus in relation to "peroneal spastic flatfoot," *J Bone Joint Surg (Br)* 36B:530, 1954.

Kashuk KB, Hanft JR, Schabler JA et al: An unusual intermetatarsal coalition, *J Am Podiatr Med Assoc* 81(7):384, 1991.

Keenleyside A, Mann RW: Unilateral ectrodactyly, metatarsal synostosis, and hypoplasia in an Eskimo, *J Am Podiatr Med Assoc* 81(1):18, 1991.

Kumar SJ, Guille JT, Lee MS et al: Osseous and non-osseous coalition of the middle facet of the talocalcaneal joint, *J Bone Joint Surg (Am)* 74A(4):529, 1992.

Lapidus PW: Congenital fusion of the bones of the foot; with a report of congenital astragaloscaphoid fusion, *J Bone Joint Surg* 14:888, 1932.

Pachuda NM, Lasday SD, Jay RM: Tarsal coalition: etiology, diagnosis, and treatment, *JFS* 29(5):474, 1990.

Page JC: Peroneal spastic flatfoot and tarsal coalitions, *J Am Podiatr Med Assoc* 77(1):29, 1987.

Palladino SJ, Schiller L, Johnson JD: Cubonavicular coalition, *J Am Podiatr Med Assoc* 81(5):262, 1991.

Pensieri SL, Jay RM, Schoenhaus HD et al: Bilateral congenital calcaneocuboid synostosis and subtalar joint coalition, *J Am Podiatr Med Assoc* 75(8):406, 1985.

Percy EC, Mann DL: Tarsal coalition: a review of the literature and presentation of 13 cases, *Foot Ankle* 9(1):40, 1988.

Perlman MD, Wertheimer SJ: Tarsal coalitions, *JFS* 25(1):58, 1986.

Person V, Lembach L: Six cases of tarsal coalition in children aged 4 to 12 years, *J Am Podiatr Med Assoc* 75(6):320, 1985.

Pontious J, Hillstrom HJ, Monahan T et al: Talonavicular coalition: objective gait analysis, *J Am Podiatr Med Assoc* 83(7):379, 1993.

Salomao O, Napoli MMM, de Carvalho AE et al: Talocalcaneal coalition: diagnosis and surgical management, *Foot Ankle* 13(5):251, 1992.

Schlefman BS, Ruch JA: Diagnosis of subtalar joint coalition, *J Am Podiatr Assoc* 72(4):166, 1982.

Takakura Y, Sugimoto K, Tanaka Y et al: Symptomatic talocalcaneal coalition, *Clin Orthop* 269:249, 1991.

Venning P: Variation of the digital skeleton of the foot, *Clin Orthop* 16:26, 1960.

Wiles S, Palladino SJ, Stavosky JW: Naviculocuneiform coalition, *J Am Podiatr Med Assoc* 78(7):355, 1988.

*Accessory Bones*

Helal B: The accessory ossicles and sesamoids. In Helal B, Wilson D, editors: *The foot*, New York, 1988, Churchill-Livingstone.

*Os Interphalangeus*

Genakos JJ: Clinical sign consistent with the hallucal interphalangeal sesamoid, *J Am Podiatr Med Assoc* 83(12):696, 1993.

*Os Intermetatarseum*

Henderson RS: Os intermetatarseum and a possible relationship to hallux valgus, *J Bone Joint Surg (Br)* 45B:117, 1963.

Scarlet JJ, Gunther R, Katz J et al: Os intermetatarseum-one, *J Am Podiatr Assoc* 68(6):431, 1978.

*Os Supranaviculare*

Miller GA, Black JR: Symptomatic os supranaviculare, *J Am Podiatr Med Assoc* 80(5):248, 1990.

Pacini AJ: Anomalies of the pedal scaphoid, *Am J Electrother Radiol* 39(6):217, 1921.

Pirie AH: A normal ossicle in the foot frequently diagnosed as a fracture, *Arch Radiol Electrother* 24:93, 1919.

*Accessory Navicular*

Anspach WE, Wright EB: The divided navicular of the foot, *Radiology* 29:725, 1937.

Chater EH: Foot pain and the accessory navicular bone, *Ir J Med Sci* 442:471, 1962.

Herrmann NP: An unusual example of a calcaneus secundarius, *J Am Podiatr Med Assoc* 82(12):623, 1992.

Mann RW: Calcaneus secundarius: Variation of a common accessory ossicle, *J Am Podiatr Med Assoc* 79(8):363, 1989.

Wood WA, Spencer AM: Incidence of os tibiale externum in clinical pes planus, *J Am Podiatr Assoc* 60(7):276, 1970.

Zadek I, Gold AM: The accessory tarsal scaphoid, *J Bone Joint Surg (Am)* 30A(4):957, 1948.

*Accessory Calcaneus*

Heller AG: Accessory calcaneus, *J Am Podiatr Med Assoc* 51:275, 1961.

*Os Trigonum*

Blake RL, Lallas PJ, Ferguson H: The os trigonum syndrome, *J Am Podiatr Med Assoc* 82(3):154, 1992.

Brodsky AE, Khalil MA: Talar compression syndrome, *Foot Ankle* 7:338, 1987.

Grogan DP, Walling AK, Ogden JA: Anatomy of the os trigonum, *J Pediatr Orthop* 10(5):618, 1990.

Hamilton, WG: Stenosing tenosynovitis of the flexor hallucis longus tendon and posterior impingement upon the os trigonum in ballet dancers, *Foot Ankle* 3:74, 1982.

Mann RW, Owsley DW: Os trigonum: variation of a common accessory ossicle of the talus, *J Am Podiatr Med Assoc* 80(10):536, 1990.

Marotta JJ, Micheli LJ: Os trigonum impingement in dancers, *Am J Sports Med* 20(5):533, 1992.

Martin BF: Posterior triangle pain: the os trigonum, *JFS* 28(4):312, 1989.

Reinherz RP: The significance of the os trigonum, *J Foot Surg* 18:61, 1979.

Wenig JA: Os trigonum syndrome, *J Am Podiatr Med Assoc* 80(5):278, 1990.

*Os Supracalcaneum*

Milgrom C, Kaplan L, Lax E: Case report 341: Quiz, *Skeletal Radiol* 15:150, 1986.

*Os Subfibulare*

Bowlus TH, Korman SF, DeSilvio M, Climo R: Accessory os subfibulare avulsion secondary to the inversion ankle injury, *J Am Podiatr Assoc* 70(6):302, 1980.

Mancuso JE, Hutchison PW, Abramow SP, Landsman MJ: Accessory ossicle of the lateral malleolus, *JFS* 30(1):52, 1991.

# CHAPTER 9

# Normal Development

ROBERT A. CHRISTMAN

The radiographic presentation, or ossification, of the pediatric foot and ankle varies considerably from patient to patient. It depends on the age and sex of the individual, and variation is frequently encountered. Ossification center time of appearance can vary not only between individuals but also within the same individual with respect to the other bones in the same extremity. The normal expectation learning curve, therefore, is much longer than that for radiographic anatomy of the adult foot and ankle, especially because pedal abnormalities are not as frequently seen in the pediatric patient as in the adult.

Evaluation of the pediatric skeleton requires observation of all the following:

1. Presence of the ossification centers
2. Orderly appearance of the ossification centers
3. Form (size and shape) of visible ossification centers
4. Relationships of one ossification center to another

Several authors have listed the time of appearance of primary and secondary ossification centers; Tables 9-1 through 9-4 summarize many of them.[1-3] In some instances you can see a range of appearance time, and these times may vary among authors. Especially note that the appearance time of ossification centers is earlier for females than for males. The sequence of fetal ossification (primary centers) of the foot bones is listed in Box 9-1.[4] Time of completion of ossification is listed in Table 9-5.

Describing the radiographic anatomy of the developing foot requires descriptions at numerous ages. However, one cannot simply show an example of a child's foot at ages 1, 2, 3, and so on, because ranges of ossification vary, as shown in Tables 9-1 through 9-4. I have reviewed numerous sets of radiographs of children at varying stages of development. Composite radiographs based primarily on the orderly appearance of primary and secondary ossification centers are illustrated in Figures 9-1 through 9-19. These examples adhere to the skeletal maturity indicators described by Hoerr, Pyle, and Francis.[5]

---

**TABLE 9-1**  Time of Appearance of Primary Ossification Centers: Male

|  | Garn | Acheson | | Sarrafian |
|---|---|---|---|---|
|  |  | Cleveland | Boston |  |
| Medial cuneiform | 11 mo-3 yr, 9 m | 1 yr, 2 mo-2 yr, 10 mo | 1 yr, 3 mo-2 yr, 11 mo | 1.9 yr |
| Intermediate cuneiform | 1 yr, 2 mo-4 yr, 3 mo | 1 yr, 8 mo-3 yr, 2 mo |  | 2.3 yr |
| Lateral cuneiform | 1 mo-1 yr |  | 0-10 mo | 4.4 mo |
| Cuboid | 1 mo-4 mo | 0-6 mo |  |  |
| Navicular | 1 yr, 1 mo-5 yr, 5 mo | 1 yr, 8 mo-4 yr | 1 yr, 10 mo-4 yr | 2.7 yr |

Compiled from Garn SM, Rohmann CG, Silverman FN: *Medical Radiogr Photogr* 43(2):45, 1967; Acheson RM: Maturation of the skeleton, in Falkner F, editor: *Human development*, Philadelphia, 1966, Saunders; and Sarrafian SK: *Anatomy of the foot and ankle*, p 32, Philadelphia, 1983, Lippincott.

**TABLE 9-2**  Time of Appearance of Primary Ossification Centers: Female

|  | Garn | Acheson | | Sarrafian |
|---|---|---|---|---|
|  |  | Cleveland | Boston |  |
| Medial cuneiform | 1.5 yr-2 yr, 10 mo | 9 mo-1 yr, 11 mo | 8 mo-2 yr | 1.3 yr |
| Intermediate cuneiform | 10 mo-3 yr | 1 yr, 1 mo-2 yr, 3 mo |  | 1.6 yr |
| Lateral cuneiform | 3 mo-1 yr, 3 mo |  | 0-8 mo | 3.8 mo |
| Cuboid | 1-2 mo | 0-4 mo |  |  |
| Navicular | 9 mo-3 yr, 7 mo | 4 yr-6 yr, 2 mo | 4 yr, 6 mo-6 yr, 5 mo | 2 yr |

Compiled from Garn SM, Rohmann CG, Silverman FN: *Med Radiogr Photogr* 43(2):45, 1967; Acheson RM: Maturation of the skeleton, in Falkner F, editor: *Human development*, Philadelphia, 1966, Saunders; and Sarrafian SK: *Anatomy of the foot and ankle*, p 32, Philadelphia, 1983, Lippincott.

**TABLE 9-3**  Time of Appearance of Secondary Ossification Centers: Male

|  |  | Garn | Acheson | | Sarrafian |
|---|---|---|---|---|---|
|  |  |  | Cleveland | Boston |  |
| Distal phalanx basal epiphysis | Hallux | 9 mo-2 yr, 1 mo | 11 mo-1 yr, 9 mo | 1 yr-1 yr, 10 mo | 1.3 yr |
|  | Toe 2 | 3 yr, 3 mo-6 yr, 9 mo | 3 yr, 9 mo-5 yr, 11 mo |  | 4.7 yr |
|  | Toe 3 | 3 yr-6 yr, 2 mo | 3 yr, 4 mo-5 yr, 6 mo |  | 4.4 yr |
|  | Toe 4 | 2 yr, 11 mo-6 yr, 5 mo | 3 yr, 5 mo-5 yr, 3 mo |  | 4.2 yr |
|  | Toe 5 | 2 yr, 4 mo-6 yr, 4 mo |  |  |  |
| Middle phalanx basal epiphysis | Toe 2 | 11 mo-4 yr, 1 mo |  |  |  |
|  | Toe 3 | 5 mo-4 yr, 3 mo |  |  |  |
|  | Toe 4 | 5 mo-2 yr, 11 yr |  |  |  |
|  | Toe 5 | 1 yr-3 yr, 10 mo |  |  |  |
| Proximal phalanx basal epiphysis | Hallux | 1 yr, 5 mo-3 yr, 4 mo | 1 yr, 11 mo-2 yr, 9 mo |  | 2.3 yr |
|  | Toe 2 | 1 yr-2 yr, 8 mo | 1 yr, 4 mo-2 yr, 2 mo |  | 1.7 yr |
|  | Toe 3 | 11 mo-2 yr, 6 mo | 1 yr, 1 mo-2 yr |  | 1.5 yr |
|  | Toe 4 | 11 mo-2 yr, 8 mo | 1 yr, 3 mo-2 yr, 1 mo |  | 1.6 yr |
|  | Toe 5 | 1 yr, 6 mo-3 yr, 8 mo | 2 yr-3 yr, 1 mo | 2 yr, 1 mo-3 yr, 5 mo | 2.2 yr |
| First-metatarsal basal epiphysis |  | 1 yr, 5 mo-3 yr, 1 mo | 2 yr-2 yr, 10 mo |  | 2.3 yr |
| First-metatarsal head epiphysis |  |  |  | 2-3 yr |  |
| Fibular sesamoid |  |  |  |  | 11 yr |
| Lesser-metatarsal head epiphysis | 2 | 1 yr, 11 mo-4 yr, 4 mo | 2 yr, 4 mo-3 yr, 6 mo |  | 2.8 yr |
|  | 3 | 2 yr, 4 mo-5 yr | 2 yr, 10 mo-4 yr, 2 mo |  | 3.4 yr |
|  | 4 | 2 yr, 11 mo-5 yr, 9 mo | 3 yr, 4 mo-4 yr, 8 mo |  | 3.9 yr |
|  | 5 | 3 yr, 1 mo-6 yr, 4 mo | 3 yr, 7 mo-5 yr, 4 mo | 3 yr, 6 mo-5 yr, 4 mo | 4.5 yr |
| Fifth-metatarsal apophysis |  |  |  |  | 11 yr-14 yr |
| Calcaneal apophysis |  | 5 yr, 2 mo-9 yr, 7 mo | 6 yr, 6 mo-8 yr, 7 mo | 6 yr, 2 mo-8 yr, 8 mo | 7.4 yr |
| Distal tibial epiphysis |  |  | 3 mo-6 mo | 2 mo-7 mo | 4.1 mo |
| Distal fibular epiphysis |  |  | 9 mo-1 yr, 5 mo | 8 mo-1 yr, 6 mo | 12.5 mo |
| Posterior talus (os trigonum) |  |  |  |  | 11.1±1.9 yr |

Compiled from Garn SM, Rohmann CG, Silverman FN: *Med Radiogr Photogr* 43(2):45, 1967; Acheson RM: Maturation of the skeleton, in Falkner F, editor: *Human development*, Philadelphia, 1966, Saunders; and Sarrafian SK: *Anatomy of the foot and ankle*, p 32, Philadelphia, 1983, Lippincott.

**TABLE 9-4** Time of Appearance of Secondary Ossification Centers: Female

| | | Garn | Acheson — Cleveland | Acheson — Boston | Sarrafian |
|---|---|---|---|---|---|
| Distal phalanx basal epiphysis | Hallux | 5 mo-1 yr, 8 mo | 5 mo-1 yr | 6 mo-1 yr, 4 mo | 10 mo |
| | Toe 2 | 1 yr, 6 mo-4 yr, 6 mo | 2 yr, 3 mo-3 yr, 9 mo | | 2.9 yr |
| | Toe 3 | 1 yr, 4 mo-4 yr, 1 mo | 2 yr, 1 mo-3 yr, 7 mo | | 3.2 yr |
| | Toe 4 | 1 yr, 4 mo-4 yr, 1 mo | 1 yr, 10 mo-3 yr, 2 mo | | 2.5 yr |
| | Toe 5 | 1 yr, 2 mo-4 yr, 1 mo | | | |
| Middle phalanx basal epiphysis | Toe 2 | 6 mo-2 yr, 3 mo | | | |
| | Toe 3 | 3 mo-2 yr, 6 mo | | | |
| | Toe 4 | 5 mo-3 yr | | | |
| | Toe 5 | 9 mo-2 yr, 1 mo | | | |
| Proximal phalanx basal epiphysis | Hallux | 11 mo-2 yr, 6 mo | 1 yr, 2 mo-2 yr | | 1.6 yr |
| | Toe 2 | 8 mo-2 yr, 1 mo | 10 mo-1 yr, 6 mo | | 1.1 yr |
| | Toe 3 | 6 mo-1 yr, 11 mo | 7 mo-1 yr, 3 mo | | 1.5 yr |
| | Toe 4 | 7 mo-2 yr, 1 mo | 7 mo-1 yr, 5 mo | | 1 yr |
| | Toe 5 | 1 yr-2 yr, 8 mo | 1 yr, 3 mo-2 yr, 3 mo | 1 yr, 4 mo-2 yr, 4 mo | 1.7 yr |
| First-metatarsal basal epiphysis | | Birth-2 yr, 3 mo | 1 yr, 3 mo-2 yr | | 1.6 yr |
| First-metatarsal head epiphysis | | | | | 2 yr-3 yr |
| Fibular sesamoid | | | | | 9 yr |
| Lesser-metatarsal head epiphysis | 2 | 1 yr, 3 mo-3 yr, 5 mo | 1 yr, 7 mo-2 yr, 5 mo | | 2 yr |
| | 3 | 1 yr, 2 mo-4 yr, 1 mo | 1 yr, 10 mo-2 yr, 11 mo | | 2.3 yr |
| | 4 | 1 yr, 9 mo-4 yr, 1 mo | 2 yr, 2 mo-3 yr, 4 mo | | 2.75 yr |
| | 5 | 2 yr, 1 mo-4 yr, 11 mo | 2 yr, 6 mo-4 yr | 2 yr, 8 mo-4 yr, 1 mo | 3.2 yr |
| Fifth-metatarsal apophysis | | | | | 9 yr-11 yr |
| Calcaneal apophysis | | 3 yr, 6 mo-7 yr, 4 mo | 4 yr-6 yr, 2 mo | 4 yr, 6 mo-6 yr, 5 mo | 5.4 yr |
| Distal tibial epiphysis | | | 2 mo-5 mo | 2 mo-7 mo | 3.7 mo |
| Distal fibular epiphysis | | | 6 mo-1 yr | 6 mo-1 yr, 1 mo | 9.1 mo |
| Posterior talus (os trigonum) | | | | | 8.1 yr ±1.3 yr |

Compiled from Garn SM, Rohmann CG, Silverman FN: *Med Radiogr Photogr* 43(2):45, 1967; Acheson RM: Maturation of the skeleton, in Falkner F, editor: *Human development*, Philadelphia, 1966, Saunders; and Sarrafian SK: *Anatomy of the foot and ankle*, p 32, Philadelphia, 1983, Lippincott.

**BOX 9-1** Sequence of Ossification of Fetal Foot

Sequence:
1st  Hallux distal phalanx and second, third, and fourth metatarsals
2nd  Second- through fifth-toe distal phalanges and the first and fifth metatarsals
3rd  Hallux and second-toe proximal phalanges
4th  Second-, third-, and fourth-toe proximal phalanges
5th  Second-, third-, and fourth-toe middle phalanges
6th  Fifth-toe middle phalanx
7th  Calcaneus
8th  Talus
9th  Cuboid

Compiled from Arey LB: *Developmental anatomy*, ed 7, p 104, Philadelphia, 1965, Saunders.

**TABLE 9-5** Completion of Ossification

| | Male (years) | Female (years) |
|---|---|---|
| Hallux distal phalanx basal epiphysis | 13.6-16 | 11.3-13.4 |
| Fifth-toe proximal phalanx basal epiphysis | 14.7-16.7 | 12.9-15.1 |
| Fifth-metatarsal head epiphysis | 14.8-16.7 | 13-15.3 |
| Medial cuneiform | 13.8-15.6 | 11.2-13.3 |
| Lateral cuneiform | 13.8-15.6 | 11-13.5 |
| Navicular | 13.8-15.6 | 11.1-13.3 |
| Calcaneal apophysis | 14.5-16.6 | 12.8-15.2 |
| Distal tibial epiphysis | 15.3-17.2 | 13.8-15.9 |
| Distal fibular epiphysis | 15.4-17.4 | 14-16.2 |

Compiled from Acheson RM: Maturation of the skeleton. In Falkner F, editor: *Human development*, Philadelphia, 1966, Saunders.

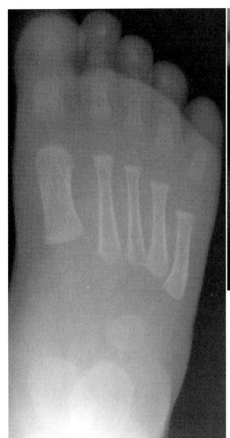

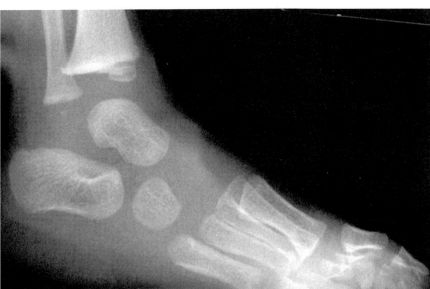

Figure 9-1   **A**, Dorsoplantar view. **B**, Lateral view. The following primary ossification centers are visible: most phalanges, all metatarsals, the cuboid, talus, calcaneus, distal tibia and fibula. The distal tibial and fibular secondary ossification centers are also visible.

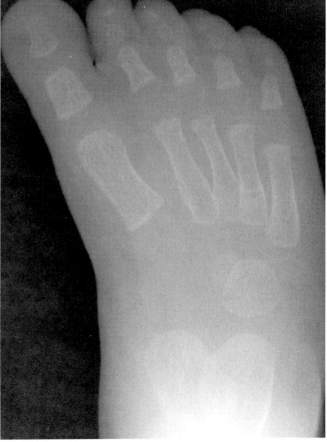

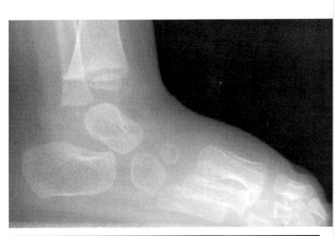

Figure 9-2   **A**, Lateral view. **B**, Dorsoplantar view. The lateral cuneiform ossification center is now visible.

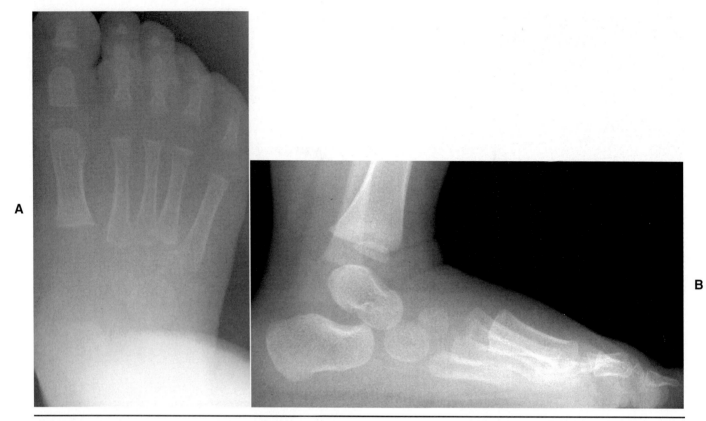

Figure 9-3    **A**, Dorsoplantar view. **B**, Lateral view. The hallux distal phalanx secondary ossification center (basal epiphysis) is visible.

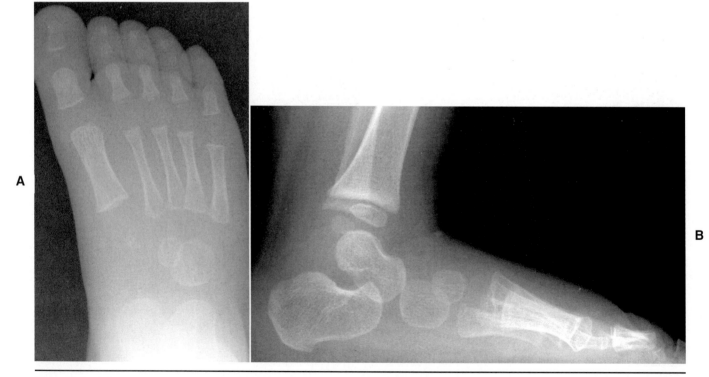

Figure 9-4    **A**, Dorsoplantar view. **B**, Lateral view. The medial cuneiform primary ossification and the lesser-toe proximal phalangeal secondary ossification centers (basal epiphyses) are now becoming visible.

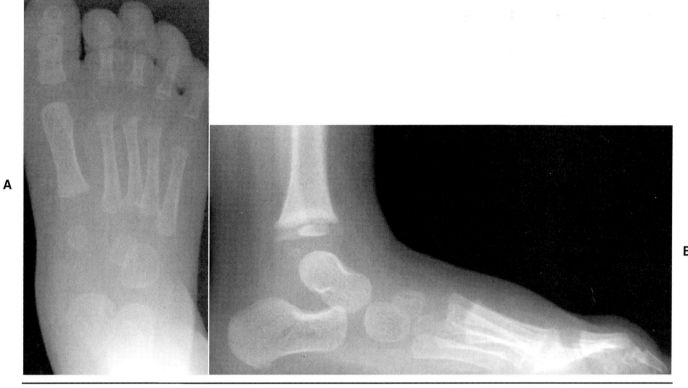

Figure 9-5    **A**, Dorsoplantar view. **B**, Lateral view. The hallux proximal phalanx and first-metatarsal secondary ossification centers (basal epiphyses) are barely visible.

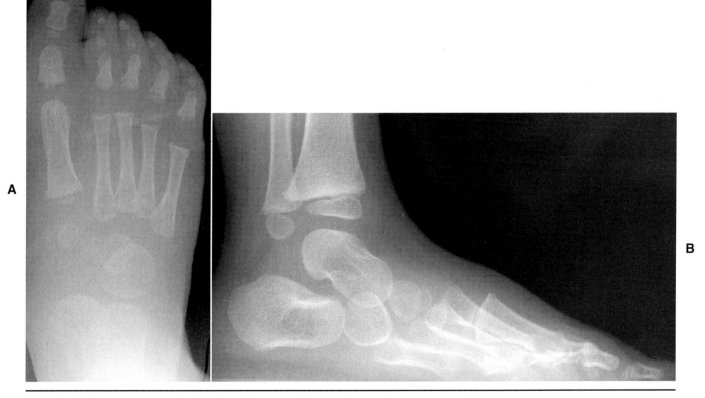

Figure 9-6    **A**, Dorsoplantar view. **B**, Lateral view. The intermediate cuneiform ossification center is visible.

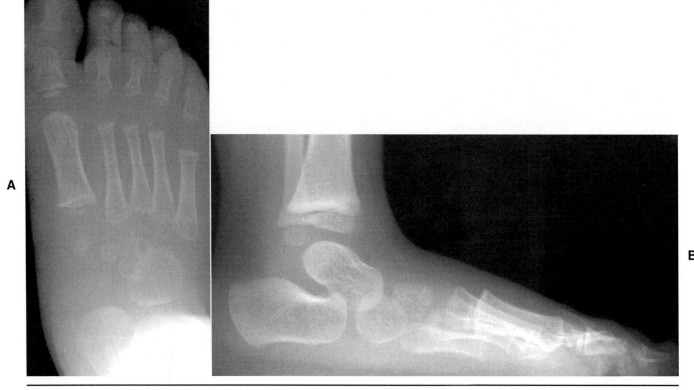

Figure 9-7   **A**, Dorsoplantar view. **B**, Lateral view. The navicular ossification center is visible.

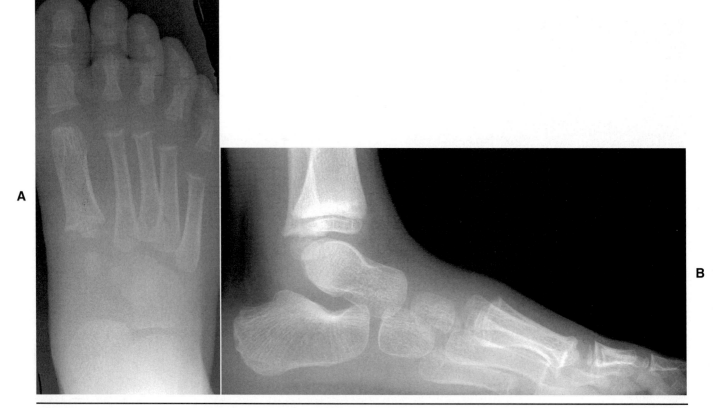

Figure 9-8   **A**, Dorsoplantar view. **B**, Lateral view. The lesser metatarsal secondary ossification centers (distal epiphyses) are beginning to ossify. The first-metatarsal distal epiphysis (sometimes referred to as the pseudoepiphysis), when present, may also be seen.

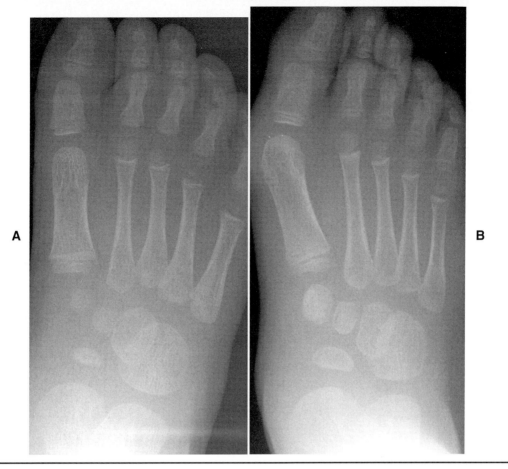

Figure 9-9  **A,** Dorsoplantar view. **B,** Lateral view. The middle phalanx secondary ossification centers (basal epiphyses) are visible.

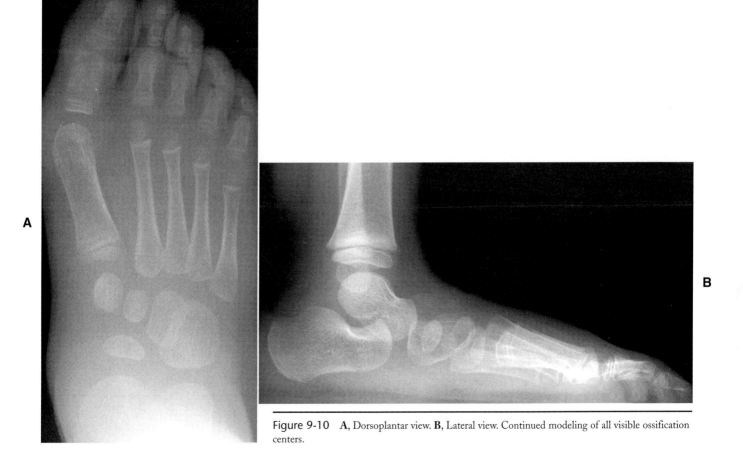

Figure 9-10  **A,** Dorsoplantar view. **B,** Lateral view. Continued modeling of all visible ossification centers.

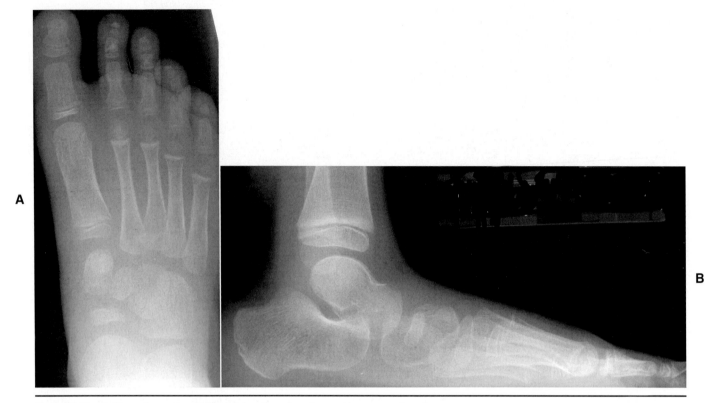

Figure 9-11   **A,** Dorsoplantar view. **B,** Lateral view. Posterior calcaneus becomes roughened.

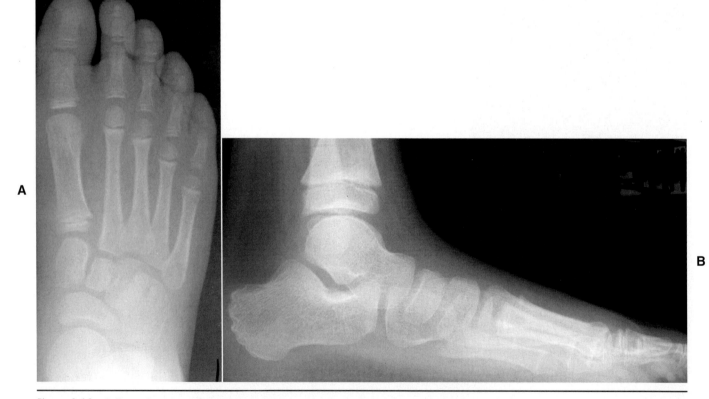

Figure 9-12   **A,** Dorsoplantar view. **B,** Lateral view. Posterior calcaneus (metaphysis) becomes jagged.

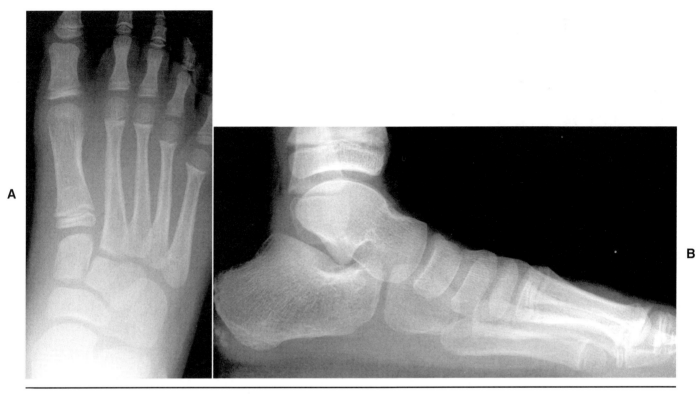

Figure 9-13   **A,** Dorsoplantar view. **B,** Lateral view. Early ossification of calcaneal apophysis (secondary epiphysis) is visible.

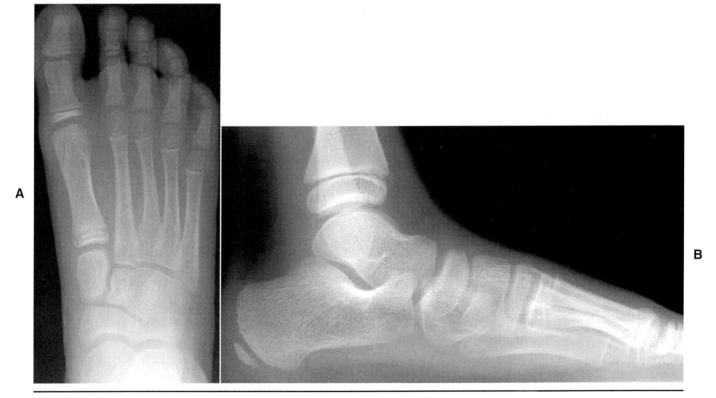

Figure 9-14   **A,** Dorsoplantar view. **B,** Lateral view. Continued ossification of calcaneal apophysis.

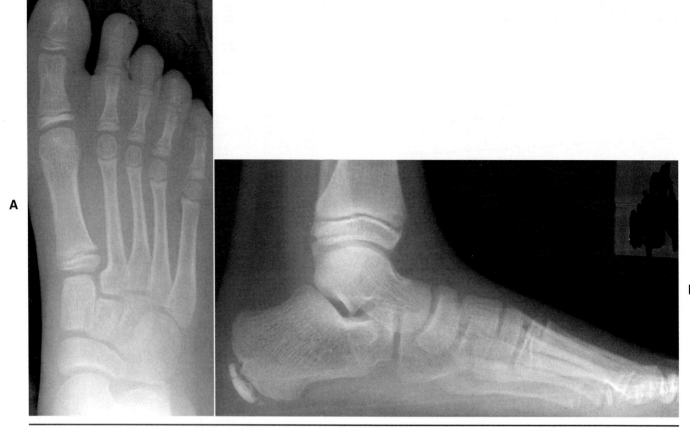

Figure 9-15   **A,** Dorsoplantar view. **B,** Lateral view. Calcaneal apophysis appears sclerotic relative to calcaneal body.

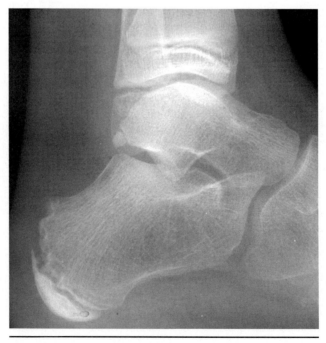

Figure 9-16   Lateral view. Ossification of os trigonum.

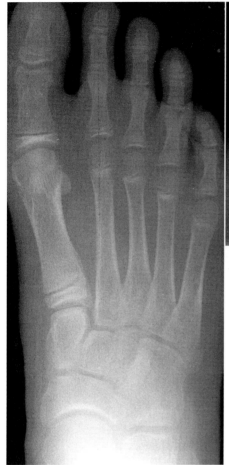

A

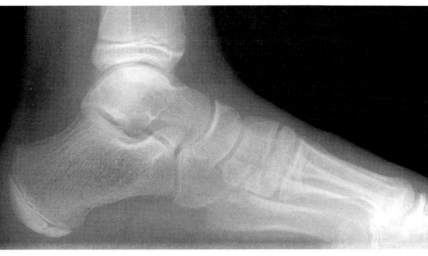

B

Figure 9-17   **A**, Dorsoplantar view. **B**, Lateral view. Fifth-metatarsal apophysis (basal epiphysis/tuberosity) is visible, as are the sesamoids.

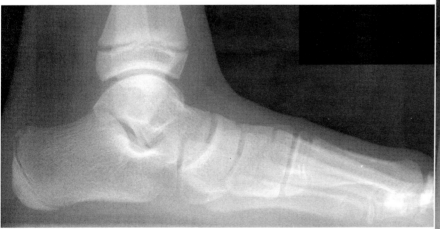

A

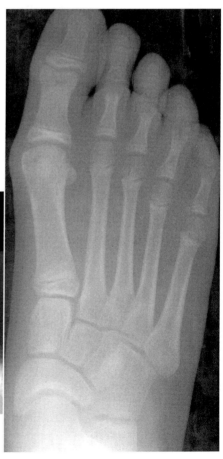

B

Figure 9-18   **A**, Lateral view. **B**, Dorsoplantar view. Continued ossification of all centers, especially calcaneal apophysis.

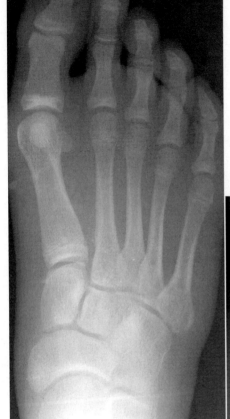

A

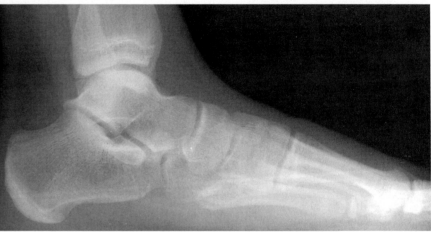

B

Figure 9-19  **A**, Dorsoplantar view. **B**, Lateral view. Physes are beginning to close at multiple sites.

## References

1. Garn SM, Rohmann CG, Silverman FN: Radiographic standards for postnatal ossification and tooth calcification, *Med Radiogr Photogr* 43(2):45, 1967.
2. Acheson RM: Maturation of the skeleton. In Falkner F, editor: *Human development*, Philadelphia, 1966, Saunders.
3. Sarrafian SK: *Anatomy of the foot and ankle*, p 32, Philadelphia, 1983, Lippincott.
4. Arey LB: *Developmental anatomy*, ed 7, p 104, Philadelphia, 1965, Saunders.
5. Hoerr NL, Pyle SI, Francis CC: *Radiographic atlas of skeletal development of the foot and ankle*, Springfield, Ill, 1962, Charles C Thomas.

## Suggested Readings

Acheson RM, Vicinus JH, Fowler GB: Studies in the reliability of assessing skeletal maturity from x-rays. III. The methods contrasted, *Human Biology* 38:204, 1966.

Bareither D: Prenatal development of the foot and ankle, *J Am Podiatr Med Assoc* 85(12):753, 1995.

Blass BC: A preliminary study of the fetal skeleton of the human foot, *J Am Podiatr Assoc* 63(1):12, 1973.

Cheng X, Wang Y, Qu H, Jiang Y: Ossification processes and perichondral ossification groove of Ranvier: a morpho-logical study in developing human calcaneus and talus, *Foot Ankle* 16(1):7, 1995.

Chung T, Jaramillo D: Normal maturing distal tibia and fibula: changes with age at MR imaging, *Radiology* 194:227, 1995.

Ferguson AB, Gingrich RM: The normal and the abnormal calcaneal apophysis and tarsal navicular, *Clin Orthop* 10:87, 1957.

Gardner E, Gray DJ, O'Rahilly R: The prenatal development

of the skeleton and joints of the human foot, *J Bone Joint Surg (Am)* 41A(5):847, 1959.

Gould N, Moreland M, Alvarez R et al: Development of the child's arch. *Foot Ankle* 9(5):241, 1989.

Graham CB: Assessment of bone maturation—methods and pitfalls, *Radiol Clin North Am* 10:185, 1972.

Harris EJ: The relationship of the ossification centers of the talus and calcaneus to the developing bone, *J Am Podiatr Assoc* 66(2):76, 1976.

Hensinger RN: *Standards in pediatric orthopedics. Tables, charts, and graphs illustrating growth*, New York, 1986, Raven Press.

Hubbard AM, Meyer JS, Davidson RS et al: Relationship between the ossification center and cartilaginous anlage in the normal hindfoot in children: study with MR imaging, *AJR* 161:849, 1993.

Keats TE, Smith TH: *An atlas of normal developmental roentgen anatomy*, ed 2, Chicago, 1988, Mosby.

Keats TE: *Atlas of roentgenographic measurement*, ed 6, St. Louis, 1990, Mosby.

Kuhns LR, Poznanski AK: Radiological assessment of maturity and size of the newborn infant, *CRC Crit Rev Diagn Imaging* 12(3):245, Jan 1980.

Meschan I: *Roentgen signs in diagnostic imaging*, ed 2, vol 2, Philadelphia, 1985, Saunders.

O'Rahilly R, Gardner E, Gray DJ: The skeletal development of the foot, *Clin Orthop* 16:7, 1960.

O'Rahilly R, Gray DJ, Gardner E: Chondrification in the hands and feet of staged human embryos, *Contrib Embryol* 36:185, 1957.

Senior HD: The chondrification of the human hand and foot skeleton, *Anat Rec* 42:35, 1929 (abstr).

Vilaseca RR, Ribes ER: The growth of the first metatarsal, *Foot Ankle* 1(2):117, 1980.

# CHAPTER 10

# Developmental Variants

ROBERT A. CHRISTMAN

The number of variations in the adult foot may appear overwhelming, but at least they are of one developmental age group, that is, mature. In contrast, consider all the variations that might occur at all different developmental stages! And the radiographic appearance of one child's foot at age 5 may be considerably different from another child's at the same chronological age. Fortunately the variants of development are not that numerous and are primarily seen during the earlier stages of development; the reader should, however, refer to Chapter 9 for the varying radiographic presentations seen during skeletal development.

Developmental variants may easily be mistaken for pathology. The more frequent variants are multiple primary or secondary ossification centers, the presence of epiphyses and physes at sites other than the expected locations, and variants of form. A jagged metaphysis adjacent to the physis, for example, may suggest abnormality. Accessory ossicles may be seen, but usually only later in skeletal development. Also, don't be surprised to see the initial appearance of an ossification center much earlier or even later than expected.

Confusion exists regarding the terms *epiphysis* and *apophysis*. An epiphysis is defined as "a part or process of a bone that ossifies separately and later becomes ankylosed to the main part of the bone."[1] This is typically seen at the end of a tubular bone. In contrast, an apophysis is "any outgrowth or swelling, especially a bony outgrowth that has never been entirely separated from the bone of which it forms a part, such as a process, tubercle, or tuberosity."[2] Although the secondary center of ossification for the calcaneus is not a tubular bone, the calcaneal "apophysis" is really an epiphysis based on the preceding definitions. The same holds true for the secondary center of ossification at the base of the fifth metatarsal.

## ◼ MULTIPLE OSSIFICATION CENTERS

Both primary and secondary (that is, epiphyseal) ossification centers can radiographically appear to ossify from multiple sites. These findings typically are asymptomatic and have been associated with a heterogeneous group of disorders known as the osteochondroses[3] (see Chapter 20). Generally speaking, the radiographic picture of multiple centers of ossification is a variant of normal and occurs frequently.

The irregular bones of the midtarsus are often affected; it is rare to see the primary centers of tubular bones ossify from multiple areas. The more commonly affected midtarsal bones are the medial cuneiform and navicular (Figures 10-1 and 10-2, respectively). Depending on the stage of development, appearance can vary considerably. The presence of multiple navicular ossification centers alone is not diagnostic of the osteochondrosis known as Kohler's disease. In fact, in most cases, radiographs of these same patients years later show normal ossification (Figure 10-3).

Rarely, the calcaneus may appear to ossify from two centers (Figure 10-4); this has been called the bifid calcaneus.[4,5] Characteristically, the calcaneus in this situation develops from a larger posterior and smaller anterior segment.[6]

The persistence of two separate primary ossification centers into adulthood is known as a bipartition. The precursor to bipartition may be seen in the developing skeleton; it not uncommonly affects the sesamoid, albeit later in development,[7] and rarely the medial cuneiform, navicular, and talus[8,9] bones.

Secondary centers (the epiphyses) frequently ossify from multiple sites, especially of the tubular bones.[10] This ossification is most evident in the metatarsals and calcaneus. Other sites affected include the fifth-metatarsal tuberosity epiphysis, the hallux proximal phalanx basal epiphysis, and the distal tibial epiphysis. Except for the lesser-metatarsal head epiphyses, partitioning of the remaining secondary ossification centers may be mistaken for fracture. Multiple secondary ossification centers seem always to coalesce into one center, although the entire center may remain separate from its adjacent primary ossification center (the persistent fifth-metatarsal tuberosity epiphysis, for example).

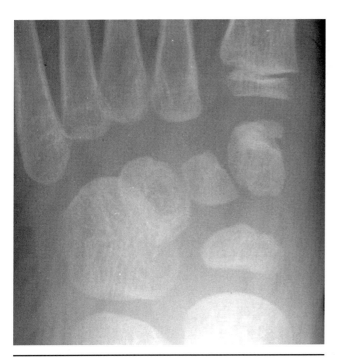

Figure 10-1    Multiple ossification centers, medial cuneiform, in a 5-year-old male.

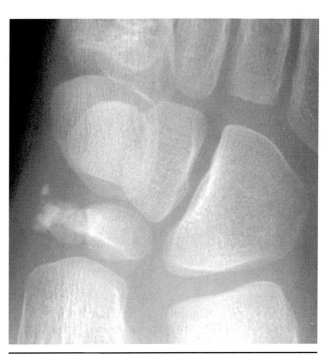

Figure 10-2    Multiple ossification centers, navicular, in a 7-year-old male (medial oblique view).

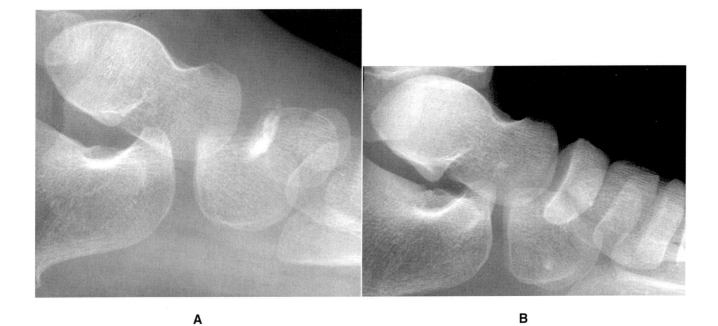

**A**                                                                                  **B**

Figure 10-3    Variant navicular ossification can easily be misdiagnosed as Kohler's disease. **A,** Sclerotic fragmented appearance at 4 years of age (asymptomatic). **B,** Normal navicular ossification at 8 years of age in the same patient.

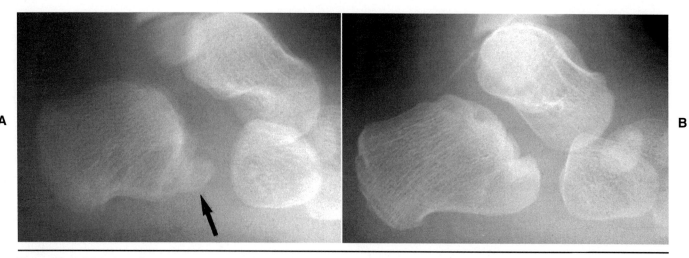

Figure 10-4    Multiple ossification centers, calcaneus. **A,** Smaller, separate ossification center anteriorly. **B,** One year later, the two ossification centers are united.

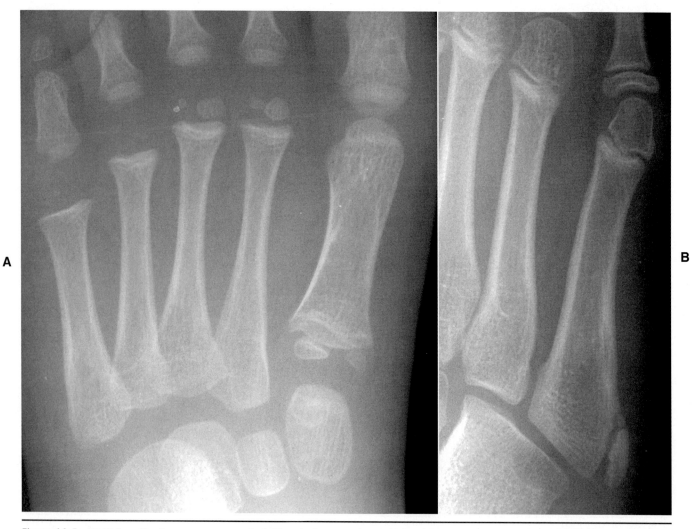

Figure 10-5    Multiple ossification centers, metatarsals. **A,** Bipartite first, second, and third metatarsals (5-year-old male). **B,** Bipartite fifth-metatarsal tuberosity epiphysis.

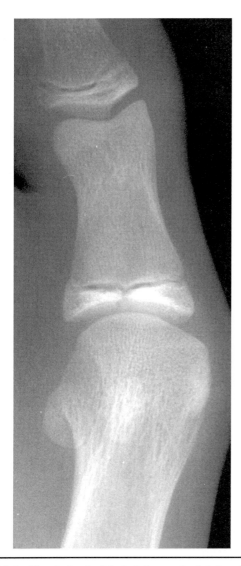

**Figure 10-6**  Bipartite basal epiphysis, hallux proximal phalanx (a unilateral finding in this patient).

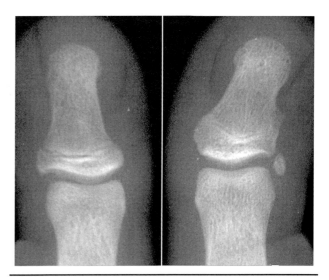

**Figure 10-7**  Bipartite basal epiphysis, hallux distal phalanx, in a 15-year-old male (unilateral finding). Note the different form of the adjacent epiphysis and metaphysis compared to the opposite foot.

It is not uncommon to see a metatarsal epiphysis ossify from two, sometimes three centers (Figure 10-5). However, not all metatarsal epiphyseal centers need be bipartite in the same foot or even bilaterally. Furthermore, their size and shape may not be symmetric.

The hallux phalangeal epiphyseal centers may develop from two ossification sites. Segmentation of the hallux proximal phalanx epiphysis is known as a bipartite basal epiphysis and can easily mimic a fracture (Figure 10-6). Typically, the bipartition is off center, the medial segment being the larger of the two. It may or may not present bilaterally. Partition of the distal phalanx basal epiphysis may be the precursor of the eccentric os interphalangeus in the adult (Figure 10-7).

The calcaneal epiphysis characteristically appears with multiple ossification centers radiographically (Figure 10-8). These centers are often irregular in outline and easily mimic fracture or osteochondrosis (so-called Sever's disease). However, this apparent "fragmentation" of the epiphysis is entirely normal. At first ossification begins postero-inferiorly; later ossification extends inferiorly to include the tuberosities and superiorly the bursal projection. At times an ossification center for the lateral tuberosity may be very large and suggest the development of an os subcalcis (Figure 10-9).

Irregular segmentation of the fifth-metatarsal tuberosity epiphysis is also frequent (Figure 10-10). And don't be quick to interpret segmentation of the distal tibial epiphysis as fracture (Figure 10-11).

## PSEUDOEPIPHYSES

Secondary ossification centers may appear to present at locations in addition to the normally expected epiphyseal sites. Typical sites in the foot include the head of the first metatarsal and the bases of the second through fourth metatarsals. The terms *pseudoepiphysis* and *supernumerary epiphysis* have been used to describe these variants in the forefoot. Lachman[11] differentiates between the two types radiographically as follows: *Pseudoepiphysis* refers to "those epiphyses that show a bony bridge connecting them with the shaft," and *supernumerary epiphysis* presents as a "truly independent center." However, these two types more likely represent the same entity at varying stages of development

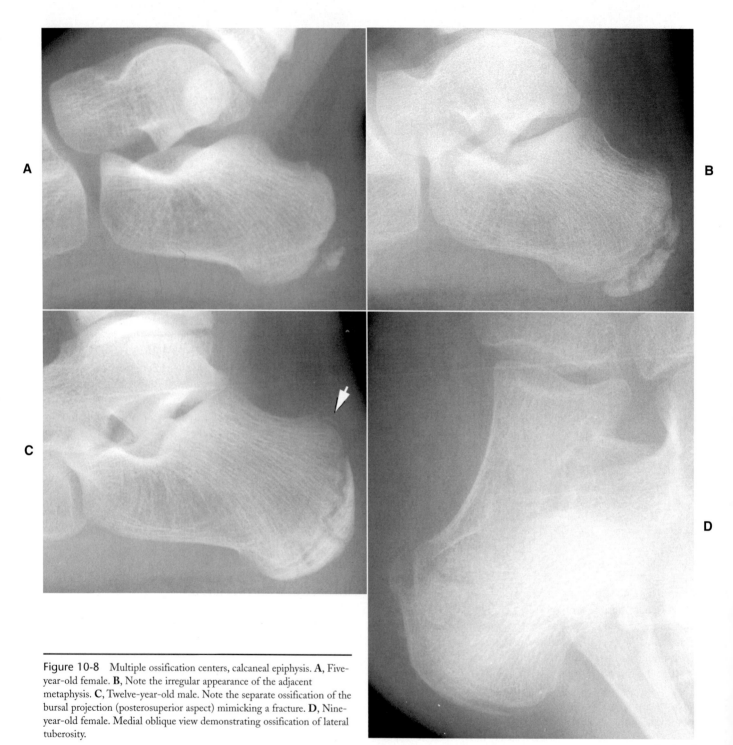

Figure 10-8  Multiple ossification centers, calcaneal epiphysis. **A**, Five-
year-old female. **B**, Note the irregular appearance of the adjacent
metaphysis. **C**, Twelve-year-old male. Note the separate ossification of the
bursal projection (posterosuperior aspect) mimicking a fracture. **D**, Nine-
year-old female. Medial oblique view demonstrating ossification of lateral
tuberosity.

*Continued*

**E**

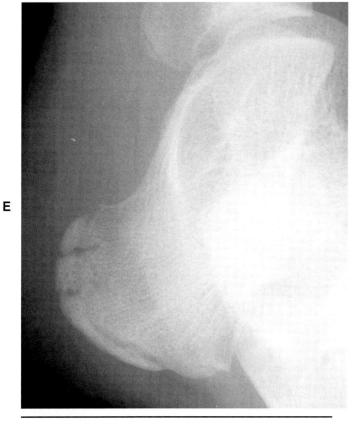

Figure 10-8, cont'd   Multiple ossification centers, calcaneal epiphysis. **E**, Thirteen-year-old male. Lateral oblique view demonstrating ossification of medial tuberosity.

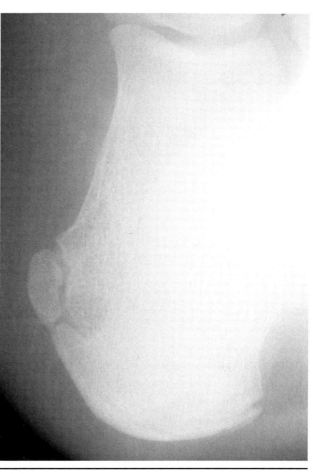

Figure 10-9   Separate, large ossification center for the lateral tuberosity in a 14-year-old male (medial oblique view) This center eventually united with the parent bone 2 years later.

(see Figure 10-16). Furthermore, discrepancy exists regarding the histology of this enigma. Ogden and associates have demonstrated that this is not a true epiphysis but an extension of the metaphysis (hence, pseudo-epiphysis).[12] In contrast, Vilaseca claims that it histologically and anatomically resembles all other physes.[13] Another study has shown that this entity is actually quite common.[14]

Radiographically, the first-metatarsal pseudoepiphysis appears to develop similar to other secondary ossification centers; however, as ossification increases, superimposition and early closure of the physis give the appearance of incomplete development (Figure 10-12). I have also noticed consistent hypertrophy of the adjacent distal metaphysis laterally and superiorly (Figure 10-13).

Pseudoepiphyses may also be seen along the bases of the second, third, and fourth metatarsals. Initially the

developing bases appear irregular; separate ossification centers may or may not be easily visualized, again depending on the amount of superimposition and the stage of development (Figure 10-14).

## ACCESSORY EPIPHYSES

Occasionally an epiphyseal accessory center of ossification may be seen for the medial malleolus (Figure 10-15).

Histologically this ossification center is continuous with the adjacent distal tibial epiphysis.[15] In his review of 100 radiographs, Powell found the incidence of a separate tibial malleolus ossification center in 20 children and a separate fibular malleolus center in 1 child.[16] Persistence of a tibial or fibular malleolus accessory ossification center is known as an os subtibiale or subfibulare, respectively.

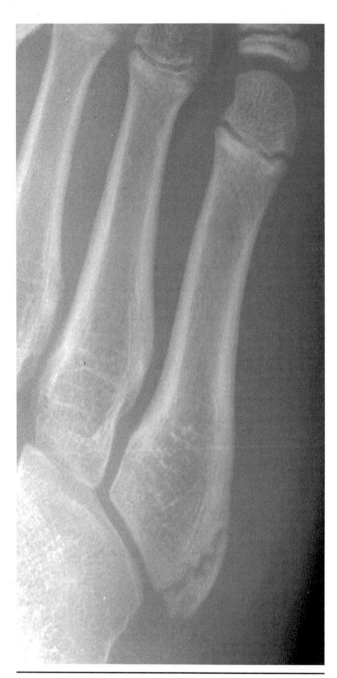

Figure 10-10   Irregular, multiple ossification centers for the fifth-metatarsal tuberosity epiphysis.

## ABSENT OSSIFICATION CENTERS

Absence of a primary ossification center, especially tarsal or metatarsal, results in an anomaly (see Chapter 8). However, it is not uncommon to have absence of secondary ossification centers in the lesser toes. Absence of the middle phalangeal basal epiphysis is most common (Figure 10-16). Absence of the distal phalanx basal epiphysis can accompany synostosis.

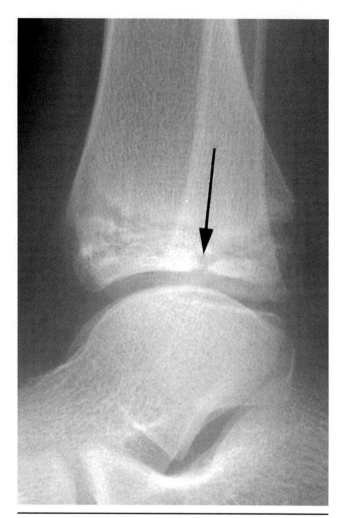

Figure 10-11   Segmentation (bipartition) of the distal tibial epiphysis, lateral view (a bilateral finding).

## ACCESSORY OSSICLES

An ossification center may be seen for any of the accessory ossicles mentioned in Chapter 8. Typically such centers appear during the later stages of development. Examples include the accessory sesamoid, os intermetatarseum, accessory navicular, and os supranaviculare.

It is not uncommon to see a separate center of ossification for the talar posterior process in the younger child. During development this center may unite with the parent bone; if it remains separate, it is known as the *os trigonum* (Figure 10-17).

The os subcalcis is extremely rare to see in the adult. Although the lateral tuberosity ossifies later in development as part of the calcaneal epiphysis (see Figures 10-8, *D*, and

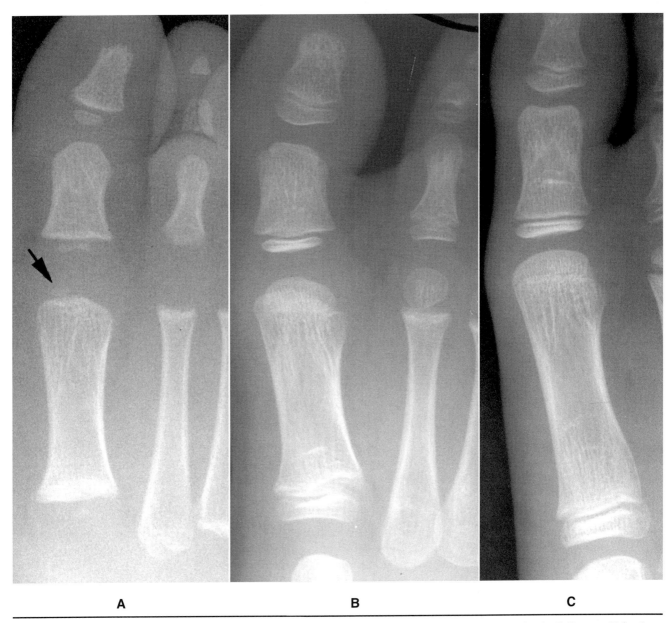

**Figure 10-12**   First-metatarsal distal epiphysis at varying stages of development. **A**, Two-year-old male. **B**, Five-year-old male. **C**, Six-year-old female.

10-9), I have seen a large, separate ossification in a young child before the calcaneal epiphysis had ossified. This example appears similar to the reverse calcaneal spur (see later) except that the outline of a superimposed ossicle can be visualized.

## TARSAL COALITION

Obvious tarsal coalition is not usually seen radiographically until the second decade, although the talonavicular coalition

can be seen earlier.[17] Coalitions have been discussed and illustrated in Chapter 8.

## VARIANTS OF FORM

### Phalanges

Clefts are frequently seen in the heads of the phalanges. They mimic the appearance of a supernumerary epiphysis, except that they are only at the margins of the phalanx and do not completely cross it. The cleft seen in the hallux

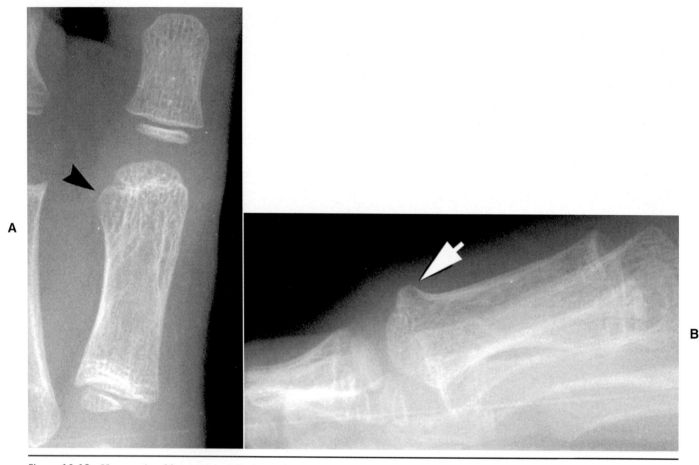

Figure 10-13 Hypertrophy of first-metatarsal distal metaphysis adjacent to distal epiphysis. **A,** Lateral hypertrophy (dorsoplantar view). **B,** Superior hypertrophy (lateral view).

proximal phalanx head is more often found only on its lateral side, although it may be seen both medially and laterally (Figure 10-18). It may either run transversely or obliquely. Clefts also are seen in the lesser-toe middle and proximal phalanges. Those in the middle phalanges more resemble that seen in the hallux (Figure 10-19); proximal phalangeal clefts are subtle in appearance.

Epiphyses of the lesser-toe phalanges occasionally are triangular in shape. They have also been called bell- or cone-shaped epiphyses. The proximal, middle, or distal phalangeal basal epiphyses may be affected (Figure 10-20).

A rare variant of form that affects small tubular bones is known as the longitudinal *epiphyseal bracket*.[18] Jones originally suggested the term "delta phalanx" to describe this deformity in the middle phalanx of a finger: "[T]he bone is triangular in shape and has a continuous epiphysis running from the proximal to the distal end along the shortened side."[19] Although this entity has been associated with anomalies such as polydactyly,[20,21] it may present solely as varus congenitus in the hallux.[22] Figure 10-21 shows an example of the longitudinal epiphyseal bracket in a second-toe middle phalanx. In this case the epiphysis is seen laterally and communicates with what could be interpreted as a cleft in the head. The lateral side of this bone is short relative to the medial side, resulting in lateral angulation of the distal phalanx at the interphalangeal joint. This may be related to the adult skeletal variant pictured in Figure 8-12 on page 150.

Other phalangeal variants include "exostoses" originating from the distal metaphyses of the proximal phalanges (Figure 10-22), short phalanges secondary to early physeal closure (Figure 10-23), absent ungual tuberosities (Figure 10-24), and circular radiolucencies in the shafts of proximal phalanges (Figure 10-25).

## Metatarsals

As noted earlier, hypertrophy along the first-metatarsal distal metaphysis has been associated with the super-numerary epiphysis. The first-metatarsal basal epiphysis can vary in its form, especially at its junction with the metaphysis (Figure 10-26). Irregular outline of the proximal

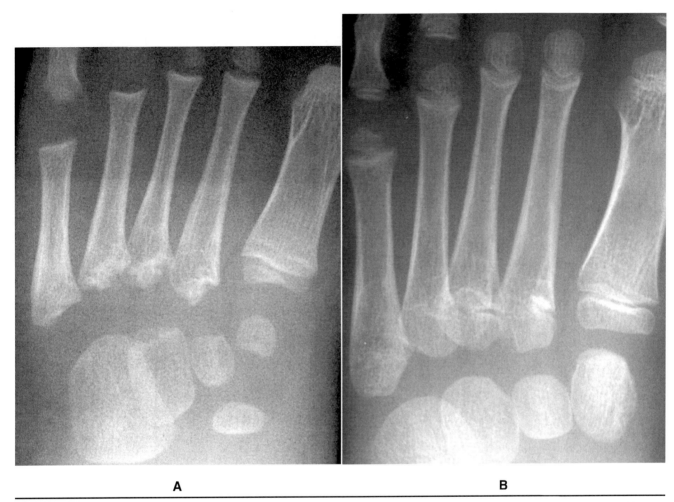

|   A   |   B   |

**Figure 10-14**  Supernumerary epiphyses at the bases of the second, third, and fourth metatarsals. **A,** Rarely, epiphyseal ossification is represented by irregular metaphyseal margins and superimposed epiphyses (2-year-old female). **B,** Epiphyses and metaphyses well defined later in development (5-year-old male).

ends of the second through fourth metatarsals is not uncommon and may indicate early ossification of supernumerary epiphyses (Figure 10-27). Early physeal closure causes short metatarsal length.

## Tarsal Bones

The metaphysis adjacent to the posterior calcaneal epiphysis frequently appears jagged (Figure 10-28). This finding is entirely normal and should not be mistaken for pathology. It typically is symmetric in presentation bilaterally. Another unusual variation is known as the *reverse calcaneal spur*. This infrequent entity is seen very early in development (within the first two years) and later disappears. It has been

described in both boys and girls.[23,24] The spur may either point posteriorly, anteriorly, or directly vertical (Figure 10-29). Other calcaneal variants include a "hole" in the neutral triangle, and unusual shape overall (Figure 10-30). Variant shape of the talus may also be seen (Figure 10-31).

The distal tibial epiphysis is very irregular in form. In both the anteroposterior (or mortise) and lateral ankle views, the physis appears widened medially and anteriorly, respectively (Figure 10-32). This common finding should not be misinterpreted as pathologic.

Occasionally a lucent defect is seen along the lateral aspect of the distal tibial metaphysis in the anteroposterior or mortise ankle views (Figure 10-33). This finding may or may not present bilaterally.

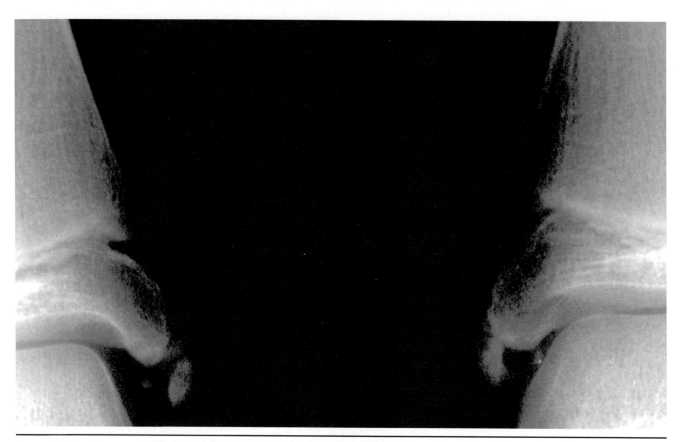

Figure 10-15    Accessory ossification center for the tibial malleolus (7-year-old female).

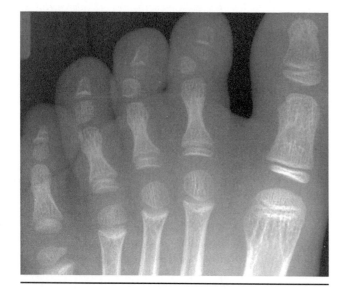

Figure 10-16    Absent phalangeal basal epiphysis. Middle phalanx epiphyses of all lesser toes are absent (5-year-old male).

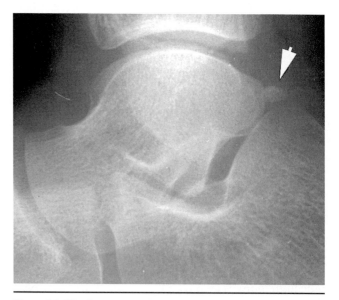

Figure 10-17    Os trigonum. Early ossification (9-year-old male).

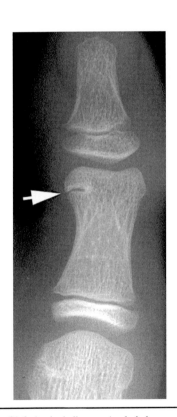

Figure 10-18   Clefts in the hallux proximal phalanx positioned laterally and oriented transversely (10-year-old male).

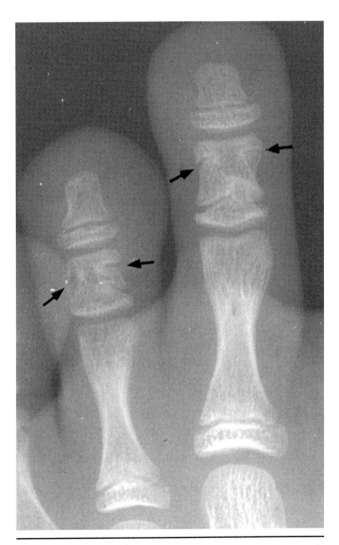

Figure 10-19   Middle phalangeal clefts second toe (medial and lateral) (10-year-old female).

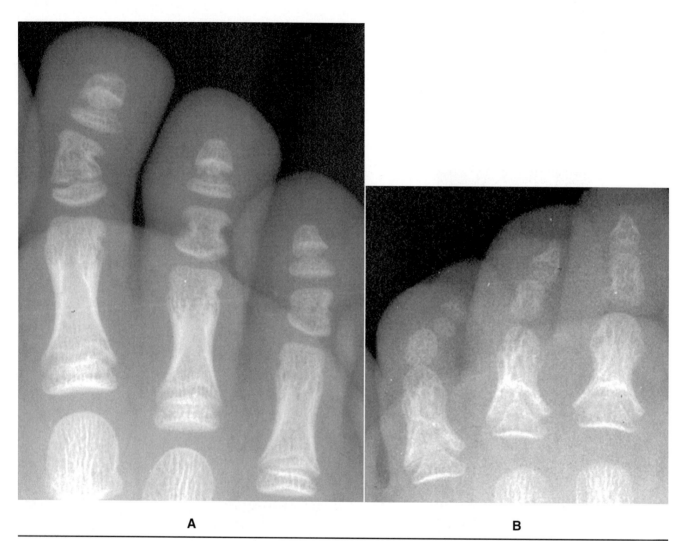

**A**                                        **B**

Figure 10-20   Triangular (bell- or cone-shaped) epiphyses. **A**, Distal phalanges (10-year-old male). **B**, Proximal phalanges (5-year-old male).

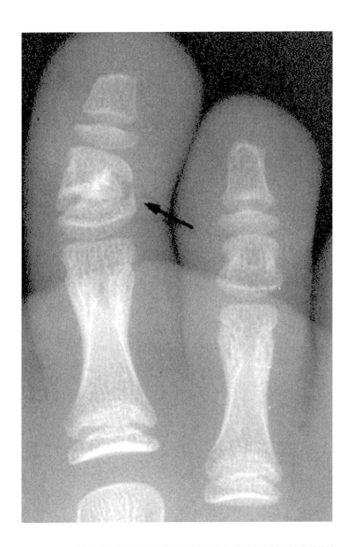

Figure 10-21   Longitudinal epiphyseal bracketing second-digit middle phalanx, a bilateral finding (11-year-old male).

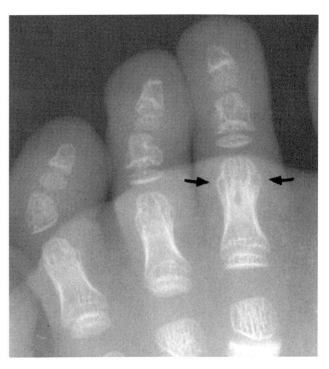

Figure 10-22   Hypertrophy of the margins of the proximal phalangeal distal metaphyses.

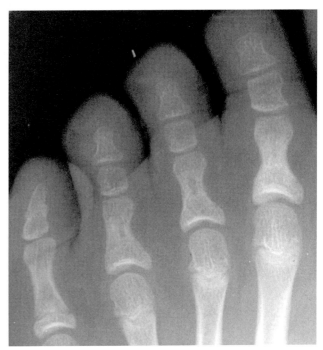

Figure 10-23   Short second-, third-, and fourth-toe proximal phalanges caused by premature physeal closure (10-year-old female).

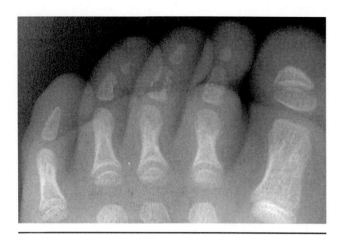

Figure 10-24    Absent ungual tuberosities (5-year-old female).

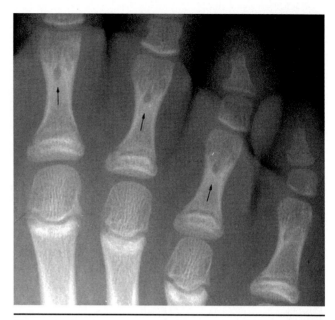

Figure 10-25    Circular radiolucencies in the diaphyses of the second-through fourth-toe proximal phalanges, a bilateral finding (10-year-old female).

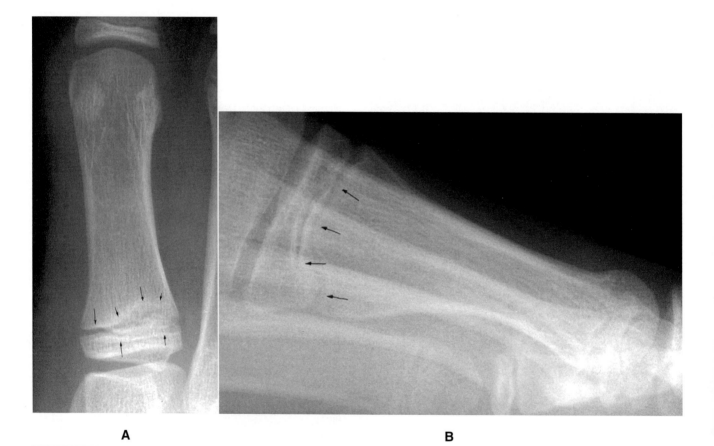

A

B

Figure 10-26    Irregular outline of first-metatarsal basal physis and adjacent metaphysis and epiphysis (12-year-old male). **A,** Dorsoplantar view. **B,** Lateral view.

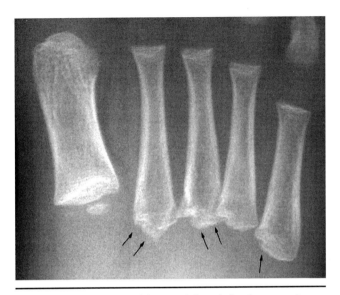

Figure 10-27   The bases of the second through fourth metatarsals are quite irregular, possibly initial ossification of supernumerary epiphyses (2-year-old male).

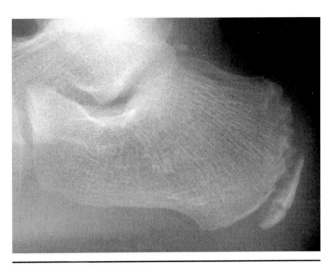

Figure 10-28   Jagged posterior calcaneal metaphysis at varying stages of development (10-year-old male).

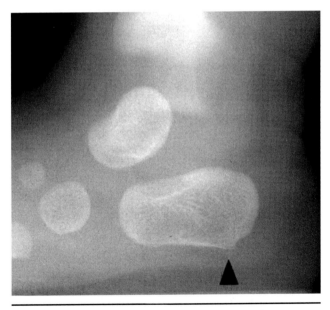

Figure 10-29   Reverse calcaneal spur (6-month-old male).

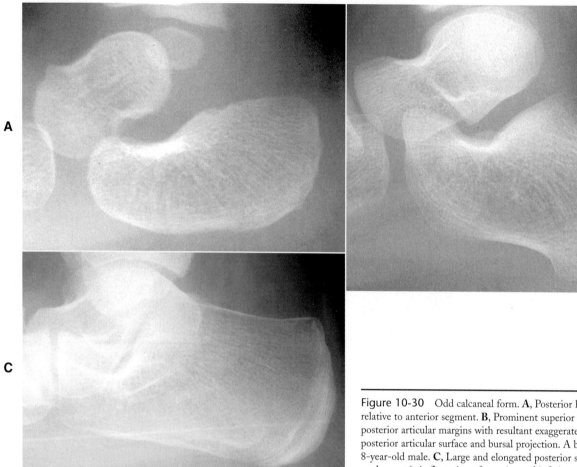

Figure 10-30   Odd calcaneal form. **A**, Posterior half is very large relative to anterior segment. **B**, Prominent superior aspects of anterior and posterior articular margins with resultant exaggerated concavity between posterior articular surface and bursal projection. A bilateral finding in this 8-year-old male. **C**, Large and elongated posterior section with uncharacteristic flattening of superior and inferior surfaces, present bilaterally.

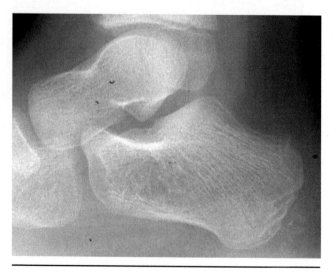

Figure 10-31   Elongated talar head and neck relative to the body in a 5-year-old female.

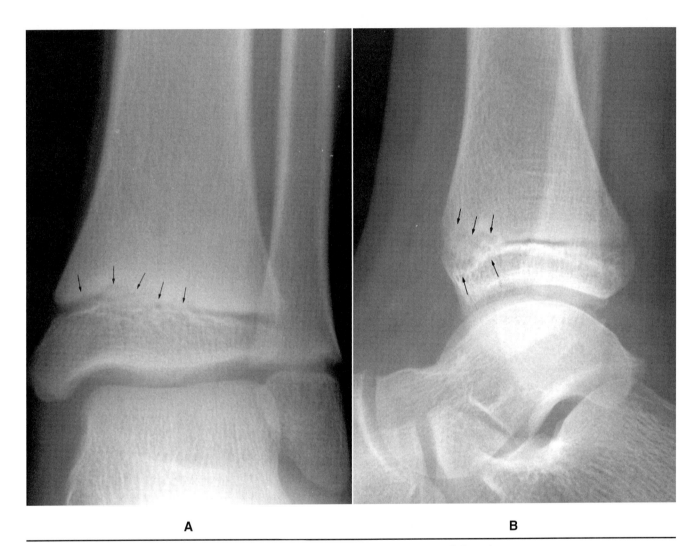

**A**                                              **B**

Figure 10-32   Irregular outline of distal tibial physis (9-year-old female). **A,** Anteroposterior view. **B,** Lateral view.

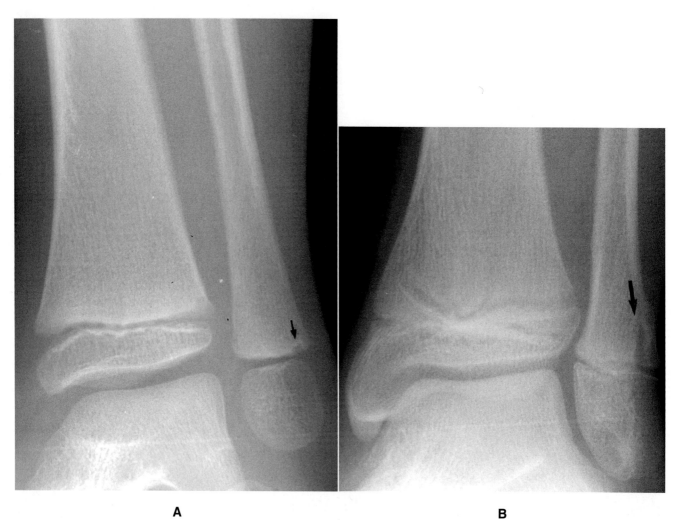

**A**                                    **B**

Figure 10-33    Lucent defect at distal fibular metaphysis. **A**, Six-year-old male. **B**, Thirteen-year-old male.

## References

1. *Webster's medical desk dictionary*, Springfield, Mass, 1986, Merriam-Webster.

2. *Dorland's illustrated medical dictionary*, ed 25, Philadelphia, 1974, Saunders.

3. Resnick D: *Bone and joint imaging*, Philadelphia, 1989, Saunders.

4. Schmidt H, Freyschmidt J: *Kohler/Zimmer borderlands of normal and early pathologic findings in skeletal radiology*, ed 4, New York, 1993, Thieme Medical Publishers.

5. Szaboky GT, Anderson JJ, Wiltsie RA: Bifid os calcis, *Clin Orthop* 68:136, 1970.

6. Ogden JA: Anomalous multifocal ossification of the os calcis, *Clin Orthop* 162:113, 1982.

7. Feldman F, Pochaczevsky R, Hecht H: The case of the wandering sesamoid and other sesamoid afflictions, *Radiology* 96:275, 1970.

8. Schreiber A, Differding P, Zollinger H: Talus partitus, *J Bone Joint Surg (Br)* 67B(3):430, 1985.

9. Weinstein SL, Bonfiglio M: Unusual accessory (bipartite) talus simulating fracture, *J Bone Joint Surg (Am)* 57A(8):1161, 1975.

10. Roche AF, Sunderland S: Multiple ossification centres in the epiphyses of the long bones of the human hand and foot, *J Bone Joint Surg (Br)* 41B(2):375, 1959.

11. Lachman E: Pseudo-epiphyses in hand and foot, *AJR* 70(1):149, 1953.

12. Ogden JA, Ganey TM, Light TR et al: Ossification and pseudoepiphysis formation in the "nonepiphyseal" end of bones of the hands and feet, *Skeletal Radiol* 23:3, 1994.

13. Vilaseca RR, Ribes ER: The growth of the first metatarsal bone, *Foot Ankle* 1(2):117, 1980.

14. Mathis SK, Frame BA, Smith CE: Distal first metatarsal

epiphysis: a common pediatric variant, *J Am Podiatr Med Assoc* 70(8):375, 1989.

15. Stanitski CL, Micheli LJ: Observations on symptomatic medial malleolus ossification centers, *J Pediatr Orthop* 13(2):164, 1993.

16. Powell HDW: Extra centre of ossification for the medial malleolus in children, *J Bone Joint Surg (Br)* 43B(1):107, 1961.

17. Person V, Lembach L: Six cases of tarsal coalition in children aged 4 to 12 years, *J Am Podiatr Med Assoc* 75(6):320, 1985.

18. Light TR, Ogden JA: The longitudinal epiphyseal bracket: implications for surgical correction, *J Pediatr Orthop* 1:299, 1981.

19. Jones GB: Delta phalanx, *J Bone Joint Surg (Br)* 46B(2):226, 1964.

20. Watson HK, Boyes JH: Congenital angular deformity of the digits, *J Bone Joint Surg (Am)* 49A(2):333, 1967.

21. Jaeger M, Refior HJ: The congenital triangular deformity of the tubular bones of hand and foot, *Clin Orthop* 81:139, 1971.

22. Neil MJ: Bilateral delta phalanx of the proximal phalanges of the great toes, *J Bone Joint Surg (Br)* 66B(1):77, 1984.

23. Robinson HM: Symmetrical reversed plantar calcaneal spurs in children, *Radiology* 119:187, 1976.

24. van Wiechen PJ: Reversed calcaneal spurs in children, *Skeletal Radiol* 16:17, 1987.

## Suggested Readings

Keats TE: *An atlas of normal roentgen variants that may simulate disease*, ed 4, St. Louis, 1992, Mosby.

Reed MH: *Pediatric skeletal radiology*, Baltimore, 1992, Williams & Wilkins.

Schmidt H, Freyschmidt J, editors: *Kohler/Zimmer borderlands of normal and early pathologic findings in skeletal radiography*, ed 4, New York, 1993, Thieme Medical Publishers.

Silverman FN, editor: *Caffey's pediatric x-ray diagnosis*, ed 8, St. Louis, 1985, Mosby.

# Systematic Approach to Bone and Joint Abnormalities

# CHAPTER 11

# View Selection for the Radiographic Study

ROBERT A. CHRISTMAN

Careful thought and consideration is necessary to select the positioning techniques that optimally demonstrate the area in question. One must be able to predict, before the study is ordered, how each bone will appear in every view. This is not easy. In addition to the differing appearances of the foot in each view, the appearance of the bones in a pronated foot, for example, is quite different from those in a supinated foot in the same view. Competency, therefore, requires continual and repetitive review of radiographs, paying special attention to the form, position, density, and architecture of each bone.

Selecting positioning techniques for a foot or ankle study should not be performed as a routine. However, it has become common practice to perform a standard set of positioning techniques for these studies; emphasis is not placed on the specific clinical area of symptomatology but on the views that show the most bones with the least amount of superimposition. They include the dorsoplantar, lateral, and medial oblique foot views and the mortise and lateral ankle views. Alternative views that may be more appropriate are not initially considered in this scenario. Because of this way of thinking, some pathologic conditions are not diagnosed.

It is not uncommon for certain practices or procedures to continue for decades without being questioned. This, unfortunately, doesn't make such procedures correct. One example is the routine bilateral radiographic foot or ankle study. Another is the number of positioning techniques performed. A third example concerns the technical aspects of a weight-bearing foot study. These are discussed in turn. I also briefly examine overutilization of radiographic studies.

The last half of this chapter concentrates on which views best demonstrate each bone and specific osseous landmarks. I present a method that simplifies the process by which views are selected. Radiographic anatomy, in contrast, is a subject of its own merit; an entire section of this book has been devoted to that topic (Chapters 6 through 10).

## ▥ BILATERAL VERSUS UNILATERAL STUDY

No written rule states that an extremity study should routinely be performed bilaterally. Many practitioners, however, commonly obtain views of both feet or ankles for every radiographic study performed. This practice has been followed to provide a comparison view of the opposite extremity, a baseline for future reference, or a means for biomechanical (orthomensurative) examination.

Use of comparison views should decrease as the practitioner's level of experience increases. The more familiar one becomes with normal radiographic anatomy, the less necessary are comparison films. Use of a reference standard, such as that provided in the radiographic anatomy section of this text, may in many instances be sufficient to replace the need for a comparison film of the opposite extremity. Furthermore, short tubular bones, such as the metatarsal and phalanx, rarely require comparison films of the opposite extremity; the remaining tubular bones of the same extremity serve as useful standards for comparison. To become familiar with the multiple superimposed shadows in the midfoot, rearfoot, and ankle regions, one must study these areas carefully and correlate them to the gross anatomic specimen routinely, not just when searching for a specific pathology.

Bilateral studies have also been advocated for the pediatric radiographic study, especially for epiphyseal injuries.[1] However, irregular ossification, multiple ossification centers, and accessory ossification centers are frequently encountered as variations of normal development; their differentiation from abnormality may be impossible, even with comparison films of the opposite extremity. Comparison films of the pediatric foot or ankle may actually be misleading more often than they are beneficial. For example, developmental variants are frequently unilateral. The absence of a variant in the opposite extremity encourages the misdiagnosis of fracture or other pathology.[2] Studies have shown that pediatric radiologists don't consider bilateral studies routinely necessary.[3,4]

The need for bilateral studies is obvious for patients who exhibit symptomatology in both extremities. They are also valuable for assessing joint disease. However, it is illogical to order and perform bilateral radiographic studies routinely for every patient. Direct trauma, for example, does not require radiographic examination of the opposite extremity if the fracture is obvious.

Comparison films of the opposite, asymptomatic extremity may be useful when a questionable lesion or finding is present in the affected extremity. In most instances the questionable finding only appears in one view. A comparison study of the opposite extremity can therefore be limited to the view in question. Other supplementary comparison views offer no additional diagnostic information and expose the patient to additional potentially harmful radiation. Ask yourself, If you were the patient, would you appreciate the physician ordering radiographic studies that were not going to contribute to the diagnosis or treatment of your condition?

Plain film radiography should not be performed until after an adequate history and physical examination has been performed on the patient and then only if clinically indicated. Baseline radiographic studies without clinical indication should therefore not be performed and are discouraged. Nor should radiography for biomechanical examination be performed routinely. The foot should first be analyzed clinically; radiographs should only be obtained if the examination suggests that an osseous structural or positional abnormality exists and could be contributing to the presenting concern and if the outcome of the study could affect the treatment rendered.

## ■ NUMBER OF VIEWS

How many views are necessary for evaluating the foot or ankle? This depends entirely on the provisional diagnosis (or diagnoses) and the area of concern. For example, when evaluating the first metatarsophalangeal joint for degenerative joint disease, only dorsoplantar and lateral views are necessary to make the general diagnosis. An oblique view ordinarily does not offer any additional information in the diagnosis of osteoarthritis unless the physician is looking for a more specific condition or lesion, such as a loose osseous body.

Controversy exists regarding the number of views necessary to assess ankle trauma. The practice of obtaining three views is advocated widely in the literature.[5-7] These views include the anteroposterior, lateral, and oblique (typically the mortise). However, others suggest that the number of ankle views be limited to two (anteroposterior

and lateral) or even eliminated in the absence of soft tissue swelling.[8-11] Studies now suggest that ankle fractures can be discriminated from nonfractures by considering specific clinical variables.[12,13]

A rational, analytic approach for selecting a radiographic study is to first obtain two or three views that best demonstrate the area in question. Typically this would include dorsoplantar (or anteroposterior) and lateral views; an oblique or axial view may be indicated if the area of concern is best seen in one. If your diagnosis is confirmed, no other views are necessary. If a unilateral study is inconclusive or a questionable lesion is seen, additional views should then be obtained of the same extremity. If comparison views of the opposite extremity are warranted, select only those views that were questionable from the initial study. Of course, conditions that can demonstrate generalized radiographic findings, such as inflammatory joint disease, requires examination of other regions and/or extremities. Because the distribution of radiographic findings and patterns of joint involvement are important aspects for the evaluation of joint disease, bilateral dorsoplantar and lateral films are advocated.

## ■ OVERUTILIZATION

Overutilization of radiography has been defined as "excessive irradiation per unit of diagnostic information, therapeutic impact or health income"; it can include excessive radiation per film, excessive films per examination, or excessive examinations per patient.[14] Regarding foot radiography, excessive radiation per film can be minimized by limiting the size of the x-ray beam to the area in question (also known as collimation), using rare-earth screen/film combinations, and shielding the patient with a lead apron; excessive films per examination can be limited by initially obtaining only the basic views to assess the area in question and by preventing repeat examinations required by poor positioning and exposure technique and faulty processing; and excessive examinations per patient can be reduced by depending more on clinical findings than relying on radiographs for follow-up examination, by educating the patient who makes demands that a study is not indicated, and by imagining that the cost of the study is being funded by the patient, not reimbursed by insurance. Examples have already been briefly addressed citing areas of potential overuse of radiographic studies, including bilateral comparison studies, the number of views selected for any particular study, and whether the study should be performed at all.

Several factors affect one's decision to obtain radiographic studies (Box 11-1).[15,16] A primary factor is the training and experience of the practitioner. Someone trained to order bilateral comparison views for every patient will certainly perpetuate this activity in practice. Experience, addressed earlier, should also have an effect: The number of studies and/or films ordered should decrease as practical experience increases. Another factor addresses the patient evaluation: Radiographs should never replace a thorough history and physical examination.

Nonclinical factors may significantly affect the practitioner's decision to perform a radiographic study. Radiographs are routinely ordered by many for patients presenting with a history of trauma, with the intent of providing medicolegal documentation. Long[15] poses this dilemma: "If the justification for ordering a radiograph is to protect the physician, one wonders what number of those radiographs are clinically necessary." Radiographic studies are also ordered for reassurance, especially after orthopedic surgical procedures and fractures. Generally speaking, most follow-up radiographic examinations only require reassessment at three- to four-week intervals, unless clinical history or physical evaluation warrants otherwise. Examples of the latter include postreduction, reinjury, and infection. Another nonclinical factor includes the patient's insistence. The practitioner should be prepared to educate the patient regarding the determination for radiographs or against their inclusion in the diagnostic workup.

The goal to controlling overutilization is learning diagnostic restraint.[17] Occasionally we need to rely on our clinical wisdom; a condition does not always have to be "ruled in or out" by performing one more test, in this case, the radiographic study. Will the outcome of the study affect the treatment instituted? We also must remember that there are possible dangers associated with low levels of ionizing radiation, including diagnostic x-ray studies.[18,19] Ask yourself, Is this radiographic study really necessary?[20,21] Finally, determine whether or not another diagnostic technique may be more appropriate to assess the underlying problem.[22]

## ■ TECHNICAL CONSIDERATIONS

Bilateral studies should be performed as individual studies of each extremity. This limits and directs the x-ray beam to the part under study. X-ray beam limitation (or collimation)

reduces scatter radiation that otherwise may be absorbed by the patient. For example, bilateral dorsoplantar views of the feet should be performed so that individual exposures of each foot are obtained. The useful x-ray beam can then be collimated to the individual foot (a 5- × 12-inch area for a 10- × 12-inch film). Exposure of both feet together requires collimation to an area that is much larger (10 × 12 inches for a 10- × 12-inch film). Scatter radiation increases when collimating to a larger area; this low-energy radiation is easily absorbed by the patient, increasing their dose of ionizing radiation, and impairs the quality of the film image. Image quality can also be affected by the direction of the central x-ray beam. A central x-ray beam that is directed to the individual foot or area in question reduces geometric blurring and distortion, resulting in an image that is truer in size, shape, and position.

A basic principle in radiography is to have the x-ray central beam directed perpendicular to both the subject and the image receptor (x-ray film). Oblique views of the feet should therefore not be performed weight bearing. Significant distortion of the image results when the central x-ray beam is directed at a 45-degree angulation to the film (Figure 11-1). Oblique foot views should be performed non–weight bearing and with the foot angulated 45 degrees so that the x-ray beam is directed perpendicular to both the foot and the film. This positioning technique minimizes distortion of the image.

A compromise in positioning technique is made with the weight-bearing dorsoplantar view. The central x-ray beam unfortunately cannot be directed perpendicular to both the foot and the film. Because the tube head physically cannot be positioned perpendicular to the film with the patient standing and because the metatarsals are declined approximately 15 degrees (when averaged together), the tubehead is directed at a 15-degree angle from perpendicular so that it is perpendicular to the osseous structures. Minimal image distortion occurs in this view.

Occasionally a question arises regarding which side of the foot should be positioned closer to the film. Generally speaking, that aspect of the body farthest from the film appears magnified and less sharp. This is especially true in the chest, which has considerable depth. The size of the heart appears larger in an anteroposterior view than a posteroanterior view. However, the foot is not very thick (relative to the chest), and size of the foot bones is not a critical aspect in their assessment. The width of the average foot is approximately 3 inches (personal observation). Magnification of that side farthest from the film is only between 1.08 and 1.14, depending on the source-to-image distance (40 and 24 inches, respectively). (Magnification factors are determined by dividing the source-to-film distance by the source-to-object distance.[23]) Chapter 4 discusses exposure techniques in more detail.

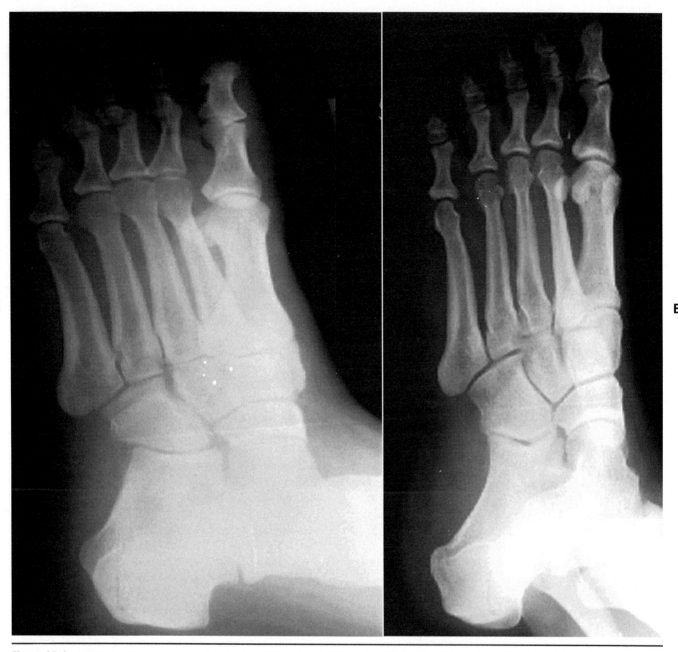

**Figure 11-1**    Weight bearing versus non–weight-bearing oblique view. **A,** Distorted weight-bearing oblique view with tube head directed at 45 degrees. **B,** Non–weight-bearing oblique view with tube head directed perpendicular to film and foot turned 45 degrees.

## ■ SELECTION OF POSITIONING TECHNIQUES

Before studying the following paradigm, it is important to understand the concept of marginal (or tangential) surfaces. A tangent is defined as a line that intersects a curved surface at a single point of intersection[24] (Figure 11-2). The outermost aspect or margin of a tubular bone, for example, seen in a two-dimensional radiograph represents the three-dimensional anatomic surface that is tangent to the primary x-ray beam. Unfortunately, bones are irregularly shaped and occasionally have flat surfaces. Furthermore, more than one point or surface may be tangent to the x-ray beam in the same plane. For these reasons, I use the word *margin*, not *tangent*, to describe the outermost aspect or outline of a bone seen in the two-dimensional radiograph.

Boxes 11-2 and 11-3 list the bone margins that are seen in each standard foot and ankle view. (All views except the

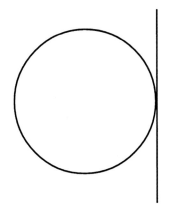

Figure 11-2    Illustration of a line tangent to a circle.

| BOX 11-2 | Marginal Bone Surfaces Seen in Each Foot View |
|---|---|

| Foot View | Marginal Surfaces |
|---|---|
| Dorsoplantar | Medial, lateral, anterior, and posterior |
| Lateral | Superior, inferior, anterior, and posterior |
| Medial oblique | Superomedial, inferolateral, anterior, and posterior |
| Lateral oblique | Superolateral, inferomedial, anterior, and posterior |
| Sesamoid axial | Superior, inferior, medial, and lateral |
| Calcaneal axial | Medial, lateral, and inferior |

| BOX 11-3 | Marginal Bone Surfaces Seen in Each Ankle View |
|---|---|

| Ankle View | Marginal Surfaces |
|---|---|
| Anteroposterior | Medial, lateral, superior, and inferior |
| Mortise | Same as anteroposterior, although slightly rotated |
| Internal oblique | Anteromedial, posterolateral, superior, and inferior |
| External oblique | Posteromedial, anterolateral, superior, and inferior |
| Lateral | Anterior, posterior, superior, and inferior |

foot obliques are weight bearing; see Chapter 3 for a description of positioning techniques.) The marginal surfaces for most views are straightforward and obvious. However, the oblique views are initially confusing. Use a foot skeleton to correlate the bone position for each positioning technique to the radiographic image. The general principle of marginal surfaces can be applied to two scenarios: the selection of an appropriate positioning technique and the interpretation of precise anatomic location in the radiograph.

Selecting the positioning technique depends on the anatomic site in question. Appropriate views are recommended that optimally demonstrate each bone. The "basic study" consists of those views that best isolate the area in question. Applicable adjunctive views are also included. However, the best view may not necessarily be the one that isolates a bone with little or no superimposition of other structures. Positioning techniques should also be selected based on the marginal surface to be examined radiographically, when appropriate.

## Hallux

The hallux (Figure 11-3) is best seen in the dorsoplantar view. It is also visible in both oblique views, if the hallux is separated from the adjacent second toe. Unfortunately, the hallux is fully superimposed on the remaining lesser digits in the weight-bearing lateral view, although the distal phalanx can be isolated if attention is paid to elevating the hallux prior to exposure or by placing dental x-ray film between the hallux and second toe. A lateral view of the isolated hallux may be better achieved with a non–weight-bearing positioning technique.

## Lesser Digits

The lesser digits (see Figure 11-3) are best seen in the dorsoplantar and both oblique views. To minimize superimposition, the digit or digits in question should be separated from the remaining adjacent digits. In the lateral view, the lesser digits are superimposed on each other. However, hammer toe deformity and/or elevation of the second digit may provide partial visibility of the phalanges.

The fourth and fifth toes are seen best in the oblique views. These digits are typically adductovarus in position, so a dorsoplantar view of these digits shows them obliquely oriented. A medial oblique view of an adductovarus digit demonstrates a true dorsoplantar perspective of the toe, and a lateral oblique view shows the digit from a lateral perspective.

## Sesamoids

The sesamoids (Figure 11-4) are isolated only in the axial view. Although the entire outline of each ossicle is seen in the dorsoplantar view, they are fully superimposed on the first metatarsal. The tibial and fibular sesamoids are superimposed on the first and second metatarsals, respectively, in the medial oblique view. Superimposition also occurs in the lateral oblique view; however, approximately a third of the tibial sesamoid is isolated and viewed clearly, its inferomedial aspect. The lateral view should not be considered when performing a radiographic study for examination of the sesamoids alone. The sesamoids are fully

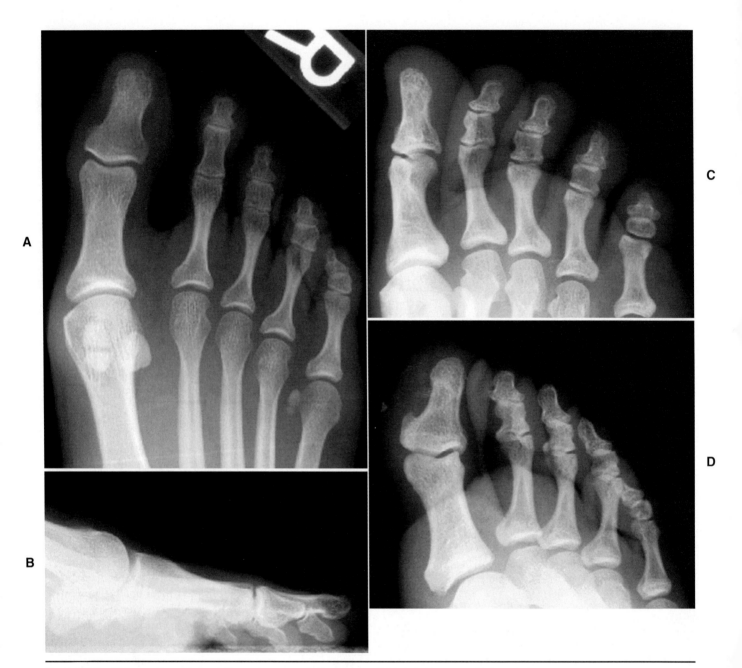

**Figure 11-3**    Hallux and lesser digits. **A**, Dorsoplantar view. **B**, Lateral view. **C**, Medial oblique view. **D**, Lateral oblique view.

superimposed on each other as well as on the lesser metatarsophalangeal joint structures in this view.

## First Metatarsal

Optimal views for examining the first metatarsal and metatarsophalangeal joint (see Figure 11-4) are the dorso-plantar and lateral views. The first metatarsal is isolated almost entirely in the dorsoplantar view; minimal super-imposition of the proximal phalanx base and medial cuneiform is found at its anterior and posterior margins,

respectively. Although the first metatarsal is superimposed on the remaining metatarsals in the lateral view, its entire outline can be traced. This should not hinder evaluating the first metatarsal. The metatarsosesamoid articulation is best seen in the axial view.

The medial oblique view demonstrates a different aspect of the articular surface from that seen in the dorsoplantar and lateral views. The superomedial and inferolateral surfaces are viewed along the margins. Examples of osseous landmarks and pathology identified in this view include the medial tubercle, inferolateral articular surface for the proximal phalangeal base, bunion hyperostosis and accompanying degenerative cysts, insertion site of the peroneus longus tendon, and gouty erosions. Although this view shifts the fibular sesamoid laterally (relatively speaking) so that it is not superimposed on the first metatarsal, it is now superimposed on the second metatarsal.

The following landmarks can be identified in the lateral oblique view: the lateral tubercle, inferomedial articular surface for the proximal phalangeal base, insertion site for the tibialis anterior tendon, as well as other structures along the inferomedial and superolateral surfaces of the first metatarsal. Osteophyte proliferation along the superolateral aspect of the first metatarsophalangeal joint are isolated in this view.

## Second Through Fourth Metatarsals

The second, third, and fourth metatarsals (see Figure 11-4) are best seen in the medial oblique view, because the

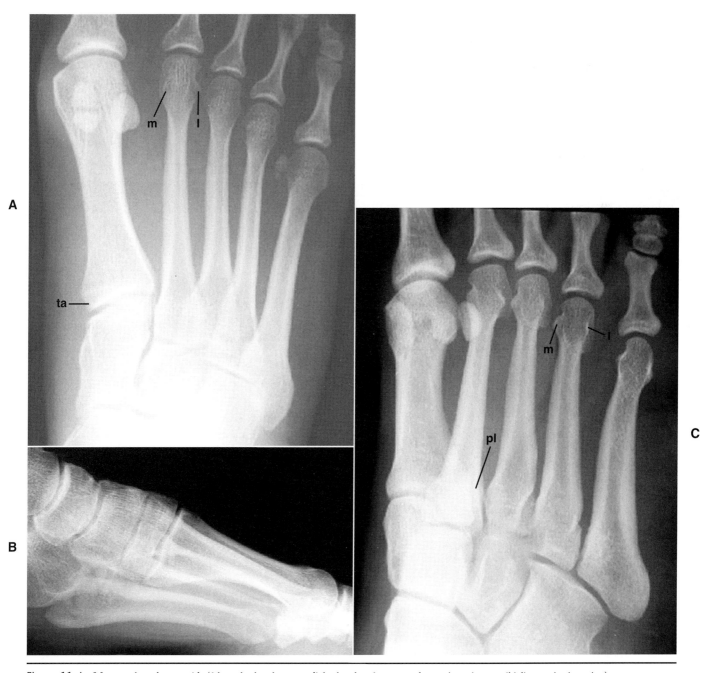

Figure 11-4    Metatarsals and sesamoids (*l*, lateral tubercle; *m*, medial tubercle; *pl*, peroneus longus insertion; *ta*, tibialis anterior insertion). **A**, Dorsoplantar view. **B**, Lateral view. **C**, Medial oblique view.

*Continued*

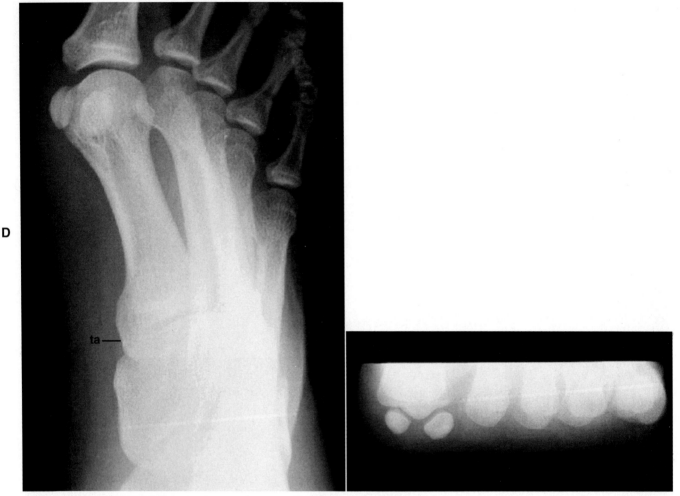

**Figure 11-4, cont'd**   Metatarsals and sesamoids (*ta*, tibialis anterior insertion). **D**, Lateral oblique view. **E**, Sesamoid axial view.

metatarsal bases are positioned obliquely in the arch of the midfoot. The metatarsal heads are occasionally viewed axially but are typically everted in this view. The inferolateral articular surface and medial tubercle are isolated at the head's margins.

The metatarsal heads are viewed axially to slightly inverted in the dorsoplantar view. When inverted, the inferomedial articular surface and lateral tubercle are visible. The bases are rotated and therefore obliquely viewed and partially superimposed.

The lateral oblique view is not very useful for evaluating the second through fourth metatarsals. However, it does provide visibility of a different aspect of the metatarsal head and neck. This can be valuable when evaluating subtle fractures or other pathology to these areas.

All three metatarsals are fully superimposed in the lateral view and cannot be easily visualized. This view, however, can be used to evaluate the positional relationships of the metatarsal heads in the sagittal plane. Obviously, excellent-quality films are necessary for this application. A smooth parabola or transition should be noted, with each metatarsal being only slightly superior to the next from lateral to medial. This view probably represents a more accurate reflection of the positioning of the metatarsal heads than does the sesamoid axial view with its overextension of the toes at the metatarsophalangeal joints. The inferior articular aspect of each metatarsal head is isolated in the axial view.

## Fifth Metatarsal

The entire fifth metatarsal (see Figure 11-4) is isolated in the medial oblique view. The tuberosity and metatarso-cuboid articulation can be seen. The fifth metatarsal is clearly visible in the dorsoplantar view except for the proximal articulation. Also, the tuberosity is partially

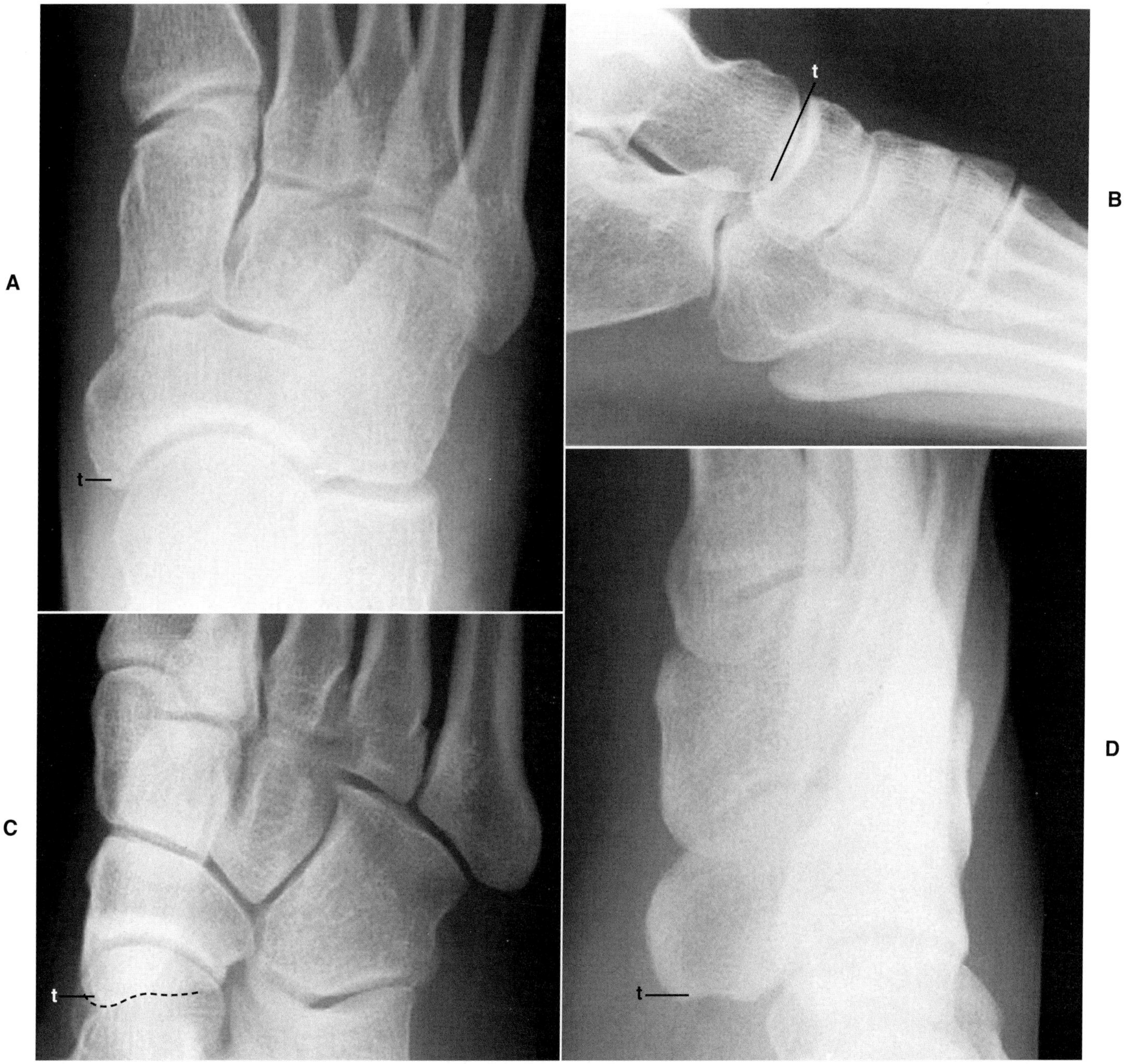

**Figure 11-5**   Cuneiforms, cuboid, and navicular (*t*, navicular tuberosity). **A**, Dorsoplantar view. **B**, Lateral view. **C**, Medial oblique view. **D**, Lateral oblique view.

superimposed on the base. The fifth metatarsal can be seen in the lateral view even though there is some super-imposition on the fourth metatarsal. The tuberosity is viewed clearly, but the metatarsocuboid joint cannot be appreciated. The lateral oblique view is not useful for evaluating the fifth metatarsal except for pathology involving the head or neck.

## Cuneiforms

The cuneiforms (Figure 11-5) are superimposed on themselves and on neighboring bones in most views. The dorsoplantar view best isolates the medial cuneiform. It can also be seen in the medial oblique view, but it is superimposed on the intermediate cuneiform. Although it is fully superimposed on the remaining cuneiforms in the lateral view, the entire outline of the medial cuneiform can be traced. Most of the medial cuneiform is superimposed in the lateral oblique view; only its inferomedial aspect is isolated.

The intermediate cuneiform can best be isolated in a modified medial oblique view. Depending on the foot structure (cavus, rectus, or planus), the foot should be slanted approximately 5 to 20 degrees. The joint between

the intermediate and lateral cuneiforms can be isolated with a 20-degree medial oblique position; the joint between the intermediate and medial cuneiforms with a 10-degree lateral oblique position.[25] Most of the intermediate cuneiform can be seen in the dorsoplantar view. Only the superoposterior aspect is isolated in the lateral view. The lateral oblique view is not useful for evaluating the intermediate cuneiform.

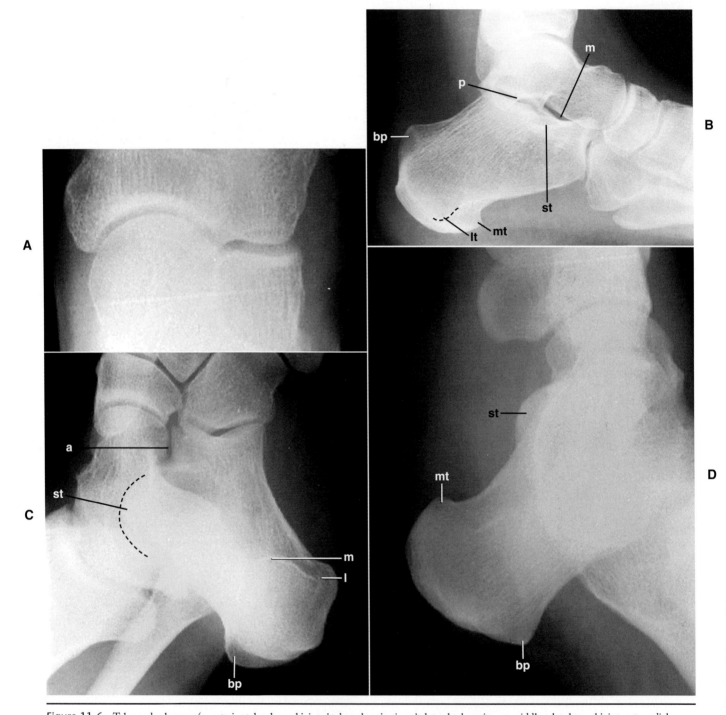

**Figure 11-6**    Talus and calcaneus (*a*, anterior talocalcaneal joint; *bp*, bursal projection; *lt*, lateral tuberosity; *m*, middle talocalcaneal joint; *mt*, medial tuberosity; *p*, posterior subtalar joint; *st*, sustentaculum tali). **A**, Dorsoplantar view. **B**, Lateral view. **C**, Medial oblique view. **D**, Lateral oblique view.

*Continued*

Figure 11-6, cont'd    Talus and calcaneus (*lt*, lateral tuberosity; *m*, middle subtalar joint; *mt*, medial tuberosity; *p*, posterior talocalcaneal joint; *st*, sustentaculum tali). **E**, Calcaneal axial view.

The lateral cuneiform is best isolated radiographically in the medial oblique view. This bone is partially superimposed in the dorsoplantar view. It is fully superimposed on neighboring bones in the lateral oblique and lateral views.

## Cuboid

The cuboid (see Figure 11-5) is fully visible in the medial oblique view. It can also be evaluated in the dorsoplantar and lateral views, although there is some superimposition. The outline of the cuboid is barely visible in the lateral oblique view; it is fully superimposed on multiple structures and cannot be assessed.

## Navicular

The navicular (see Figure 11-5) can be assessed in all foot views except the axial views. Evaluation is best accomplished using both the dorsoplantar and lateral views. The tuberosity can be partially seen in the dorsoplantar view. Although the tuberosity is fully superimposed in the lateral view, its outline can still be identified; this view can prove quite valuable when evaluating tuberosity fractures. The navicular tuberosity is best seen in the lateral oblique view. The dorsomedial aspect of the navicular is isolated in the medial oblique view.

## Talus

The entire talus (Figure 11-6) can be identified only in the lateral view. Superimposition prevents adequate visibility in the oblique views. However, the anterior articular facet for the calcaneus is isolated in the medial oblique view. Occasionally the posterolateral trigonal process can be identified with this view, although it is superimposed. Only the talar head and neck are visible in the dorsoplantar view.

## Calcaneus

The entire calcaneus (see Figure 11-6) can be seen in the lateral and medial oblique views. The medial tuberosity is isolated in the lateral oblique and lateral views. The sustentaculum tali is visible in the lateral, axial, medial oblique, and lateral oblique views. The middle and posterior talar articular surfaces can be seen in the lateral and axial views. The lateral tuberosity, anterior talar articular facet, and bursal projection are isolated in the medial oblique view. Only the lateral and anterior aspects of the anterior calcaneus are visible in the dorsoplantar view.

## Distal Tibia

The tibial malleolus (Figure 11-7) can be identified in all ankle views, although it is best seen in the anteroposterior view. The lateral view is useful for distinguishing between the anterior and posterior colliculi and differentiating between avulsion fractures of the anterior colliculus versus the os subtibiale. The articular surfaces are seen best in the anteroposterior, mortise, and lateral views.

## Distal Fibula

The fibular malleolus (see Figure 11-7) is isolated in the mortise view. It is also visible, with only slight superimposition, in the anteroposterior and internal oblique views. Although the malleolus is fully superimposed on the tibia in the lateral view, its entire outline can still be seen. The lateral view is extremely valuable for evaluation of distal fibular fractures. The articulation between the distal fibula and the talus is best viewed in the mortise view.

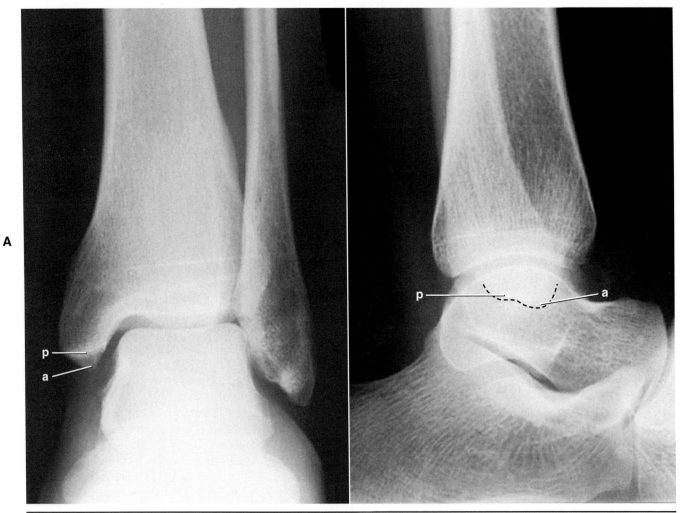

Figure 11-7   Distal tibia and fibula (*a*, anterior colliculus; *p*, posterior colliculus). **A,** Anteroposterior view. **B,** Lateral view.

*Continued*

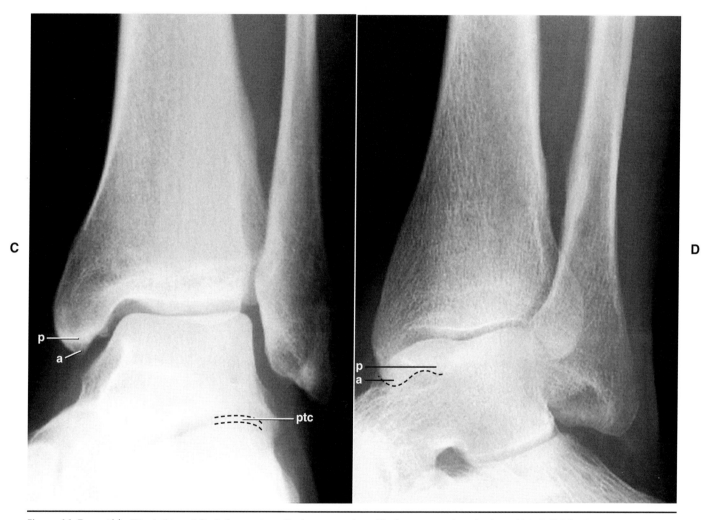

**Figure 11-7, cont'd**  Distal tibia and fibula (*a*, anterior colliculus; *p*, posterior colliculus; *ptc*, posterior talocalcaneal joint). **C**, Mortise view. **D**, Internal oblique view.

*Continued*

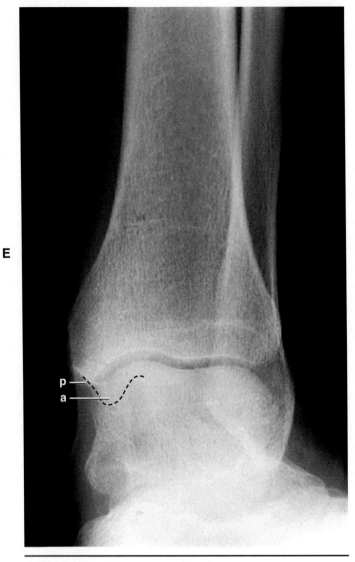

**Figure 11-7, cont'd**  Distal tibia and fibula (*a*, anterior colliculus; *p*, posterior colliculus). **E**, External oblique view.

## References

1. Oloff, J: Radiology of the foot in pediatrics. In Weissman SD, editor: *Radiology of the foot*, ed 2, Baltimore, 1989, Williams & Wilkins.
2. Ozonoff MB: *Pediatric orthopedic radiology*, Philadelphia, 1979, Saunders.
3. McCauley RGK, Schwartz AM, Leonidas JC et al: Comparison views in extremity injury in children: an efficacy study, *Radiology* 131:95, 1979.
4. Merten DF: Comparison radiographs in extremity injuries of childhood: current application in radiological practice, *Radiology* 126:209, 1978.
5. Weissman BNW, Sledge CB: *Orthopedic radiology*, Philadelphia, 1986, Saunders.
6. Berquist TH, Johnson KA: Trauma. In Berquist TH, editor: *Radiology of the foot and ankle*, New York, 1989, Raven Press.
7. Conrad JJ, Tannin AH: Trauma to the ankle. In Jahss MH, editor: *Disorders of the foot*, Philadelphia, 1982, Saunders.
8. Garfield JS: Is radiological examination of the twisted ankle necessary? *Lancet* 2:1167, 1960.

9. de Lacey GJ, Bradbrooke S: Rationalizing requests for x-ray examination of acute ankle injuries, *BMJ* 1:1597, 1979.

10. Cockshott WP, Jenkin JK, Pui M: Limiting the use of routine radiography for acute ankle injuries, *CMAJ* 129:129, 1983.

11. Wallis MG: Are three views necessary to examine acute ankle injuries? *Clin Radiol* 40:424, 1989.

12. Diehr P, Highley R, Dehkordi F et al: Prediction of fracture in patients with acute musculoskeletal ankle trauma, *Med Decis Making* 8:40, 1988.

13. Stiell IG, Greenberg GH, McKnight RD et al: Decision rules for the use of radiography in acute ankle injuries, *JAMA* 269:1127, 1993.

14. Abrams HL: The "overutilization" of x-rays, *N Engl J Med* 300:1213, 1979.

15. Long AE: Radiographic decision-making by the emergency physician, *Emerg Med Clin North Am* 3(3):437, 1985.

16. Hall FM: Overutilization of radiological examinations, *Radiology* 120:443, 1976.

17. Reuben DB: Learning diagnostic restraint, *N Engl J Med* 310:591, 1984.

18. Boice JD: The danger of x-rays: real or apparent? *N Engl J Med* 315:828, 1986.

19. Upton AC: The biological effects of low-level ionizing radiation, *Sci Am* 246:41, 1982.

20. Rigler LG: Is this radiograph really necessary? *Radiology* 120:449, 1976.

21. McClenahan JL: Wasted x-rays, *Radiology* 96:453, 1970.

22. Palmer PES, Cockshott WP: The appropriate use of diagnostic imaging, *JAMA* 252:2753, 1984.

23. Bushong SC: *Radiologic science for technologists*, ed 4, St. Louis, 1988, Mosby.

24. *Funk and Wagnall's new comprehensive international dictionary of the English language*, Newark, NJ, 1982, Publisher's International Press.

25. Montagne J, Chevrot A, Galmiche JM: *Atlas of foot radiology*, New York, 1981, Masson.

# CHAPTER 12

# Systematic Evaluation of Bone and Joint Abnormalities

ROBERT A. CHRISTMAN

A planned, routine methodology is needed when viewing radiographs. The reason for this is obvious: Following a habitual sequence of events during the review process helps avoid the omission of any necessary aspects of film evaluation.

Routinely assess all imaged structures in every available view. Avoid the timesaving technique of honing in on the area of question. If only the symptomatic area is evaluated, abnormalities may be missed. Analysis of all anatomic structures also serves as a form of continuing education: Interpretation skills are enhanced as one becomes more familiar with the normal and variant presentations.

The primary features of film evaluation include position, form, density, and architecture. The soft tissue and osseous elements of the foot and ankle have consistent radiographic appearances based on these features. A firm knowledge and understanding of normal radiographic anatomy are necessary before abnormalities of position, form, density, and architecture can be identified. If not, normal and variant features of a structure are misinterpreted as abnormal. (Familiarity with normal radiographic anatomy cannot be emphasized enough.)

Abnormalities are recognized and appreciated more readily if judged against the normal expected appearance of each structure. One could rely on memorizing each and every pathologic picture; however, several varying radiographic presentations are seen with many disorders. To complicate matters, different pathologic entities may have similar radiographic presentations. The interpretation process is greatly simplified by first identifying abnormal radiographic findings and by then associating these findings with applicable disorders. (This process is exactly like that used by the emergency room physician, the general practitioner, or specialist evaluating a patient. Each

---

**BOX 12-1**  **Primary Features of Film Evaluation**

Position
Form
Density
Architecture

---

physician compiles data or findings based on the patient's history and physical examination and considers disorders—that is, differential diagnoses—that may apply to these findings.)

The challenge initially is to recognize that an abnormality exists. At the outset of film evaluation, consider all radiographic shadows normal anatomy until proven otherwise. If a shadow cannot be explained as normal radiographic anatomy, it is either variant or abnormal. Then the appropriate terminology must be applied to the abnormality. Finally, diagnoses are considered that can demonstrate the finding or findings encountered.

Few authors have described methods for evaluating a radiograph.[1-4] Most of these approaches have compiled long lists to emulate and have concentrated on the characteristics of abnormal lesions. The following method emphasizes the identification of abnormal findings by comparing to normal anatomy and variants. It uses multiple short lists that are categorized topically. First the four primary features of film evaluation (Box 12-1) are discussed. They are then incorporated into a method for assessing all soft tissue and skeletal structures. Applicable disorders associated with these findings are discussed in individual chapters that follow.

## ■ PRIMARY FEATURES OF FILM EVALUATION

### Position

Position initially entails a general overview of the foot and is assessed with the planar views, that is, dorsoplantar (anteroposterior) and lateral views. Sit back and gain an overall impression of the foot type. Appreciate the position of each bone relative to the remaining structures (a precursory biomechanical/orthomensurative evaluation). (This is best performed with a weight-bearing study and the foot positioned in angle and base of gait as described in Chapter 3.) The axis of each bone has a characteristic position in the foot relative to neighboring bones. Primarily, the angulation between the two bones is assessed and compared to the rectus foot. For example, in the dorsoplantar view the talar axis is mildly adducted (or angulated medially) relative to the calcaneal axis in the rectus foot, greatly adducted in the pes planovalgus foot, and nearly parallel to the calcaneal axis in the pes cavus foot (Figure 12-1). Abnormalities of position may develop in utero or over the lifetime of the patient. Representative examples include clubfoot and hallux abductovalgus, respectively. Appropriate terminology should be used to

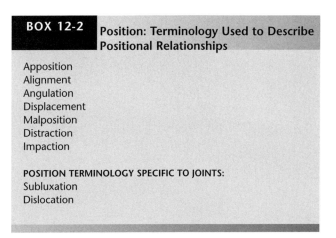

**BOX 12-2    Position: Terminology Used to Describe Positional Relationships**

Apposition
Alignment
Angulation
Displacement
Malposition
Distraction
Impaction

**POSITION TERMINOLOGY SPECIFIC TO JOINTS:**
Subluxation
Dislocation

describe position abnormalities (Box 12-2). If it is a bilateral study, compare symmetry between both feet.

The position of adjacent articular surfaces is also assessed. The two surfaces should normally show 100% apposition. Partial apposition is a sign of subluxation, and 0% apposition represents dislocation (Figure 12-2).

Positioning terminology is especially useful when describing the position of a fracture fragment relative to

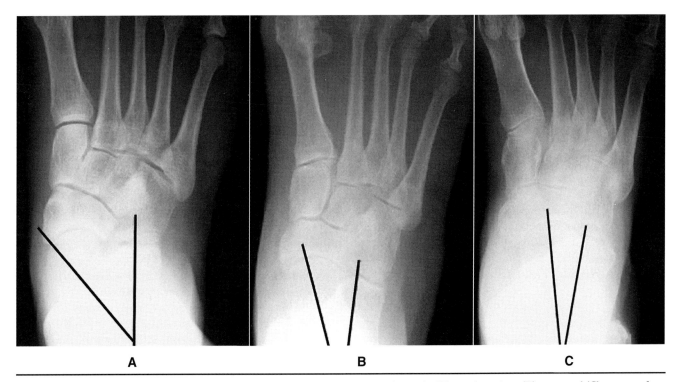

Figure 12-1    Changes in the position of the talar and calcaneal axes relative to one another in the (**A**) pes planovalgus, (**B**) rectus, and (**C**) pes cavus foot.

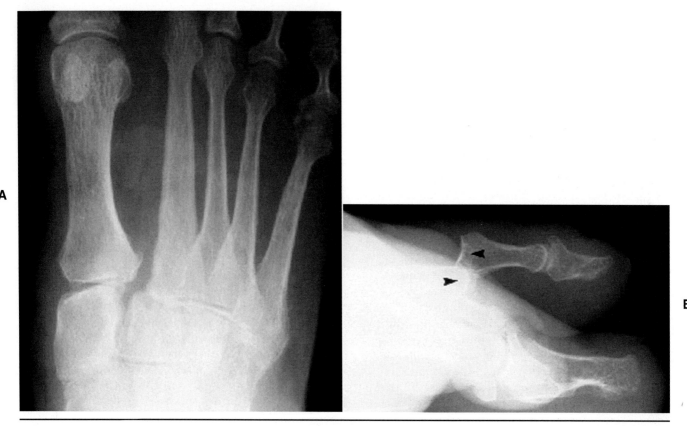

**Figure 12-2** Position: Apposition between two articular surfaces. **A,** Partial apposition (subluxation of the first and second metatarsocuneiform joints); **B,** 0% apposition (dislocation of the second-toe proximal interphalangeal joint).

another. Alignment conveys the degree of parallelism of the two fragments.[1] Angulation is a lack of alignment or parallelism of the two segments and can be described in two ways: by the tilt of the distal segment relative to the proximal segment, or by the direction pointed to by the apex formed between the two segments.[1] The degree of bony contact (touching) between the two fracture fragments is referred to as apposition.[1] If the two fragments show total (or 100%) apposition, there is no displacement. If the two fragments show partial or no apposition, displacement exists (Figure 12-3). The preceding positional terms must be described in two perpendicular planes to fully appreciate three-dimensional position (Figure 12-4).

## Form

Assess for abnormalities or variations of the form or shape and size of each bone, including girth, tubulation, length, contour, and growth (Box 12-3). The form of identifiable soft tissue shadows (the Achilles tendon, for example)

> **BOX 12-3**  **Form (size and shape): Terminology Used to Describe Characteristics of Form**
>
> Girth (increased or decreased)
> Tubulation (over- or under-)
> Length (short or long)
> Contour (irregular, expanded, deformed, scalloped)
> Growth (over-, under-)

should also be evaluated. The girth of a short tubular bone (such as the metatarsal or phalanx) is affected by subperiosteal remodeling: Apposition increases the girth; resorption decreases it. Decreased girth or overtubulation of short tubular bones, for example, is seen with the variant spool-shaped phalanx and pathologic states such as osteogenesis imperfecta (Figure 12-5). Increased girth is frequently secondary to periosteal apposition of bone,

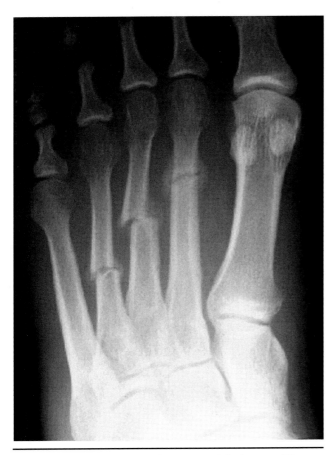

**Figure 12-3** Fracture position: Angulation and displacement. The dorsoplantar radiograph of this popular music artist demonstrates three different examples of fracture position in the transverse plane. *Second metatarsal:* The distal segment shows no angulation or displacement relative to the proximal segment. *Third metatarsal:* The distal segment is displaced laterally (50% apposition) and angulated medially. *Fourth metatarsal:* The distal segment is displaced laterally (75% apposition), but no angulation is apparent.

although undertubulation may be a variation of skeletal development (Figure 12-6). Increased and decreased bone length should also be noted (Figure 12-7). Irregularity or deformity of the bone's contour may be caused by periosteal apposition, an exostosis along the outer aspect of a bone, or by an internal "expansile" lesion (Figure 12-8). The growth of a bone or bones can be increased or decreased by hyper- or hypothyroid conditions, respectively.

## Density

Density is the degree of blackness seen on the radiograph. The term is relative; that is, increased or decreased density depends on the blackness of surrounding structures. Differing degrees of subject radiodensity are what constitute

the radiographic image. Therefore some decreased densities are normal findings, and others are abnormal (Figure 12-9). The same holds true for increased densities (Figure 12-10). You must become familiar with the normal radiographic anatomy of all soft tissue and osseous structures before you can differentiate between normal and abnormal radiodensities.

Recall that subject radiodensity depends on the thickness, atomic number, and compactness of the tissue being imaged. An area of increased radiodensity, such as cortical bone, is radiopaque—absorbs x rays—and appears white in the radiograph. Air, in contrast, is radiolucent—transmits x rays—and appears blacker. In contrast, optical density, also known as radiographic or film density, is the overall blackening of the finished radiograph.[1] A blacker film has increased optical density and is therefore opaque (it absorbs light); a lighter film is lucent (transmits light) and demonstrates decreased optical density.

Abnormal radiodensity may be either an isolated finding (local), distributed in one extremity or a segment of the extremity (regional), or found throughout the entire skeleton (diffuse). The finding is primarily described as an increased or decreased density; applicable adjectives should be used when appropriate (Box 12-4). For example, in bone an ill-defined decreased density may have a *permeative* or *moth-eaten (spotty or mottled)* appearance; a well-defined, localized decreased density that has form (or sharply delineated margins) can be described as being *geographic* (Figure 12-11). An abnormal decreased density seen in soft tissues is air (especially gas produced by some anaerobic

| **BOX 12-4** | **Density (degree of blackness): Synonyms Used in Place of and Adjectives in Conjunction with Relative Increased and Decreased Densities** | |
|---|---|---|
| | **INCREASED DENSITY** | **DECREASED DENSITY** |
| **SYNONYMS** | Radiopaque | Radiolucent |
| | Sclerosis* | Rarefaction* |
| | Eburnation* | Osteopenia* |
| | | Osteolysis* |
| **ADJECTIVES** | Cloudlike | Geographic |
| | Solid | Mottled |
| | Ivorylike | Spotty |
| | Stippled | Motheaten |
| | Speckled | Permeative |
| | Rings and arcs | |
| | Flocculent | |
| | Hazy | |
| | Ground glass | |

*Specific to bone.

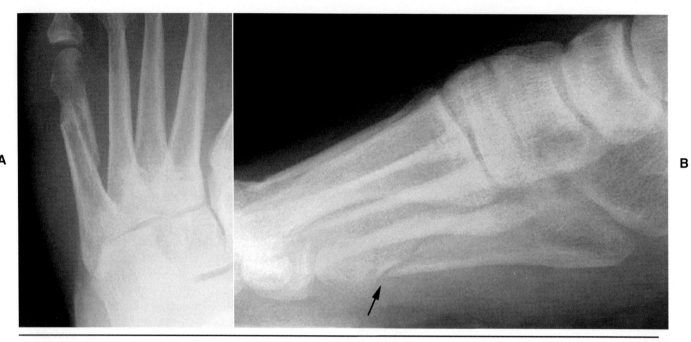

**Figure 12-4**    Fracture position: Two perpendicular planar views of a fifth-metatarsal diaphyseal fracture. **A,** Dorsoplantar view: The distal fracture segment is displaced medially and slightly angulated medially relative to the proximal segment. **B,** Lateral view: The distal segment is displaced superiorly and angulated inferiorly.

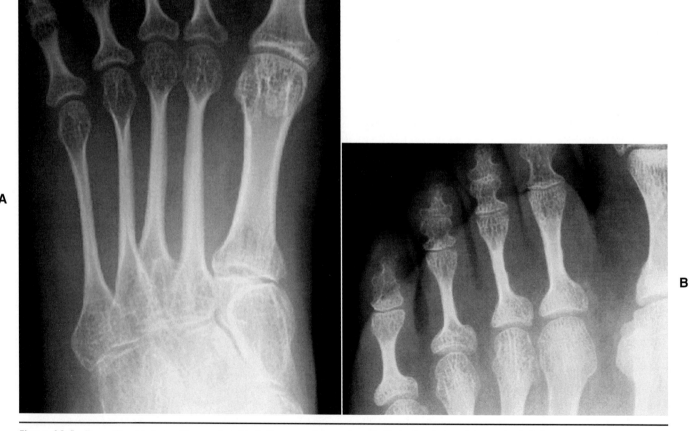

**Figure 12-5**    Form: Overtubulation (decreased girth). **A,** Osteogenesis imperfecta. **B,** Skeletal variation of the proximal phalanges.

**Figure 12-6**    Form: Undertubulation (increased girth). Periosteal bone apposition of the second, third, and fourth metatarsals (unknown etiology). **B,** Skeletal variation affecting all metatarsals.

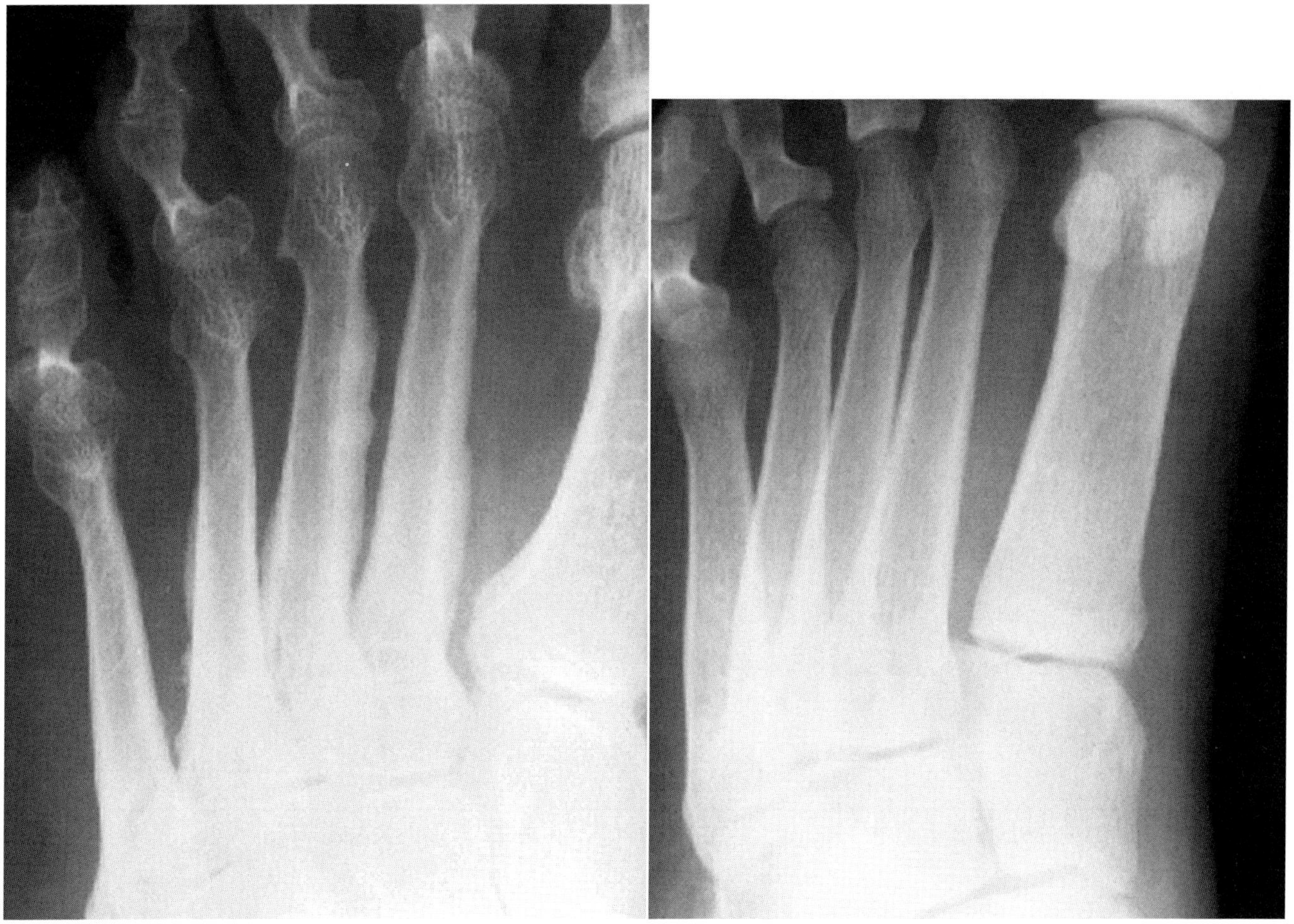

bacteria). It also may be localized or regional (Figure 12-12). Increased soft tissue densities may be related to ectopic calcification or ossification (Figure 12-13). The earliest finding of a periosteal reaction is a localized increased density at the interface between the bone's outer margin and adjacent soft tissue (Figure 12-14). Joint effusion appears as a fairly well-defined increased soft tissue density adjacent to an articulation (Figure 12-15).

Several terms are used interchangeably to describe subject radiodensity in the radiograph (see Box 12-4). For example, the terms *sclerosis, eburnation,* and *radiopacity* are used to denote increased bone density. Abnormal increased density in bone usually indicates reactive new bone or tumor bone formation. Other names for decreased bone density are *osteopenia, radiolucency,* and *rarefaction.* The terms *osteoporosis, demineralization, undermineralization,* and *deossification* should not be used for describing relative radiodensities, because they imply specific etiologies.[1]

The radiodensity of anatomic structures on the radiograph can also be influenced by the film's optical density, which depends heavily on technical factors. For example, increased or decreased kilovoltage (kVp), milliampere-seconds (mAs), and processing time and temperature, to name a few, can result in an overall blacker or less black radiograph, respectively. These factors not only can impair the quality of the image but also can give the wrong impression of subject density.

Generalized loss of bone density is a feature of the metabolic bone diseases (for example, osteoporosis). Unfortunately, diffuse decreased bone density can easily be misjudged in the plain x-ray film. Its appearance is quite subjective and depends on several factors, such as the

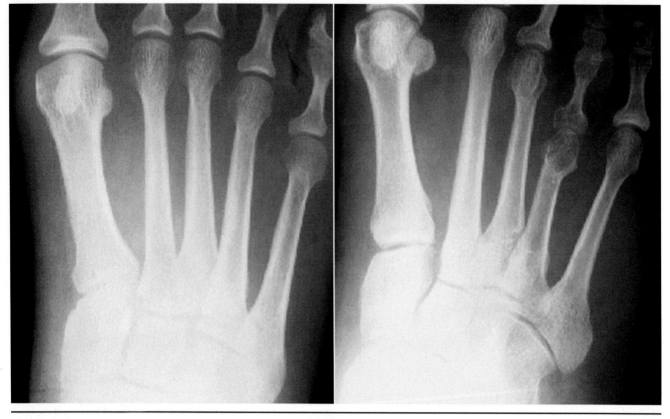

**Figure 12-7**    Form: Increased and decreased bone length. **A,** Elongated third metatarsal. **B,** Short fourth metatarsal.

superimposition of other tissues, bone position, and, most importantly, exposure and processing techniques. It is therefore recommended that the interpreter not rely on the appearance of diffuse decreased bone density alone for evaluating osteopenia. Examination of architectural features is useful for assessing osteopenia and is more objective (see the next section).

## Architecture

Each bone has its own characteristic appearance or structure. The architecture of each bone viewed in a radiograph can be divided into external and internal aspects. The outer margin is the bone's external architecture. It consists of the subperiosteal surface of the cortex, entheses (where tendon, muscle, and joint capsule insert), and the subchondral bone plate. The internal architecture consists of multiple textures, including cortex, spongiosa, and the shadows of normal osteologic landmarks. In the pediatric

| BOX 12-5 | Terminology Used to Describe Findings Related to Architecture |

**EXTERNAL ARCHITECTURE: THE OUTLINE OR MARGIN OF EACH BONE (INCLUDES THE SUBPERIOSTEAL SURFACE AND SUBCHONDRAL BONE PLATE)**
Discontinuous
Ill defined
Erosion
Subperiosteal bone resorption
Dot-dash or skip pattern (subchondral bone plate)
Periosteal reaction

**INTERNAL ARCHITECTURE (INCLUDES CORTEX AND SPONGIOSA)**
Intracortical tunneling or striations
Endosteal scalloping
Cortical thinning
Cortical thickening
Trabecular thinning
Trabecular coarsening

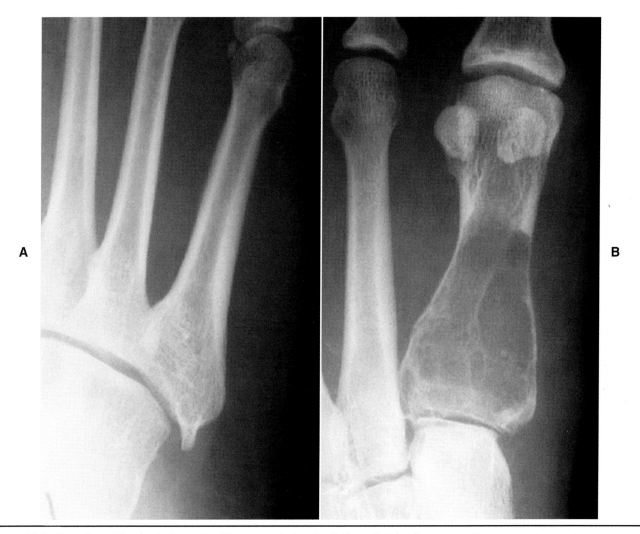

Figure 12-8    Form: Bone deformity. **A,** Spur at the fifth-metatarsal tuberosity. **B,** Expansile lesion (first metatarsal).

patient, the metaphysis, zone of provisional calcification, physis, and epiphysis are additional aspects of internal architecture.

Definition and continuity are two important attributes to consider when evaluating a bone's external architecture (Box 12-5). The margins of the subperiosteal and subchondral surfaces should be well defined and continuous. Discontinuity and/or loss of definition of the subperiosteal aspect of the cortex is an abnormal finding; it can represent fracture or bone resorption (erosion) (Figure 12-16). Periosteal new bone formation may present as an ill-defined thickening of the involved margin. Entheses, although they may appear irregular, should be well defined and continuous.

Erosion and/or calcification/ossification may occur at these sites (Figure 12-17). Discontinuity of the subchondral bone plate is seen with joint disorders (Figure 12-18). A "dot-dash" appearance or "skip" pattern of the bone plate is considered a pre-erosive finding (Figure 12-19) and is associated with inflammatory joint disorders. Generalized subperiosteal bone resorption throughout the skeleton is characteristic of hyperparathyroidism (Figure 12-20).

The periosteum is defined as "a specialized connective tissue covering all bones of the body, and possessing bone forming potentialities."[1] This connective tissue membrane envelops all bones except at entheses and where bones are covered by cartilage.[1] The periosteum is only a few cell layers

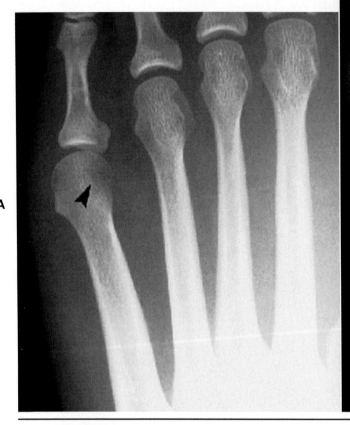

**Figure 12-9**    Examples of normal and abnormal decreased bone density. **A,** The decreased density (*arrow*) seen in the medial aspect of the fifth-metatarsal head is a normal finding. **B,** The decreased density in the medial aspect of the first-metatarsal head is an abnormal finding secondary to intraosseous deposition of gouty tophi.

| BOX 12-6 | Types of Periosteal Reaction |
|---|---|

**CONTINUOUS**
Solid (elliptical, undulating)
Shell ("expansion")
Lamellated ("onion-skin")

**DISCONTINUOUS (OR, INTERRUPTED)**
Buttress
Codman angle
Interrupted lamellar

**COMPLEX**
Spiculated
Radiating
Sunburst

thick. The adult periosteal sheath is thinner in the adult, and more firmly bound to the underlying bone, than in the child.[5] It also is quite vascular.

Histologically, the periosteum consists of two layers. The outer fibrous layer is composed of dense fibrous tissue, blood vessels, and nerve filaments. The inner osteogenic, or cambium, layer is made up of more loosely arranged tissue.[1] These two layers are distinct in the child. However, they become fused in the adult. On stimulation by outside influences, such as trauma, connective tissue cells become activated and osteoblasts appear.

Anything that physically lifts the periosteum from the underlying bone can result in the formation of periosteal new bone formation.[4] Examples include blood, pus, and tumor cells. Other terms synonymous with periosteal new

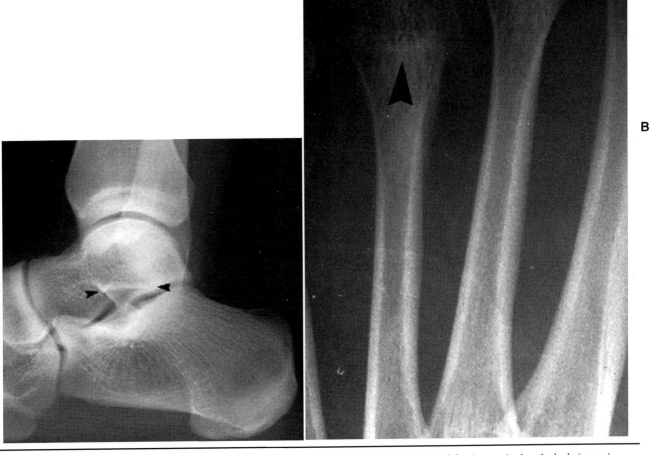

Figure 12-10    Examples of normal and abnormal increased bone density. **A,** The linear, transverse increased density seen in the talar body (*arrows*) corresponds to the superimposed ridge along the medial surface of the talar body for insertion of the deltoid ligament. **B,** The ill-defined increased density viewed in the fourth-metatarsal head (*arrow*) represents a healing stress fracture.

bone formation include *periostitis* and *periosteal reaction.* Its presentation is highly variable[1] (Box 12-6, Figure 12-21). Initially it may only appear as an ill-defined increased density adjacent to the cortex. As it remodels, it can deform the contour of the bone. In either case, periosteal reaction is best appreciated while examining the continuity and definition of the external bone margin.

Cortical bone and spongiosa constitute the greater part of internal architecture. The cortex normally is radiopaque

and homogeneous (Figure 12-22, *A*). Linear radiolucent striations within the cortex of a long bone that run parallel to its long axis suggests intracortical tunneling, a finding associated with osteopenia (Figure 12-22, *B*). The endosteal margin of the cortex should be well defined. A scalloped appearance or loss of definition along the endosteal margin and subsequent thinning of the cortex indicate bone resorption (Figure 12-22, *C*). Cancellous bone (spongiosa) consists of a honeycomb-like mesh of trabeculae. Trabeculae

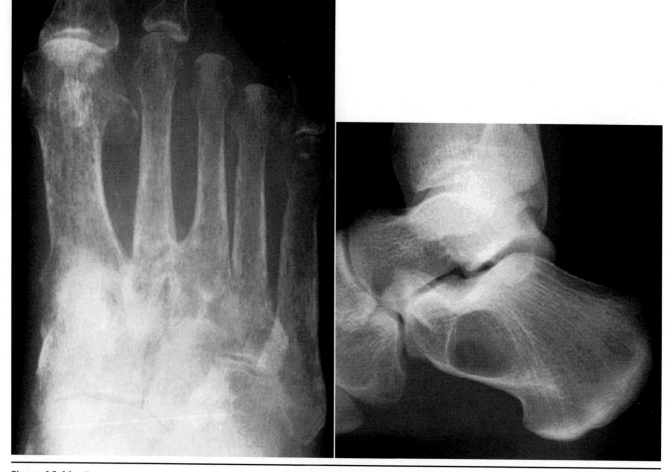

Figure 12-11    Examples of adjectives used to describe decreased bone density. **A,** Mottled (acute osteopenia affecting all metatarsals). **B,** Geographic (solitary bone cyst).

can be subdivided into primary and secondary trabeculae. The primary trabeculae are found along the lines of stress and are easily identified; secondary trabeculae run at angles to the lines of stress and have a fine appearance, giving an overall meshlike appearance to normal spongiosa. With osteopenic conditions, resorption of secondary trabeculae leaves the primary trabeculae to stand out in relief. Subsequent compensatory apposition of new bone onto the remaining primary trabeculae may occur, appearing as trabecular coarsening or thickening[1] (Figure 12-23). It has been suggested that the appearance of calcaneal trabecular patterns provides an index for assessing osteoporosis.[1] However, controversy exists as to whether or not these trabecular patterns correlate with actual bone density.[2]

The superimposed shadows of osseous landmarks and adjacent tissues compose the remainder of the internal architecture of a given bone. These shadows can easily be mistaken for abnormal findings (Figure 12-24).

In the pediatric patient the metaphysis, zone of provisional calcification, physis, and epiphysis must also be assessed (Figure 12-25). The metaphysis, found at the end of the diaphysis of a tubular bone, primarily consists of spongiosa and has a characteristic density. The zone of provisional calcification is located at the junction of the metaphysis and physis (or growth plate). It may be smooth or irregular (but well defined) in contour and is sclerotic relative to the neighboring metaphysis. The physis is wholly cartilaginous and appears radiolucent. It separates the metaphysis and zone of provisional calcification from the epiphysis. The epiphysis has a well-defined sclerotic margin around its entire circumference. In its center it is composed of spongiosa and has a characteristic density.

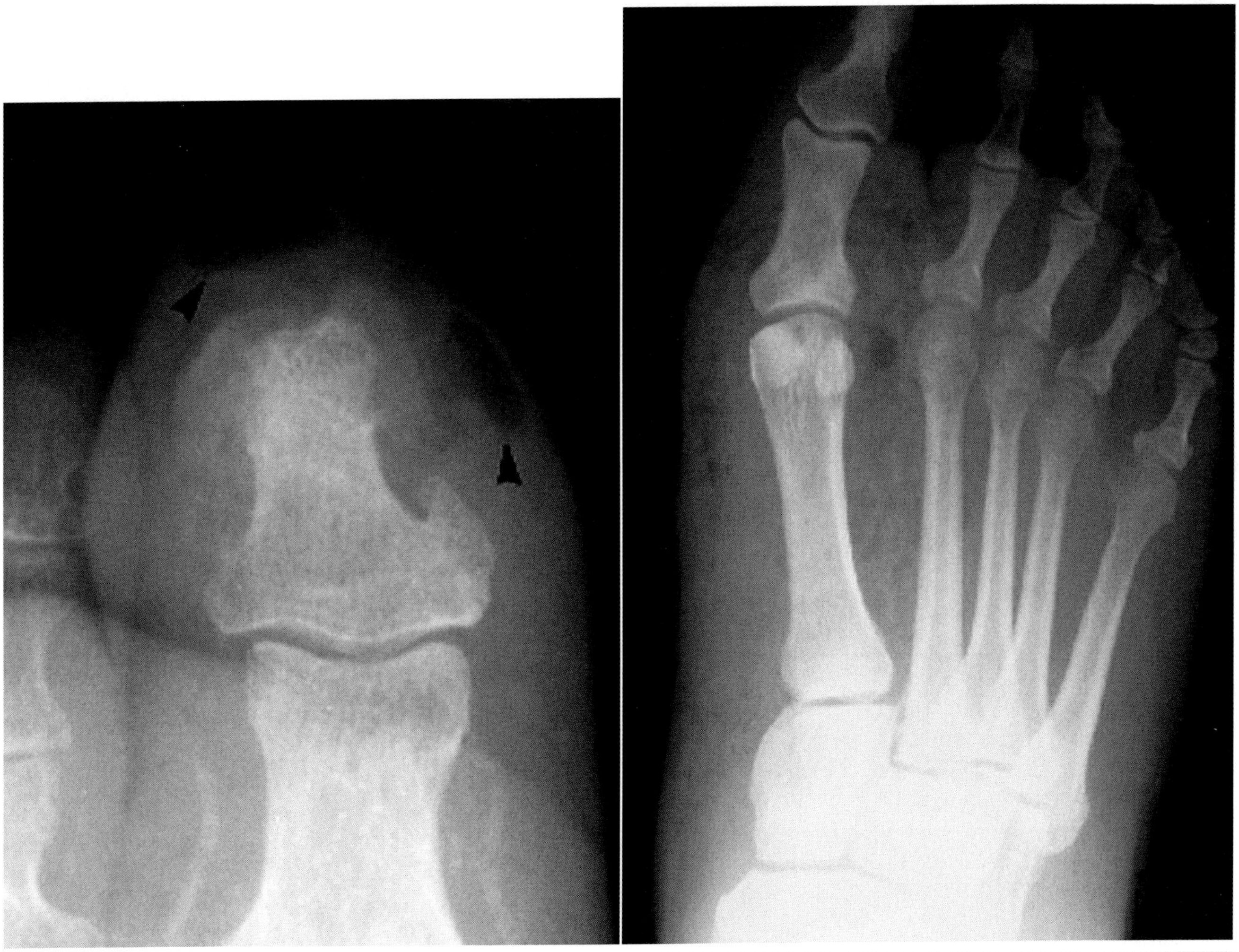

Figure 12-12  Decreased density in soft tissue: Air produced by gas-forming bacteria. **A,** Localized. **B,** Regional (gas gangrene).

## ▓ METHOD OF ASSESSMENT

Each of the preceding criteria must be evaluated on all applicable anatomic structures. The actual order of assessment is not as important as is the consistent use of a system. The following method for analyzing foot and ankle radiographs provides a means for evaluating all anatomic structures in an order that the interpreter can easily follow and, more importantly, repeat. This method focuses on examination of the skeletal system; for a thorough evaluation, however, the soft tissues must also be included (Box 12-7). Each abnormality should be described in detail, using any appropriate adjectives. The specific location of any particular finding should also be described.

## General Overview

Sit back and look at the entire film. Evaluate the overall blackness of each film (that is, optical density), and determine whether or not the blackness (or lack of blackening) of the image is influenced by technical factors. Observe the positional relationships of osseous structures to one another, and compare to normal expectations.

## Soft Tissue Examination

It is recommended that the soft tissues be observed before the individual bones. Radiographs of the foot or ankle are primarily obtained for assessing bone or joint pathology; the

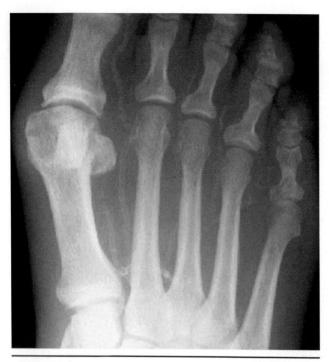

Figure 12-13    Increased density in soft tissue: Vessel calcification.

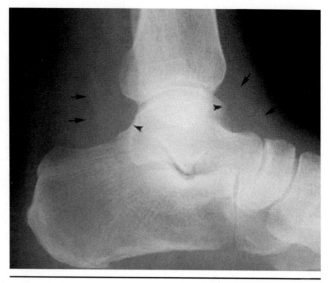

Figure 12-15    Increased soft tissue density at a periarticular location: Joint effusion.

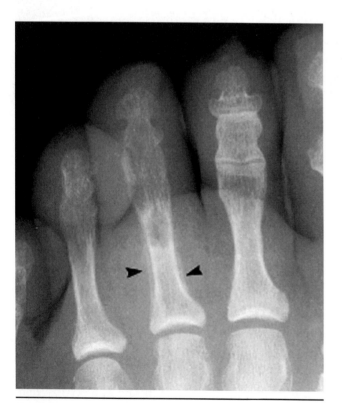

Figure 12-14    Increased soft tissue density along the outer margin of a bone: Periosteal reaction.

soft tissues, therefore, are easily overlooked. A system that evaluates the soft tissues first prevents this inadvertent omission. Evaluate the form and density of all soft tissue shadows, comparing to the normal expected image. Search for abnormalities of soft tissue density and/or volume. Identify any aberrant increased or decreased densities seen in the soft tissues (foreign bodies, for example). Are there calcifications, ossifications, or gas in the soft tissues?

---

**BOX 12-7**    Method of Assessment

**GENERAL OVERVIEW**
Overall degree of blackness (film density)
Positional relationships

**SOFT TISSUE EXAMINATION**
Density
Position
Form

**EXAMINATION OF BONE AND CONTIGUOUS STRUCTURES**
Density
Position
Form
Architecture

**JOINT EVALUATION**
Position (space, apposition)
Review adjacent bone architecture, form, and density
Periarticular soft tissues

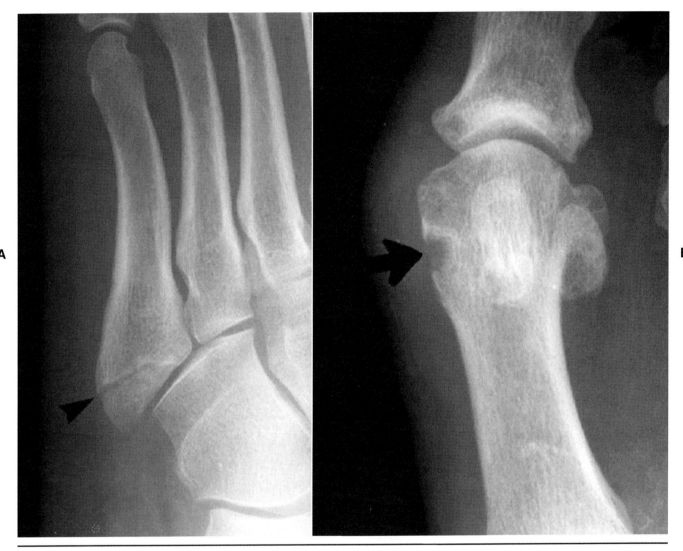

**Figure 12-16**    External architecture abnormality. **A,** Discontinuity (fracture). **B,** Ill defined (loss of definition): Erosion.

## Examination of Bone and Contiguous Structures

Examine the individual bones in each view. Proceed from the digits to the tarsus (recommended) or vice versa, or from medial to lateral or lateral to medial. Whichever way you choose, do it in the same fashion each and every time. This sounds like a long, tedious exercise, and initially it is. However, with practice all structures in a foot and/or ankle study can be assessed expeditiously.

First, examine the bone's overall form. Second, identify any abnormal densities. Third, evaluate the cortex, including its subperiosteal and endosteal surfaces. Look at the medullary canal, spongiosa, and the articular surfaces (subchondral bone plates). Assess all entheses. Periosteal and periarticular

contiguous structures should be examined closely. If the patient is a child, also examine the metaphysis, zone of provisional calcification, physis, and epiphysis. Perform this examination on each and every bone (Box 12-8).

## Joint Evaluation

Finally, all articulations are evaluated (see Chapter 22). The joint spaces are examined for width, parallelism, and apposition between the opposing subchondral bone plates. Assess the periarticular soft tissues for increased density (joint effusion) and calcifications. Any erosions or periarticular bone production should already have been recognized while assessing bone architecture.

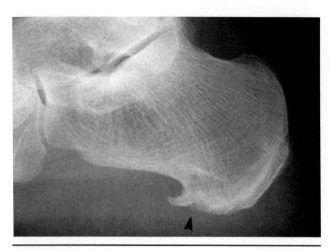

**Figure 12-17**  Mixed erosive and spurlike enthesopathy, calcaneal medial tuberosity.

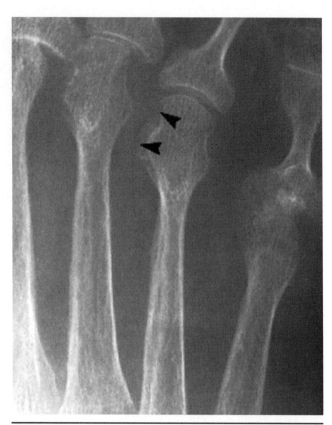

**Figure 12-19**  External architecture: Dot-dash or "skip" pattern in a patient with rheumatoid arthritis.

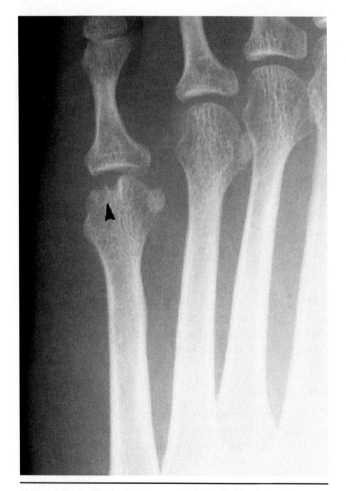

**Figure 12-18**  External architecture: Subchondral bone plate. Erosion (rheumatoid arthritis).

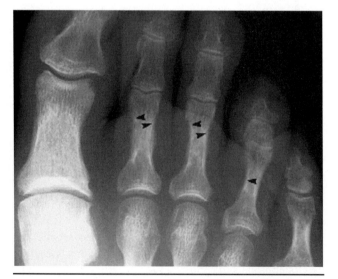

**Figure 12-20**  External architecture: Phalangeal subperiosteal bone resorption.

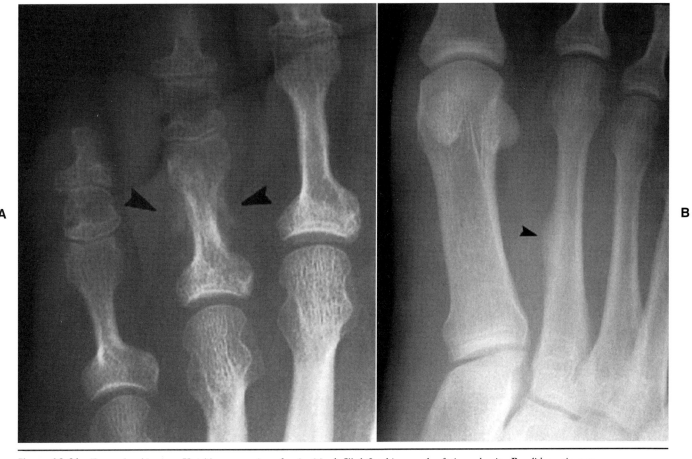

Figure 12-21   External architecture: Variable presentation of periostitis. **A,** Ill-defined increased soft tissue density; **B,** solid, continuous.

*Continued*

---

**BOX 12-8**   **Evaluation of Bone and Contiguous Structures**

| TUBULAR BONES | IRREGULAR BONES |
|---|---|
| **EXTERNAL MARGIN** | **EXTERNAL MARGIN** |
| Periosteal surface of cortex | Periosteal surface of cortex |
| Entheses | Entheses |
| Subchondral bone plate | Subchondral bone plate |
| | |
| **INTERNAL ARCHITECTURE** | **INTERNAL ARCHITECTURE** |
| Cortex | Spongiosa |
| Endosteal surface of cortex | |
| Medullary canal | **CONTIGUOUS STRUCTURES** |
| Spongiosa | Joint space |
| Metaphysis* | Periarticular soft tissues |
| Zone of provisional calcification* | |
| Physis* | |
| Epiphysis* | |
| | |
| **CONTIGUOUS STRUCTURES** | |
| Joint space | |
| Periarticular soft tissues | |

*Before closure of growth plate.

C

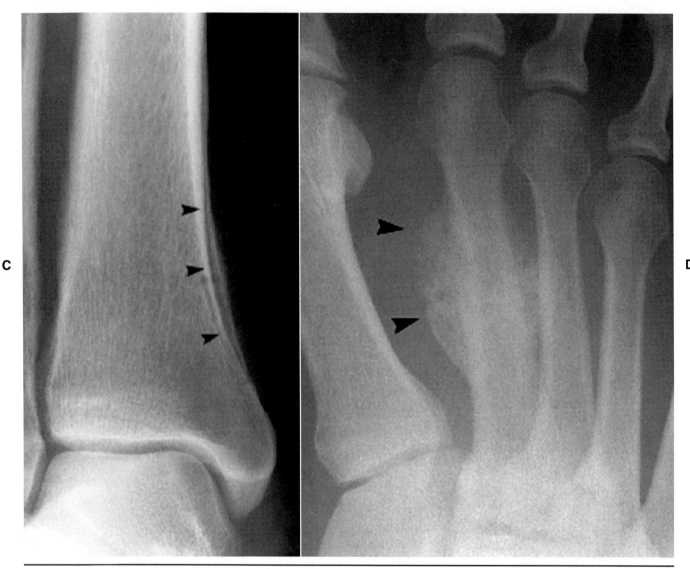

D

Figure 12-21, cont'd   External architecture: Variable presentation of periostitis. **C**, solid, lamellated; **D**, complex (spiculated and radiating). (**D**, Courtesy Louis P. Zulli, D.P.M., Philadelphia).

## ■ SUMMARY

A common pitfall when interpreting foot and ankle radiographs is mistaking normal anatomic shadows for pathology. It is therefore strongly recommended that the clinician keep at hand a loosely articulated set of foot and ankle bones when viewing radiographs of the same. The reader is encouraged to study Chapter 7 for further information on this topic.

The system for evaluating foot and ankle radiographs discussed in this chapter emphasizes the recognition of an abnormality set apart from the normal expectation. Each and every abnormal finding is recognized in all instances if the interpreter (1) is familiar with the normal radiographic anatomy and variations of the foot and ankle, and (2) evaluates the density, position, form, and architecture of all structures. The next step requires using the appropriate terminology to describe the abnormal finding. Finally, select applicable differential diagnoses. All available data should be considered, including history of the present illness, patient medical history, clinical presentation, radiographic findings, and the results of laboratory tests and other diagnostic procedures.

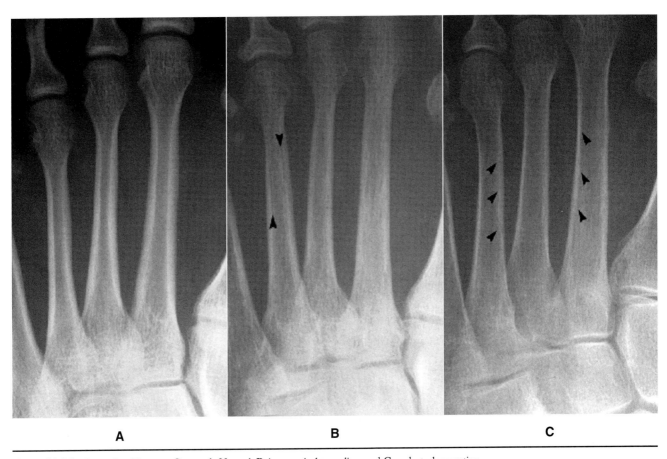

Figure 12-22   Internal architecture: Cortex. **A**, Normal; **B**, intracortical tunneling; and **C**, endosteal resorption.

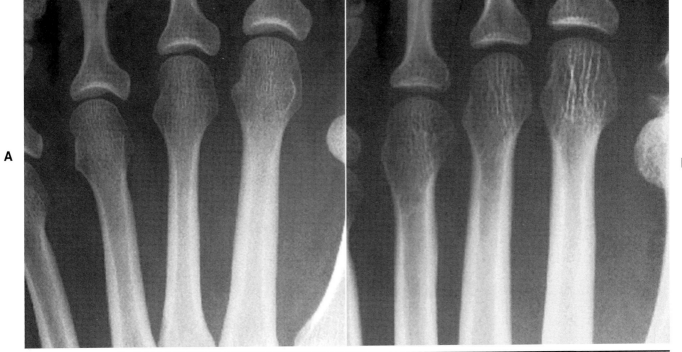

Figure 12-23   Internal architecture: Trabecular bone resorption. **A**, Normal metatarsal head. **B**, Osteopenia.

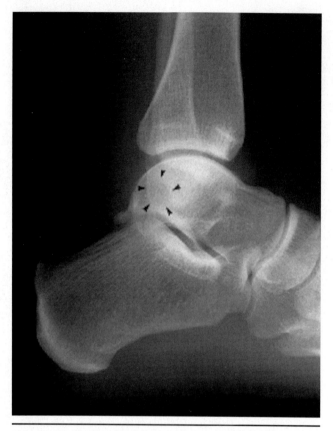

**Figure 12-24** Internal architecture: Misinterpretation. The radiolucency *(arrow)* in the talar body represents the superimposed fibular notch, not a solitary bone lesion.

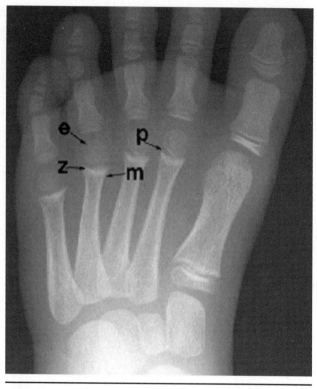

**Figure 12-25** The normal growing long bone (*e*, epiphysis; *m*, metaphysis; *p*, physis; *z*, zone of provisional calcification).

## References

1. Meschan I: *Roentgen signs in diagnostic imaging*, ed 2, Philadelphia, 1985, Saunders.

2. Squire LF, Novelline RA: *Fundamentals of radiography*, ed 4, Cambridge, Mass, 1988, Harvard University Press.

3. Bonakdarpour A: A systematic approach to skeletal radiology. Temple University School of Medicine, Philadelphia, unpublished.

4. Greenfield, GB: *Radiology of bone diseases*, ed 4, Philadelphia, 1986, Lippincott.

5. Cimmino CV: The radiologist and the orthopedist, *Radiology* 97:690, 1970.

6. Pitt MJ, Speer DP: Radiologic reporting of orthopedic trauma, *Med Radiogr Photogr* 58:14, 1982.

7. Renner RR, Mauler GG, Ambrose JL: The radiologist, the orthopedist, the lawyer and the fracture. *Sem Roentgenol* 13(1):7, 1978.

8. Bushong SC: *Radiologic science for technologists*, ed 5, St. Louis, 1993, Mosby.

9. Resnick D, Niwayama, G: *Diagnosis of bone and joint disorders*, ed 2, Philadelphia, 1988, Saunders.

10. *Dorland's illustrated medical dictionary*, ed 27, Philadelphia, 1988, Saunders.

11. Jaffe HL: *Metabolic, degenerative, and inflammatory diseases of bones and joints*, Philadelphia, 1972, Lea & Febiger.

12. Leeson CR, Leeson TS: *Histology*, ed 3, Philadelphia, 1976, Saunders.

13. Ragsdale BD, Madewell JE, Sweet DE: Radiologic and pathologic analysis of solitary bone lesions. II. Periosteal reactions, *Radiol Clin North Am* 19(4):749, 1981.

14. Bullough PG, Vigorita VJ: *Atlas of orthopaedic pathology with clinical and radiologic correlations*, Baltimore, 1984, University Park Press.

15. Jhamaria NL, Lal KB, Udawat M et al: The trabecular pattern of the calcaneum as an index of osteoporosis, *J Bone Joint Surg* 65B(2):195, 1983.

16. Cockshott WP, Occleshaw CJ, Webber C et al: Can a calcaneal morphologic index determine the degree of osteoporosis? *Skeletal Radiol* 12:119, 1984.

# Radiographic Biomechanical Analysis

# CHAPTER 13

# Principles of Biomechanical Radiographic Analysis of the Foot

WILLIAM H. SANNER

The purposes of using radiographs to analyze foot biomechanics are to determine foot stability and individual joint stability, to evaluate the foot as a tool for locomotion, to correlate to the physical exam, and to plan surgery.[1,2] This chapter describes a system based on the concepts of stability that can be used to analyze the biomechanics of the foot.

## ■ REVIEW

The majority of foot radiographs used to assess foot mechanics are weight bearing so as to more closely approximate osseous relationships in gait.[3] Approximating gait and standardization are also why foot radiographs are taken in the angle and base of gait.[3–5] The forces are not the same, because midstance is dynamic and radiographs represent a static situation. Nevertheless, radiographs demonstrate how the weight-bearing foot reacts in a closed kinetic-chain environment as the foot interacts with ground reactive forces.

Although specialty views are used, such as Harris-Beath[6] and anterior axial view of the foot,[7] the primary views used are the dorsoplantar and lateral.[2–4] The dorsoplantar view represents the transverse-plane relationships within the foot, and the lateral view represents the sagittal-plane relationships.[2,3,7,8] The dorsoplantar and lateral views are used together to infer frontal-plane relationships. The anteroposterior axial views of the foot provide direct frontal-plane relationships.[7,9]

Positioning the weight-bearing patient is very important, because the osseous relationships represented by the radiograph and then analyzed by the clinician can be changed dramatically if the patient is not relaxed in his or her angle and base of gait.[10–14] Standardized positioning is essential for reproduction and accuracy of the radiograph representing the foot's interaction with ground reactive forces.

The foot bones have a genetically predetermined shape and alignment, which can be modified secondarily by stress created by force that originates intrinsically and extrinsically to the foot.[15] This phenomenon is generally referred to as Wolff's law. The clinician can assess these stresses by observing the trabeculae and bone shapes.[16,17] The trabeculae are created parallel to the direction of stress. Bone shape evolves as the result of compression and tension experienced by the bone when standing and walking. Thus if compression is not even across a joint, the bones of the joint change shape, reflecting the abnormal application of force on the joint. What may begin as a minor asymmetry of force applied through a joint may result in the bones of the joint developing a shape that perpetuates the reduced efficiency of the joint. The shape of the foot bones is crucial—the foot is like a bridge that must carry the body.[18,19]

To meet the requirements of gait, the foot bridge bones must be well aligned to provide stability, yet allow just enough motion to help absorb shock and adapt to terrain while walking. The foot must also not become so flexible that it is not stable during midstance and propulsion, to allow timely first-metatarsophalangeal joint dorsiflexion.[20–22] The ideal foot is not the most stable or the most unstable, but rather is balanced between the two conditions.

When clinicians review foot radiographs and examine the foot for the purpose of analyzing the foot as a tool for locomotion, they are looking for signs of stability. When describing foot radiographs, evaluators compare the alignment of one segment to another and always describe the distal relative to the proximal segment. Keep in mind that the distal part cannot be stable unless the proximal segment is stable.[21,23]

## TERMINOLOGY

Throughout this chapter the terms *position, stability*, and *alignment* are used. The key to understanding the concepts described in this chapter is to have a sound understanding of these terms.

### Position

According to *Webster's New World Dictionary of the American Language*, position means "the place where a thing is … in relationship to others."[24] Position of a joint describes where in the range of motion of that joint the respective bones are placed or situated. Therefore, to give the position of a joint a reference must be provided. The reference may be degrees or angulation relative to a proximal segment (for example, the calcaneus is 5 degrees inverted relative to the leg), relative to an end range of motion (such as maximally pronated), or relative to a neutral position (for example, the ankle is 10 degrees dorsiflexed). Position does not imply motion or direction of motion. For example, an ankle may be 10 degrees dorsiflexed, but this does not imply that it is dorsiflexing, plantarflexing, or stationary, these being terms of motion.

If the clinician does not have a reference to which to compare the relative position of two bones, then the position of that joint or series of joints cannot be determined. For example, you must first determine the subtalar joint neutral position before you can determine if the position of the subtalar joint is pronated, neutral, or supinated. The terms *plantarflexed/dorsiflexed, abducted/adducted*, and *varus/valgus* can be used when describing radiographs of the foot, because these terms compare one foot segment to another.

The subtalar joint neutral position cannot be determined radiographically, as it can in a clinical exam. Because no reference exists for subtalar neutral position on foot radiographs, the terms *supinated, neutral*, and *pronated* should not be used to describe foot position. Instead, terms referring to alignment and stability must be used to describe foot morphology.

### Stability

Stability of an object is the "state of being fixed," "resistant to change," and the "ability to return to its original position."[24] Thus a stable object is "not easily moved or thrown off balance," "is not likely to break down or fall apart," is "lasting and enduring," and "is able to return to its original position after being displaced."

Similarly the foot must for many years be able to adapt to uneven terrain, be a rigid lever for propulsion, and yet return to its original position at the beginning of each step.[2] A foot that is too stable could not adapt to uneven terrain because it would be too "resistant to change." A foot that is not stable cannot act as a rigid lever or return to its original position once displaced. The degree of stability is a quality important to proper foot mechanics and is a quality that can be inferred in radiographs based on the alignment of weight-bearing bones.

### Alignment

The term *alignment* means "arrangement in a straight line," and *to align* means "to bring into a straight line."[24] Thus in an aligned foot the bones have straight linear relationships. When performing biomechanical radiographic evaluation of the foot, the term *alignment* should be used instead of *position*. This is because a straight line can be used as a reference and because the concept of linearity is the foundation for the concept of stability.

In general, most objects are more stable when they are well aligned (linear), that is, they bear loads better (Figure 13-1). The linear relationship of a well-aligned load-bearing object allows even distribution of the stress of the load and reduces the tendency for bending. In the foot we evaluate the relative stability of joints. When a joint is loaded, the joint has more inherent stability when the joint is arranged in a straight line.

The foot must not have perfect linear relationships because such alignment would provide too much stability. As described earlier, a foot that is too stable cannot serve all the functions required for normal locomotion. In contrast, a foot that has its respective bones angled too much is too unstable and collapses under the load.

## PRINCIPLES OF STABILITY

Joints are the most stable when they are compressed and are subject to no moments, that is, rotational forces.[21] The most stable joint is one that is linear and has force directed at the joint axis, and the compression is distributed evenly and perpendicular to the joint surface.[21] (Figure 13-2). This creates maximum compression and stability. A stable joint must have even compression across the joint surface. The radiograph should show the joint space (surface) to be congruent for the joint to have even transmission of compression. An angled, subluxated, or dislocated joint does not have even compression across the joint surface and is not stable.

Thus the most stable foot would be one that has only straight joints, no angulation of the various osseous

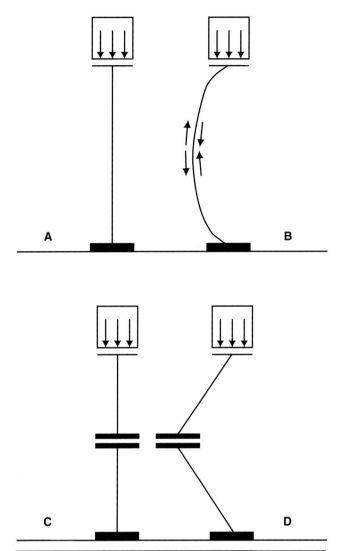

Figure 13-1   In general, a straight load-bearing column (**A**) is more stable than one that is curved (**B**) or angled (**D**). A curved or angled load-bearing column structure when compressed by the load develops a compression side and a tension side. Even if the nonlinear load-bearing column is stable, the uneven load borne through the nonlinear structure is more likely to result in fatigue of the column and eventually may lead to collapse. If the linear column has a joint that is properly aligned with the loading force (**C**) (perpendicular with the loading force vector and the loading force vector passes through the joint), the column continues to support the load because no rotational force (moment) is exerted at the joint.

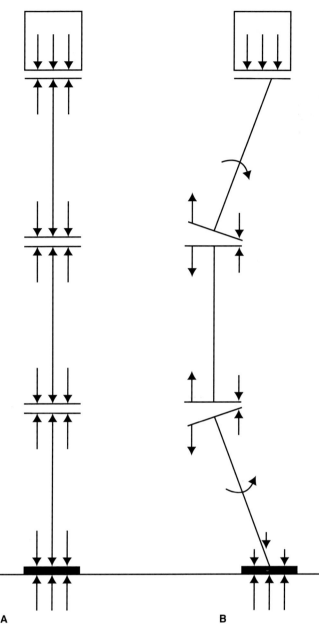

Figure 13-2   A column that has a series of segments is stable so long as the joints between the segments have even compression across the joint surface (**A**). Even compression is achieved when the joints are aligned so that the joint surface is perpendicular to the compressive force vector and the force vector passes through the joint. When the joints are not aligned linearly with the compressive force, a moment (rotational force) is created at the joint and the joint rotates instead of bearing the load (**B**).

segments, even joint spaces, and perpendicularity of all forces to the joint axes and surfaces. Because each osseous segment would be well aligned relative to its neighbor and thus stable, the entire foot would be stable.

A force vector that creates rotation at a joint is called a *moment*. Moments and the resulting rotation are the opposite of stability. The most unstable foot is one that has much angulation between the osseous segments, uneven

joint spaces, uneven compression of the joints, and a net force vector that is not perpendicular to the joint axes, so that a moment is created. The joint angulation (lack of alignment) and nonperpendicularity of the net force to the joint surface and axis results in rotation, which is the opposite of stability.

When the foot pushes down on the ground, the ground pushes upward; this is ground reactive force.[25,26] The majority of ground reactive forces are not directed toward most of the nearly vertically oriented foot joint surfaces or joint axes[27] (Figure 13-3). The foot develops stability although the net force vector acting on the foot is not directed perpendicular to most of the joint surfaces. The foot tension bands (more correctly called a *truss*) are the key elements in changing how the vertical (sagittal plane) force, which is the largest component of ground reactive force, is directed through the foot.[19,28–36] The plantar fascial and ligament tension band system converts the vertically directed forces into compression of a series of straight, self-locking wedges by not allowing the rotation to occur.[28,29,34–39] The rotation prevented is forefoot dorsiflexion on the rearfoot.

First-metatarsophalangeal joint dorsiflexion during propulsion winds the plantar aponeuros is around the first-metatarsal head, effectively shortening the plantar aponeurosis in wrenchlike fashion. The winding of the plantar aponeurosis around the first-metatarsal head plantarflexes the forefoot on the rearfoot (supinates the foot), reduces the angles between segments of the foot, and increases foot stability by resisting rotation of the forefoot on the rearfoot (dorsiflexion). This wrenchlike mechanism is called the *windlass effect*.[28] Timely first-metatarsophalangeal joint dorsiflexion during propulsion increases foot stability at a time when ground reactive forces are the greatest. The extrinsic and intrinsic foot muscles aid the plantar aponeurosis in stabilizing the forefoot on the rearfoot, specifically the medial longitudinal arch. Thus the foot was designed to function well in the face of large vertical forces, as long as the foot is well aligned.

The foot is not as well designed to resist the influences of transverse- and frontal-plane forces, because there is no tension band mechanism designed for these forces. Instead, muscles and ligaments must resist transverse- and frontal-plane forces. Only when the foot is well aligned and inherently stable, with ground reactive forces that are

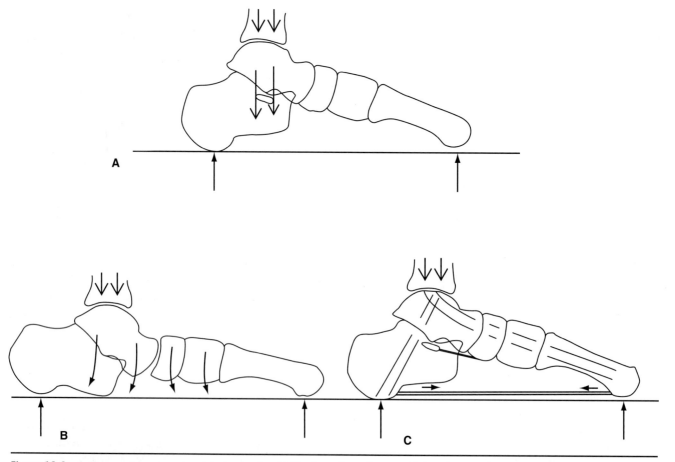

Figure 13-3   **A,** Forces acting on a static weight-bearing foot. **B,** The foot collapses because it did not have an effective plantar truss mechanism. As the foot collapses, it elongates. **C,** The plantar truss prevents elongation of the foot as the loading forces try to collapse the foot. Instead of collapsing the foot, the force created by the load is translated into compression of the midfoot and subtalar joints. If the joints being compressed are well aligned (straight), the compression increases stability of the joints as opposed to resulting in an unstable rotational force (moment).

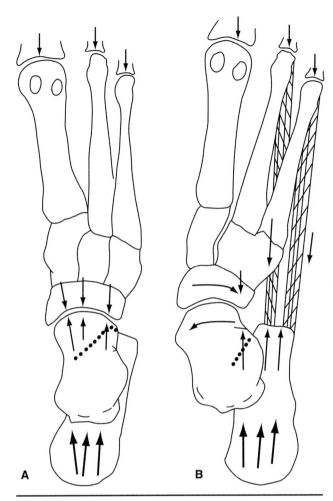

**Figure 13-4   A,** Dorsal view of a rectus (straight) medial column with the plantar fascia and ligaments under the bones and not visible. The resulting vectors of force *(arrows)* are shown as creating compression and thus stability at the joints. **B,** Dorsal view of a pronated medial column with the plantar fascia and ligaments now lateral to the medial column. Because of the pronated position, the proximal medial column is largely medial to the plantar fascia and ligaments. The compression is translated into rotation at the talonavicular joint, which exacerbates the pronated position.

principally sagittal plane in nature and are not converted into transverse- and frontal-plane moments, can the muscles and ligaments adequately decelerate the resulting transverse- and frontal-plane joint motion, and convert the rotational potential into compressive forces in the joints (Figure 13-4). When the foot is unstable, more muscle activity is necessary to improve stability.[40]

Thus the ideal foot has a slight angulation, which allows for motion and transmission of force consistent with stability, yet is not so straight as to be rigid. The ideal foot has forces acting on it, which principally oriented toward the sagittal plane, and the tension band mechanism can convert the forces into compression instead of moments. The

frontal- and transverse-plane moments must be small in magnitude so that the resulting motion can be decelerated by the muscles. Dynamically, most of the motion should be in the sagittal plane. The ankle and first-metatarsophalangeal joints must be able to function with appropriate alignment relative to the line of progression, and have timing of motion to allow smooth, nonhalting, forward progression.[22]

## ■ NORMAL (RECTUS) FOOT ALIGNMENT BASED ON PRINCIPLES OF STABILITY

Although the theme has variations, all descriptions of the normal (ideal) lower extremity are based on alignment of the various segments to promote stability during gait. The normal (ideal) lower extremity places the knee and first-metatarsophalangeal joint axes approximately perpendicular to the line of progression and the ankle only slightly externally rotated to facilitate motion in the sagittal plane.[2,11] The tibia and calcaneus are vertical, like a weight-bearing column, and the forefoot is well aligned anterior to the rearfoot and is not contributing either pronatory or supinatory retrograde force.

The distal segment must be able to be compressed onto the proximal segment for stability.[21,23] The talus is locked in the ankle mortise and thus is an extension of the leg.[41] As an extension of the leg, the talus is the most proximal portion of the foot. It is appropriate to use the talus as the proximal reference when evaluating foot mechanical stability with radiographs, because the foot must align so as to be able to be compressed onto its most proximal segment. For stability and efficient transmission of force, the foot should be under and immediately anterior to the ankle.[19]

The normal rearfoot should be an extension of the straight weight-bearing column of the leg.[42] Therefore the calcaneus must be under the talus in the frontal plane (anterior axial view of the foot) to minimize inversion/eversion moments (Figure 13-5), and in the transverse plane (dorsoplantar view talocalcaneal angle and superimposition) to support the talus (Figure 13-6).

In the sagittal plane the calcaneus medial tubercle needs to be far enough posterior to the ankle axis so as to create a plantarflexion moment at the ankle. This translates heel contact shock into ankle plantarflexion, which in turn is decelerated by the anterior compartment muscles. If the calcaneal contact point is moved anteriorly by a high-pitched calcaneus, the calcaneal contact point is close to the ankle axis, and a sharp increase in ground reactive force is transmitted up the leg instead of absorbed by ankle plantarflexion deceleration (Figure 13-7).

The calcaneus should be inclined (lateral view, calcaneal inclination angle) to the supporting surface to lift the talus so that an arch is created to facilitate the tension band

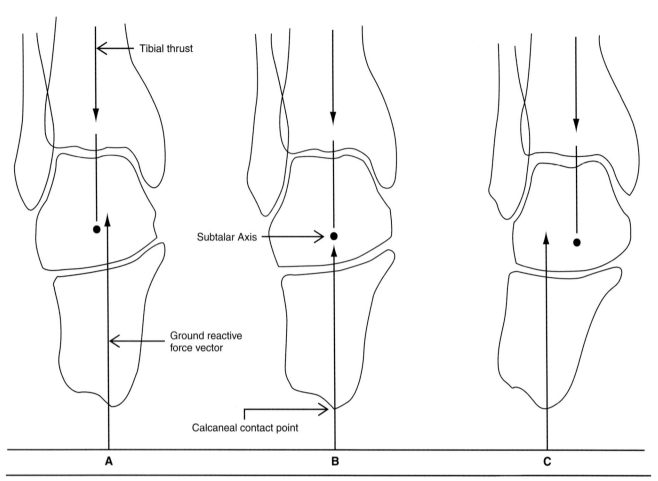

**Figure 13-5** The subtalar axis is approximately inferior to the center of the ankle. The subtalar joint is influenced by the forces acting from superiorly (tibial thrust) and inferiorly (ground reactive forces). The ground reactive forces have vectors of force pointing superiorly and are equal and opposite to the downward force that the body exerts on the supporting surface at the calcaneal contact point. Because the tibial thrust is usually directly superior to the subtalar axis, the tibial thrust has a very short moment arm and minimal influence on the subtalar. The calcaneal contact point, in contrast, is further away from the subtalar axis, and thus has a longer moment arm and greater influence on the subtalar. **A,** The contact point is medial to the subtalar axis. Thus the ground reactive force is a supinatory influence on the subtalar. **B,** The calcaneal contact point ideally should be directly inferior to the center of the ankle (tibial thrust) to minimize pronatory or supinatory moments acting at the subtalar axis. **C,** The calcaneal contact point is lateral to the subtalar axis, and thus the ground reactive force has pronatory influence on the subtalar.

mechanism. The arch moves the plantar fascia away from the midfoot joints, thus providing a longer lever to resist forefoot ground reactive forces and to prevent overextension (dorsiflexion) of the forefoot.

The normal forefoot in the transverse plane should be placed anterior to the rearfoot such that the first-metatarsophalangeal joint plane of motion is parallel to the line of progression to facilitate timely dorsiflexion, and the ankle rests within the triangular base of support created by the heel and medial and lateral forefoot columns (see Figure 13-6). If the ankle is not centered over the foot, then the weight (tibial thrust) will be tilting toward and overloading one side of the foot.[43] Thus the forefoot cannot be overly adducted or abducted. The forefoot-to-rearfoot transverse-plane relationship is assessed on the dorsoplantar view with

the talocuboid angle, forefoot angle, and talar longitudinal axis relative to the longitudinal bisection of the first ray.[2,21,44]

Likewise, if the calcaneus is too far laterally displaced relative to the talus, the net moment will evert the rearfoot (see Figure 13-5). This eversion moment over time may lead to subtalar subluxation and to instability in the forefoot.[45] Having the calcaneus too far medially, relative to the ankle and talus, results in increased shock because of the reduced subtalar motion during the contact period of gait, and lateral ankle instability.

In the sagittal plane the proximal portion of the medial column is raised away from the supporting surface by the calcaneus, and the talocalcaneal angle defines the relationship of the calcaneus to the medial column in the normal foot (see Figure 13-3). The medial column should be

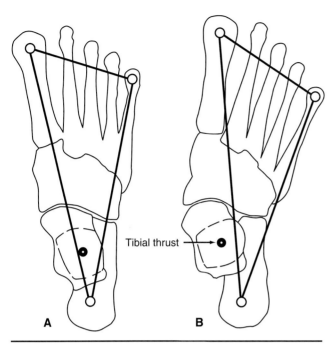

**Figure 13-6    A,** The rectus foot depicted has the tibial thrust (superior center of force) within the weight-bearing triangle of the foot. **B,** The overpronated foot depicted has talar adductus and forefoot abductus. Thus the tibial thrust is medial to the weight-bearing triangle of the foot and becomes a pronatory influence on the subtalar.

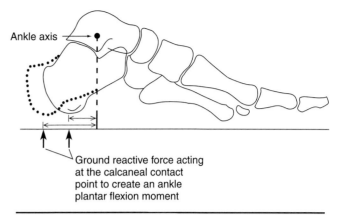

**Figure 13-7**    The normal calcaneus (*dotted lines*) has a calcaneal contact point that is further posterior to the ankle axis than is a short or highly inclined calcaneus. The longer the moment arm of the normal calcaneus means that at heel contact the vertical force results in a rotation (plantarflexion) of the ankle. This rotation is decelerated by the anterior compartment muscles during the contact period, which contributes to shock absorption. When the calcaneus is short or vertical, the ground reactive force at heel contact is transmitted up the leg as shock (rapid deceleration) instead of attenuated by the ankle plantarflexion decelerators.

aligned as a series of straight bones for optimal stability when compressed by the tension band (lateral view, longitudinal axis of the talus bisecting the medial column), and should be angled to the supporting surface (talar declination angle) such that rotational moments can be translated into compression by the plantar aponeurosis, which is removed from the midfoot joints. The forefoot must not be so vertical that intrinsic muscle balance is disturbed or that the plantar fascia can make the metatarsus too rigid.

The frontal-plane alignment of the foot is created by extrapolating from the dorsoplantar and lateral views. Frontal-plane alignment is viewed as superimposition (stacking) of bones on the dorsoplantar view (talocalcaneal, navicularcuboid, and metatarsal base) and lateral view (navicularcuboid). The ideal foot has the rearfoot stacked enough (dorsoplantar view talocalcaneal superimposition) to minimize frontal-plane moments and to take advantage of the midtarsal self-locking mechanism inherent to the talonavicular and calcaneocuboid joints sitting one above the other,[21] which complements the divergent axis mechanism proposed by Hicks.[46] The ideal frontal-plane–aligned forefoot, when weight bearing, should not be creating an inversion or eversion moment, which would result in the forefoot (1) rolling medially (forefoot varus), creating reduced stacking, or (2) rolling laterally (forefoot valgus), resulting in increased stacking and in the respective reduced and increased stability.

Radiographic evaluation of the first-metatarsophalangeal joint for stability is primarily a transverse-plane assessment. The hallux must be less than 15 degrees abducted relative to the first metatarsal for the six muscles and plantar aponeurosis to be able to compress the proximal phalanx on the metatarsal without creating an abductory moment that cannot be neutralized by the medial structures. This compression of the proximal phalanx on the first metatarsal is a key component in compression of the medial column.

In the sagittal plane, the ideal first-metatarsophalangeal joint dorsiflexes as the heel lifts during propulsion. This allows for uninterrupted anterior motion of the body,[22] and for the windlass mechanism described by Hicks to further stabilize the foot for propulsion by winding the plantar aponeurosis around the first-metatarsal head.[28,29] The lateral view should demonstrate the longitudinal axis of the hallux proximal phalanx to bisect the head of the first metatarsal and should be parallel to the supporting surface. If the proximal phalanx is translated plantarly or is plantarflexed, the first metatarsophalangeal joint will not dorsiflex in a timely fashion, if it dorsiflexes at all, and will create a significant retrograde extension (dorsiflexion) force to the forefoot.

## ■ FOOT RADIOGRAPHS DO NOT HAVE A NEUTRAL POSITION FOR REFERENCE

The subtalar neutral position is a reference position to facilitate examination and the theorized position of best function for a foot that meets the criteria of an ideal lower extremity.[2,21] It is reasonable to assume for a moment that if there were not a subtalar neutral position, the criteria for an ideal lower extremity would remain virtually the same. The nonsubtalar criteria would be the same, with a vertical tibia and calcaneus and with the calcaneus positioned directly under the leg (ankle) so as to not create a large frontal-plane moment. The forefoot would be aligned so as to be directly anterior to the ankle and the midtarsal joint maximally pronated. The angle of gait would still be 5 to 10 degrees abducted so that the first-metatarsophalangeal joint is aligned with its axis perpendicular to the line of progression.[47]

When evaluating foot radiographs for the purpose of classifying feet, there is no subtalar neutral position to which the clinician can refer. Instead, there are degrees of stability. (Figures 13-8 and 13-9). Foot structure is a spectrum of morphologic variations and does not lend itself well to strict classification systems, because of the large variety of exceptions. In addition, most feet when in relaxed weight bearing assume a subtalar position that is pronated from the neutral position with the calcaneus approximately vertical, as opposed to the 6 to 12 degrees inverted neutral calcaneal stance position observed for most of the population.[42] Because the talus is the most proximal portion of the foot and is an extension of the leg, the talus is used as the reference for determining foot alignment and thus stability, instead of the subtalar neutral position. The following is a classification system, based on stability, that broadly organizes feet into three levels of stability.

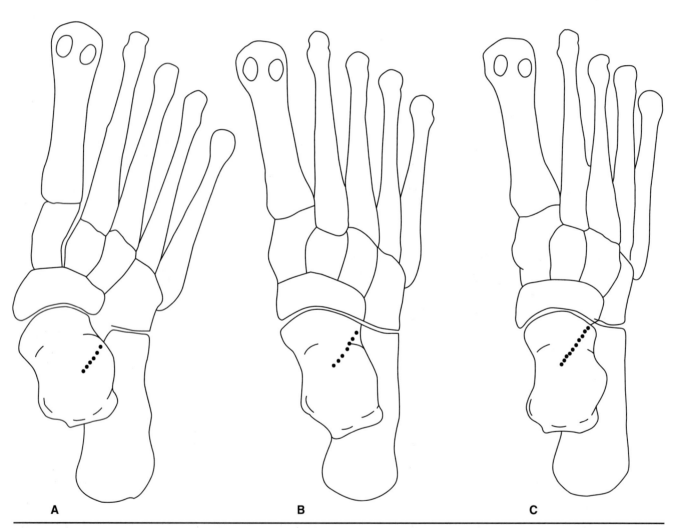

**A**                                        **B**                                        **C**

Figure 13-8  Feet can be classified by level of stability. The dorsoplantar view offers the clinician the opportunity to view the foot's transverse plane ability to compress the forefoot on the talus and the degree of stacking of the forefoot and rearfoot. The greater the angles between segments, the greater are the moments and the less is the compression that is associated with stability. The dorsoplantar views depicted are as follows: **A,** Overpronated foot with above-normal angles and reduced stacking. **B,** Rectus foot with normal, mild angulation and stacking of segments. **C,** Pes cavus foot with smaller-than-normal angles and reduced stacking because it is not pronated enough.

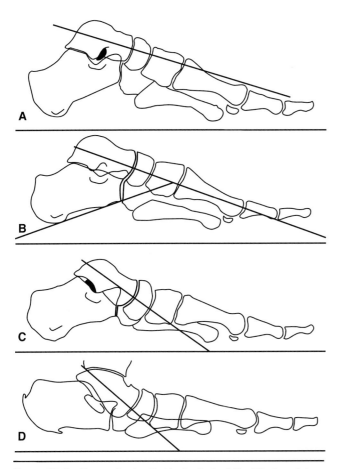

Figure 13-9   Feet can be classified by level of stability. The lateral view offers the clinician the opportunity to view the foot's sagittal-plane ability to compress the medial column on the talus and the ability of the calcaneus to lift the proximal portion of the medial column. The following lateral views are depicted: **A,** Pes cavus with higher-than-normal calcaneal inclination and plantarflexed medial column, making the foot too vertical and rigid. **B,** Rectus foot with the talar longitudinal bisection line bisecting the medial column and the calcaneus lifting the medial column so that the truss effect of the plantar soft tissue is effective. **C,** Overpronated foot with the medial column angled dorsally on the talus as noted with the medial column fault and the reduced calcaneal inclination compromising the ability of the plantar truss mechanism resistance of forefoot dorsiflexion. **D,** Subluxated overpronated foot, showing complete failure of the plantar truss to convert vertical forces into medial column compression and stability.

Feet that are relatively straight and have angular relationships that fall within the ranges considered normal are classified as rectus (Figures 13-8, *B,* and 13-9, *B*). These feet are stable but have enough angulation among the segments to provide the motion necessary for shock absorption and adaption to terrain variations. Rectus feet have normal angular relationships, as described by several authors.*

The second group of feet have larger-than-normal angulation between the osseous segments and thus are not

*References 2, 3, 8, 11, 44, 48, 49.

as stable as the rectus group. These feet are obviously pronated, and are referred to as *overpronated* (Figures 13-8, *A,* and 13-9, *A*). Remember that rectus feet also have pronated subtalar joints in relaxed stance but maintain less angulation between the osseous segments and thus have an acceptable level of static stability. The overpronated foot cannot create the joint compression necessary to resist the moments that result from ground reactive force. This is because of the increased angulation of the osseous segments and because the joint surfaces are poorly interfaced. Thus the self-locking mechanism of the medial column is compromised,[50] as is that of the lateral column and rearfoot.

The third group of feet in the spectrum of stability have angles that are too small; that is, they are not pronated enough to have normal angular relationships and thus are too rigid to provide the motion necessary for normal gait. Feet that are insufficiently pronated are described as *pes cavus*.[51] Pes cavus feet may stand in relaxed stance with the subtalar joint in neutral (talocalcaneal congruency)[52] or supinated from neutral. However, most pes cavus feet stand with the subtalar joint pronated from the neutral position. The pes cavus foot is overly vertical (stacked) and straight in its orientation to ground reactive forces, and thus is overly stable. It has reduced ability to absorb shock or adapt to terrain variations. The overeffective tension banding mechanism contributes to the overrigidity of the pes cavus foot.[19]

The preceding classification is deliberately broad, and the degree of stability within each classification has a range. In addition, the forefoot and rearfoot can be classified separately. Radiographic classification and assessment of foot pathology is meant to complement history, physical examination, and gait analysis and should not be used as a substitute for clinical evaluation.

## ■ SUMMARY

Biomechanical analysis of weight-bearing foot radiographs taken in the patient's angle and base of gait is done for the purpose of assessing foot stability. The bone shapes, trabecular patterns, and alignment all give information as to the degree of the foot's stability. A foot must be flexible enough to adapt to uneven terrain yet rigid enough to act as a lever and allow timely first-metatarsophalangeal joint dorsiflexion during propulsion.

Joint stability is affected by the compression of the joint surface. The forces acting on the joint should be directed toward the joint axis and provide even compression across the joint surface for maximum compression. Instability is created by rotation forces (moments) and angled joints, which are not conducive to compression. The foot is made stable by the plantar aponeurosis truss mechanism converting vertical ground reactive forces into compression of the forefoot on the rearfoot.

The foot can be classified by levels of stability using the talus as the primary reference. The talus is the most proximal portion of the foot and is an extension of the leg. Rectus feet are aligned relative to the talus so that their various osseous segmental angular relationships fall into ranges generally accepted as normal. Pes cavus feet have smaller angular relationships, are insufficiently pronated, are overly stacked, and thus overrigid. Overpronated feet are less stable because their osseous segments have larger angular relationships relative to the talus. The first-metatarsophalangeal joint must be aligned relative to the first metatarsal in the sagittal and transverse planes and the line of progression so that it can dorsiflex in a timely manner.

## References

1. Kaschuk TJ, Laine W: Surgical radiology. *Clin Podiatr Med Surg* 5(4):797-830, Oct 1988.

2. Sgarlato TE et al: *A compendium of podiatric biomechanics,* San Francisco, 1971, California College of Podiatric Medicine.

3. Gamble FO, Yale I: *Clinical foot roentgenology,* ed 2, Huntington, NY, 1975, Krieger Publishing.

4. Weissman SD: *Radiology of the foot,* Baltimore, 1989, Williams & Wilkins.

5. Johnson RE: Podiatric radiology. In Levy LA, Hetherington VJ, editors: *The principles and practice of podiatric medicine,* pp 231-271, New York, 1990, Churchill-Livingstone.

6. Harris RI, Beath T: *Army foot survey,* Ottawa, 1947, National Research Council of Canada.

7. Kirby KA, Loendorf AJ, Gregorio R: Anterior axial projection of the foot, *J Am Podiatr Med Assoc* 78(4): 159-170, 1988.

8. Weissman S: Standard radiographic techniques of the foot and ankle, *Clin Podiatr Med Surg* 5(4):767-775, Oct 1988.

9. Cobey JC: Posterior roentgenogram of the foot, *Clin Orthop* 118:202, 1976.

10. Hlavac HF: Differences in x-ray findings with varied positioning of the foot, *Journal of the American Podiatry Association* 57(10):465-471, 1967.

11. DiGiovanni JN, Smith S: Normal biomechanics of the adult rearfoot, a radiographic analysis, *Journal of the American Podiatry Association* 66:812-824, 1976.

12. Sanner WH, Page JC, Tolboe HR, Blake R, Bax CA: A study of ankle joint height changes with subtalar motion, *Journal of the American Podiatry Association* 71(3):158-161, 1981.

13. LaPorta GA, Scarlet J: Radiographic changes in the pronated and supinated foot, *Journal of the American Podiatry Association* 67(5):334-338, 1977.

14. Cobey JC, Sella E: Standardizing methods of measurements of foot shape by including the effects of subtalar rotation, *Foot & Ankle* 2:30, 1980.

15. Salter RB: *Textbook of disorders and injuries of the musculoskeletal system,* ed 2, p 9, Baltimore, 1983, Williams & Wilkins.

16. Hall MC: The trabecular patterns of the normal foot, *Clin Orthop* 16:15, 1960.

17. Lelievre J: *Pathologie du pied,* p 43, Paris, 1971, Masson et Cie.

18. Snell RS: *Clinical anatomy for medical students,* ed 3, Boston, 1986, Little, Brown.

19. Vogler HW: Biomechanics of talipes equinovalgus, *Journal of the American Podiatry Association* 77(1):21-28, 1987.

20. Wright DG, Desai SM, Henderson WH: Action of the subtalar and ankle joint complex during the stance phase of walking, *J Bone Joint Surg* 46A:36, 1964.

21. Root ML, Orien WP, Weed JH: *Normal and abnormal function of the foot,* Los Angeles, 1977, Clinical Biomechanics Corporation.

22. Dananberg HJ: Functional hallux limitus and its relationship to gait efficiency, *Journal of the American Podiatry Association* 76(11):648-652, 1986.

23. Winter DA: *The biomechanics and motor control of human gait,* Waterloo, Ont., 1987, [Monograph], University of Waterloo Press.

24. Guralnik DB: *Webster's New World dictionary of the American language,* New York, 1970, World Publishing.

25. Braune W, Fischer O: *The human gait,* p 264, New York, 1987, Springer. (Translated by P Maquet, R Furlong).

26. Kirby KA: Methods for determination of positional variations of the axis of the subtalar joint, *Journal of the American Podiatry Association* 77:228, 1987.

27. Hiss JM: *Functional foot disorders,* Los Angeles, 1937, University Publishing Co.

28. Hicks JH: The mechanics of the foot. II. The plantar aponeurosis and arch, *J Anat* 88:25, 1954.

29. Bojsen-Moeller F: Calcaneocuboid joint and stability of the longitudinal arch of the foot at high and low gear push off, *J Anat* 129:165-176, 1979.

30. Simon SR, Mann RA, Hagy JL et al: Role of the posterior calf muscles in normal gait, *J Bone Joint Surg* 60A:465-472, 1978.

31. Nuber GW: Biomechanics of the foot and ankle during gait, *Clin Podiatr Med Surg,* edited by Lepow GW, 5(3):615-627, July 1989.

32. Schoenhaus HD, Gold M, Hylinski J, Keating J: Computerized analysis of gait, clinical examples relating to torque, *J Am Podiatr Med Assoc* 69:11-16, 1979.

33. Cochran G, Van B: *A primer of orthopaedic biomechanics*, p 268, New York, 1982, Churchill-Livingstone.

34. Katoh Y, Cao, EY, Laughman RK, Schneider E, Morrey BF: Biomechanical analysis of foot function during gait and clinical applications, *Clin Orthop* 177:23, July-Aug 1983.

35. Cerny K: Pathomechanics of stance: clinical concepts for analysis, *Physical Therapy* 64(12): 1851-1859, 1984.

36. Nigg BM, Skleryk BN: Gait characteristics of the elderly, *Clin Biomech* (Bristol, Avon) 3(2):79-87, 1988.

37. Manter JT: Distribution of compressive forces in the joints of the human foot, *Anat Rec* 96:313, 1946.

38. Hicks JH: The foot as a support, *Acta Anatomica* 25:34, 1955.

39. Pauwel F: *Biomechanics of the locomotor apparatus*, New York, 1982, Springer.

40. Basmajian JM, Stecko G: The role of muscles in the arch support of the foot: an electromyographic study, *J Bone Joint Surg* 45A:1184-1190, 1963.

41. Ganley JV: Theory of the two unit tarsus, Philadelphia, 1984 (seminar presentation), Pennsylvania College of Podiatric Medicine.

42. Sanner WH: The functional foot orthosis prescription. In Jay RM, editor: *Current therapy in podiatric surgery*, pp 301-307, Philadelphia, 1989, Decker.

43. Rose GJK: Pes planus. In Jahss MH, editor: *Disorders of the foot*, pp 486-520, Philadelphia, 1982, Saunders.

44. Greenberg GS: Relationship of hallux abductus angle and first metatarsal angle of to severity of pronation, *Journal of the American Podiatry Association* 69:29-34, 1979.

45. Sanner WH: Midtarsal joint contribution to transverse plane leg rotation. In Pratt DJ, Johnson, GR, editors: *The biomechanics & orthotic management of the foot*, vol 1, Darby, Eng., 1987, Biological Engineering Society.

46. Hicks JH: Mechanics of the foot. I. The joints. *J Anat* 87:345, 1953.

47. Sgarlato TE: The angle of gait. *J Am Podiatr Med Assoc* 55:645, 1965.

48. Altman MI: Sagittal plane angles of the talus and calcaneus in the developing foot, *J Am Podiatr Assoc* 58:463, 1968.

49. Lewis MR: *Roentgen foot diagnosis*, pp 269-275, Chicago, 1967, Von Schill Memorial Press.

50. Zitzlsperger S: The mechanics of the foot based on the concept of the skeleton as a statically indetermined space framework, *Clin Orthop* 16:47, 1960.

51. Sayre LA: *A practical manual of the treatment of clubfoot*, ed 3, 1875, Appleton.

52. Root ML, Orien WP, Weed JH, Hughes RJ: *Biomechanical examination of the foot*, Los Angeles, 1971, Clinical Biomechanics Corporation.

# CHAPTER 14

# Foot Segmental Relationships and Bone Morphology

WILLIAM H. SANNER

The purpose of this chapter is to provide a basic understanding and basis for interpretation of the mechanics represented by weight-bearing foot radiographs. This chapter also demonstrates how radiographs can be used to complement the physical, biomechanical (range of motion and morphologic observations), and gait analysis portions of an examination. Two basic radiographic views are used for mechanical evaluation of feet: the dorsoplantar (or anteroposterior) and lateral.

Both radiographic views have value for evaluating the biomechanics of the foot. The dorsoplantar foot view provides information primarily about transverse-plane relationships seen in the foot.[1-4] Any transverse-plane foot deformity or transverse-plane component of compensation by the foot can be observed with a dorsoplantar x-ray study. The lateral view x-ray study provides information primarily about sagittal-plane structural relationships and compensation within the foot. The dorsoplantar and lateral radiographic views are used to infer frontal-plane relationships.

Both the lateral and dorsoplantar radiographs are performed with the patient in the relaxed calcaneal stance. In other words, the major requirements for weight-bearing dorsoplantar and lateral x-ray views are that the patient be standing in his or her angle and base of gait and that the foot be placed appropriately relative to the film.[2,3] (See radiographic positioning technique Chapter 3). Failure to position the patient properly significantly alters the information provided by the radiograph.[5,6]

Specialty views also allow the clinician to make specific assessments. Examples are sesamoid axial and anterior axial views.

When using a radiograph to assess the mechanics and morphology of a foot, the clinician must keep in mind that each radiograph depicts osseous alignments and shapes that represent the net result of a variety of influences on the foot. Examples of these influences are genetic information influencing bone shape, and morphologic variations of the entire body, which create a variety of normal and abnormal interacting forces (such as functional equinus, forefoot valgus, muscle strength, and weight of individual). Thus radiographs infer foot mechanics and the morphologic influences that affect the foot mechanics but do not absolutely represent specific morphologic types. Foot radiographs are not a substitute for examination of the patient and are only meaningful when the radiographic and physical exams correlate. The wise clinician uses radiographs as a supplement to the physical exam and treats people, not radiographs.[7]

This chapter seeks to provide the clinician with insights on interpreting some of the most common radiographic representations of foot alignment and mechanics. The basic tools are reference lines, angles between segments, and the shape of the foot and its individual bones. Reference lines are created so as to measure the orientation of a foot segment or bone to another foot segment, bone, or the supporting surface. As with position and motion, the distal segment is always described relative to the proximal segment. Angles made by the reference lines between segments and bones are a reflection of foot linearity. Bone and joint shape are the net result of ontogeny and the forces acting on the bones. The angles, shapes, and relative position of one bone to another as represented on the radiographic shadow allow clinicians to infer static foot mechanics and the influence of dynamic forces on the foot during ambulation.

## ◼ DORSOPLANTAR RADIOGRAPHIC ANALYSIS

### Longitudinal Axis of the Rearfoot

The longitudinal axis of the rearfoot (Figures 14-1 and 14-2) is a reference line also known as the longitudinal axis of the calcaneus.[1,2,8] On the DP radiograph a dot is placed in the center of the posterior surface of the calcaneus and at the anterior medial edge of the calcaneus. A straight edge is used to connect these two points, the line being equivalent to the longitudinal axis of the rearfoot. The difficulty with this method of radiographic charting is that because of the angle of the x-ray beam, the beam must pass through the tibia, talus, and calcaneus and the posterior surface of the calcaneus is obscured. In this case, the clinician uses the lateral border of the calcaneus to aid in drawing this axis and should refer to it as the longitudinal rearfoot reference line.[9] The lateral calcaneal border is approximately parallel to the longitudinal rearfoot axis but averages 5 degrees abducted from the longitudinal axis of the rearfoot. To use the lateral border of the calcaneus, measure the distance from the lateral calcaneal border to the anterior, medial, distal point of the calcaneus. This distance is used to place a second point in the body of the calcaneus so that a line representing the longitudinal axis of the rearfoot can be drawn. This line should pass distally and approximate the longitudinal bisection of the fourth metatarsal.[2] The longitudinal axis of the rearfoot has historically been considered a stable reference to which other parts of the foot should be compared.[1] A good argument can be made for the talus being the major reference point of the foot, because the talus is more proximal and stable.[10]

The distal calcaneal articular surface should be facing anteriorly and perpendicular or slightly laterally directed relative to the longitudinal axis of the calcaneus so that the cuboid is not placed in an abducted position.

### Longitudinal Axis of the Talar Neck and Head

The longitudinal axis of the talar neck and head (see Figure 14-1) is a reference line that represents the leg. To draw the longitudinal axis of the talar neck and head, a line is drawn across the widest dimension of the head of the talus. A point is then found at the exact midpoint of this line. After this point is marked, a second line is drawn across a consistent point of the talar neck. The exact midpoint of this line is then determined and marked. The two midpoints are then connected, and this line is the longitudinal axis of the talar neck and head.[1,2] The longitudinal axis of the talar neck and head extends distally and should be an approximate longitudinal bisection of the first metatarsal.[2] The longitudinal axis of the talar neck and head should be the

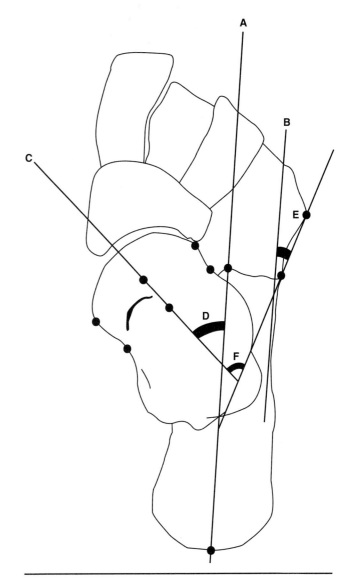

Figure 14-1    The dorsoplantar view allows evaluation of transverse-plane relationships of the rearfoot. The following axes and angles allow quantification of these relationships. *A*, Longitudinal axis of the rearfoot (calcaneus); *B*, alternative longitudinal rearfoot reference line (parallel to lateral calcaneus); *C*, longitudinal axis of talar neck and head; *D*, talocalcaneal angle; *E*, calcaneocuboid angle; *F*, talocuboid angle.

proximal reference line to which more distal segments of the foot are compared for the purpose of assessing foot linearity and level of stability. The longitudinal axis of the rearfoot (calcaneus) has traditionally been the proximal reference.

The talar neck and head bisection is adducted slightly from the body of the talus and is not perpendicular to the ankle joint axis. This adduction is necessary for the talus to be the proximal portion of the medial column of the foot, particularly so that it is well aligned for compression from the first metatarsal.

## Longitudinal Axis of the Lesser Tarsus

The longitudinal axis of the lesser tarsus (see Figure 14-2) is a reference line representing the general orientation of the midfoot in the transverse plane.[1,2,7] Many lines are drawn to determine the longitudinal axis of the lesser tarsus. First, a point is drawn at the anterior lateral extent of the calcaneus. A second point is drawn at the lateral proximal corner of the base of the fourth metatarsal. A line is then drawn connecting these two points. The midpoint of this line is then found and marked. Next, a point is placed on the talus at the anterior medial aspect of the effective talar articular surface with the navicular. A second medial point is drawn at the proximal medial corner of the base of the first metatarsal. The midpoint of a line connecting the talar and first metatarsal points is then determined and marked. The midpoint dots of the medial and lateral lines are then connected with a line that is called the transection of the midfoot. Finally, a perpendicular line is drawn relative to the transection line. The perpendicular line is the longitudinal axis of the lesser tarsus. The longitudinal axis of the lesser tarsus approximately parallels the longitudinal bisection of the second cuneiform (see Figure 14-2).[11]

Longitudinal axis of the lesser tarsus is used to assess the linearity of the lesser tarsus relative to the segments proximal and distal.

## Longitudinal Axis of the Metatarsus (and Forefoot)

The longitudinal axis of the metatarsus is a longitudinal bisection of the second metatarsal (see Figure 14-2), and is a reference line representing the orientation of the metatarsals and forefoot in the transverse plane.[1,2,7] The second metatarsal is used because it is the most stable metatarsal and its position is the least variable. The other metatarsals flair away from the second metatarsal.

Classical anatomic definition defines motion moving toward the second metatarsal as being adduction and motion moving away as abduction. This explains the name of the hallux adductus and abductus muscles. Radiographic analysis uses the midline of the body as the central reference. Thus the term *metatarsus primus adductus*, meaning first metatarsal positioned angled toward the midline of the body and away from the second metatarsal.

The first line that is drawn to determine the longitudinal axis of the metatarsus is one that extends across the widest portion of the base of the second metatarsal. The midpoint of this line is then determined and marked. A second line is drawn across the neck of the second metatarsal. The midpoint of this line is then connected to the midpoint of the proximal line. The line that connects the bisections of the base and neck of the second metatarsal is used as the

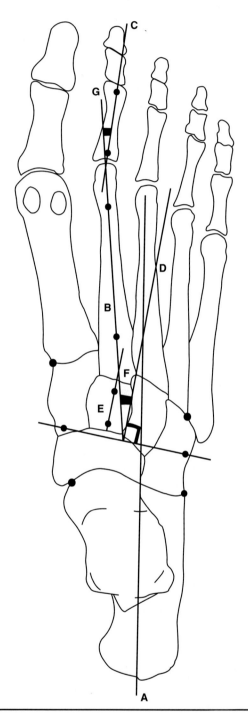

**Figure 14-2**  The forefoot angle can be determined using the longitudinal axes of the rearfoot and forefoot. *A,* Longitudinal axis of rearfoot; *B,* longitudinal axis of metatarsus and forefoot; *C,* longitudinal axis of the digits; *D,* longitudinal axis of the lesser tarsus, a line perpendicular to the transection of the midfoot; *E,* longitudinal bisection of the second cuneiform; *F,* metatarsus adductus angle; *G,* digital angle.

longitudinal axis of the metatarsus and the longitudinal axis of the forefoot.

The longitudinal axis of the metatarsus and forefoot is used as a reference for the orientation of these segments relative to the distal and proximal segments.

## Longitudinal Axis of the Digits

Lines are also used to chart the longitudinal axis of the digits (see Figure 14-2) relative to the metatarsals.[1,2,7] The longitudinal bisection of the proximal phalanx of the second toe is used as the longitudinal axis of the digits. The first of the lines used to define the axis is drawn across the base of the second proximal phalange. A second line is drawn across the head of this phalange. The midpoint of the head and base of the proximal phalanx are determined and connected. The resulting line is the longitudinal axis of the digits.

The longitudinal axis of the digits should be approximately parallel to the longitudinal axis of the rearfoot.

## Talocalcaneal Angle

The talocalcaneal angle on a DP radiograph is defined as the angulation made by the longitudinal axis of the rearfoot and the longitudinal axis of the talar neck and head.[1,2,7,12,13] The talocalcaneal angle (see Figure 14-1) is a transverse plane representation of subtalar position. In a normal lower extremity this angle is approximately 15 to 18 degrees. If the lateral border of the calcaneus is used as the longitudinal reference line of the rearfoot, the normal range for the talocalcaneal angle increases to 20 to 23 degrees.[14] Weissman[7] reports 17 to 21 degrees as normal, and based on linearity for stability, this appears a reasonable range as compared to Rowland's[14] 20 to 23 degrees.

The talus "corkscrews" around the sustentaculum tali as it adducts and plantarflexes during subtalar pronation, and it abducts and dorsiflexes during supination.[1,15] With this closed kinetic-chain motion the talus moves while the calcaneus remains relatively stable in these directions of motion, but the calcaneus does pivot on its medial tubercle to accommodate midtarsal motion.[16] Thus subtalar pronation results in the longitudinal axis of the talar neck and head pointing more toward the midline of the body and deviates from the longitudinal axis of the rearfoot, thereby increasing the talocalcaneal angle. The opposite is true during dorsiflexion and abduction of the talus when the subtalar supinates as the two axes move closer together and the angulation decreases.

Although the talus does adduct and plantarflex relative to the calcaneus in closed kinetic-chain subtalar pronation, an argument can be made conceptually that the foot has abducted relative to the talus.[17] This change in description

of the same motion is helpful when considering reconstruction of a flatfoot.

The foot is realigned relative to the talus and not the calcaneus. Because the talus moves in closed kinetic-chain foot mechanics and the calcaneus appears stable, the calcaneus has heretofore been erroneously used as the most proximal reference of the foot. The calcaneus does rotate in the transverse plane as the result of midtarsal motion.[16]

An increase in the talocalcaneal angle means that the ankle's plane of motion cannot be oriented in the same general direction as the foot. This reduces the efficiency with which the foot can act as a lever for the ankle and places excess stress on the foot because the foot joints are forced to perform functions not consistent with their design. As the talocalcaneal angle increases, the head of the talus can be seen protruding medially when the foot is observed in a weight-bearing position.

## The Lesser Tarsus Angle

The lesser tarsus angle on a dorsoplantar radiograph is defined as the angulation between the longitudinal bisection of the rearfoot and the longitudinal bisection of the lesser tarsus.[1,2,7] In a normal lower extremity, the longitudinal axis of the lesser tarsus is abducted slightly in relation to the longitudinal axis of the rearfoot. No specific value has been determined, but 10 ± 5 degrees is a reasonable range. Because the forefoot abducts on the rearfoot when the midtarsal joint pronates, the abducted lesser tarsus angle can become excessive. The opposite is true with midtarsal joint supination. With forefoot adduction the lesser tarsus axis comes to lie more parallel to the longitudinal axis of the rearfoot, and the angulation decreases.

As the foot moves, a greater relative positional change occurs between the lesser tarsus and the talus, as opposed to the calcaneus. There are two reasons for this. First, the design of the calcaneocuboid joint means that the midfoot and calcaneus tend to move together. Second, because of the ball-and-socket design of the talonavicular joint, more motion can occur between the talus and midfoot. In addition, talar and lesser tarsus relative position changes as the result of motion at both the subtalar and midtarsal joints. The distal opening osteotomy of the calcaneus (Evans procedure[18]) is designed to place the midfoot/forefoot anterior to the talus and ankle[17] and thus to reduce the deformity created by the midfoot and forefoot abducting with the calcaneus away from the talus.

## The Metatarsus Adductus Angle

The metatarsus adductus angle (see Figure 14-2) on a dorsoplantar radiograph is defined as the angulation between the longitudinal axis of the lesser tarsus and the longitudinal axis of the metatarsus.[1,2,7,19] In a normal lower extremity, the metatarsus angle is 10 to 20 degrees adducted in relation to the lesser tarsus axis and is frequently referred to as the metatarsus adductus angle. If the adduction is greater than 20 degrees, a deformity is present known as metatarsus adductus. Metatarsus adductus creates problems of digital alignment relative to the metatarsals. For example, as the digits are more abducted relative to the metatarsals as the metatarsus adductus angle increases, the likelihood of developing hallux abductus increases.

Less frequently one finds less than 10 degrees of metatarsus adduction. This deformity is known as metatarsus abductus, even though the axis of the metatarsus may still be adducted in relation to the axis of the lesser tarsus. For example, if the metatarsus axis is 5 degrees adducted to the lesser tarsus axis, then metatarsus abductus deformity is present. The metatarsus abductus deformity places the forefoot weight-bearing surface farther lateral relative to the rearfoot joint axes, and thus ground reactive forces on the metatarsal heads have a greater pronatory influence on the foot.[20]

The final point to be made about the metatarsus angle is that it remains unchanged with pronation and supination. Both axes move together as components of the forefoot during pronation and supination of the foot.

An alternate method for determining the metatarsus adductus angle is to measure the angle between the longitudinal axis of the metatarsus, and the longitudinal axis of the second cuneiform, instead of the lesser tarsus.[1,11] The second cuneiform is stable and rectangular (see Figure 14-2). Engel found that using the longitudinal axis of the second metatarsal yields an angle 3 degrees higher than using the longitudinal axis of the lesser tarsus. Thus the normal range is 13 to 23 degrees when the second cuneiform is used as the proximal reference.

## The Z Foot Situation

In the Z foot concept, three segmental reference lines are used to roughly assess foot linearity. The closer the three reference lines are to being parallel, the more stable the foot. The first of the reference lines is the base of the Z represented by the longitudinal axis of the rearfoot. The center portion of the Z is represented by the longitudinal axis of the lesser tarsus. The third and final reference line forming the Z is the longitudinal axis of the metatarsus.

In a normal foot the longitudinal axes of the rearfoot, lesser tarsus (midfoot), and metatarsus all fall within the normal values described earlier. In the Z foot deformity the lesser tarsus is severely abducted, and the metatarsus is adducted.

A Z foot is unstable because of the large angles made by three major segments of the foot. As the distal segments are compressed on the proximal segments, there compression of the joints is reduced because the angular relationships make the joints nonperpendicular to the compressive force vector.

## Forefoot Angulation

The forefoot angle on a dorsoplantar radiograph is defined as the angulation between the longitudinal axis of the rearfoot and the longitudinal axis of the forefoot.[1,2,7] A normal lower extremity, generally has more metatarsus adduction than lesser tarsus abduction. Therefore it is normal for the forefoot to be slightly adducted relative to the rearfoot (calcaneus). No normal angular value has been determined, but roughly 8 to 12 degrees is acceptable.[7]

The forefoot in a stable rectus foot should be slightly abducted relative to the longitudinal axis of the talar neck and head. Thus the forefoot is aligned roughly in the same direction as the leg, allowing sagittal-plane motion at the knee, ankle, and metatarsophalangeal joints to occur in approximately the same direction.

When the forefoot is abducted relative to the direction of gait, the metatarsophalangeal joints do not dorsiflex as much, because the metatarsals roll around their longitudinal axes, as opposed to the metatarsophalangeal joint axes. This reduces foot stability, because the plantar fascia is not adequately tightened.

## Proximal Articular Set Angle

The proximal articular set angle, or PASA (Figure 14-3), is defined as the angulation between a line perpendicular to the first-metatarsal articular cartilage and the longitudinal axis of the first metatarsal.[1,2,7,21] A perpendicular is drawn to a line that extends across the widest margin of the articular area of the first-metatarsal head. Because the cartilage cannot be visualized, the margins of the denser subchondral bone that outline the cartilage are used.[22] A second line is drawn as a longitudinal bisection of the first metatarsal. The angulation between these two lines is equal to the proximal articular set angle. In a normal lower extremity, the proximal articular set angle is usually 0 to 8 degrees abducted in relation to the first-metatarsal bisection.[7,23] The slight lateral deviation of the articular cartilage in a normal lower extremity places the plane of motion of the first-metatarsophalangeal joint approximately parallel to the line of progression. The proximal articular set angle may become greatly increased through remodeling that occurs via Wolff's law (1884) as the hallux drifts laterally and becomes abducted relative to the first metatarsal with development of the hallux abductovalgus deformity and the associated bunion.

Amarnek[24] compared the PASA measured radiographically to that measured by direct visualization of the first-metatarsal distal cartilage at the time of surgery. The conclusion was that the first-metatarsal head articular carti-

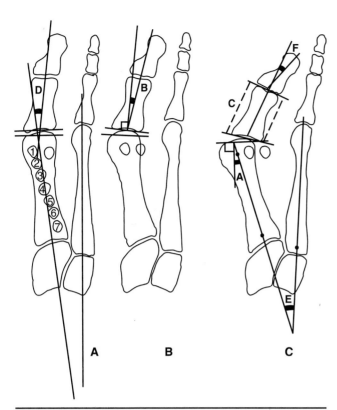

Figure 14-3  Quantitative methods used to evaluate first-ray osseous relationships. First-metatarsal phalangeal joint articular cartilage relationships are described as congruous (**A**), deviated (**B**), and subluxated (**C**) based on the lines connecting the medial and lateral extent of the joint cartilage. First-metatarsal cuneiform joint angle and shape (**A** has small angle and relatively flat shape; **C** has oblique angulation and round shape). *A*, Proximal articular set angle (PASA); *B*, distal articular set angle (DASA); *C*, proximal phalanx medial and lateral length comparison; *D*, hallux abductus angle; *E*, metatarsus primus adductus angle; *F*, hallux interphalangeus abductus angle; *1–7*, sesamoid positions.

lage on average deviated laterally 7 degrees more than was demonstrated radiographically. Therefore, because of individual variation between radiographs and actual articular direction, the surgeon should use intraoperative judgment to determine how much reduction of the PASA may be necessary.

Another manner to assess the direction of the first-metatarsal head articular surface is based on the concept that all the metatarsophalangeal joints should have roughly parallel planes of motion. With this concept in mind, Shechter[25] developed the tangential angle of the second axis (TASA). TASA is the angle made by the cartilage on the head of the first metatarsal relative to a line perpendicular to the long axis of the second metatarsal. The normal angulation is 0 ± 5 degrees. The TASA is frequently increased in hallux abductus deformities, just as the PASA is increased. Generally the TASA equals the PASA minus the metatarsus primus adductus angle.

## Distal Articular Set Angle

The distal articular set angle (DASA) is defined as the angulation between a perpendicular to the proximal articular surface and the longitudinal bisection of the hallux proximal phalanx.[1,2,7,21,26] DASA (see Figure 14-3) represents the proximal phalanx longitudinal axis relative to its proximal articular cartilage. A perpendicular is first drawn to a line that extends across the widest margin of the proximal articular surface of the hallux proximal phalanx, just as was done for the PASA. Then the angle between the longitudinal bisection of the proximal phalanx and the perpendicular to the proximal articular cartilage is measured. The shaft of the proximal phalanx normally is 7 to 9 degrees abducted in relation to the articular cartilage.[2,26,27]

Balding[27] found an inverse relationship between (1) the DASA and (2) the hallux abductus and metatarsus primus adductus angles. He rationalized this relationship developed from the increase in the DASA being caused by ground reactive forces during gait and by shoe pressure. For example, as a shoe applies an abductory force on the hallux, if the first-metatarsophalangeal joint is stable, it will be the proximal phalanx that remodels consistent with Wolff's law. If the first-metatarsophalangeal joint is unstable, the abductory force increases the hallux abductus angle and secondarily the metatarsus primus adductus angle. As hallux abductus increases, less force is exerted on the proximal phalanx and the DASA is less likely to increase.

Christman[28] measured the DASA of the same digit in varus and valgus positions relative to normal. He found that as the proximal phalanx valgus rotates, as in hallux abductovalgus, the DASA decreases, and it increases as the proximal phalanx is varus rotated—an unusual occurrence. Thus the DASA may not be a true representation of the proximal articular cartilage relative to the shaft if the proximal phalanx is rotated.

Instead of measuring the DASA, an alternative is to measure the medial and lateral sides of the proximal phalanx.[29] Lines are drawn across the most proximal and distal portions of the proximal phalanx, and then the sides are measured (see Figure 14-3). This measurement is helpful for the clinician who is considering straightening the proximal phalanx by removing a wedge of bone (e.g., distal Akin procedure).

## Hallux Abductus Angle

The hallux abductus angle (see Figure 14-3) is defined as the angulation between the longitudinal bisection of the first metatarsal and the longitudinal bisection of the first-toe proximal phalanx (hallux).[1,2,7,21,26] In a normal lower extremity the hallux is approximately parallel to the second toe, and 15 degrees or less abducted relative to the first metatarsal. (The range of acceptable values may be as wide as 0 to 20 degrees depending on foot morphology.[22] Ideally the hallux abductus angle should equal the sum of the PASA and DASA.

In assessing the hallux abductovalgus deformity, the sum of the PASA and the DASA equals the hallux abductus angle if the deformity is purely osseous in nature; that is, the articular surfaces are well aligned.[26] Recall that the proximal and distal articular set angles indicate the direction in which the articular surfaces of the bones face in relation to the long axis of the respective bones. For example, if the PASA equals 8 degrees, then the direction of articulation of the head of the first metatarsal is abducted 8 degrees to the long axis of the first metatarsal. Therefore, if the DASA was zero, we would expect the long axis of the first proximal phalange to be directly in the line with the direction of articulation of the head of the first metatarsal. The hallux abductus angle would be expected to be equal to 8 degrees in this case, provided that only an osseous relationship existed.

If the sum of the PASA and the DASA do not equal the hallux abductus angle, then a soft tissue component must be part of the deformity.[26] The soft tissue component maintains the hallux in relation to the first-metatarsal shaft in a manner not consistent with the expected angulation based on how the articular surfaces would normally allow the bones to relate.

In those strictly osseous relationships where the articular cartilages are well aligned, articular set lines will be parallel, and the joint is referred to as being congruous.[22,26] If the lines representing the proximal and distal first-metatarsophalangeal joint articular surfaces are not parallel, and cross outside of the joint, the joint is said to be deviated. If the lines cross within the joint, the joint is said to be subluxated.[30] Both deviated and subluxated joints have soft tissue components of the deformity.

According to Wolff's law, tension stress affects bone growth and trabecular alignment. Because of this phenomenon congruous and deviated first-metatarsophalangeal joints have different subchondral structure.[31] A congruous first-metatarsophalangeal joint is superior to a subluxated joint both functionally and structurally as determined by gross and microscopic examination. The congruous joint has smooth, intact articular surface and demonstrates signs of uniform stress and strain. The subchondral junction finds the cartilage and osseous tissue parallel, and the trabecular pattern is arranged evenly and perpendicular to the articular surface. The subluxated joint has uneven articular surface, indicating uneven stress. The subchondral junction has compaction and fissuring instead of a uniform pattern. The trabecular pattern is not perpendicular to the joint surface and is distributed unevenly, with thickening in areas of greatest stress.

Consistent with this observation, Miller[32] demonstrated congruous joints have more even stress, and incongruity of the first-metatarsophalangeal joint creates uneven stress across the joint and decreased joint surface contact. Specifically, congruous joints have 100% contact, whereas 10 degrees of deviation between the proximal and distal articular surfaces resulted in only 50% surface area contact.

As the hallux abductus deformity increases, one frequently finds a simultaneous valgus rotation of the hallux. The clinician finds the plantar surface of the proximal phalanx partially visible and erroneously identified as the lateral aspect.

Researchers have long suspected that rounder first-metatarsal heads (higher radius of curvature of the articular cartilage relative to the width of the first metatarsal with one being normal) are more likely to have an increased hallux abductus angle than are flatter first-metatarsal heads.[26,33-35] Brahm[35] notes that this finding is not consistent. Brahm theorized that when an abnormal abductory force is applied to the first-metatarsophalangeal joint, an unstable joint subluxes (abducts) and a stable joint destroys itself.

McCrea found an explanation for why flatter first-metatarsophalangeal joints are not necessarily more stable than round heads.[36] He found that changing the central x-ray angle from 5, 15, and 25 degrees to the supporting surface, makes a first-metatarsophalangeal joint head look round, square, and square with a ridge, respectively. Thus if all dorsoplantar radiographs are taken at 15-degree central beam angle, the declination of the metatarsal may change the shape of the metatarsal head on the radiograph, depending on whether the dorsal (round), central (square), or plantar surfaces (square with ridge) are represented on the radiograph.

The development of hallux abductus and metatarsus adductus has been attributed to first-metatarsal hypermobility (dorsiflexion of the first ray by ground reactive forces during gait at a time when the first ray should be stable) as the result of foot pronation. Greenberg[37] found no correlation to subtalar pronation as reflected by talocalcaneal angle when measured on the dorsoplantar and lateral views, talar declination, or calcaneal inclination. He did find, however, that when abduction of the cuboid was included as an indicator of midtarsal pronation with subtalar pronation, hallux abductus and metatarsus primus adductus angle correlated to increases in the talocuboid angle.

## Metatarsus Primus Adductus Angle

The metatarsus primus adductus (MPA) angle (see Figure 14-3) is defined as the angulation between the longitudinal bisections of the first and second metatarsals. In a normal lower extremity, the first-metatarsal longitudinal axis is approximately 8 degrees adducted relative to the longitudinal axis of the second metatarsal.[38] The metatarsus primus adductus angle is not considered pathological until it becomes 12 degrees adducted in a rectus foot and 10 degrees adducted in an adductus foot, namely metatarsus adductus.[38]

It is generally accepted that the retrograde force created by an abducted hallux, once the hallux abuts against the second toe, is the cause for first-metatarsal adduction and the initiation of the third stage of hallux abductovalgus deformity, or metatarsus primus adductus.[15,38,39] The retrograde force is created by the proximally directed pull by muscles inserting or positioned on the lateral side of the hallux dominating those on the medial side that are responsible for resisting hallux abduction. The hallux proximal phalanx is abducted, while the muscles of the foot maintain a posterior lateral retrograde pull on this phalange. The proximal phalanx pushes the first metatarsal medially, away from the second metatarsal in a bowing, reverse buckling action.[38] The hallux abductus angle does not appear correlated with the development of metatarsus primus adductus.[39]

The reason why the hallux abductus angle increase does not correlate with metatarsus primus adductus may be because of the association of metatarsus adductus with hallux abductus and inversely related to metatarsus primus adductus. Griffiths and Palladino[40] reconfirmed an increased incidence of increased metatarsus adductus angle in feet with increased hallux abductus angles and a lower incidence in feet with normal hallux abductus angles. In addition, they found that as the metatarsus adductus increases, the proximal articular set angle increases and a slight tendency appears toward a lower metatarsus primus adductus angle than one would expect in feet with hallux abductus and normal metatarsus adductus angles.

Several authors have suggested that the direction of the first-metatarsal cuneiform joint influences the tendency for first-metatarsal adduction deformity (see Figure 14-3). McCrea and Lichty[41] confirmed numerically the observations of others[42-44] by concluding that the more oblique— that is, medially directed—the first-metatarsal cuneiform joint, the greater the metatarsus primus adductus. McCrea and Lichty observed that the first-metatarsal cuneiform angle was increased and the lateral side of the first metatarsal was longer relative to the medial side in feet with increased metatarsus adductus angle, as compared to feet with normal metatarsus adductus angles. Therefore children with longer lateral sides of their first metatarsals may be candidates for epiphysiodesis.

Medial cuneiform articular shape also affects the tendency for metatarsus adductus. A square articular surface is generally thought to be more stable than a round one. LaPorta[21] and Fenton[38] observed, and Pressman[45] confirmed, that when doing soft tissue hallux abductus correction a round first-metatarsal cuneiform joint allows 2 to 4 degrees of reduction of the metatarsus primus adductus angle and that less reduction occurs if the joint is square.[38]

The term *atavistic cuneiform* refers to the space between the first and second cuneiforms seen in some feet. The term *atavistic* was used to describe the split between the cuneiforms as remnants of a thumblike appendage.[46] However, the visibility of this space is positional; the more pronated the foot becomes, the more likely the space is observed. Pressman[45] has found that feet with a space between the first and second cuneiform have a soft tissue component to their metatarsus primus adductus deformity and that in these feet correction of the hallux abductus is more likely to reduce some of the metatarsus primus adductus angle as well. Therefore it appears that an atavistic cuneiform is a sign of an overpronated foot, and one subsequently finds that the first ray is unstable (hypermobile) in gait.

## Sesamoid Position

The sesamoids should sit directly under the first metatarsal head and articulate with the first metatarsal in their respective sesamoidal grooves. As the first metatarsal adducts the sesamoids do not move, because they are anchored to the second metatarsal by the transverse metatarsal ligament. As the first metatarsal moves medially, the sesamoids are positioned lateral to their ideal position.

The tibial sesamoidal position (see Figure 14-3) is a descriptive way to communicate sesamoid position relative to the first metatarsal.[1,26] The longitudinal bisection of the first metatarsal is used as the reference. There are seven tibial sesamoidal positions. Normally the tibial sesamoid is medial to the first metatarsal bisection, and this is called Position 1. Position 4 is when the tibial sesamoid is centered on the bisection, and there is likely to be crista erosion present as well. Position 7 is when the sesamoid is completely lateral to the first metatarsal bisection, and the fibular sesamoid is in the first metatarsal interspace. From Position 3 and higher there is likely to be erosion of the first metatarsal articulation with the sesamoids.[47] The sesamoid axial view should be correlated with the dorsoplantar view to assess sesamoid articulation. The sesamoids as viewed on the sesamoid axial view are frequently more laterally displaced than one might expect from a dorsoplantar view alone.

The further lateral the sesamoids are positioned relative to the first metatarsal, the greater the abductory force the flexor hallucis brevis exerts on the hallux, and the less effectively the windlass mechanism performs. Poor function of the windlass mechanism is also observed when the sesamoids drop proximally after injury or surgery.

## First-Metatarsal Length

The changing relative length of the first metatarsal has been attributed to a variety of secondary deformities. The length

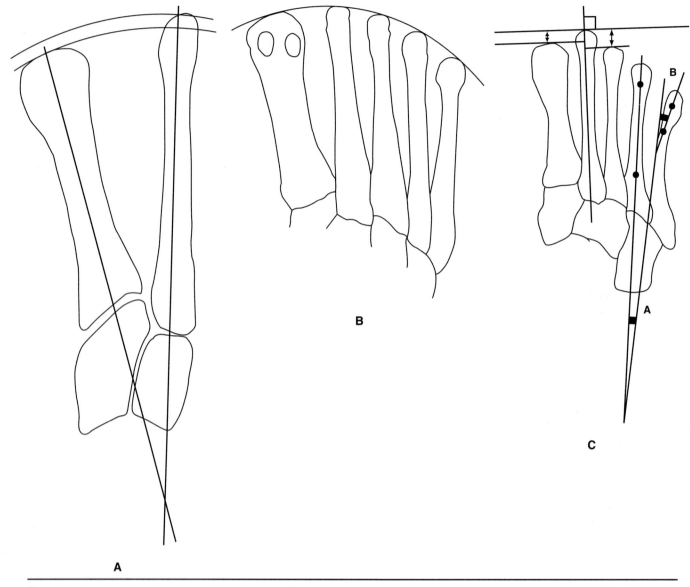

**Figure 14-4**   **A,** Uses the relative length of the radius created by the distance from the intersection of the longitudinal bisections of the first and second metatarsals to their respective distal aspects where the bisections exist. **B,** Demonstrates the distal metatarsal break pattern as a curve and not as straight lines that make an angle with the second metatarsal at the apex. **C,** Individual relative metatarsal length is measured using lines tangential to the distal end of the metatarsals being evaluated and perpendicular to the longitudinal bisection of the second metatarsal. *A,* Fifth intermetatarsal angle; *B,* fifth-metatarsal lateral-deviation angles are depicted.

of the first metatarsal is measured relative to the length of the adjacent second metatarsal (Figure 14-4). The longitudinal bisections of the first and second metatarsals are extended proximally until they intersect.[21] The distance from the intersection of the first- and second-metatarsal longitudinal bisections to the end of each metatarsal is measured and compared. Although ±2 mm is generally accepted as normal, the first metatarsal from a functional perspective should not be longer. As the metatarsus adductus angle increases, the first metatarsal measures and is

functionally longer than in a foot with a lower metatarsus adductus angle.[48] Zlotoff[49] found in a study of weight-bearing radiographs that of the first metatarsals he measured 40% were longer, 38% were shorter, and 22% were the same length as the second metatarsals.

Heden[50] suggested that most hallux abductus deformities have relatively longer (protruding) first metatarsals (and longer hallux), and that those people with higher metatarsus primus adductus angles also have protruding first metatarsals. In a study of people with hallux abductus, Duke[48] found that subluxated first-metatarsophalangeal joints were more often associated with first metatarsals over 1 mm longer than the second, whereas congruous and deviated joints were more often associated with first metatarsals that protruded less than 1 mm or were shorter than the second metatarsal. Duke also noted a tendency for hallux abductus angles over 20 degrees to be associated with longer first metatarsals. Increased hallux interphalangeal abductus may also be associated with longer first metatarsals because there is more shoe pressure.[48] Hallux varus has also been associated with relatively longer first metatarsals, as well as hallux limitus.[51]

In separate studies, Zlotoff[49] and Schweitzer[52] found that the most commonly performed first metatarsal osteotomies shorten the bone by 2 to 4 mm, with a range of 0.5 to 6 mm, and that the shortening also dorsiflexes the first metatarsal because of the declination of the bone.

Short metatarsals are also associated with pathology. Morton[53] described the short first metatarsal as bearing less weight, and subsequently the second metatarsal as bearing more weight, as indicated by its increased cortical thickness.[54] Reduced weight bearing by the first metatarsal is frequently the etiology of second-metatarsal stress fractures. Hardy and Clapham[55] observed that less metatarsus primus adductus was associated with short first metatarsals.

It is common that preoperative and postoperative radiographs are taken at different angles relative to the metatarsals because the postoperative radiographs are frequently taken nonweight bearing. Because of the difference in angulation of the central beam relative to the metatarsals, the metatarsals measure different lengths whether or not they have been operated on. A simple algebraic formula can be used to determine what length each metatarsal should have been if the metatarsal had not been operated.[49]

$$\frac{\text{Preoperative length of first metatarsal}}{\text{Preoperative length of second metatarsal}} = \frac{\text{Postoperative length of first metatarsal}}{\text{Postoperative length of second metatarsal}}$$

The actual amount of shortening is the difference between the expected length of the operated metatarsal and the length actually measured.

An alternative method for measuring relative first- and second-metatarsal length is to draw lines, at the ends of the first and second metatarsals, that are perpendicular to the second-metatarsal longitudinal bisection (see Figure 14-4,C). A first metatarsal that is 2 to 4 mm shorter is appropriate.

The significance of relative first metatarsal length is related to timely dorsiflexion of the first-metatarsophalangeal joint in early propulsion, and overload of the second metatarsal. It should be remembered that the first-metatarsal plantar weight-bearing surface is the plantar surface of the sesamoid bones, which are not located at the distal end of

the first metatarsal unless the first-metatarsophalangeal joint dorsiflexes in a timely fashion during propulsion. Thus delay or lack of first-metatarsophalangeal dorsiflexion during propulsion effectively shortens the first metatarsal.

The first metatarsal must plantarflex in order for the first-metatarsophalangeal joint to dorsiflex adequately during gait.[15] To plantarflex during propulsion, the first metatarsal must be shorter than the second metatarsal, hence the increased incidence of hallux valgus and limitus/rigidus associated with long first metatarsals.

The appropriate length for a first metatarsal must be taken into consideration with its position relative to the second metatarsal in the sagittal plane. A short first metatarsal that cannot reach the ground functions as if it were dorsiflexed and results in overload of the second metatarsal.[53] A short, plantarflexed first metatarsal may bear adequate weight to prevent second-metatarsal overload.

## Hallux Limitus and Rigidus

The term *hallux limitus* refers to reduced first-metatarsophalangeal joint dorsiflexion available during gait. Hallux limitus may result from a structural or functional restriction of motion. Hallux rigidus is the end stage of structural hallux limitus, and no dorsiflexion is available, because of degenerative joint disease.[50] Hallux limitus and rigidus are frequently associated with long first metatarsals.

The dorsoplantar radiograph provides limited information concerning hallux limitus and a bit more concerning hallux rigidus. Because functional and early stages of structural hallux limitus do not have gross morphologic changes of the first-metatarsophalangeal joint, minimal radiographic signs can be observed.

Because hallux rigidus is the end stage of hallux limitus and represents degeneration of the joint, signs of joint degeneration can be observed on the dorsoplantar view. Thus signs of hallux rigidus are broadening of the first-metatarsal head and narrowing of the joint space. Unless the etiology is traumatic, the etiology of hallux rigidus and hallux valgus are the same (first-ray/medial-column hypermobility, elevated or long first ray). Hallux rigidus occurs instead of hallux abductus in those joints that are too stable to abduct, and whose lower extremities have minimal transverse-plane variation from normal. In some instances hallux abductus and rigidus both exist at the same location.

## Hallux Interphalangeal Angle (Hallux Abductus Interphalangeus)

The hallux interphalangeal angle (see Figure 14-3) is defined as the angle between the longitudinal bisections of the hallux proximal and distal phalanges. In a normal lower extremity, the first distal phalange is 13 degrees abducted in relation to the first proximal phalange.[57] This angulation is created by an oblique orientation of the proximal phalanx cartilage and/or asymmetrical form of the distal phalanx.[58] In unshod people of Papua New Guinea, Barnett[58] found the hallux abductus interphalangeus angle is 9.[58]

Sorto[57] found that when the hallux abductus angle was under 8 degrees, implying a stable first-metatarsophalangeal joint, the hallux abductus interphalangeus angle increased to an average of 16 degrees. He also found that when the hallux abductus angle is over 25 degrees, implying an unstable first-metatarsophalangeal joint, the hallux abductus interphalangeus angle reduces to an average of 9 degrees, just like the unshod individuals mentioned above. Given this information, Sorto theorized that when the first-metatarsophalangeal joint is unstable, shoe pressure will abduct the entire great toe. When the first-metatarsophalangeal joint is stable, the shoe pressure creates a bend more distally in the toe. Based on the observations of Christman[28] the question can be asked, Is hallux interphalangeus abductus less because the hallux is abducted and there is less pressure to create the deformity, or does the hallux abductus interphalangeus appear reduced because of the valgus rotation associated with hallux abductus?

The total lateral deviation (TLD) of the hallux is calculated by adding the hallux abductus angle and hallux abductus interphalangeus angles. Robbins[39] found that when the hallux TLD is greater than 31 degrees, the development of metatarsus primus adductus (MPA) is accelerated. Conversely, when the total lateral deviation of the hallux is less than 31 degrees, the TLD increases at a faster rate than the MPA. Robbins hypothesized that when the hallux abuts the second toe, the abduction forces become retrograde forces that push the first metatarsal medially, instead of abducting the hallux.

## The Digital Angle

The digital angle on a dorsoplantar radiograph (see Figure 14-2) is defined as the angulation between the longitudinal bisections of the second proximal phalange and second metatarsal.[1,2] The longitudinal axis of the digits and rearfoot (calcaneus) are approximately parallel in a normal foot.

Variations from normal in the transverse plane can be caused by hallux abductus pressure on the lesser digits, intrinsic muscle atrophy (such as in rheumatoid arthritis), and misalignment of the flexor and extensor tendons. As the foot pronates and supinates, the forefoot abducts and adducts, respectively. This results in misalignment of the flexor and extensor tendons, which results in adduction or abduction of the digits. The most common example of this occurrence is the adductovarus fifth toe. As the forefoot abducts, the long flexor tendon pulls from medial as opposed to from directly proximal.[1] This misalignment results in adduction and varus rotation of the fifth toe.

When a digit becomes adducted or abducted relative to its metatarsal, the metatarsal will frequently move in the opposite direction because of the retrograde force. Just as in hallux abductus and the secondary metatarsus primus adductus, correction of the digital misalignment necessitates soft tissue and possibly osseous surgical attention to correct the lesser metatarsal adduction or abduction, and the proximal articular set angle.[59]

In addition, midfoot stability is reduced as the flexor and extensor muscles attempt to compress the proximal phalanx onto the metatarsal head but result in adduction or abduction of the digit instead, because of the misalignment.

Sagittal-plane contractures of the digits are recognized on the dorsoplantar view as reduction of metatarsophalangeal joint space because of overlap of the proximal phalanx on the respective metatarsal head, intermediate phalanx foreshortening of each phalange, gun barrel sign (a circular appearance of the phalange, caused by the radiographic shadow, that represents looking through the longitudinal axis of the long bone instead of looking down onto the bone), and loss of interphalangeal joint space. Observation of any of these signs indicates an extension contracture of the metatarsophalangeal joint and/or flexion contracture of the interphalangeal joint(s). With signs of metatarsophalangeal joint contracture (proximal phalanx foreshortening, reduced metatarsophalangeal joint space), a retrograde force may be significant enough to create a downward push on the metatarsal head, resulting in corresponding increased plantar pressure. Sagittal-plane digital contracture signs are usually associated with feet most likely to have shoe-fitting problems and associated pain from excess friction on the toe box.

Because digital pathology generally becomes symptomatic as the result of wearing shoes that do not accommodate the digits and that affect digital alignment, it can be very informative to the physician and patients to take a dorsoplantar radiograph with the shoe on. This may reveal the fifth toe to underlap the fourth and may show other dramatic changes in transverse-plane digital alignment resulting from shoe pressure that may not be fully appreciated with the shoes off.

## Metatarsal Break and Curve

The significance of the geometric shape created by the distal ends of the metatarsals has been discussed by several authors, and to date is not well understood. Two basic principles need to be applied when evaluating the shape created by the distal metatarsals. First, the difference in length created by metatarsals 1 and 2, versus 2 through 5, serves a function.[60] The shorter metatarsals 2 through 5 act to stabilize the lateral midfoot and functions like a low gear early in propulsion as the center of force travels laterally and anteriorly through the foot in midstance and early propulsion. Once up to speed, the longer high gear of metatarsals 1 and 2 is used during propulsion as the center of force passes through the first metatarsal interspace. The longer lever created by metatarsals 1 and 2 increases the tension on the plantar fascia. Thus the compression and associated stability within the midfoot increases at a time when ground reactive forces are the greatest.[61]

The second principle is related to the shape created by the gentle curve described by the distal extreme of the metatarsals. The metatarsal length pattern should be a curve that allows hinge motion at the metatarsophalangeal joints without imposing excessive force on any one metatarsal.[62] The longer metatarsal, which does not fit the gentle curve pattern, usually bears the greatest load.[62] Thinking of the distal metatarsal relative length pattern as a curve is a fairly new concept.

The distal metatarsal length pattern was originally described as an angle created by the line described by connecting the most distal point of metatarsals 1 and 2, and the line created by the line created by connecting the most distal points of metatarsals 2 and 5.[1,2,62a] The average angle of 142.5 degrees was considered normal for the metatarsal break angle. An angle lower than 142 may function fine, but larger angles mean that the second metatarsal is long and is likely to become overloaded. The concept to remember about this manner of assessment is that if metatarsal 2 is too long relative to the other metatarsals, the angle increases and metatarsal 2 bears too much weight.

The next concept to evolve was describing the distal metatarsal pattern as a parabola, a constant radius curve. This was later challenged and described as a different type of symmetric curve, a conic curve.[63]

A more accurate description of the distal metatarsal length pattern is that of an asymmetric curve (see Figure 14-4.), that is, radius changes like a French curve.[64] Robbins[64] found that the distal metatarsals lie on a nonlinear curve and are related to one another semilogarithmically. He also found that all feet are on the same curve, but on different places along the curve. Thus the metatarsal curve is not unique for each person. Weight distribution is disturbed when a metatarsal does not conform to its place on the curve. Too short, and the adjacent metatarsals are at risk for excessive weight bearing. Too long, and the long metatarsal bears excessive weight for a prolonged period of time.

The formula for describing the appropriate metatarsal length as determined by Robbins is as follows:

$-y = 6.18 - 2.44 (\ln X)$ = optimal forefoot point on the curve centered

$y$ = $y$ coordinate of a metatarsal point

$X$ = natural logarithm of the $x$ coordinate

$2.44$ = average slope

$6.18$ = average regression constant that is equal to $y$ when $\ln X = 0$

Those metatarsals whose distal ends do not lie on the semilogarithmic curve are more likely to develop or be next to a metatarsal that develops pathology. As a goal, surgical solutions may consider placing the metatarsals on the curve.

The sesamoid axial view (see Figure 14-9) provides the clinician with a rough approximation of the semilogarithmic (linear) relationship of relative metatarsal length. The sesamoid axial view evaluation is explained later in this chapter.

## Relative Metatarsal Length and Height

The significance of relative metatarsal length is related to the weight bearing performed by each metatarsal. In general, if a metatarsal is too long, it bears too much weight during propulsion and possibly during midstance.[62] A long metatarsal also bears weight for a longer period of time than a short metatarsal, because of its protrusion during propulsion. A short metatarsal generally bears less weight, because the metatarsal declination makes the short metatarsal actually dorsiflexed relative to the adjacent metatarsals. Also, during propulsion, the short metatarsal comes off the ground earlier than a normal-length metatarsal, leaving the relatively longer metatarsals to bear more weight for a longer period when the forefoot is subjected to the greatest ground reactive forces.

Metatarsal length can be measured relative to the adjacent metatarsals using lines perpendicular their respective longitudinal bisections (Figure 14-4, C). Normal values are 3 mm second metatarsal, 2 mm third metatarsal, and 1 mm fourth metatarsal, all ± 1 millimeter.[65] Another method is to draw a reference line from the most distal points of metatarsals 1 and 5, and then measure the central metatarsal's protrusion distal to the reference line.[65] Valley and Reese[65] found that the second and third metatarsals should protrude 10 mm ± 3 mm and the fourth metatarsal, 7 mm ± 3 mm distal to the reference line.

Before shortening a metatarsal, its sagittal-plane position relative to the adjacent metatarsals must be considered. In general, every 4 mm of metatarsal shortening entails 1 mm of elevation. This ratio varies depending on the individual metatarsal's declination angle. The steeper the declination angle, the more elevation that occurs with shortening.[65]

Individual metatarsals that bear excessive load relative to their neighbors may have increased cortical thickening in reaction to the increased stress.[53,54] Once the overloaded metatarsals have been identified radiographically, the clinician should correlate this finding to other signs such as skin changes (to confirm overload) and to physical examination (to determine why the metatarsal is overloaded).

Determining which metatarsal is long depends on the relative metatarsal length compared to the adjacent metatarsals, as well as on the curve created by the distal metatarsals.[64]

Determining relative metatarsal length, cortical thickening, and distal metatarsal curve on the dorsoplantar view is helpful but must be correlated to the lateral and axial views and to the clinical exam before one can visualize the relative metatarsal relationships in three dimensions. Lesser metatarsal osteotomies only have a 50% success rate, largely because the clinician has only considered whether the metatarsal is plantarflexed and has neglected a variety of possible, complicated morphologic variations.

## Fifth-Metatarsal Relationships

The distal lateral curve of the fifth metatarsal requires two measurements to assess the fifth metatarsal's transverse-plane relationship relative to the adjacent fourth metatarsal.[66] The fifth intermetatarsal angle (see Figure 14-4, *C*) is created by measuring the angle made by the medial border of the proximal portion of the fifth metatarsal relative to the adjacent fourth-metatarsal longitudinal bisection. In the normal population, the fifth intermetatarsal angle is 6.5 degrees. Feet with bunionettes average 9 degrees. Eversion of the foot with pronation increases the intermetatarsal angle, so a positional component contributes.

To distinguish fifth-metatarsal splaying from the fourth metatarsal (fifth intermetatarsal angle) and distal lateral curving of the fifth-metatarsal head on the proximal metatarsal, the lateral deviation angle was developed.[66] The lateral deviation angle (see Figure 14-4, *C*) is the angle made by the longitudinal bisection of the fifth-metatarsal head and neck, and the line drawn parallel to the proximal medial border of the fifth metatarsal. Normally this angle is 2 to 3 degrees but averages 8 degrees in feet with bunionettes. Pronation of the foot does not change this angle, so it is structural.

The dorsoplantar assessment of the fifth metatarsal allows the clinician to determine the level of the fifth metatarsal abduction deformity, making it possible to design specific therapy to correct the deformity.

The proximal portion of the fifth metatarsal may also be prominent laterally because of hypertrophy but more commonly because metatarsus adductus has left the fifth-metatarsal base exposed laterally, as it lies at the apex of the metatarsus adductus deformity.

## Talar Superimposition on the Calcaneus (Talocalcaneal Superimposition)

On a dorsoplantar radiograph, the talus should be found superimposed on the calcaneus by approximately 50%,[1] and the medial side of the talus should align with the medial border of the sustentaculum tali.[2] This superimposition is considered to be a transverse-plane indicator of transverse-plane and frontal-plane (calcaneal everted or inverted) deformity. The degree of calcaneal inversion or eversion that is present directly influences the amount of superimposition.

Recall that calcaneal inversion and eversion occurs in response to closed kinetic-chain supination and pronation, respectively. An inverted calcaneus is oriented such that the plantar plane of the calcaneus begins to face toward the midline of the body. As the calcaneus inverts further and moves toward the midline, more and more of the calcaneus becomes superimposed under the talus. Therefore it can be said that talocalcaneal superimposition increases with supination (reduction of pronation) or supinated deformities. The opposite is true for pronation. As the calcaneus everts (becomes less inverted), the subtalar becomes less supinated (or more pronated), and the talus is less superimposed on the calcaneus.

Examples of radiographic evidence indicating deformity in this manner are as follows: In partially compensated rearfoot varus, the calcaneus is inverted relative to the sagittal plane when the subtalar joint is maximally pronated and the patient is standing in his or her angle and base of gait. Despite the subtalar joint being maximally pronated, we see greater than 50% superimposition because the calcaneus is inverted. In a compensated rearfoot varus, the foot can pronate to place the calcaneus in a vertical position. The vertical position of the calcaneus is associated with approximately 50% superimposition.

Talocalcaneal superimposition is also affected by transverse-plane translation between the talus and calcaneus. Translation in a joint usually occurs at its end range of motion. In the subtalar joint it occurs at the end range of pronation, particularly if the subtalar is being forced beyond its normal range of motion. Subtalar translation usually means that the talus moves medial to its normal position on the calcaneus. This can be observed clinically by observing a weight-bearing rearfoot pronate. In many feet when the calcaneus stops everting, the talus and ankle continue to move medially relative to the calcaneus. Some of the medial talar motion is subtalar joint, and some is coming from the midtarsal joint as well.

Talocalcaneal superimposition is a reflection of where the calcaneus sits under the talus. The talus sits on top of the calcaneus and depends on the calcaneus for support. The more medial the talus is positioned relative to the calcaneus, the more likely that the talus will plantarflex (fall off medially) as the sustentaculum tali and spring ligament become less effective as talar supports.

Ideally, the calcaneus should sit slightly lateral to the talus, making the center of force from the leg and the ground reactive force from the calcaneus minimal eversion torques on the rearfoot.[15] As the calcaneus is displaced further laterally relative to the talus, the eversion torque on the rearfoot increases and a corresponding reduction in rearfoot stability occurs. This is why a partially compensated rearfoot varus is usually associated with a rearfoot that is more stable (less pronated) than one in which the calcaneus can evert to a vertical position, and both these situations are much more stable than a rearfoot with an everted calcaneus. These are different levels of stability reflected in feet that are all maximally pronated.

Instability may also develop when the calcaneus is too far medial to the subtalar axis as well. An underpronated or oversupinated rearfoot results in lateral ankle instability because of subtalar supinatory influences from the ground reactive force medial to the subtalar axis. The different levels

of stability seen by talocalcaneal superimposition are directly related to how far lateral or medial the calcaneal contact point moves relative to the subtalar axis.

## Talonavicular Articulation and Wedge-Shaped Navicular

The talonavicular articular assessment on a dorsoplantar radiograph is a reflection of deformities in the midfoot or midtarsal joint (Figure 14-5). In a normal lower extremity, 75% of the articular surface on the head of the talus articulates with the navicular and the navicular is roughly rectangular in shape.[1,2]

The ideal value is 75%, with values ranging between 75% and 80% being normal. The percentage of the articu-

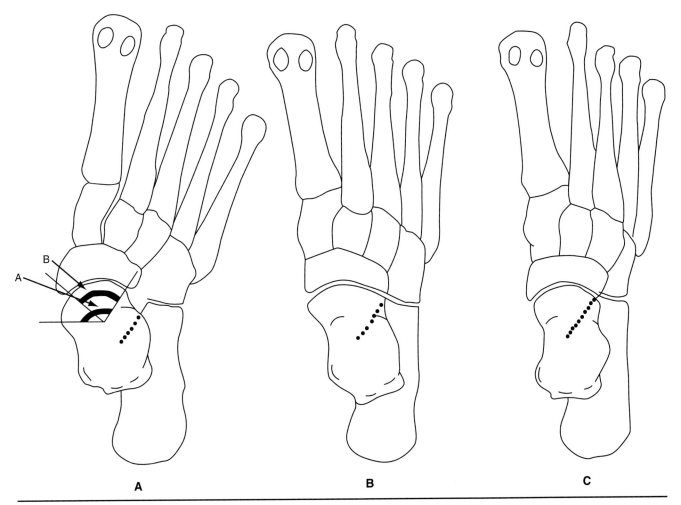

**A**                                    **B**                                    **C**

Figure 14-5   The transverse-plane relationships of overpronated (**A**), rectus/normal (**B**) and underpronated (**C**) feet are depicted. These are not meant to be the same foot positioned differently. As the foot is less pronated, the segments become less angulated and the midfoot has reduced width with greater overlapping of the bones as the foot assumes a more stacked dorsoplantar relationship. **A** shows the talonavicular articulation percentage using angles *A* and *B*. Angle *A* is the angle made by the lines marking the medial and lateral extent of the talar head articular cartilage, and angle *B* that portion of the talus that is articulating with the navicular. Thus angle *B* divided by angle *A* give the percentage of the talus articulating with the navicular.

lar surface that articulates with the navicular changes with pronation and supination. Deformities that cause excessive midtarsal pronatory compensations decrease this articulation value below 70%. Deformities that cause excessive midtarsal supinatory compensation increase this articulation percentage to greater than 80%. How much of the talus articulating with the navicular depends on transverse-plane midfoot position relative to the rearfoot.

The percentage is derived by picking a random point proximal to the talonavicular joint, and extending lines from this random point to the medial and lateral extent of the talar articular surface. This creates an angle. Next, lines are extended to the medial and lateral extent of where the navicular articulates with the talus. The percentage is derived from the navicular angle divided by the talar angle.

As the forefoot abducts (and the talus adducts) in closed kinetic-chain pronation, the navicular moves laterally on the talar articular surface. This leaves a large portion of the medial talar articular surface not articulating with the navicular, hence the reduction in the percentage of talar articular surface articulating with the navicular. As the navicular moves laterally, the posterior tibial muscle pulls very forcefully to try to reduce or slow the lateral movement (abduction). Pulling of the posterior tibial on the navicular during the early years of life stimulates the medial side of the navicular to grow and can be seen as hypertrophy of the proximal medial aspect of the navicular.

Abduction of the navicular also results in increased compression along the joint line laterally and reduced compression medially, instead of even compression across the entire talonavicular joint surface. The increased lateral compression during the developmental years results in a narrower lateral navicular and a laterally deviated talar articular surface (Wolff's law). With reduced medial compression and increased pull by the posterior tibial tendon, the medial side of the navicular will enlarge. The result of reduced lateral navicular size and increased medial navicular size is a wedge-shaped navicular (apex lateral).[1,2] The wedged navicular perpetuates the pronated position by maintaining the forefoot in an abducted position.

## Accessory Navicular

The accessory bone, accessory navicular, is located at the proximal medial plantar aspect of the navicular and is invested within the posterior tibial insertion. The os accessory navicular has a synovial joint with the navicular that can become symptomatic.[67] The insertion of the posterior tibial muscle has generally been assumed to be less effective with an accessory navicular placing the insertion more proximal, thereby lengthening the tendon.

## Calcaneocuboid Angle

The calcaneocuboid angle on a dorsoplantar radiograph (see Figure 14-1) indicates deformities of the midtarsal joint, and infers subtalar joints position. The calcaneocuboid angle is formed by two lines. The first line is a tangent drawn along the lateral side of the cuboid. The second line is drawn as a tangent along the lateral border of the calcaneus. In a normal lower extremity, the angulation of these two lines lies between 0 and 5 degrees.

Increases occur for three reasons. The first cause is forefoot abduction on the rearfoot with midtarsal pronation. As the subtalar allows more midtarsal pronation, the cuboid appears to be more abducted relative to the calcaneus. Over time the calcaneocuboid joint is redirected by chronic lateral compression (Wolff's law).

The second cause occurs indirectly as a result of calcaneal eversion with excessive subtalar pronation. As the calcaneus everts, the cuboid is able to drift laterally, and this lateral position allows the cuboid to escape dorsal laterally around the calcaneal anterior process (beak) as it is pushed by the vertical ground reactive forces.[68] The result is that the cuboid can become more abducted, that is, laterally positioned, relative to the calcaneus.

The third reason why the cuboid may appear more abducted on the calcaneus is that eversion of the calcaneus means that the dorsoplantar view is now looking slightly at the plantar lateral surface of the calcaneus and cuboid. Thus what is represented on the dorsoplantar radiograph is in part the normal plantarflexed position of the cuboid on the calcaneus. This change of perspective makes the cuboid appear very abducted in feet with an everted calcaneus. Regardless of the reason, an abducted cuboid usually means an everted calcaneus is present and considerable midfoot instability exists and is likely to worsen.

As vertical ground reactive forces develop more influence in the transverse plane of the foot because of calcaneal eversion, the foot assumes a much more pronated position with subluxation of the subtalar and midtarsal joints over a prolonged period of time. This is because the foot is ill prepared to counter transverse plane forces the magnitude of vertical ground reactive forces. Also, as the calcaneus everts and the cuboid escapes laterally the talus is forced medially.[68] Eventually the spring ligament and posterior tibial tendon allow the talus to move further medially.

## Talocuboid Angle

The talocuboid angle on a dorsoplantar radiograph (see Figure 14-1) is unique in that it is both a midtarsal joint and subtalar joint determination. Thus the talocuboid angle could be considered the most important angle with regard to evaluating foot linearity and stability. The talocuboid angle is equal to the sum of the talocalcaneal angle and the calcaneocuboid angles.[37] The talocuboid angle is the angulation between the talar neck and head longitudinal bisection and a tangent along the lateral side of the cuboid.

In a normal lower extremity, this angulation lies in a range between 15 and 20 degrees. Values of greater than 25 degrees are considered pathologic. This can be understood when it is recalled that a normal talocalcaneal angle range is between 15 and 18 degrees, whereas normal calcaneocuboid angle range is between 0 and 5 degrees. The normal maximum sum of these two angles should therefore never be greater than 23 degrees. Large values for this angle indicate transverse-plane pronatory compensations or deformities causing subtalar (talocalcaneal) and midtarsal (calcaneocuboid) angular increases. Talocuboid angle of less than 15 degrees is a reflection of an underpronated (oversupinated) foot.

Normal talocuboid angles of 15 to 20 degrees reflect moderate divergents of the talus and lateral column of the triangular foot. They are not too angulated, which would reduce the ability of joint compression to create stability.

Greenberg[37] compared the amount of hallux abductus and metatarsus primus adductus to a variety of sagittal- and transverse-plane rearfoot angular measurements, most of which were subtalar oriented. Only when he compared the transverse plane first-ray deviations to a subtalar-midtarsal transverse-plane measurement, talocuboid angle, was there a correlation. The more pronated the rearfoot in the transverse plane, as represented by the talocuboid angle, the higher was the first-ray transverse-plane deviations.

## Other Dorsoplantar Radiographic Signs

Two final dorsoplantar radiographic signs (see Figure 14-5) are metatarsal-base superimposition and midfoot width (naviculocuboid superimposition). Normally the metatarsal bases are superimposed one on another by 50%. In general, metatarsal-base superimposition increases with inversion of the midfoot as the midfoot assumes a less pronated position. For example, this may be seen with midfoot compensation (supination) for a rigid forefoot valgus. In contrast, as the forefoot pronates, metatarsal-base superimposition decreases as the forefoot assumes a position closer to being parallel to the transverse plane (unstacked) as the forefoot becomes less inverted in the midfoot. An example is a compensated forefoot varus. As the medial forefoot of a compensated forefoot varus comes down to the ground, the medial side of the arch moves closer to the ground, and the midfoot assumes a position closer to being parallel to the supporting surface. Thus there is less vertical stacking in the radiographic representation, or superimposition.

Consistent with the metatarsal-base observations, the width of the midfoot generally increases with pronation and decreases with supination. These two statements are

**TABLE 14-1   Dorsoplantar Radiographic Changes with Motion**

| Radiographic Morphologic Observation | Motion | | |
|---|---|---|---|
| | Pronate | Rectus | Supinate |
| Talocalcaneal angle | I | 17–21 | D |
| Lesser tarsus angle | I | 10 ± 5 | D |
| Metatarsus adductus angle | — | 10–20 | — |
| Forefoot angle | D | Slight Add. | I |
| Talocalcaneal superimposition | D | Approx. 50% | I |
| Talonavicular articulation | D | 75%–80% | I |
| Calcaneocuboid angle | I | 0–5 | D |
| Talocuboid angle | I | 15–20 | D |
| Metatarsal base superimposition | I | Approx. 50% | I |

I, Increase; D, decrease, —, no change.

consistent with our observation of how the midfoot looks broader as viewed from dorsally with excessive pronation and appears stacked and narrower with excessive supination (Table 14-1).

## LATERAL RADIOGRAPHIC ANALYSIS

The lateral radiograph is the sagittal-plane shadow of the foot. The trabecular pattern observed on the lateral radiograph parallels the force transmitted through the foot.[69] The force created by the body standing on the foot is transmitted through the talus and then to the weight-bearing areas of the foot, metatarsal heads and medial calcaneal tubercle. Linear relationships are important for the transmission of this force and to resist the equal and opposite ground reactive force.

To properly and consistently evaluate the sagittal-plane relationships and bone morphology of the foot, the lateral radiograph should be taken with the patient standing in his or her angle and base of gait, and the film parallel to the medial side of the foot. A properly positioned patient's lateral radiograph should demonstrate a talotrochlear surface that has the medial and lateral contours superimposed so that it appears to be one curve and not two. This is difficult with people whose forefoot is very abducted or adducted, because the film cannot parallel markedly deviated anatomy.

## The Calcaneal Inclination Line and Angle

The calcaneal inclination line on a lateral view radiograph (Figure 14-6) can be drawn on the plantar surface of the

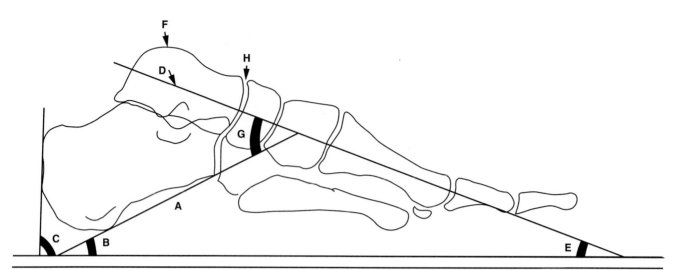

**Figure 14-6**   The lateral view allows evaluation of sagittal-plane alignment of the various foot segments. The posterior calcaneal angle is normally less than 90 degrees. *A*, Calcaneal inclination line; *B*, calcaneal inclination angle; *C*, posterior calcaneal angle of Ruch; *D*, talar declination line; *E*, talar declination angle; *F*, talotrochlear surface shape; *G*, lateral talocalcaneal angle; *H*, cyma line.

calcaneus by connecting two points. The first point is drawn at the anterior, plantar extent of the calcaneal tuberosity. The second point is drawn at the most plantar point of the calcaneocuboid articulation.[1,7] The angulation of the line connecting these points in relation to the supporting surface is equal to the calcaneal inclination angle.[2] The horizontal reference has also been a line connecting the plantar surface of the calcaneal tubercle and the fifth-metatarsal head.[1,15] In a normal lower extremity, this angle is equal to 18 to 20 degrees.[2,70,71]

The calcaneal inclination angle is normally not affected by pronation or supination of the foot.[2,72,73] However, long-term pronation of the foot when bearing weight can cause the calcaneal inclination angle to decrease as the forefoot is subluxated dorsally by a deformity that creates a sagittal-plane force, such as congenital equinus. A low calcaneal inclination angle is not pathognomonic for equinus deformities, because forefoot varus and obesity may also reduce the angle over time. Also, a normal or increased calcaneal inclination angle does not mean that a congenital functional equinus is present or not. Functional equinus must be evaluated independent of calcaneal inclination.

Normal calcaneal inclination places the talus far enough away from the plantar fascia to enhance the tension band's ability to compress the forefoot onto the rearfoot, and ability to resist hyperextension (dorsiflexion) of the forefoot on the rearfoot. A low calcaneal inclination angle reduces the stability of the forefoot and increases the likelihood that the rotational vector of force (moment) from the ground reactive force pushing upward on the metatarsal heads will not be adequately resisted. This moment dorsiflexes the forefoot on the rearfoot, thus creating greater plantar fascial tension and increasing likelihood of plantar fascial injury as the foot flattens.[74]

An increase in the calcaneal inclination angle has the effect of foreshortening the calcaneus, that is, placing the calcaneal contact point closer to the ankle axis. Thus the ground reactive force at heel contact has a reduced plantar-flexory moment at the ankle and increased shock. The higher calcaneal inclination may also result in ankle instability as the talus and subtalar joint are raised away from the supporting surface, creating a longer frontal-plane moment arm. The longer moment arm increases the likelihood of inversion ankle trauma, because it is more difficult for the peroneal muscles to resist the proportionately increased inversion moment.

## Haglund's Deformity

Haglund's deformity[75] is a posterosuperior prominence of bone on the calcaneus, which may rub the shoe heel counter or create pressure on the Achilles tendon.[76,77] Synonyms include *pump bump, winter heel, retrocalcaneal bursitis,* and *Achilles bursitis.*[7] Radiographically it is viewed as an osseous prominence extending dorsal and/or posterior to the dorsal and posterior surfaces of the calcaneus respectively. Two methods are used to determine if a deformity is present. If the posterior surface of the calcaneus is tilted posteriorly, then the posterosuperior surface of the calcaneus will be prominent, and motion of the calcaneus will create irritation of the overlying soft tissue.[78–80] The Phillip and Fowler angle (posterosuperior surface line and plantar calcaneal line) does not take into consideration calcaneal inclination and thus is not adequate alone.[81,82]

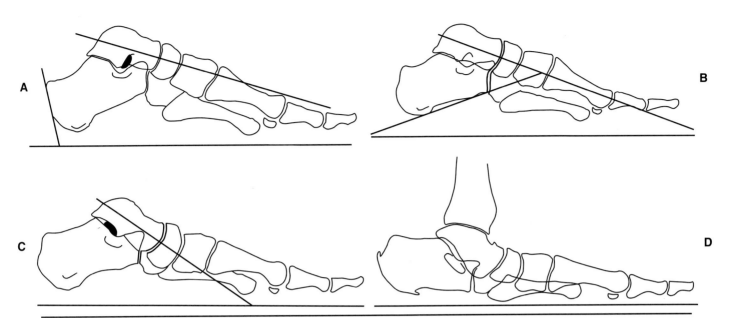

**Figure 14-7**    Lateral views of underpronated pes cavus (**A**), normal/ rectus (**B**), overpronated (**C**), and grossly overpronated and subluxated (**D**) feet are depicted. Underpronated pes cavus feet (**A**) have many of the following signs: talar declination line passing dorsal to the first metatarsal, exaggeration of the sinus tarsi, increased calcaneal inclination angle, posterior facet of the subtalar frequently has a flattened appearance, sustentaculum tali is closer to being horizontal. Reduced naviculocuboid superimposition is a reflection of midtarsal position and is also associated with underpronated pes cavus feet but may be present in overpronated feet that have forefoot valgus. The normal/rectus foot (**B**) demonstrates moderate calcaneal inclination to lift the talus from the supporting surface, but the hallmark is the bisection of the medial column by the talar declination line. The more pronated feet (**C** and **D**) have increased plantarflexion of the talus, adduction of the talus making the head appear foreshortened, sustentaculum tali has increased angulation to the plane of support, allowing the talus to move anteriorly, anterior displacement of the talus breaks the cyma line anteriorly and opens the posterior facet, creating the appearance of the pseudo-sinus tarsi, increased naviculocuboid superimposition as the arch collapses (medial column dorsiflexes), wedge-shaped navicular created by prolonged increased dorsal compression, and medial-column faults. As the calcaneus assumes a less inverted or more pronated position, the lateral calcaneal tubercle moves further from the weight-bearing surface. The grossly overpronated foot has all the signs of the overpronated foot just listed, but exaggerated. In addition, **D** depicts posterior and plantar calcaneal spurring, calcaneocuboid fault, increased weight bearing of the fifth-metatarsal base, flat talotrochlear surface, and talar neck dorsal exostosis associated with an osseus equinus. The most obvious sign is that of hyperextension of the medial column, which alignment makes it impossible for the plantar truss to create the compression necessary for stability.

The posterosuperior surface of the calcaneus must be evaluated for its protrusion posteriorly by comparing the posterior surface plane to a line vertical to the supporting surface.[78,79] The protrusion of the calcaneus posteriorly results in rubbing on shoes and is treated by calcaneal osteotomy to bring the posterior surface anteriorly.[80]

The second method of radiographic assessment are parallel pitch lines. A line parallel to the calcaneal inclination line is drawn from the posterior lip of the posterior facet in a posterior direction. If the posterosuperior portion of the calcaneus extends superior to the dorsal line, it should be considered enlarged.[79,80,83] The dorsal protrusion of the posterior calcaneus evaluated by the parallel pitch lines is of much less importance clinically than the posterior protrusion of the superioposterior surface relative to a vertical line.

## Calcaneal Spurring

The calcaneus has two places where spurs develop most frequently as the result of excessive tension. These are (1) the posterior surface of the calcaneus at the insertion of the Achilles tendon and (2) the anterior surface of the medial calcaneal tubercle (see Figure 14-7). The spurs may first be viewed as periosteal lifting. This ill-defined, radiolucency on the calcaneal surface, or at the end of the spur, is frequently associated with pain created by the inflamed periosteum.

The retrocalcaneal and plantar calcaneal spurs are mostly frequently caused by obesity or a form of equinus creating the excessive tension. Calcification of the Achilles tendon is much more likely to be associated with pain than a spur at the insertion.[84] The plantar calcaneal spur is most commonly associated with overpronation and the accompanying lengthening of the foot, but is also found in rectus and cavus feet, which have a lot of plantar soft tissue tension. Scherer and co-workers[85] associated dorsiflexion of the medial column that accompanies longitudinal midtarsal supination as frequently involved, because of the simultaneous lengthening of the foot. The tension itself is thought to be related to the plantar fascia. Forman and Green[86] found the plantar calcaneal spur at the origin of the flexor digitorum brevis, and McCarthy and Gorecki[87] found them at the origin of the intrinsic muscles, specifically the flexor digitorum brevis, as well as the plantar fascia.

Besides tension, direct pressure on the plantar or retrocalcaneal spurs can cause discomfort. Direct pressure on the plantar spur occurs most often plantarly when the spur is located very low on the medial calcaneal tubercle, when calcaneal inclination has reduced over time, making the spur point slightly plantar as opposed to horizontal, and when wearing high-heeled shoes, which also reduces the calcaneal inclination relative to the supporting surface.

In a broad cross section of people with foot pathology requiring radiographs, 13% had plantar calcaneal spurs and only 39% of those with spurs had ever experienced heel pain.[88] Although only 50% of the feet with plantar calcaneal spurs also showed radiographic signs of foot pronation, 81% of the heels that had a history of pain were overpronated. This is consistent with Jacoby's[74] mathematical model demonstrating that the flatter the foot, the greater the plantar tension. In Shama's study, heel pain was not subdivided into smaller groups, such as those not related to the spur, such as contusion, bursa, and neuroma. Therefore a patient experiencing pain in the plantar heel region does not necessarily have the pain emanating from the calcaneal spur. The radiographic signs must be corroborated by physical examination before diagnosing a calcaneal spur as responsible for pain.

## Boehler's Angle

Boehler's angle is a measure of the angulation between the anterior dorsal and posterior dorsal aspects of the calcaneus.[84] It is used primarily to determine if there has been a compression fracture of the calcaneus with a depressed posterior facet. Normally there is a 0- to 6-degree difference between the limbs, and the normal Boehler's angle range is 20 to 45 degrees.[90] This angle has erroneously been used to classify feet; that is, to say that higher the calcaneal inclination, the larger Boehler's angle. No correlation exists between calcaneal inclination and Boehler's angle.[90]

## Talar Declination Line and Angle

The talar declination line on a lateral view radiograph, (see Figure 14-6) is drawn as a perpendicular to a line connecting two points on the talar head.[1,2] The first point is the superior articular point of the head of the talus with the navicular. The second point is drawn at the anterior inferior superimposition of the articular surface of the talus by the calcaneus. A line drawn perpendicular to the line made by connecting these two points is then drawn as the talar declination line. The talar declination line usually parallels the trabecular pattern in the head and neck of the talus.

Normally the talar declination line parallels the lateral longitudinal bisection of the navicular and first metatarsal,[8] and ideally should bisect the first metatarsal in people over 3 years of age.[71] When the talar declination line projects superior to the first metatarsal, the subtalar or midtarsal joints are usually not pronated enough, and a plantarflexed medial column is frequently associated. When the talar declination line projects inferior to the first metatarsal, the subtalar is overpronated, and the medial column of the foot is frequently dorsiflexed, with a medial column fault present radiographically.

The angulation of the talar declination line with the supporting surface is known as the talar declination angle (see Figure 14-6). In a normal lower extremity, this angle averages 21 degrees. It increases with pronation as the talus plantarflexes and decreases with supination as the talus dorsiflexes.

## Dorsiflexed Talus: Pseudoequinus

The talus and calcaneus may be dorsiflexed by a retrograde force from a plantarflexed forefoot. Dorsiflexing the talus in the ankle may reduce the available dorsiflexion. Thus a patient may have an equinus, inadequate foot-to-leg dorsiflexion range available with the subtalar neutral and the midtarsal maximally pronated. However, the lack of dorsiflexion stems from a plantarflexed forefoot creating the need for more than the usual amount of ankle dorsiflexion instead of from an intrinsic lack of ankle dorsiflexion.[91]

Pseudoequinus may be present whenever the talar declination line passes dorsal to the first metatarsal.

## Talar Trochlear Surface Shape

Normally the trochlear surface of the talus has a round surface profile when viewed from laterally (see Figures 14-6 and 14-7). In some feet with severe equinus deformity, the trochlear surface appears flattened as compared to a normal radius curve (see Figure 14-7). This flattening is caused by the forceful pulling downward of the leg by the triceps surae, in addition to the weight of the body compressing the talus. The resulting larger radius of curvature cannot allow as much dorsiflexion, which further contributes to the equinus.

## Talar Neck Dorsal Exostosis

Hypertrophy of the dorsal surface of the neck of the talus (see Figure 14-7) or anterior surface of the tibia may obstruct ankle dorsiflexion, osseous equinus.[1] The stress lateral radiograph provides the clinician with a pictorial representation of osseous obstruction if it exists, and with the use of the tibiotrochlear angle can assess the degree of limitation.

The tibiotrochlear angle is the angle made by the longitudinal axis of the tibia, and the transtrochlear axis. The longitudinal axis of the tibia is created by a line connecting the bisections of tibial metaphyseal-diaphyseal junction, and the anterior and posterior limits of the distal tibial articular surface. The transtrochlear axis is a line connecting the anterior and posterior limits of the trochlear surface.

Normally the ankle should allow 10 degrees of dorsiflexion when the relaxed and stress lateral views are compared. Less than 10 degrees of dorsiflexion is highly suggestive that the talar neck is obstructing ankle dorsiflexion. A talar neck dorsal exostosis that is touched by the tibia in the stress view is pathognomonic for osseus ankle equinus.

## Talar Head Shape

Normally the lateral view provides a silhouette of the talar head with a normal-length neck. When the foot becomes very pronated, the talus adducts and the lateral radiograph represents the talus from a slightly anterior position.[62] This change of perspective projects as a rounder, ball-like appearance to the talar head and foreshortening of the talar neck. This is usually a sign of severe transverse-plane subtalar pronation, that is, talar adduction, which should be confirmed on the dorsoplantar view.

## Lateral Talocalcaneal Angle

The talocalcaneal angle on a lateral-view radiograph (see Figure 14-6) is defined as the angulation between the calcaneal inclination line and the talar declination line.[1,2,7] In a normal lower extremity, this angulation is found to range between 35 and 40 degrees. Because the calcaneal inclination line does not move as the foot pronates and supinates, the lateral talocalcaneal angle changes with the talar declination line. Therefore as the talus plantarflexes with subtalar pronation the talocalcaneal angle increases, and it decreases with subtalar supination as the talus dorsiflexes. The dominance of the talar component of subtalar sagittal-plane motion, and talar linkage to midtarsal medial-column motion, is why foot orthoses that support the arch (talonavicular joint) have altered foot mechanics and provided comfort.

## Subtalar: Sustentaculum Tali Changes

On a lateral-view radiograph in a normal lower extremity, the sustentaculum tali is found to parallel the supporting surface and functions as a support for the talus.[2] With prolonged pronation the sustentaculum tali may remodel and begin to slope plantarly (see Figure 14-7). The plantar slope makes it easier for the talus to adduct and slide anteriorly that perpetuates closed kinetic-chain subtalar joint pronation. Therefore feet that have a sustentaculum tali that slopes toward the plantar surface are structurally predisposed to pronate. A downward-facing sustentaculum tali is a sign of a chronically pronating subtalar.

As the calcaneus everts, the sustentaculum tali becomes less obvious radiographically.

## Subtalar: Sinus Tarsi and Posterior Articular Facet Alignment

On a lateral-view radiograph in a normal lower extremity, a moderately sized sinus tarsi can be visualized at the level of the talar neck, and the posterior articular facets of the calcaneus and talus are congruent (see Figure 14-7). The posterior facet may appear as a round curvature from laterally, or flat and parallel with the middle facet. The flat posterior facets are sometimes associated with subtalar joints having reduced ranges of motion. The appearance of the sinus tarsi and posterior facet change as the subtalar joint position changes.

In a normally aligned subtalar joint the majority of compressive forces created by body weight are carried by the large posterior facet.[62a] The sustentaculum tali middle facet acts as a guidepost, and the anterior facet and spring ligament offer support for the talar head.

With subtalar joint pronation, the talus appears to move anteriorly in a "corkscrew" fashion. As the talus appears to move anteriorly on the calcaneus, it is moving in a plantar and medial direction around the calcaneal sustentaculum tali while the calcaneus everts. At the end of the pronatory range, the sinus tarsi is visually obliterated (or twisted into nonexistence by talar adduction) as the talus moves forward, while a pseudo–sinus tarsi has been created from the pulled-apart posterior subtalar articulation. Because the posterior facet is distracted as opposed to compressed, the majority of subtalar joint compression must be occurring at the middle facet, particularly its lateral portion, with the spring ligament providing a greater supporting role for the head of the talus. In addition, the lateral process of the talus is compressed into the calcaneus, which is seen as sclerosis (increased density) of the calcaneus and rounding of the lateral process. This increased calcaneal sclerosis on the lateral view is superimposed on the sustentaculum tali.

In severely overpronated feet that have had the foot placed parallel to the film, the talus is adducted relative to the foot and appears foreshortened, with the head looking round. This is usually accompanied by superimposition of the talar head over the anterior process of the calcaneus (beak).

The anterior position of the talus associated with subtalar joint pronation moves a large overlapping talar posterior process anteriorly into the calcaneal posterior facet, creating eventual degenerative signs and symptoms.

With subtalar joint supination, the talus "corkscrews" posteriorly in a dorsiflexion, abduction motion. This causes the talar posterior articular facet to protrude posteriorly as the talus moves posteriorly on the calcaneus and the sinus tarsi becomes exaggerated. The posterior facet will appear less curved as the subtalar joint becomes supinated. Posterior facets that appear to have less curve when viewed laterally, usually have less subtalar joint range of motion than the average.

## Signs of Restricted Subtalar Joint Range of Motion

Restricted subtalar joint range of motion, that is, under 15 degrees frontal- and transverse-plane motion, has several causes. Tarsal coalitions and bars usually come to mind first, but some subtalar joints that have restricted ranges of motion or that do not pronate adequately may manifest the same signs. Signs of restricted subtalar joint range of motion (see Figure 14-7) include narrowing of the posterior facet joint space, broadening of the lateral talar process secondary to calcaneal eversion, sclerotic circle around the sustentaculum tali called a halo effect or sign,[1] and talar beaking.[92]

Talar beaking is frequently misinterpreted as pathognomonic for tarsal coalitions. Talar beaking is hypertrophy of the superior lateral aspect of the talar head and is not a sign of talonavicular joint degeneration.[92] Talar beaking is also seen in rheumatoid arthritis, acromegaly, hypermobile flatfoot, overzealous clubfoot correction, and post-Grice extra-articular arthroresis.[93]

## The Cyma Lines

Cyma lines appear in both lateral (see Figure 14-6) and dorsoplantar radiographic views. The cyma line is a lazy S-shaped line that runs through the joint spaces of well-aligned calcaneocuboid and talonavicular joints. Pronation and supination of the foot results in changes in the continuity of the cyma line. Excessive pronatory movement of the talus on the calcaneus causes an anterior break in the cyma line as the talus appears to move anteriorly. Excessive supinatory movement or positioning of the talus on the calcaneus causes the cyma line to be broken posteriorly. The cyma line is influenced by both subtalar and midtarsal positions.

The anteroposterior break in the cyma line is thought to be caused by the talus moving anteriorly or posteriorly on the calcaneus as the foot pronates and supinates.[1] Also contributing to the anterior break is the adduction (medial rotation) of the talus that would make the anterior lateral portion of the talus more prominent anteriorly as viewed laterally.[10]

## The Foot-Arch Formula

Both *pes planus* and *pes cavus* are terms that relate to the height of the medial longitudinal arch of the weight-bearing foot. To proportionally describe arch height of feet with varying-length feet, a formula was developed by Demp[94] based on principles of stability. This formula relates arch height to foot length. Foot length is defined as the distance between the calcaneal tuberosity and the first-metatarsal head. In a normal lower extremity, the high point (height) of the arch of a foot is equal to 40% of the length. The high point of the bottom of the arch is measured at the base of the navicular on a lateral-view radiograph to the line connecting the calcaneus to the first metatarsal.

## The Talonavicular, Naviculocuneiform, and Calcaneocuboid Faults

A fault is when a segment of the foot hyperextends, that is, shows excessive dorsiflexion. Hyperextension is viewed as a collapse of a portion of the arch of the foot. No matter which joint(s) is involved, as the forefoot is dorsiflexed, the dorsal surfaces of the joints may appear compressed, the plantar joint space appears wider, and a sag in the involved segment is perceived.

The talonavicular or naviculocuneiform fault is a feature that appears on a lateral radiograph view when an unstable medial column is present (see Figure 14-7). The medial column is usually unstable as a result of excessive pronation causing the medial column to be overloaded and excessively dorsiflexed on the rearfoot. With continued dorsiflexion and ground reactive force pressure, tension bands and muscles are not able to stabilize the medial column from being bent dorsally. Another frequent contributing factor is the retrograde force created by delayed first-metatarsophalangeal joint dorsiflexion in early propulsion, functional hallux limitus.[95]

The bend (subluxation) occurs as the medial column is forcefully dorsiflexed on the rearfoot. Subsequently the talonavicular or naviculocuneiform joints are remodeled. The hallmarks of a medial-column fault are an increased declination of that portion of the medial-column posterior to the fault and a rather obvious nonlinear appearance of the medial-column bones. A medial-column fault is a sign of medial-column hypermobility and is an indication that the foot is very unstable. Whenever a medial-column fault is present, a supinatus is also present.[96]

The calcaneocuboid fault[62a] is less easily described and more difficult to recognize. The dominant features are increase in plantar joint space width, suggestion of plantar displacement of the cuboid (plantar surfaces do not align), and reduced congruity of the superior portions of the joint. The basic mechanism is also overdorsiflexion (hyperextension) as the result of overloading. Equinus deformities and obesity are the most common factors contributing to the overload. Abduction of the cuboid, allowing the cuboid to escape dorsal laterally,[68] makes the calcaneocuboid joint more susceptible to faulting.

In some instances involving severe lateral-column overload, the fifth-metatarsal base is separated plantarly from the cuboid instead of closely approximated. When this is the case, usually the fifth-metatarsal head is dorsiflexing as the result of bearing excessive ground reactive forces, and the fifth-metatarsal base becomes a weight-bearing surface. Radiographically the fifth-metatarsal base appears closer to the supporting surface than is usual compared to the plantar surface of the calcaneus and metatarsal heads.[2]

Bearing excessive weight on the fifth-metatarsal base may lead to a painful contusion as the result of repeated microtrauma and provides a very effective pronatory moment arm to the midtarsal and subtalar joints. The result is gradual increase in the pronated position of the foot. The situation can be aggravated by wearing shoes that have a slight curve in the shank, not straight as in a wedge-shaped shoe.

## Cuboid Declination (Plantarflexed Cuboid)

The plantarflexed cuboid places excessive weight-bearing responsibility on the lateral column and creates one of the forefoot varus deformities.[96] The results are an exaggerated pronatory moment and excessive weight bearing by the fifth metatarsal.

On the lateral view the cuboid may assume a variety of shapes, hindering a description of the plantarflexed cuboid as a unique morphology. In general the plantarflexed cuboid extends further plantar than usual from the anterior plantar surface of the calcaneus and may appear slightly shorter in its anteroposterior dimension. The trabecular pattern in the plantarflexed cuboid may assume a more vertical orientation than in normal-shaped cuboids because of the change of weight-bearing pattern, that is, the fifth-metatarsal base bearing weight. The vertically oriented trabecular pattern is not unique, because equinus and forefoot varus also have this change of direction.

## Fifth Metatarsal

Normally the lateral column of the foot has an arch contour whereby the fifth-metatarsal base is above the level created by a line connecting the plantar surfaces of the calcaneus and fifth-metatarsal head. Thus the fifth-metatarsal base generally bears relatively little weight during ambulation and stance. The closer the fifth-metatarsal base is to the ground, the more likely that it will bear weight (see Figure 14-7).

Weight bearing by the fifth-metatarsal base, when excessive, can lead to contusion of the base from the repetitive microtrauma and to overpronation of the foot. The fifth-metatarsal base has a long and effective pronatory moment arm to the subtalar and midtarsal joints because it is lateral to these axes by a considerable distance.[97] Significant weight bearing by the fifth-metatarsal base results in overpronation of the foot and is identified clinically by lateral displacement of the soft tissue plantar to the fifth-metatarsal base in stance. Merely adding a heel lift off-loads the fifth-metatarsal base and can reduce foot pronation.

The fifth-metatarsal base can also become weight bearing when excessive ground reactive force subluxes the distal fifth metatarsal dorsally. This usually is accompanied by a fault at the articulation between the cuboid and the fifth metatarsal.

## Wedge-Shaped Navicular

Forceful dorsiflexion of the medial column produces greater dorsal compression of the medial-column bones. This may lead to a narrower dorsal surface than plantar surface of the navicular. Thus the navicular may assume a wedge shape, with apex dorsal, on the lateral view in feet with severely overpronated positions.[68] This wedge shape of the navicular helps to perpetuate the overpronated position of the foot and holds a poor prognosis for significantly altering foot position with foot orthoses. The wedge-shaped navicular is observed most frequently associated with functional equinus and forefoot varus deformities.

## Naviculocuboid Superimposition

Superimposition of the navicular and cuboid is an indicator of midtarsal position and frontal-plane deformity. In a normal lower extremity, the navicular is superimposed on 50% (or slightly less) of the cuboid. The amount of superimposition increases with midtarsal pronation as the medial column moves closer to the ground. Superimposition decreases with midtarsal supination as the medial column moves away from the ground and the navicular obstructs less of the side view of the cuboid (see Figure 14-7).

Naviculocuboid superimposition can also be used as an indicator of forefoot deformity. For example, in forefoot varus the midtarsal is forced to pronate to bring the medial column down to the ground and generally results in increased naviculocuboid superimposition. Compensation for forefoot valgus involves midtarsal supination, which reduces the amount of naviculocuboid superimposition. In fact, it is fairly common to find feet that are excessively pronated but have reduced naviculocuboid superimposition because a forefoot valgus is present. A foot that has an approximately perpendicular forefoot to rearfoot relation has approximately 50% (or slightly less) naviculocuboid

**TABLE 14-2** Lateral View Changes in Osseous Alignment with Motion

| Observation | Motion | | |
|---|---|---|---|
| | Pronate | Rectus | Supinate |
| Calcaneal inclination angle | — | 18–20 | — |
| Talar declination angle | I | 21 | D |
| Talar declination line | Plantar | Bisect | Dorsal |
| Talocalcaneal angle | I | 35–40 | D |
| Sinus tarsi | Pseudo | Half | Open |
| Cyma line | Anterior | Curve | Posterior |
| Foot/arch ratio | D | 40% | I |
| Naviculocuboid superimposition | I | Approx. 50% | D |

*I*, Increase; *D*, decrease; —, no change.

superimposition, if no other morphologic variation present is affecting arch height.

Naviculocuboid superimposition can also be used as a guide when assessing the vector of pull of the peroneus longus on the first ray. The peroneus longus uses the cuboid as a pulley so that it may pull the first ray plantarly. This can only occur if the proximal portion of the first ray is farther from the supporting surface than the cuboid.[15] With increased naviculocuboid superimposition the peroneus longus has a decreasing plantar vector of pull to stabilize the first ray. In addition, as the plantar vector of pull decreases the lateral vector increases, and the peroneus longus becomes more of a forefoot pronator.[68]

Table 14-2 summarizes the radiographic finding associated with motion in the lateral view.

## Congenital Versus Acquired Arch Deformities

The difference between congenital and acquired arch deformities can be seen on the lateral-view radiograph. In general, congenital arch deformities have their bones giving a linear appearance, although the bones may be in abnormal configurations. For example, in congenital pes planus the talar declination line may still bisect the medial column although the talar declination angle would be much decreased from normal. With an acquired pes planus, the bones may have normal configurations but they would not have a linear appearance. The same generalizations can be made for pes cavus.

## First Ray

On the lateral-view radiograph the first-ray longitudinal bisection (axis, declination line) should parallel the talar declination line, and the medial column should have a linear appearance (see Figure 14-6 and 14-7). The first-ray

declination line (bisection) is created by drawing a line through the bisections of the proximal and distal diaphysis of the first metatarsal. When the first ray has a congenital deformity, the linear appearance may be disturbed if the deformity is significant. A foot with a congenital plantar-flexed first-ray deformity may have a first ray that appears from a lateral perspective to have increased declination. The first-ray portion of the medial column appears plantarflexed relative to the talus and navicular, particularly if the first ray has forced the midtarsal and subtalar to supinate.

A congenital metatarsus primus elevatus may have a linear or nonlinear medial column lateral appearance with the first ray dorsiflexed relative to the proximal portion of the medial column. Reduced declination angle is also seen, and most importantly, the head of the metatarsal appears further from the supporting surface than is usual. If the head of the metatarsal is not raised farther than usual from the supporting surface, it is difficult to differentiate a hyper-mobile medial column or a pronated foot from metatarsus primus elevatus.

When evaluating first-ray sagittal plane position (plantarflexed, elevatus, or hypermobile), comparing the dorsal cortex of the first and second metatarsals can be helpful. Normally the first- and second-metatarsal dorsal cortexes are parallel. If the first-ray dorsal cortex is angle up or down, you should suspect elevatus or hypermobility and plantarflexed variations from normal, respectively.

The medial oblique view can suggest metatarsal mis-alignment. Using the medial oblique radiograph to assess first-ray sagittal-plane position is fraught with error, and the clinician should put minimal faith in this technique. The reason for the reduced confidence is that the first metatarsal is adducted from the second metatarsal and normally appears slightly splayed from the second metatarsal on the medial oblique view. This can easily be erroneously interpreted as a dorsiflexed first ray, particularly with metatarsus primus adductus present.

It is often difficult to assess first-metatarsal declination after a proximal first-metatarsal osteotomy. An alternative to the longitudinal bisection of the first metatarsal is to use the angle made by the dorsal or plantar surface of the first- and second-metatarsal diaphyses to assess relative preoperative and postoperative change.[98]

## First-Metatarsophalangeal Joint

### Stages of Hallux Limitus. 
A normal first-metatarso-phalangeal joint has a round joint curvature with the dorsal surface of the first metatarsal sloping posteriorly, and the longitudinal bisections of the first metatarsal and proximal phalanx should intersect in the middle of the first-metatarsal head (Figure 14-8). First-metatarsophalangeal joint deformities of hallux valgus and hallux limitus each

begin with functional limitation of dorsiflexion and may result in combined deformity.

The first radiographic sign of functional limitation of dorsiflexion is a plantar shift of the proximal phalanx relative to the first-metatarsal head. This is observed by the longitudinal bisection of the proximal phalanx intersecting the longitudinal bisection of the first metatarsal in the plantar half of the metatarsal head and anterior to its center point.[56] This is classified as stage I hallux limitus, functional hallux limitus, and does not demonstrate any signs of joint degeneration.

Stage II hallux limitus is the beginning of structural restriction of first-metatarsal dorsiflexion, and signs of joint degeneration can be observed. Radiographic signs consistent with stage II hallux limitus are hyperextension of the hallux interphalangeal joint, and hypertrophy of the dorsal surface of the first-metatarsal head. The interphalangeal hyperextension is caused by forceful subluxation of this joint in propulsion by the ground reactive forces that should be dorsiflexing the first-metatarsophalangeal joint. When the first-metatarsophalangeal joint does not dorsiflex, the dorsiflexion force eventually forces the interphalangeal joint to dorsiflex (hyperextend).

Hypertrophy of the dorsal surface of the first-metatarsal head and subchondral sclerosis are signs of joint degeneration as the result of the dorsal surface of the proximal phalanx focally compressing and eventually eroding the dorsal articular surface. This is caused by a plantar shift of the proximal phalanx creating a noncongruent joint surface accompanied by dorsiflexory ground reactive forces attempting to dorsiflex the joint, plantar fascia restricting the joint's dorsiflexory range of motion, and the dorsiflexory force excessively compressing the dorsal portion of the joint. In severe cases the dorsal proximal aspect of the proximal phalanx also has signs of joint degeneration.

When first-metatarsophalangeal joint dorsiflexion needs to be assessed radiographically to determine if hypertrophy of the dorsal surface of the first metatarsal is obstructing motion, the lateral-stress view can be helpful. Caution must be applied when interpreting a lateral stress view. When the lateral-stress radiograph is made, the first ray may have plantarflexed more than it does when walking. Increased dorsiflexion made available by plantarflexion of the first ray while taking the radiograph may not occur when walking. Thus increased dorsiflexion motion may be viewed in the lateral-stress view, which is not available in gait because of first-ray hypermobility.

The end stage of hallux limitus is hallux rigidus. The stage III deformity shows a dramatic loss of first-metatarsophalangeal joint dorsiflexion from joint degeneration. Radiographically the first-metatarsophalangeal joint space may appear absent, and the joint margins show hypertrophy.

## Hallux

The hallux in the lateral view should parallel the supporting surface, the proximal and distal phalanx should make a straight column, and the longitudinal axis of the proximal phalanx should pass proximally through the center of the head of the first metatarsal (see Figure 14-8). Interphalangeal joint hyperextension, plantarflexed proximal phalanx from its horizontal position and plantar translation of the proximal phalanx with its bisection passing below the first-metatarsal head center, are all signs of functional hallux limitus and rigidus.

None of the signs of functional hallux limitus may be present in the lateral view, particularly in less severe instances, because the first-metatarsophalangeal joint is not stressed as much in relaxed stance as during propulsion. The clinician needs to correlate the clinical signs of plantar hallux hyperkeratosis, late midstance and early propulsion pronation, radiographic signs of medial-column fault, and dorsal first-metatarsal cuneiform dorsal exostosis to the radiographic signs of functional hallux limitus.

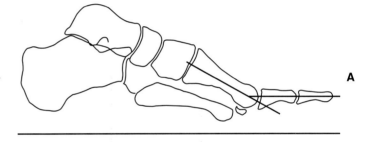

A

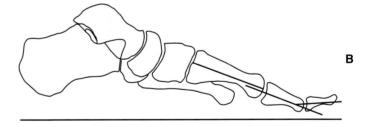

B

Figure 14-8   Normal first-metatarsophalangeal joint alignment and functional hallux limitus. **A,** Normal sagittal-plane first-ray alignment with the proximal phalanx longitudinal axis approximately bisecting the first-metatarsal head and paralleling the supporting surface. **B,** Common radiographic signs that are associated with functional hallux limitus and hallux rigidus: plantarly translated and plantarflexed proximal phalanx; hyperextended hallux interphalangeal joint; the proximal phalanx longitudinal axis passes through the plantar portion of the first-metatarsal head and does not intersect the first-metatarsal longitudinal axis in the center of the metatarsal head; and in advanced stages, hypertrophy of the dorsum of the first-metatarsal head. This illustration shows a medial column fault, which is the equivalent of a dorsiflexed (hyperextended) medial column. The dorsiflexed medial column is unlikely to plantarflex in a timely fashion during gait, and thus results in restriction of first-metatarsophalangeal joint dorsiflexion.

## Digital Contractures

In the normal foot, the lateral view demonstrates the digits to be linear and parallel to the supporting surface, with the longitudinal bisections passing through the center of their respective metatarsal heads. Radiographs document the level of deformity and provide information as to the dorsal or plantar prominence of those digits that have metatarsophalangeal joint contracture. Of course, the radiographs must be correlated to the weight-bearing digital exam to determine the reducibility of each level of the deformity.

A mallet toe is a plantarflexion deformity of the distal interphalangeal joint. Mallet toes frequently develop after shortening or amputation of an adjacent ray. Pain or ulceration develop on the distal end of the toe because of the contusion created by the repeated microtrauma associated with weight bearing on the distal toe surface instead of on the well-cushioned plantar pad.

Claw toe consists of flexion contractures at the interphalangeal joints of the digit, and most characteristically, extension deformity at the metatarsophalangeal joint. Claw toe deformity is frequently associated with pes cavus and extensor substitution as the extensors attempt to dorsiflex the foot against equinus, either forefoot (pseudoequinus), or ankle. Having the proximal phalanx on top of the respective metatarsal creates a retrograde force on the metatarsal that may result in overload of the metatarsal, and commonly the head of the proximal phalanx rubs dorsally in shoes.

Hammer toe deformity has proximal interphalangeal joint flexion contracture and frequently has either distal interphalangeal joint hyperextension or flexion deformity. Flexor stabilization is usually the etiology as the overactive flexors attempt to reduce pronation of the foot. Also, flexor substitution can lead to hammer toes as the deep posterior muscles assist weak triceps surae with ankle plantarflexion.

## ■ RADIOGRAPHIC ANALYSIS USING OTHER VIEWS

### Lateral-Stress View of the Ankle

The lateral-stress view of the foot and ankle is used to determine if the dorsal surface of the neck of the talus is obstructing the anterior movement of the tibia as the ankle is dorsiflexed. As described, the standard lateral view and stress lateral views are compared to determine the amount of ankle dorsiflexion available. The amount is determined not just by the tibia touching the talar neck but also by the range of motion available before contact. At least 10 degrees should be available.

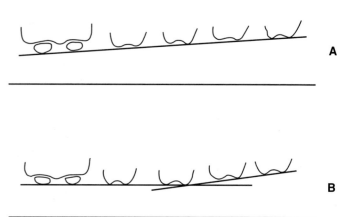

Figure 14-9    Sesamoid axial view. **A,** Normal plantar metatarsal relationship with all the metatarsals on the same plane. **B,** Abnormal plantar metatarsal relationship with metatarsals creating two planes. Excessive weight bearing is most likely to occur at the intersection of the two planes, the third metatarsal.

## Sesamoid Axial View

The sesamoid axial view provides the clinician with information regarding the planar relationships of the plantar surfaces of the metatarsals during early propulsion.[99]

A normal foot has the plantar surface of the metatarsals in the same plane (Figure 14-9). This is evaluated by placing a mark on the most plantar aspect of each metatarsal. The marks are connected and straight lines drawn from each mark to the adjacent mark. In a normal foot with metatarsal lengths that have a semilogarithmic relationship as described by Robbins,[64] the marks make a straight line. This does not mean that the plantar plane of the metatarsals must be parallel to the supporting surface, merely a straight line. A foot that has a metatarsal bearing more weight as the result of an abnormal metatarsal length pattern has the marks make two lines and intersect plantar to the overloaded metatarsal. The overloaded metatarsal may be long, or the adjacent metatarsal may be too short. The sesamoid axial view must be correlated to the dorsoplantar view and clinical exam in order to develop a three-dimensional representation of the relative metatarsal position.

The sesamoid axial view has been erroneously used to evaluate relative metatarsal height instead of length. The sesamoid axial view does not represent the metatarsals in midstance and thus should not be used to evaluate relative metatarsal height. Instead, metatarsal protrusion is evaluated.

Lesion markers at sites that show signs of excessive weight bearing can be helpful in locating the involved metatarsal. This should be correlated to the dorsoplantar view.

Identification of enlarged or sharp plantar metatarsal condyles is possible if the condyle is of adequate size and/or positioned far enough anteriorly to be viewed. It must be remembered that the clinician is not viewing the plantar metatarsal surface but rather the distal plantar surface of the metatarsal.

And of course, the sesamoid axial view provides information about the sesamoids and plantar surface of the first metatarsal. Normally the sesamoids rest in grooves on either side of the first-metatarsal crista. As metatarsus primus adductus increases, the stationary sesamoids assume a position lateral to their normal position plantar to the first metatarsal. The tibial sesamoid frequently erodes the crista, and the fibular sesamoid may articulate with the lateral side of the first metatarsal or in the first metatarsal interspace. Between the inversion associated with first ray dorsiflexion and the eversion associated with foot pronation, either sesamoid may be plantar positioned relative to the other and bear excessive weight.

Sesamoiditis may be extra-articular in the form of contusion from the repeated microtrauma associated with excessive focal pressure associated with abnormal position or irregular sesamoid surface. Intra-articular sesamoiditis is caused by erosion of the plantar surface of the first metatarsal by the sesamoid. The sesamoid axial view usually cannot provide the diagnosis of intra-articular or extra-articular sesamoiditis but must be correlated to the physical exam and to whether or not intra-articular anesthesia relieves the pain. Bipartite sesamoids have been found to have an increased incidence of sesamoiditis, both intra-articular and extra-articular.

Landsman and associates[47] used the sesamoid axial view and direct observation of the sesamoid articulation with the first metatarsal to correlate sesamoid position. They found that in sesamoid positions 3 and higher there generally were erosive changes observed on the first metatarsal plantar articular surface. When they compared the standard dorsoplantar sesamoid position, which uses the longitudinal axis of the first metatarsal as reference for the sesamoid position, to the sesamoid axial view, which uses the bisection of the crista as reference, it was determined that on average the sesamoids are actually two positions higher on the sesamoid axial view as opposed to the dorsoplantar view.

## Anterior Axial Projection of the Foot

The anterior axial projection of the foot was developed by Kirby and associates[4] as a modification of Cobey's[100] posterior view. The anterior axial view (Figure 14-10) provides the clinician with an anterior view of the ankle and the plantar surface of the calcaneus. Kirby and associates placed the center of the heel and the second metatarsal on a line perpendicular to the film sitting behind the ankle. The foot is on a raised radiopaque device, and the central beam is angled 10 degrees from plantar to dorsal. Because the central beam is inclined slightly, what is visualized is actually the calcaneal surface immediately posterior to the actual plantar weight-bearing surface.

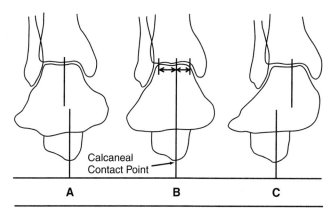

Calcaneal
Contact Point

**A**          **B**          **C**

Figure 14-10    Anterior axial projection. **A,** Calcaneal contact point medial to the middle of the ankle mortise creates a supinatory moment at the subtalar joint. **B,** Normal alignment finds the calcaneal contact point approximately centered under the middle of the ankle mortise. **C,** Calcaneal contact point lateral to the middle of the ankle mortise creates a pronatory moment at the subtalar joint.

The most plantar portion of the calcaneus is the calcaneal balance point and is always on the medial calcaneal tubercle, because the lateral calcaneal tubercle is always superior to the medial tubercle and bears insignificant weight in relaxed stance. The rearfoot ground reactive forces enter the foot at the calcaneal balance point, and it is helpful to be able to determine if the calcaneal balance point is centered, medial, or lateral relative to the center of the ankle mortise. The subtalar axis passes roughly inferior to the center of the ankle mortise. When the calcaneal balance point is lateral to the center of the ankle (and the subtalar axis), a valgus/eversion moment is experienced by the rearfoot. A medially oriented calcaneal balance point provides an inversion moment and may result in lateral ankle instability as the result of excessive subtalar supination. Based on the orientation described by Kirby and associates, the position of the calcaneus is rotated medially or laterally as the forefoot is abducted or adducted, respectively. Nevertheless, the normal orientation based on this method is to have the calcaneal balance point slightly medial of the center of the ankle. It has generally been accepted that the calcaneus should sit slightly lateral of the center of the ankle for stability and thus varies slightly from the conclusion based on Kirby and associates' positioning method.[15,101]

As the rearfoot supinates, the calcaneal balance point moves medially relative to the resting position and moves laterally with pronation.

The position of the calcaneal balance point relative to the ankle can also be approximated during the physical exam by measuring the lateral malleolar index (horizontal distance from the lateral border of the lateral calcaneal fat pad to the lateral aspect of the lateral malleolus) or by approximating the center of the ankle relative to the center of the posterior plantar portion of the heel. When the lateral malleolar index equals zero, the lateral malleolus lateral border is approximately directly superior to the lateral border of the heel fat pad, and the anterior axial projection has the calcaneal contact point approximately centered under the ankle. It also holds true that when the calcaneal balance point is too far medial on the anterior axial projection, there is usually lateral ankle instability and the heel fat pad lateral border will be medial to the lateral malleolus.

The anterior axial view of the foot can be helpful when performing calcaneal osteotomies that move the posterior portion of the calcaneus medially or laterally, such as described by Dwyer.[102] It has been erroneously accepted that such calcaneal osteotomies invert or evert the calcaneus. Instead they merely change the alignment of the posterior calcaneus and calcaneal balance point relative to the ankle and subtalar joint axis, and create the illusion of the calcaneus having been inverted or everted. If the posterior calcaneus has had any inverting or everting, it is only because of the change in position of the calcaneal balance point relative to the subtalar joint axis and thus has altered the influence of ground reactive forces at the subtalar.

## Limb Length Inequality

It is well accepted that weight-bearing foot pronation and supination lower and raise the height of the medial longitudinal arch respectively. The raising and lowering of the arch also raises and lowers the height of the ankle, and thus alters the functional length of the leg.[103] Thus asymmetric foot position may contribute to or compensate for limb length inequalities.

Foot contribution to limb length is evaluated by creating a weight-bearing mortise, lateral, or anteroposterior radiograph of the ankle with the central beam at ankle level and parallel to the supporting surface. Behind the ankle a radiopaque etched ruler is placed so that it is superimposed on the film. The left and right talar dorsotrochlear surface heights are compared (Figure 14-11). Changing foot position with a foot orthosis or surgery can alter the relative lengths of the legs.

Signs of specific foot morphology—never a pure representation (always combinations)—ff varus,[96] ff valgus,[96] equinus, STJ, everted/inverted calcaneus, transverse plane deformity.

## ◼ CORRELATION OF FOOT RADIOGRAPHIC SIGNS TO FOOT MORPHOLOGY

Some foot morphologic (biomechanic) relationships have definite radiographic correlation. The trouble with assuming that a particular morphologic relationship always results in a

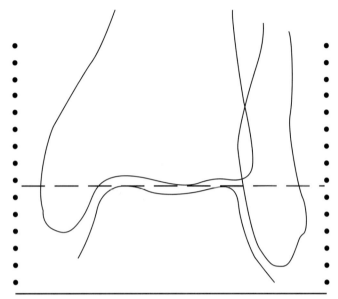

**Figure 14-11**    Ankle height changes with foot position and may contribute to limb length inequality if the feet are asymmetric.

specific radiographic sign is that the foot frequently has several morphologic relationships influencing foot morphology. Thus foot morphology is the net result of the force created by several morphologic characteristics.

Several examples can be given of morphologic relationships influencing radiographic representaions. Forefoot varus is usually identified when naviculocuboid superimposition on the lateral radiograph considerably increases. This is caused by the lowering of the medial column of the foot as it moves plantarly to make contact with the weight-bearing surface. Also associated with forefoot varus are low calcaneal inclination angle, and reduced superimposition of the metatarsal bases. Functional equinus has the same radiographic signs as forefoot varus except that the trabecular pattern in the cuboid is more vertically oriented than seen when forefoot varus is the primary influence on foot morphology.

Forefoot valgus is generally associated with reduced naviculocuboid superimposition as the retrograde supinatory force created by the plantar plane of the metatarsals supinates the midtarsal joint. The condition also shows increased superimposition of the metatarsal bases.

A foot with significant forefoot valgus and functional equinus develops a morphology dependent on the net resultant force influencing the midtarsal joint. The naviculocuboid superimposition may be increased, decreased, or normal depending on the net influence.

Another example is the cavovarus foot morphology. The forefoot varus does not create increased naviculocuboid superimposition, because the rearfoot raises the medial column far from the supporting surface. The net result is a lateral view with the increased calcaneal inclination angle contributed by the forefoot varus, and the medial column appears elevated far from the supporting surface because of the uncompensated forefoot varus.

An increase in the dorsoplantar talocalcaneal angle is associated with transverse-plane deformity in the lower extremity. Any lower-extremity transverse-plane deformity may result in an increase in the talocalcaneal angle. Location of the level of the transverse-plane deformity is accomplished with a thorough range of motion and morphologic exam (biomechanical exam).

Subtalar and midtarsal joint position may be classified based on radiographic signs and alignment. When evaluating these joints, consider their position in the sagittal and transverse planes. It should not be assumed that the subtalar and midtarsal joints are in the same position.

As the subtalar joint is evaluated in a spectrum of feet from the underpronated to the overpronated alignment, the lateral and dorsoplantar talocalcaneal angles increase, reduced superimposition of the talus on the calcaneus, the lateral calcaneal tubercle moves further from the supporting surface, the sustentaculum tali becomes less clear in its outline, the sinus tarsi reduces and the pseudo–sinus tarsi

appears, and the talus appears foreshortened on the lateral radiograph. As the midtarsal joint is evaluated in a spectrum of feet from the underpronated to the overpronated alignment, naviculocuboid superimposition is reduced on the lateral and dorsoplantar views, and on the lateral view, reduced metatarsal base superimposition. In some feet the subtalar joint can be overpronated with the midtarsal underpronated. An example is a forefoot valgus reducing the midtarsal pronated position and low malleolar torsion creating a very pronated subtalar joint alignment.

Foot alignment is the net result of forces created by several morphologic variables. Although tendencies appear, so do exceptions, because any one morphologic influence can be altered by another significant morphologic influence.

## ■ ACKNOWLEDGMENTS

Much of the information presented in this chapter that is not referenced to other authors was taught me by John Weed, D.P.M. Without Dr. Weed's tutelage this chapter would not have been possible. If only I had taken the opportunity to thank him.

## References

1. Sgarlato TE et al: *A compendium of podiatric biomechanics*, San Francisco, 1971, California College of Podiatric Medicine.
2. Gamble FO, Yale I: *Clinical foot roentgenology*, ed 2, Huntington, NY, 1975, Krieger Publishing.
3. Weissman S: Standard radiographic techniques of the foot and ankle, *Clin Podiatr Med Surg* 5(4):767-775.
4. Kirby KA, Loendorf AJ, Gregorio R: Anterior axial projection of the foot, *J Am Podiatr Assoc* 78(4):159-170, 1988.
5. Hlavac HF: Differences in x-ray findings with varied positioning of the foot, *J Am Podiatr Assoc* 10:465, 1965.
6. LaPorta GA, Scarlet J: Radiographic changes in the pronated and supinated foot, a statistical analysis, *J Am Podiatr Assoc* 76(5):334-338, 1977.
7. Weissman SD: *Radiology of the foot*, Baltimore, 1989, Williams & Wilkins.
8. Whitney AK: *Radiographic charting technic*, Philadelphia, 1978, Pennsylvania College of Podiatric Medicine.
9. Solomon MG: Roentgenographic biomechanical evaluation of the foot, pp 21-22, Cleveland, 1973, Jonathan Douglass.
10. Ganley JV: Theory of the two unit tarsus, Wednesday Evening Seminar series, Philadelphia, 1984 (seminar presentation), *Pennsylvania College of Podiatric Medicine*.
11. Engle E et al: A simplified metatarsus adductus angle,

*J Am Podiatr Assoc* 73:620-627, 1983.
12. Kite JH: *The clubfoot*, New York, 1964, Grune & Stratton.
13. Harris RI, Beath I: Hypermobile flatfoot with short tendoachilles, *J Bone Joint Surg* 30A:116, 1948.
14. Rowland RA, Ferris TL, Dobas DC: A study of the metatarsal break, *J Am Podiatr Assoc* 69(1):47-51, 1979.
15. Root ML, Orien WP, Weed JH: *Normal and abnormal function of the foot*, Los Angeles, 1977, Clinical Biomechanics Corporation.
16. Sanner WH: Midtarsal joint contribution to transverse plane leg rotation. In Pratt DJ, Johnson GR, editors: *The biomechanics & orthotic management of the foot*, vol 1, Darby, Engl, 1987, Biological Engineering Society.
17. Ganley JV: Calcaneo valgus deformity in infants, *J Am Podiatr Assoc* 5:405-421, 1975.
18. Evans D: Calcaneovalgus deformity, *J Bone Joint Surg* 57B:270-278, 1975.
19. Kellikan H: *Hallux valgus: allied deformities of the forefoot and metatarsalgia*, Philadelphia, 1965, Saunders.
20. Kirby KA: Methods for determination of positional variations of the axis of the subtalar joint, *J Am Podiatr Med Assoc* 77:228, 1987.
21. LaPorta G, Melillo T, Olinsky D: X-ray evaluation of hallux abducto valgus deformity, *J Am Podiatr Assoc* 64:544-566, 1974.

22. Shaw AH, Pack LG: Osteomies of the first ray for hallux abducto valgus deformity, *J Am Podiatr Assoc* 64(8):567-580, 1974.

23. Haas M: Radiographic and biomechanical considerations of bunion surgery. In Gerbert J, Sokoloff TH, editors: *Textbook of bunion surgery*, pp 23-62, Mt. Kisco, N.Y., 1981, Futura.

24. Amarnek DL, Mollica S, Jacobs AM, Oloff LM: A Statistical analysis on the reliability of the proximal articular set ankle, *JFS* 25(1):39-43, 1986.

25. Shechter DZ, Doll PJ: Tangential angle to the second axis: a new angle with implications for bunion surgery, *J Am Podiatr Med Assoc* 75(10):505-512, 1985.

26. Gerbert J, Sokoloff TH, editors: *Textbook of bunion surgery*, pp 23-62, Mt. Kisco, N.Y., 1981, Futura.

27. Balding, MG, Sorto LA: Distal articular set angle: etiology and x-ray evaluation, *J Am Podiatr Med Assoc* 75(12):648-652, 1985.

28. Christman RA: Radiographic evaluation of the distal articular set angle, *J Am Podiatr Med Assoc* 78(7):352-354, 1988.

29. Gohil P, Cavolo DJ: A simplified preoperative evaluation of Akin osteotomy, *J Am Podiatr Assoc* 72(1):44-45, 1982.

30. Piggott H: The natural history of hallux valgus in adolescence and early adult life, *J Bone Joint Surg* 42B:749, 1960.

31. Jaworek TE: The histological patterns in functional bony adaptation as applied to congruous and subluxed joints, *J Am Podiatr Assoc* 65(10):953-962, 1975.

32. Miller F, Arenson D, Weil LS: Incongruity of the first metatarsophalangeal joint: the effect on cartilage contact surface area, *J Am Podiatr Med Assoc* 67(5):328-333, 1977.

33. Mann RA, Coughlin MJ: Hallux valgus: etiology, anatomy, treatment and surgical considerations, *Clin Orthop* 157:31, 1981.

34. Du Vries HL: *Surgery of the foot*, p 365, St. Louis, 1957, Mosby.

35. Brahm SM: Shape of the first metatarsal head in hallux rigidus and hallux valgus, *J Am Podiatr Assoc* 78(6):301, 1988.

36. McCrea JD, Clark WD, Fann T, Venson J, Jones CL: Effects of radiographic technique on the metatarsophalangeal joints, *J Am Podiatr Med Assoc* 67(12):837-840, 1977.

37. Greenberg GS: Relationship of hallux abductus angle and metatarsal angle to severity of pronation, *J Am Podiatr Assoc* 69(1):29-34, 1979.

38. Fenton CF, McGlamery ED: Reverse buckling to reduce metatarsus primus varus: a preliminary investigation, *J Am Podiatr Med Assoc* 72(7):342-346, 1983.

39. Robbins HM: The unified forefoot. II. The relationship between hallux valgus and metatarsus primus adductus, *J Foot Surg* 22(4):320-324, 1983.

40. Griffiths TA, Palladino SJ: Metatarsus adductus and selected radiographic measurements of the first ray in normal feet, *J Am Podiatr Med Assoc* 82(12):616-622, 1992.

41. McCrea JD, Lichty TK: The first metatarsocuneiform articulation and its relationship to metatarsus primus adductus, *J Am Podiatr Med Assoc* 69(12):700-706, 1979.

42. Haines R, McDougall A: The anatomy of hallux valgus, *J Bone Joint Surg* 36B:2, 1954.

43. Ewald P: Die aetiologie des hallux valgus, *Dtsch Ztschr Chir* 114:90, 1912.

44. Berntsen J: De l'hallux valgus contribution a son etiologie et a son traitment, *Rev Orthop* (series 3e) 17:101, 1930.

45. Pressman MM, Rice AH: Correction of hallux valgus: tendoligamentous sling procedure. In Jay RM, editor: *Current Therapy in Podiatric Surgery*, pp 181-187, Philadelphia, 1989, Decker.

46. Deleted in proofs.

47. Landsman AS, Hanft JR, Levy A, Mason T, Kashuk KB: A comprehensive study of the correlation between radiographic and surgical sesamoid positions, American College of Foot and Ankle Surgeons, 51st Annual Meeting and Scientific Seminar, San Diego, Feb 1993.

48. Duke H, Newman LM, Bruskoff BL, Daniels R: Relative metatarsal length patterns in hallux abducto valgus, *J Am Podiatr Assoc* 72(1):1-5, 1982.

49. Zlotoff H: Shortening of the first metatarsal following osteotomy and its clinical significance, *J Am Podiatr Assoc* 67(6):412-426, 1977.

50. Heden RI, Sorto LA: The buckle point and the metatarsal protrusion's relationship to hallux valgus, *J Am Podiatr Assoc* 71(4):200-208, 1981.

51. Bonney G, Macnab I: Hallux valgus and hallux rigidus, *J Bone Joint Surg* 34B:366, 1952.

52. Schweitzer DA, Lew H, Shiken J, Morgan J: Central metatarsal shortening following osteotomy and its clinical significance, *J Am Podiatr Assoc* 72(1):6-10, 1982.

53. Morton D: Structural factors in static disorders of the foot, *Am J Surg* 9:315, 1930.

54. Kravitz SR, Fink K, Huber S, Bohanske L, Cicilioni S: Osseous changes in the second ray of classical ballet dancers, *J Am Podiatr Med Assoc* 75(7):346-348, 1985.

55. Hardy RH, Clapman JCR: Observations of hallux valgus, *J Bone Joint Surg* 33B:366, 1951.

56. Rzonca E, Levitz S, Lue B: Hallux equinus: the stages of hallux limitus and hallux rigidus, *J Am Podiatr Assoc* 74(8):390-393, 1984.

57. Sorto LA, Balding MG, Weil LS, Smith SD: Hallux abductus interphalangeus: etiology, x-ray evaluation and treatment, *J Am Podiatr Assoc* 66(6):384, 1976.

58. Barnett CH: Valgus deviation of the distal phalanx of the great toe, *J Anat* 96:171, 1962.

59. Weissman, Donnelley 1979.

60. Bojsen-Møeller F: Calcaneocuboid joint and stability of the longitudinal arch of the foot at high and low gear push off, *J Anat* 128:165-176, 1979.

61. Nuber GW: Biomechanics of the foot and ankle during gait, *Clin Podiatr Med Surg* 6(3):615-627, 1989.

62. Gamble FO: *Applied foot roentgenology*, Baltimore, 1957, Williams & Wilkins.

62a. Gamble FO, Yale I: *Clinical foot roentgenology: an illustrated hand book*, Baltimore, 1966, Williams & Wilkins.

63. Demp PH: A mathematical model for the study of metatarsal length patterns, *J Am Podiatr Assoc* 54:107, 1964.

64. Robbins, HM: The unified forefoot: a mathematical model in the transverse plane, *J Am Podiatr Assoc* 71(9):465-471, 1981.

65. Valley BA, Reese HW: Guidelines for reconstructing the metatarsal parabola with the shortening osteotomy, *J Am Podiatr Med Assoc* 81(8):406-413, 1991.

66. Fallat LM, Buckholtz J: An analysis of the tailor's bunion by radiographic and anatomical display, *J Am Podiatr Assoc* 70(12):597-603, 1980.

67. Lemont H, Travisano VL, Lyman J: Accessory navicular: appearance of a synovial joint, *J Am Podiatr Assoc* 78(8):423, 1981.

68. Vogler HW: Biomechanics of talipes equinovalgus, *J Am Podiatr Med Assoc* 77(1):21, 1987.

69. Sarafian SK: *Anatomy of the foot and ankle: description, topographical, function*, Philadelphia, 1983, Lippincott.

70. Altman MI: Sagittal plane angles of the talus and calcaneus in the developing foot, *J Am Podiatr Assoc* 58:11, 1968.

71. Pressman MM: Biomechanics and surgical criteria for flexible pes valgus, *J Am Podiatr Assoc* 77(1):7-13, 1987.

72. Whitney AK, Green DR: Pseudoequinus, *J Am Podiatr Assoc* 72(7):365-371, 1982.

73. DiGiovanni J, Smith S: Normal biomechanics of the adult rearfoot, a radiographic analysis, *J Am Podiatr Assoc* 58:11, 1968.

74. Jacoby M: More than you ever wanted to know about physics and whither biomechanics? *J Am Podiatr Assoc* 65(7):689-707, 1975.

75. Haglund, P: Beitrag zur Klinik der Achillessehne, *Z Orthop Chir* 49:49, 1928.

76. Yale I: *Podiatric medicine*, p 224, Baltimore, 1974, Williams & Wilkins.

77. Berlin D, Coleman W, Nickamin A: Surgical approaches to Haglund's disease, *JFS* 21(1):42-44, 1982.

78. Ruch JA: Haglund's disease, *J Am Podiatr Assoc* 64(12):1000-1015, 1974.

79. Vega MR, Cavolo DJ, Green R, Cohen SC: Haglund's deformity, *J Am Podiatr Assoc* 74(3):129-135, 1984.

80. Le TA, Joseph PM: Common exostectomies of the rearfoot. *Clin Podiatr Med Surg* 8(3):601-623, 1991.

81. Fowler A, Phillip JF: Abnormality of the calcaneus as a cause of painful heel, *Br J Surg* 32:494, 1945.

82. Notari MA, Mittler BE: An investigation of Fowler-Phillip's angle in diagnosing Haglund's deformity, *J Am Podiatr Assoc* 74(10):486-489, 1984.

83. Pavlov H, Heneghan MA, Hersh A et al: Haglund syndrome: initial and differential diagnosis, *Radiology* 144:83, 1982.

84. Fiamengo SA, Warren RF, Marchal JL et al: Posterior heel pain associated with a calcaneal step and Achilles tendon calcification, *Clin Orthop* 167:203, 1982.

85. Scherer PR: Heel spur syndrome. Pathomechanics and nonsurgical treatment. Biomechanics Graduate Research Group for 1988, *J Am Podiatr Med Assoc* 81(2):68-72, 1991.

86. Forman WM, Green MA: The role of the intrinsic musculature in the formation of inferior calcaneal exostoses, *Clin Podiatr Med Surg*, 7(2):217-223, 1990.

87. McCarthy DJ, Gorecki GE: The anatomical basis of inferior calcaneal lesions, *J Am Podiatr Assoc* 69:527, 1979.

88. Shama SS, Kominsky SJ, Lemont H: Prevalence of non-painful heel spur and its relation to postural foot position, *J Am Podiatr Assoc* 73(3):122-123, 1983.

89. Boehler L: Diagnosis, pathology, and treatment of fractures of the os calcis, *J Bone Joint Surg* 13:75-89, 1931.

90. Hauser ML: Boehler's angle, a review and a study, *J Am Podiatr Assoc* 65(6):517-521, 1975.

91. Whitney AK, Green DR: Pseudoequinus, *J Am Podiatr Med Assoc* 72(7):365, 1982.

92. Berkey SF, Clark B: Tarsal coalition, case report and review of literature, *J Am Podiatr Assoc* 74(1):31-37, 1984.

93. Stoller MI: Tarsal coalitions—a study of surgical results, *J Am Podiatr Assoc* 64(12):1004, 1974.

94. Demp PH: A mathematical taxonomy to evaluate the biomechanical quality of the human foot, *Int J Math Comput Modeling* 12(7):777-790, 1989.

95. Dananberg HJ: Functional hallux limitus and its relationship to gait efficiency, *J Am Podiatr Med Assoc* 76(11):648-652, 1986.

96. Grumbine NA: The varus components of the forefoot in flatfoot deformities, *J Am Podiatr Med Assoc* 77(1):14-20, 1987.

97. Kirby KA: Methods for determination of positional variations of the axis of the subtalar joint, *J Am Podiatr Med Assoc* 77:228, 1987.

98. Schuberth JM, Reilly CH, Gudas CJ: The closing wedge osteotomy, a critical analysis of first metatarsal elevation, *J Am Podiatr Assoc* 74(1):13-24, 1984.

99. Crystal L, Orminski D: Axial views and angle and base of

gait, review of a new technique, *J Am Podiatr Assoc* 71(6):31-32, 1981.

100. Coby JC: Posterior roentgenogram of the foot, *Clin Orthop* 118:202, 1976.

101. Sanner WH: The functional foot orthosis prescription, *Curr Ther Podiatr Surg* 302, 1989.

102. Dwyer FC: Osteotomy of the calcaneum in the treatment of grossly everted feet with special reference to cerebral palsy. In *Hiutieme Congres International de Chirurgie Orthopedique*, p 892, New York, Bruxelles, 1960, Imprimerie Liebens.

103. Sanner WH, Page JC, Talboe HR, Blake R, Bax CA: A study of ankle joint height changes with subtalar motion, *J Am Podiatr Assoc* 71(3):158-161, 1981.

# CHAPTER 15

# Pediatric Abnormalities of Position

PHILIP J. BRESNAHAN

Radiography is a valuable tool for evaluating the pediatric patient. The musculoskeletal nature of the foot and ankle lends itself very well to evaluation with radiographs. Many clinical conditions can be easily visualized with radiographs. However, radiographs often tend to be underused in the pediatric patient. This underuse may be prompted by strong concern over the greater sensitivity of the pediatric patient to ionizing radiation. In addition, the radiation exposure a person receives from x rays has a cumulative effect over a lifetime. Therefore the more exposures one receives, the greater is the potential risk of future pathology. However, with high-speed x-ray film/screen combinations currently available for skeletal radiography radiation exposure is very low for foot and ankle studies. Thus the risk in failing to diagnose a condition in a child is greater than is the radiation exposure.

Also, some practitioners believe that because many bones of the child's foot and ankle have not fully ossified, a radiograph may not provide useful information. However, the relationships among the bones of the foot are well established and can be identified by using the visible ossified portions of the bones. Radiographs can easily detect abnormalities early in the child's development.

Radiographs can also be used to monitor and document the progress of a patient's condition. Clinical signs of improvement or lack of change in the severity of the deformity determine the frequency with which radiographs should be performed in children.

To determine what constitutes a radiograph of an abnormality, we must first review what we would normally expect to see in the radiograph of a normal pediatric patient (see Chapter 9). Although many bones in the newborn and infant are in a preossification state at first, they do exist in their cartilaginous form. What appears as a blank space on a radiograph is less dense cartilaginous tissue. It is also generally in its adult shape and form, however, just in its cartilaginous nature, which is more radiolucent.

Radiographs in children are valuable for assessing orthopedic, biomechanical, and congenital abnormalities. Analysis of the osseous axes and associated angles is also valuable for determining the pathology present. The normal angular values and their applications to deformities are discussed later in this chapter.

When possible, weight-bearing (standing) foot and ankle radiographs are preferred for the pediatric patient. The weight-bearing study reveals the functional anatomic relationship of the bones under the influence of body weight. This relationship frequently is the primary cause of the deformity. Weight-bearing views are also the best method for reproducibility.[1,2] Weight-bearing views are not possible in infants, because obviously they are unable to stand erect.

Some references relate to a change in some of these angles from birth to approximately 6 years of age.[3,4] After this age, most sources state, these angles remain relatively unchanged through adulthood. The researchers feel this change is a direct effect of weight bearing and ambulation as the child grows. Although it is difficult to dispute that this apparent change in the relationship between the bones of the foot is partially caused by weight bearing, I feel more significant factors are creating this effect.

Primarily, I believe it is difficult to determine if these measurements actually represent a true change in the relationship between the bones themselves and to the weight-bearing surface. It is more likely caused by the fact that the points used to draw axes on the radiograph change as the bones ossify and grow from their cartilaginous precursors. In other words, lines drawn on a radiograph in an infant are drawn in a different location on the bones in the same child at 2 or 3 years of age. This is not an accurate method of determining a change in the bony relationships.

For example, Vanderwilde and associates[3] measured and statistically analyzed several angles and axes in children from 6 to 127 months. The dorsoplantar measurements were made using the midline of the long axis of the ossified portion of bone at the time of the study. The lateral views included measurements using a line along the plantar surface of the calcaneus. Although the midline bisection may be more consistent as the bones ossify, the measurements are not consistent at the different ages and should not be used in comparison.

Although Vanderwilde and associates did not draw any conclusions in their article, this result can lead the reader to presume that an infant with an abnormally low calcaneal inclination angle clinically representing a flatfoot deformity will improve with age and the child will have a normal foot in later childhood. This is a dangerous conclusion to reach, because a large number of children may therefore be left untreated at an early age and be left through adulthood with the same deformity they were born with.

## AXES AND ANGULAR RELATIONSHIPS

To properly evaluate a child's radiograph, it is frequently necessary to make an objective analysis of the presence, severity, and progress of the deformity. A radiograph is a verifiable means of evaluating the condition at a particular point in time. In a majority of congenital deformities, we can measure the severity of the condition in a reproducible manner that allows other observers to visualize the deformity. A radiograph also provides objective evidence about the success or lack of progress that clinical treatment is having in regard to the child's condition.

We can measure a number of axial and angular relationships in the child's foot. Axes are the lines that are drawn to determine the angular bony relationships seen on the radiographs. These axes are well described by Whitney.[5] The best way to perform this analysis clinically is to use a clear acetate sheet overlying the x-ray film. The observer can either draw the lines on the acetate, which can be preserved for later measurements, or can purchase rub-off art lines, which are placed on the acetate so that they can be reused.

### Axes: Dorsoplantar View

**Talar Axis.** The talar axis (Figure 15-1) is the bisection of the long axis of the head and neck of the talus in the dorsoplantar view. With talipes equinovarus deformity, the bisection of the body of the talus is used to measure the deviation of the head and neck of the talus relative to the talar body.

**Calcaneal Axis.** The calcaneal axis in the dorsoplantar view (see Figure 15-1) is the bisection of the long axis of the ossified portion of bone.

**First- and Second-Metatarsal Axes.** An axis for the metatarsal is made from a line connecting several midpoints

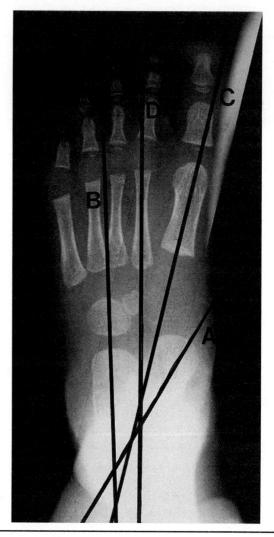

Figure 15-1   Dorsoplantar view of the foot. *A*, Talar axis, *B*, calcaneal axis; *C*, first-metatarsal axis; *D*, second-metatarsal axis. Angles formed between the following two axes form their respective angles: *AB*, talocalcaneal angle; *BD*, metatarsus adductus angle; *AC*, talar–first-metatarsal angle; *CD*, intermetatarsal angle.

along the length of the metatarsal on both radiographic views (see Figure 15-1).

### Axes: Lateral View

**Talar Axis.** The talar axis (Figure 15-2) in the lateral view is measured the same way as in the dorsoplantar view. (In an infant, the axis is drawn through the midline of the ossified portion of visible bone.)

**Calcaneal Axis.** In the lateral view, the calcaneal axis (see Figure 15-2) is a line formed by connecting the two most plantar points at the proximal and distal ends of the calcaneus. (In the infant, this axis is drawn through the midline of the ossified portion of bone.)

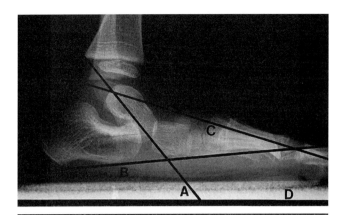

**Figure 15-2**   Lateral view of the foot. *A*, Talar axis, *B*, calcaneal axis, *C*, first-metatarsal axis, *D*, plane of support. Angles formed between the following two axes form their respective angles: *AB*, talocalcaneal angle; *AC*, talar–first-metatarsal angle; *AD*, talar declination angle; *BD*, calcaneal inclination angle.

**First-Metatarsal Axis.**   An axis for the metatarsal is made from a line connecting several midpoints along the length of the metatarsal on both radiographic views (see Figure 15-2).

## Angles: Dorsoplantar (Anteroposterior) View

The dorsoplantar view (see Figure 15-1) is perhaps the most useful foot radiograph in the child. In this view, the observer can examine the anatomy of all the visible foot bones to the greatest extent. It also reveals the attitude and relationship of the foot bones underneath the talus and leg bones in a weight-bearing view. The weight-bearing radiograph gives a "real-time" picture of how the foot bones are functioning under the influence of gravity on the body weight as well as any superimposed structural abnormalities.

**Talocalcaneal Angle.**   The main feature of the dorsoplantar radiograph is the relationship between the talus and the calcaneus. This represents the attitude of the rearfoot and its relationship of the foot to the leg. In the infant, it is measured by the angle formed by the midline bisections of the long axes of the ossified portion of the talus and calcaneus. The normal range for the talocalcaneal angle is 30 to 40 degrees.

The significance of this view includes the transverse-plane relationship of the talus over the calcaneus. The talus itself is locked in the ankle mortise, and it should be generally above the calcaneus. An increase in the talocalcaneal angle indicates the calcaneus and the remainder of the foot has moved out and away (abducted and everted) from underneath the talus in the transverse and frontal body planes. This is seen clinically as a planovalgus (flatfoot or calcaneovalgus) deformity. A decreased

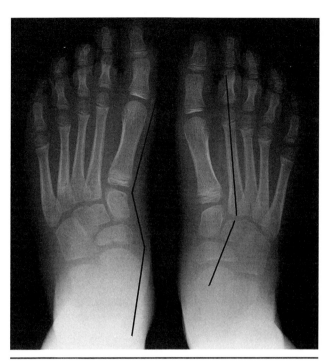

**Figure 15-3**   This is a typical metatarsus adductus deformity in an older child that was not treated earlier in life. Although the outline of the soft tissue of the foot appears generally straight as a whole, the forefoot, midfoot, and rearfoot components take a serpentine (*Z*) alignment (*black lines, left foot*). This alignment is caused by the rearfoot compensating for adduction in the forefoot. The talocalcaneal angle is mildly increased, and the talus and navicular are less articulated. The second-metatarsal and second-cuneiform axes are drawn on the right foot. The angle created by these two axes is Engel's angle.

talocalcaneal angle indicates the calcaneus and remainder of the foot is directly underneath the talus and leg. A clinical example of this is the equinovarus deformity in the child.

**Metatarsus Adductus Angle.**   This angle reveals the relationship between the five metatarsal bones and the midtarsal bones of the foot at Lisfranc's joint. An increase of the angle generally reveals a metatarsus adductus deformity, which is clinically seen as a form of in-toeing, referred to as "pigeon-toed." In infants, this angle is best determined by the angle formed by the lines representing the midline bisections of the long axes of the ossified portions of the calcaneus and the second metatarsal. The normal value for this angle is 10 degrees. The calcaneus is the best rearfoot bone to use for this measurement in infants and young children. It is more closely linked to the metatarsals than is the talus, and most cases show little motion between the bones at these joints.

In older children, the metatarsus adductus angle can be determined by the angle formed by the axes of the second metatarsal and the middle (second) cuneiform bone (see Figure 15-3) as described by Engel and associates.[3] These

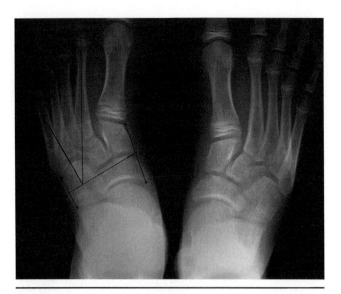

**Figure 15-4**  Metatarsus adductus is still evident in these dorsoplantar views of both feet in a 12-year-old child. Although the metatarsal bones are clearly adducted relative to the midtarsal bones, the foot appears somewhat straight overall because of the compensatory abduction/pronation in the subtalar joint. This gives the clinical appearance of a foot that has "outgrown" its intoeing that was present at birth. The second-metatarsal and lesser-tarsus axes are illustrated in the left foot.

authors consider an angle greater than 24 degrees indicative of metatarsus adductus deformity. Root and Sgarlato described the relationship between the second-metatarsal and the lesser-tarsal bones (Figure 15-4). The normal metatarsus adductus angle with this method is approximately 21 degrees.[3-5] (See Chapter 14 for further discussion of these methods.)

**Talar–First-Metatarsal Angle.**  The talar–first-metatarsal angle is measured using the bisection of the long axes of the ossified portions of the talus and first metatarsal. The talar–first-metatarsal angle reveals the relationship between the forefoot and the rearfoot. Ideally, the talus and first metatarsal should line up with each other. This indicates how the foot lines up with the leg. This alignment helps us determine how our body weight is carried over from the leg to the foot. This is very valuable, because these are the main bones that have ossified sufficiently at birth to evaluate. Simons is credited with the first study and description of this angle.[7] He used it to evaluate the equinovarus deformity. The normal value is minus 20 to 0 degrees.

## Angles: Lateral View

The lateral x-ray view (see Figure 15-2) is best for viewing rearfoot deformities. Again, this view is mainly important for revealing the relationship between the talus and calcaneus. A minimal "overlap" of the bones should be evident in normal feet where the talus rests over the posterior calcaneal facet and the sustentaculum tali. An increase in the "overlap" or "superimposition" of the bones on the lateral view indicates that the talus must have abducted away from underneath the talus, allowing the talar head to plantarflex beside the calcaneus.

**The Talocalcaneal Angle.**  The talocalcaneal angle is determined in infants by the angle formed by the lines representing the bisection of the long axes of the ossified portions of the talus and calcaneus. The normal talocalcaneal angle is 35 to 40 degrees. An increased talocalcaneal angle generally indicates the talus has plantarflexed relative to and alongside the calcaneus as in calcaneovalgus or congenital pes valgus. A decreased angle indicates the talus is "riding" on top of the calcaneus as is seen in equinovarus deformity.

**Talar–First-Metatarsal Angle.**  The lateral view also reveals the relationship between the first metatarsal and the talus. The long axis of the talus should pass through the long axis of the metatarsal. The talar and first-metatarsal axes should therefore overlap or coincide. This angle reveals the sagittal-plane relationship of the forefoot and the rearfoot. When the talar axis is below the first-metatarsal axis, the talus must be in a plantarflexed position clinically. That means that the talus is not directly over the calcaneus in its normal position. The calcaneus has moved out away from underneath the talus. This indicates a flatfoot deformity.

**Calcaneal Inclination Angle.**  The lines representing the bisection of the long axis of the ossified portion of the calcaneus and the weight-bearing surface form the calcaneal inclination angle. In infants, weight bearing is not always necessary, but can be simulated. This represents the attitude of the calcaneus to the ground in stance. It provides more information about the effects of weight bearing on the foot than does a non–weight-bearing radiograph. The normal range for this angle is 35 to 40 degrees. An increased angle indicates a cavus or high-arched foot, whereas a decreased calcaneal inclination angle indicates a low arched foot, as in pes planovalgus or flatfoot deformity.

**Talar Declination Angle.**  The talar declination angle is determined by the angle formed by the lines representing the bisection of the long axis of the ossified portion of the talus and the weight-bearing surface. It should be taken with the patient in a weight-bearing attitude. The normal angle is 30 degrees. It represents the position of the talus relative to the ground in stance. As with the talocalcaneal angle, an increase in the declination of the talus indicates the calcaneus is not in position underneath the talus, allowing it to "drop" down.

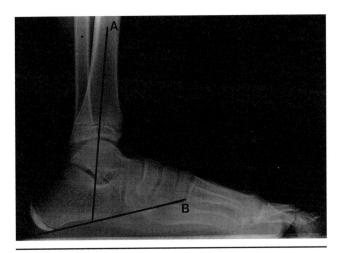

Figure 15-5    Tibiocalcaneal angle. *A*, Tibial axis; *B*, calcaneal axis.

## Talocalcaneal Index and Tibiocalcaneal Angle.

The talocalcaneal index and tibiocalcaneal angle have been described by Vanderwilde and associates.[3] They recommend these measures for assessing initial and residual deformity in patients with clubfoot, vertical talus, metatarsus adductus, or other deformities. The talocalcaneal index is the sum of the dorsoplantar talocalcaneal angle and the lateral talocalcaneal angle. A broad normal range of 45 to 103 degrees has been described. The tibiocalcaneal angle is the angle formed by the bisection of the long axis of the tibia and a line drawn along the plantar aspect of the calcaneus (Figure 15-5). With age this angle slightly decreases from approximately 77 to 70 degrees.

## ■ SPECIAL RADIOGRAPHIC VIEWS

There are some special radiographic views that can be obtained with the child's foot carefully positioned. These views provide additional information about the deformity. I frequently use subtalar joint neutral views, forced plantarflexion, and forced dorsiflexion lateral radiographic views.

### Subtalar Neutral Views

A subtalar neutral radiograph is a weight-bearing radiograph taken with the foot being held in a subtalar joint in neutral position. This may be a dramatically different foot position from the standard weight-bearing view. Dorsoplantar and lateral radiographic views both may be taken with the foot in this position. The foot can be held in a subtalar joint neutral position by the radiology technician or by the patient him- or herself. This position restores the foot to a more normal position that can be repetitively used as a reference for subsequent radiographs. While the child is ambulating

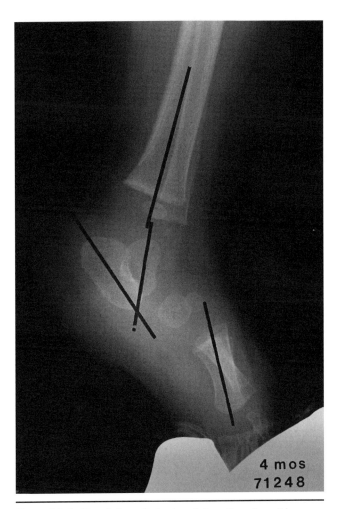

4 mos
71248

Figure 15-6    Forced plantarflexion lateral view of a patient with congenital pes valgus (vertical talus) deformity. In this example, the foot is forcibly plantarflexed and the long axis of the talus does not line up with the long axis of the metatarsals. This misalignment confirms the diagnosis of convex pes valgus as opposed to calcaneal valgus (compare to Figure 15-8). The misalignment appears because when the foot is forcibly plantarflexed, the navicular simply pushes the head and neck of the talus down even further.

with a biomechanical deformity, the foot frequently compensates for that deformity with a change in the relationship between the bones of the foot. When a radiographic study is taken with the foot in a relaxed position, the x-ray film reveals different surfaces of the bone, because the x-ray beam effectively passes at a different angle through the bones themselves. The subtalar neutral joint view consistently reveals the full extent of the bony deformity undisturbed by compensatory changes caused by ambulation. It frequently unmasks the severity of most deformities. In addition, this view is frequently more significant in older children who have been ambulating with a primary deformity for many years.

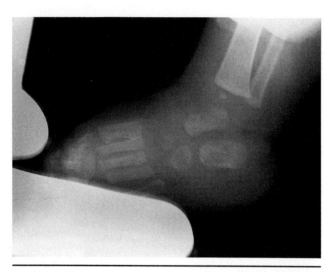

**Figure 15-7**   Forced dorsiflexion lateral view of a patient with talipes equinovarus deformity. This view helps determine the severity of clubfoot deformity. In the normal foot, the talocalcaneal angle increases as the foot is forcibly dorsiflexed. However, with talipes equinovarus the talocalcaneal angle changes very little, because the calcaneus is directly under the talus.

## Forced Plantarflexion Lateral View

A forced plantarflexion lateral radiograph view (Figure 15-6) is taken with the foot held by a technician with the ankle joint maximally plantarflexed. In a normal foot, this position changes the relationship between the talus and the calcaneus as well as between the long axis of the talus and the metatarsals. This can be valuable in determining a true congenital pes valgus foot deformity.

## Forced Dorsiflexion Lateral View

A forced dorsiflexion lateral radiograph (Figure 15-7) is a lateral x-ray view taken with the foot held maximally dorsiflexed at the ankle joint by a technician. This positioning should change the relationship between the talus and the calcaneus, that is, the talocalcaneal angle, in the normal individual. This change is caused by the effect of the Achilles tendon on the calcaneus. This view is significant when attempting to diagnose a talipes equinovarus deformity.

## ◼ CONGENITAL ABNORMALITIES AND ANOMALIES

A number of congenital pedal abnormalities and their radiographic appearance are reviewed in this section. Several congenital anomalies are also included; however, it is impossible to list every conceivable genetic deformity that affects the lower extremity. As previously mentioned, it is my opinion that radiographs should be performed for a majority of the congenital abnormalities before treatment. It is necessary to fully and objectively document the severity of deformity as well as to evaluate the progress of care throughout the course of treatment.

Radiographs need to be repeated regularly, to evaluate the progress or lack thereof of a patient's condition during treatment. Although the physician's clinical impression provides a great deal of information regarding the patient's progress, radiographs provide more specific and objective measurable information regarding the progress of treatment. The actual frequency varies depending on the nature of the deformity, its severity, and the perception of lack of improvement in the deformity.

## Calcaneovalgus

Calcaneovalgus is the most common congenital abnormality. Its incidence has been estimated at 30 to 50%,[7] although (depending on one's definition) it is probably even greater. It is most likely a result of the intrauterine position and pressure on the fetal foot. With this deformity, in the later stages of fetal development the intrauterine tissues press the foot up and against the anterior aspect of the leg. Clinically, the foot maintains a position of abduction, eversion, and dorsiflexion. More significantly, in severe cases the foot cannot plantarflex at the ankle joint past 90 degrees. This is caused by contracted anterior leg and ankle soft tissues. Treatment should include manipulation and clubfoot casting, except in the mildest of cases, to prevent excessive pronation with the onset of weight bearing.

Both dorsoplantar and lateral x-ray views should be performed in moderate to severe cases to rule out the possibility of convex pes valgus (Figure 15-8). On the dorsoplantar view, the calcaneus, midtarsal, and metatarsal bones all appear normal in anatomic form. However, these bones are abducted relative to the talus, as reflected by a greatly increased talocalcaneal (Kite's angle). This angle reflects the position of the foot relative to the talus and leg.

On the lateral view the calcaneal inclination angle is decreased and the talar declination angle is increased. Superimposition of the talar head and the anterior aspect of the calcaneus in the lateral view reflects the fact that the foot bones are abducted away from underneath the talus. In severe cases this condition can easily be confused with a congenital pes valgus deformity (vertical talus).

A forced plantarflexion lateral x-ray view (Figure 15-9) is recommended in these cases to determine if the remainder of the foot bones plantarflex in line with the long axis of the talus. This test confirms a lack of true talonavicular dislocation.

As calcaneovalgus progresses from its infant state to the pes planovalgus (flatfoot) deformity in the older child, the effects of weight bearing and ambulation become more

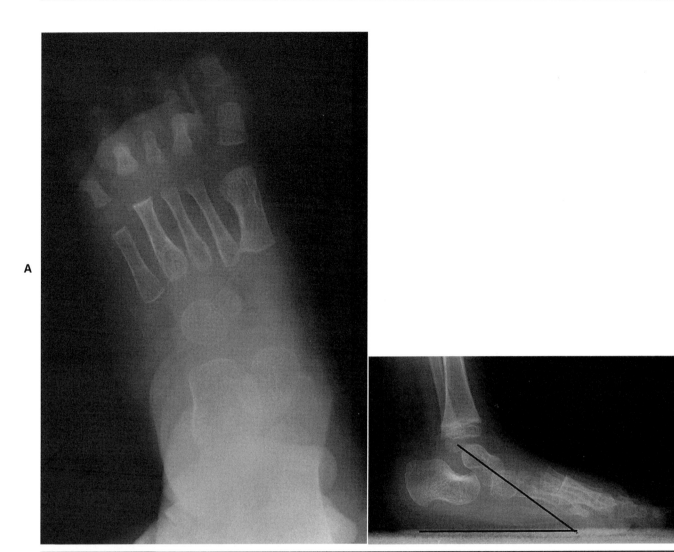

**Figure 15-8** Severe calcaneovalgus deformity. **A,** Dorsoplantar view. The talocalcaneal angle is markedly increased. Although it appears that the long axis of the talus is medially rotated relative to the foot, the reverse is actually true. The calcaneus, midtarsal bones, and metatarsals are abducted from underneath the talus. Note that the calcaneus, midfoot, and forefoot all appear to have a normal relationship relative to each other. **B,** Lateral view. The talar declination angle is increased, and the calcaneal declination angle is decreased to nearly zero degrees.

apparent and severe on radiographs (Figure 15-10). As the foot continues to adapt, the calcaneal inclination angle tends to decrease. The talar declination angle increases on the lateral view. On the dorsoplantar view, the talocalcaneal angle increases as the foot continues to abduct from underneath the leg.

## Congenital Pes Valgus

Congenital pes valgus (Figure 15-11) is frequently referred to as *vertical talus*. This descriptive term alludes to the position of the talus relative to the leg and remainder of the foot. This congenital abnormality is generally a more severe and very rigid condition, as opposed to other congenital abnormalities. The dorsoplantar view does not look much

different from the calcaneal valgus deformity. Generally the talocalcaneal angle is increased, with the entire foot abducted relative to the leg. The lateral radiograph, however, reveals the talus in a straight line with the tibia (see Figure 15-9). More significantly, the metatarsals are dorsally displaced relative to the talus. In infancy the navicular bone is not seen; however, its cartilage precursor is dorsally dislocated on top of the head of the talus.

A forced plantarflexion lateral view (see Figure 15-6) demonstrates the dislocation of the talonavicular joint. In a normal foot, forcibly plantarflexing the foot lines up the long axis of the metatarsal bones with the long axis of the talus. However, with the congenital pes valgus deformity plantarflexing the foot simply forces the navicular to push the head of the talus even further into plantarflexion. With

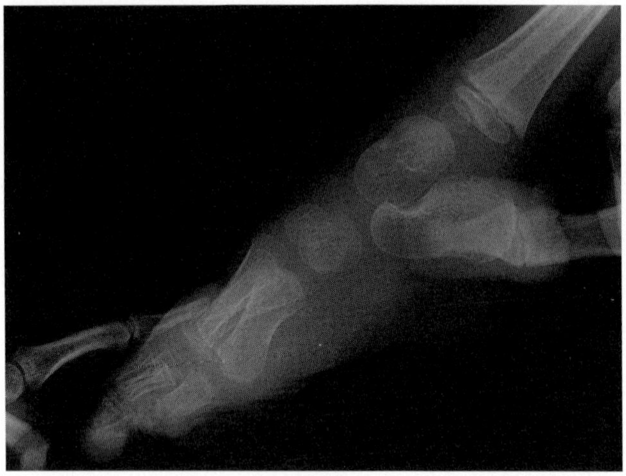

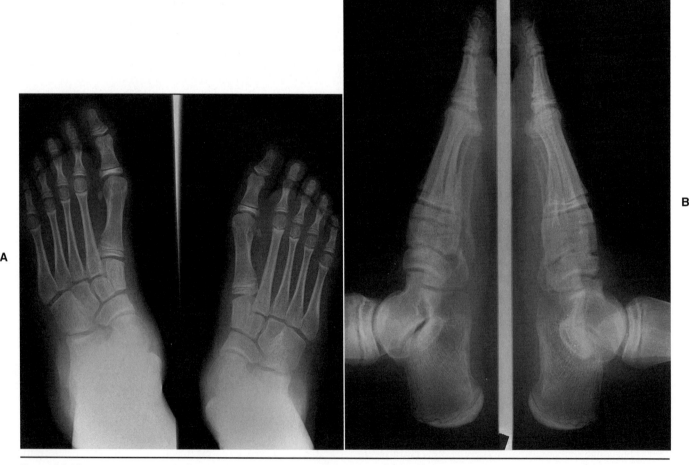

Figure 15-9    Severe calcaneal valgus, forced plantarflexion lateral view. This special view distinguishes calcaneal valgus deformity from a more rigid convex pes valgus (vertical talus) deformity. In calcaneal valgus, if the foot is forcibly plantarflexed the long axis of the talus lines up with the long axis of the metatarsals.

this condition no change should be seen between the relationship of the metatarsals and the long axis of the talus on the lateral view.

## Accessory Navicular

Children frequently demonstrate a severe flatfoot deformity clinically. Another etiology to consider is the accessory navicular or hypertrophic navicular deformity. There is an associated malinsertion of the tibialis posterior tendon into the accessory navicular bone, decreasing its supinatory effect on the foot. In infants the accessory navicular is not visible on radiographs, because it does not ossify until several years of age. However, a magnetic resonance image demonstrates the accessory navicular and malinsertion of the tendon well.

In older children the accessory navicular is frequently completely separate from the main body of the navicular and is seen radiographically (Figure 15-12).

Generally the radiograph reveals a severe flexible type of flatfoot deformity. The calcaneal inclination angle is

Figure 15-10    Pes planovalgus in an older child. **A,** Dorsoplantar view; **B,** lateral view. Note the greatly increased talocalcaneal and talar declination angles and decreased calcaneal declination angles.

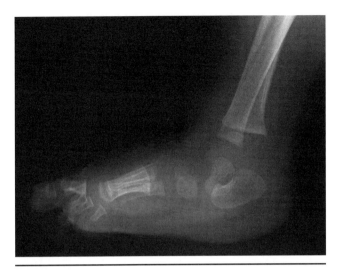

**Figure 15-11** Convex pes valgus (vertical talus) deformity, lateral view. The long axis of the talus lines up more closely with the leg bones than the metatarsals. This can be confused as a severe calcaneal valgus deformity. The calcaneus is also grossly plantarflexed.

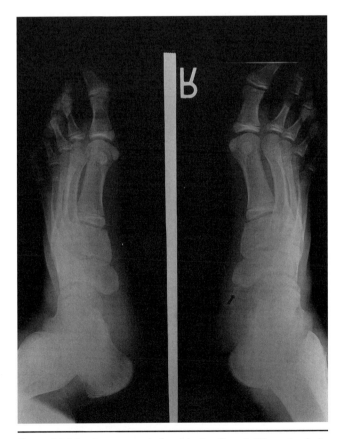

**Figure 15-12** Accessory navicular, right foot (lateral oblique views). A hypertrophic navicular and accessory navicular bone are common findings in children, as well as adults. A typical presentation shows a well-rounded ossicle, just inferior and proximal to the navicular tuberosity in the right foot only. This oblique view is best at visualizing this ossicle. It may or may not be bilateral. Clinical history is therefore very important in ruling out the possibility of fracture.

decreased; the talar declination angle is increased. The Kite's angle is increased on the dorsoplantar view.

The presence of an accessory navicular can make a diagnosis of fracture difficult, even with a history and clinical signs of trauma. Bilateral views are frequently necessary to aid the diagnosis.

## Metatarsus Adductus

Metatarsus adductus is primarily a transverse-plane deformity of the metatarsals relative to the midtarsal bones. The metatarsals are adducted at Lisfranc's joint relative to the midfoot. In severe cases a frontal-plane forefoot varus component may be present. Clinically, this deformity reveals itself as a foot with a C-shape. The lateral border of the foot is convex, and the medial border of the foot is concave.

Figure 15-13 demonstrates a dorsoplantar radiograph of a metatarsus adductus deformity. Although the midtarsal bones are radiographically invisible because of their cartilaginous nature, the metatarsal bones are obviously adducted relative to the long axis of the calcaneus. A relationship between the metatarsals and calcaneus can be used in infants and very young children to determine the severity of metatarsus adductus. It is determined using a bisection of the long axis of the calcaneus and the angle it forms with the bisection of the long axis of the second metatarsal. The normal value is less than 22 degrees. The

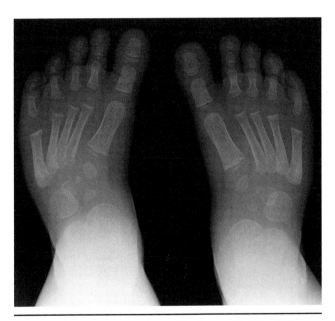

**Figure 15-13** Metatarsus adductus. This 3-year-old child exhibits changes typical of the metatarsal adductus deformity. The talocalcaneal angle is normal or slightly increased. However, the metatarsals are adducted relative to the calcaneus. The metatarsus adductus angle is greatly increased bilaterally. The lack of osseous maturity and the lack of visible midfoot bony reference points make this more difficult to measure.

values in Figure 15-13 are 52 degrees on the left and 39 degrees on the right. The lateral radiograph generally reveals very little change in the structure of the foot. This reflects the primarily transverse-plane nature of the deformity.

In the older child, metatarsus adductus deformity can be evaluated by measuring the angle between the long axis of the second metatarsal relative to the second cuneiform (see Figure 15-3, Engel's angle) or to the lesser tarsus (see Figure 15-4). The normal mean value of Engel's angle is approximately 18 degrees. A metatarsus adductus angle greater than 24 to 25 degrees using this method indicates deformity. Also, in the older child uncorrected metatarsus adductus deformity remains apparent on the dorsoplantar x-ray view. However, frequently on clinical examination the foot generally appears to have "straightened out" overall. This is due to the fact that although the metatarsus adductus deformity continues to exist and is not outgrown, the foot pronates at the subtalar joint and the midtarsal joints, giving it a straighter appearance clinically.

## Tibial Torsion

Tibial torsion is a transverse-plane twist of the long axis of the tibia bone itself. Most often medial (internal) tibial torsion is seen clinically. This torsion can create a mild-to-severe medial foot position on stance and throughout gait. Attempts have been made to identify the amount of tibial torsion by radiography.[6] Most of these methods are not wholly accurate, because it is difficult to evaluate the proximal and distal portions of the tibia. In addition, the relationship between the tibial and fibular malleoli is controversial.

Another radiographic method permits us to indirectly measure the tibial position. With the child seated and the thigh and leg flexed, a dorsoplantar radiograph can be taken. The thigh and leg should be straight ahead, and the foot should rest in its relaxed position on the x-ray film plate. The radiographic study reveals the long axis of the talus in relationship to a straight line, which is the edge of the x-ray film itself. This method reveals the medial position of the talus and the ankle mortise and reflects the twist within the tibia itself, compared to normal feet (Figure 15-14). This radiograph can be repeated during and following therapy to evaluate the progress of the treatment.

## Talipes Equinovarus

Talipes equinovarus (clubfoot) is a complex triplane deformity of the foot. This congenital abnormality is still commonly seen in about 1 in 1000 live births. Four major areas of abnormal bony relationship are visible on the radiograph:

Adduction component of the entire foot relative to the talus and leg

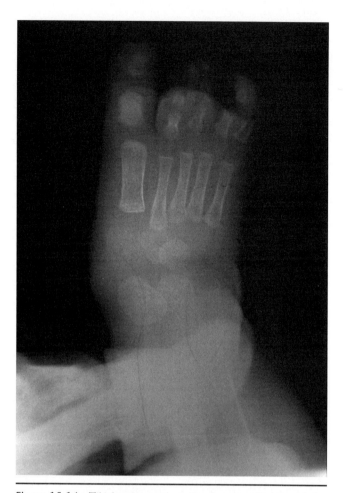

**Figure 15-14** Tibial torsion can be indirectly measured by determining the angle of the long axis of the talus relative to a perpendicular of the x-ray film when the thigh and knee are held straight ahead while the exposure is made. In this case the talus is medially deviated 43 degrees relative to the perpendicular. This reflects its position within the ankle mortise. A normal angle is 16 degrees from the sagittal plane. This method is valid only when the talus itself has no primary bone abnormality.

Adduction of the forefoot relative to the rearfoot
Varus component of the entire foot relative to the leg
Equinus position of the entire foot relative to the leg

The radiographs reveal a decreased talocalcaneal angle both on the dorsoplantar and lateral views (Figures 15-15 and 15-16). This decrease results from the adduction and varus of the calcaneus and the remainder of the foot underneath the talus. An adduction of the metatarsals is also present. A decreased or negative angle appears between talus and first metatarsal, as related by Simons.[7] The navicular is seen to be medially located relative to the head of the talus and in some instances articulates the medial malleolus. On the lateral view a decrease in the talocalcaneal angle is present. In addition, the calcaneus is plantarflexed because of the equinus position.

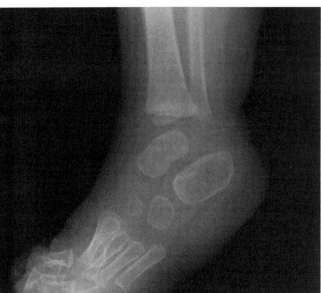

**Figure 15-15**    Talipes equinovarus deformity. **A,** Dorsoplantar view. The talus and calcaneus appear to be a single unit. However, the calcaneus is rotated directed underneath the long axis of the talus so that they appear to coincide. The metatarsals are markedly adducted relative to the rearfoot. The talocalcaneal angle is 0 degrees in the left foot and 4 degrees in the right. **B,** Lateral view. It is apparent that this child cannot bring his heel all the way to the ground because of his posterior leg muscle contracture. This same contracture forcibly plantarflexes the calcaneus. A negative calcaneal inclination angle is produced relative to the weight-bearing surface. In addition, the talocalcaneal angle in this example is 0 degrees, because the calcaneus is directly beneath the talus.

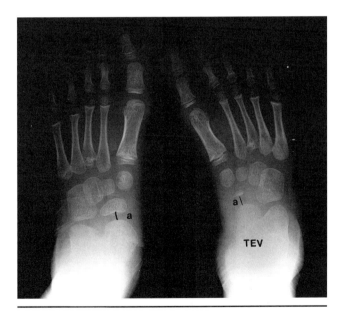

**Figure 15-16**    Talipes equinovarus. In this older child, a poorly developed navicular bone is demonstrated in the right foot as compared to the left. This is caused by a lack of physiologic contact from the talus, producing a delay in development.

## References

1. Templeton A et al: Standardization of terminology and evaluation of osseous relationships in congenitally abnormal feet, *AJR* 9:374, 1965.
2. Altman MI, Sagittal plane angles of the talus and calcaneus in the developing foot, *J Am Podiatr Assoc* 58(11):463, 1968.
3. Vanderwilde R, Staheli LT, Chew DE et al: Measurements on radiographs of the foot in normal infants and children, *J Bone Joint Surg* 70A(3):407, 1988.
4. Engel E, Erlick N, Krems I: A simplified metatarsus adductus angle, *J Am Podiatr Assoc* 73(12):620, 1983.
5. Whitney A: *Radiographic charting technic,* Pennsylvania College of Podiatric Medicine, 1978, Philadelphia.
6. Lang LMG, Volpe RG: Measurement of tibial torsion, *J Am Podiatr Med Assoc* 88(4):160, 1998.
7. Simons GW: Analytical radiography and the progressive approach in the treatment of clubfeet, *Orthop Clin North Am* 9(1):187, 1978.
8. Tachdjian MO: *The child's foot,* Philadelphia, 1985, Saunders.

## Suggested Readings

Blakeslee TJ: Comparative radiographic analysis of congenital idiopathic talipes equinovarus (clubfoot) in infancy: a retrospective study, *JFS* 27(3):188, 1988.

Bowlus TH, Dobas DC: Congenital vertical talus, *J Am Podiatr Assoc* 67(9):609, 1977.

Freiberger RH, Hersh A, Harrison MO: Radiologic study of foot deformities, *Braces Today,* August 1971.

Freiberger RH, Hersh A, Harrison MO: Roentgenology of the deformed foot, *Braces Today,* July 1971.

Miller JH, Bernstein SM: The roentgenographic appearance of the "corrected clubfoot," *Foot Ankle* 6(4):177, 1986.

Oestrich AE: *How to measure angles from foot radiographs: A primer,* New York, 1990, Springer.

Simons GW: Analytical radiography of clubfeet, *J Bone Joint Surg* 59B:485, 1977.

Simons GW: A standardized method for the radiographic evaluation of clubfeet, *Clin Orthop* 135:107, 1978.

# Special Imaging Procedures

# CHAPTER 16

# Overview of Special Imaging Studies

### ROBERT A. CHRISTMAN

Special imaging studies have proven quite valuable for the evaluation of certain foot pathologies. Most important are bone scintigraphy, computed tomography (CT), and magnetic resonance imaging (MRI). Ultrasonography is increasingly being used. Stress ankle and contrast studies, such as arthrography and tenography, play a minor role. Other procedures, including magnification radiography, low-kilovoltage radiography, and xeroradio-graphy, show some usefulness; however, they are rarely used in practice. Special imaging studies can be divided into five categories as follows: stress studies, contrast studies, nuclear medicine studies, cross-sectional imaging studies, and miscellaneous studies (Box 16-1). In almost all instances, standard plain film radiography of the area in question is performed before a special imaging study.

It is necessary not only to fully understand the indications for each of the following special studies but also to be knowledgeable as to what is involved and how the studies are performed. The practitioner who orders a radiograph must educate patients about the prescribed study to alleviate any fears or apprehensions that they might experience before and during the procedure.

The following provides an overview of special imaging studies applicable to foot and ankle disorders. For greater detail on cross-sectional imaging, please refer to Chapter 17.

## ■ STRESS STUDIES

Sprains and strains of the ankle are common. The lateral ligaments, especially the anterior talofibular and calcaneofibular ligaments, are frequently injured. Routine plain film radiography alone yields little or no information regarding the status of these structures.[1] Stress studies of the ankle are performed to assess the integrity of the lateral and medial ankle ligaments. They should be performed on both extremities, the uninjured limb serving as a "normal" comparison.

All stress studies are properly performed non–weight bearing, on a radiography examination table. The usual technique requires one experienced radiographer (or the ordering practitioner)[2] to physically hold the extremity in position during the exposure and a second radiographer to push the exposure control button. The former must wear a lead apron and gloves. However, inconsistent results can

---

| BOX 16-1 | Special Studies Applicable to the Foot and Ankle |
|---|---|

**STRESS STUDIES (ANKLE)**
  Inversion stress
  Eversion stress
  Anterior stress

**CONTRAST STUDIES**
  Arthrography
  Tenography
  Angiography
  Sinography

**NUCLEAR MEDICINE**
  Technetium scan
  Gallium scan
  Indium scan

**CROSS-SECTIONAL IMAGING**
  Conventional tomography
  Computed tomography (CT)
  Magnetic resonance imaging (MRI)

**MISCELLANEOUS PROCEDURES**
  Magnification radiography
  Ultrasonography
  Xeroradiography
  Fluoroscopy
  Low-kilovoltage radiography

occur when manually performing stress studies. For example, unequal stress may inadvertently be applied to one limb and not to the other, resulting in asymmetric radiographic findings. Furthermore, the patient's extremity may not be positioned properly. Finally, patient guarding from pain or muscle spasm may prevent adequate performance of the stress study. In these cases, infiltration of local anesthetic or a nerve block may help.

The preceding variables can be better controlled by using a mechanical apparatus specifically designed to measure the stress applied to the extremity[3] (see Figure 2-16 in Chapter 2). The stress study can thus be (1) performed uniformly bilaterally, (2) reproducibly performed on the same patient at a later date, and (3) made comparable among different patients. A stress apparatus also eliminates exposure to the radiographer, facilitates reproducible patient positioning, and gradually applies stress in an attempt to reduce guarding by the patient.[4] Sauser and associates also found, however, that even with a stress apparatus, stress radiography did not have the diagnostic accuracy of arthrography performed

within 72 hours of the injury.[4] Nevertheless, stress studies are useful for the examination of chronic ankle instability.[5]

## Inversion and Eversion Stress Studies

The inversion stress study examines the integrity of the anterior talofibular and lateral calcaneofibular ligaments; the eversion stress study investigates the status of the deltoid ligament. The extremity is positioned as it would be for the standard anteroposterior (AP) ankle view. The radiographer stands facing the medial side of the extremity to be studied for the stress inversion study and facing the lateral side for the eversion stress study. The hand that is closer to the foot cups the heel, and the other hand is placed along the distal leg. The radiographer must be careful to position his or her hands so that the lead gloves are not superimposed on the ankle joint. With the foot held perpendicular to the leg, the heel is forcibly inverted or everted (depending on which study being performed), while the opposite hand braces the leg. (Perpendicular positioning of the ankle joint primarily

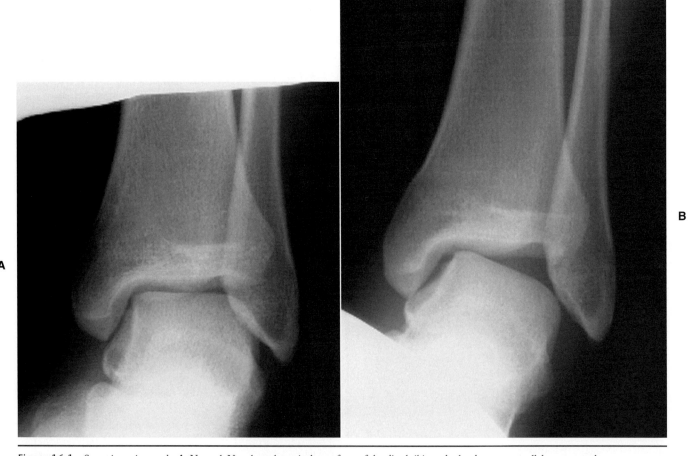

**Figure 16-1**   Stress inversion study. **A,** Normal. Note how the articular surfaces of the distal tibia and talar dome are parallel to one another. **B,** Abnormal. Note the significant degree of talar tilt.

stresses the calcaneofibular ligament; the anterior talofibular ligament contributes more in plantarflexion.[6]) The second radiographer is then signaled to push the exposure button, while the first radiographer holds the extremity steady in the stress position.

Radiographically, lines are drawn across the tibial and talar articular surfaces. In a "normal" AP ankle view, these two lines are parallel or nearly parallel to one another (Figure 16-1, *A*). A positive (or abnormal) inversion or eversion stress study is depicted by a "tilt" of the talar dome relative to the tibial plafond (Figure 16-1, *B*).

Controversy exists concerning the degree of inversion talar tilt that should be considered "abnormal." Rubin and Witten have shown that talar tilts of up to 23 degrees may be seen in an unaffected ankle.[7] However, Cox and Hewes concluded that a talar tilt greater than 5 degrees would signify injury to the lateral ligaments.[8] Generally speaking, a positive talar tilt is suggested if the measured angulation is greater than 10 degrees[9] or if the talar tilt of the affected ankle is 5 degrees or greater than that of the normal ankle.[10] Talar tilt can also increase if the foot is plantarflexed from perpendicular at the ankle joint. In contrast, talar tilt may be lower than expected because of muscle spasm or patient guarding, if prior local anesthetic or nerve block is not applied.

Partial deltoid ligament tears may produce a 10-degree talar tilt with the eversion stress study or 35 to 45 degrees tilt if completely torn.[11]

## Anterior Stress Study

The anterior stress study evaluates the anterior talofibular ligament. It is believed that this study evaluates ligament integrity more critically than the stress inversion study.[6] The anterior stress study, also known as the "push-pull" study and the anterior drawer test, is an attempt to subluxate the talus anteriorly. Technically, the extremity is positioned as it would be for a non–weight-bearing mediolateral ankle projection. The radiographer stands facing the toes. The hand that is closer to the foot cups the heel, and the other is placed along the anterior aspect of the distal leg. The radiographer must be careful to position his or her hands such that the lead gloves are not superimposed on the ankle joint. With the foot held perpendicular to the leg, the heel is forcibly pulled anteriorly, while the opposite hand pushes against the leg posteriorly. The second radiographer is then signaled to push the exposure button, while the first radiographer holds the extremity steady in the stress position.

In the lateral ankle view, the tibial plafond normally parallels the talar dome and apposes it 100%. The "positive" finding, known as the anterior drawer sign, is noted by a lack of parallelism between the tibial plafond and talar dome articular surfaces (Figure 16-2). Grace found that anterior talofibular ligament disruption was suggested if the distance between the posterior lip of the tibia and the nearest part of the talar dome was greater than 6 millimeters.[12]

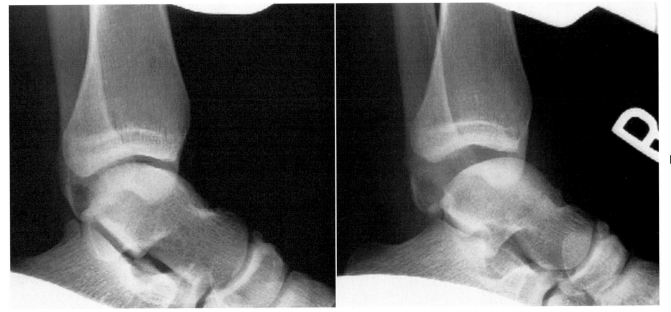

A                                                                                                                                    B

**Figure 16-2**   Anterior stress study. **A,** Normal. Note how the articular surfaces of the distal tibia and talar dome are parallel to one another. **B,** Abnormal. The foot has been subluxated anteriorly, indicating a rupture of the anterior talofibular ligament.

## ■ CONTRAST STUDIES

Most soft tissue structures in the foot are of a similar radiographic density and normally cannot be distinguished from one another in plain films. These structures include joint cartilage, synovium, and capsule. Although tendons can occasionally be identified, their outlines are typically not sharp; it is impossible to see the tendon sheath. Bursae and arteries are "invisible" and also cannot be identified in the plain film. Even soft tissue pathology, such as the ganglion cyst and the sinus associated with ulcer and infection, is not visible in most cases.

Contrast studies afford the physician an opportunity to visualize some soft tissue structures that otherwise are "invisible" in the plain film. Typically, a radiopaque, iodinated contrast agent is injected into the part in question, be it a joint, tendon, bursa, or artery. (Patients sensitive to iodine are not candidates for iodinated contrast studies.) Most contrast studies are best performed with fluoroscopic guidance. The structure is then assessed by the use of plain film radiography. After injection of the contrast agent, the structure is seen as an increased density relative to adjacent tissues. The contrast studies performed on lower-extremity structures include arthrography (joint), tenography (tendon), bursography (bursa), and angiography (blood vessel). Contrast study of pathologic entities includes sinography (sinus) and gangliography (ganglion).

In recent years, contrast agents have been used to enhance CT and MRI.[13,14] Boxes 16-2 and 16-3 list potential uses in the foot and ankle.

## Arthrography

Arthrography, although it could be performed in any pedal joint, is almost exclusively used in the ankle joint. Pedal joints are rarely studied, the exception being the subtalar joint. Applications for ankle arthrography are primarily for,

---

> ### BOX 16-3    Potential Uses for Contrast-Enhanced MRI with Gadopentetate Dimeglumine[13]
>
> 1. Infection delineation
> 2. Tumor characterization and evaluation
> 3. Pannus versus joint effusion
> 4. Articular[15,16] and tendon injuries
> 5. Fracture healing
> 6. Osteonecrosis revascularization

but not limited to, assessment of ligament damage. It can also be performed to evaluate the integrity of articular cartilage; locate loose bodies and meniscoid lesions, adhesive capsulitis, and capsular rupture[17]; and evaluate for rheumatic disease.[18] After trauma, arthrography should ideally be performed right away or at least within 1 week.[19] Indications for metatarsophalangeal joint arthrography include arthritis, integrity of joint implants,[20] plantar plate abnormalities, and capsulitis, synovitis, and metatarsalgia.[21]

Radiopaque ("positive") or radiolucent ("negative") contrast agents can be used for arthrography. Radiolucent contrast agents include air or carbon dioxide. The negative contrast study is especially useful for patients sensitive to iodine (positive contrast agents typically are iodinated). For assessing cartilage integrity, radiopaque and radiolucent contrast agents can also be injected in combination. This is known as a double-contrast study.

For an ankle arthrogram, after a sterile preparation of the site, 5 to 10 milliliters of contrast agent is injected into the anteromedial aspect of the ankle. Mortise, AP, and lateral ankle views are then obtained.

Three recesses normally fill with contrast material: the anterior recess, the posterior recess, and the region of the syndesmosis between the distal fibula and tibia.[22] The ankle joint capsule fills as a well-defined sac or pouch both anterior and posterior to the ankle joint in the lateral view.[23] In the AP view the contrast appears as an "umbrella" surrounding the talus; pouches of contrast can be seen medially and laterally but do not extend below and around the malleoli (Figure 16-3). Slight visualization of dye is normally seen in the distal tibiofibular synovial recess. As a variation of normal, the posterior subtalar joint fills in 10% of the population[24] (Figure 16-4, *A*). In the AP view this appears as a "double umbrella sign." In addition, the flexor hallucis longus and flexor digitorum longus tendons fill in patients with no underlying pathology in 20% of the normal population[25] (Figure 16-4, *B*).

Positive (abnormal) findings include absence of a well-defined joint capsule extending anteriorly or posteriorly, the presence of dye inferior to the tips of either malleolus,

---

> ### BOX 16-2    Potential Uses for Computed Tomography (CT) Imaging with Iodinated Contrast Agents[13]
>
> **INTRAVENOUS ENHANCED CONTRAST**
> 1. Osteomyelitis (soft tissue extent)
> 2. Primary soft tissue abscess
> 3. Soft tissue component of bone tumors
>
> **INTRA-ARTICULAR CONTRAST**
> 1. Osteochondritis dissecans
> 2. Loose bodies
> 3. Synovial chondromatosis
> 4. Pigmented villonodular synovitis

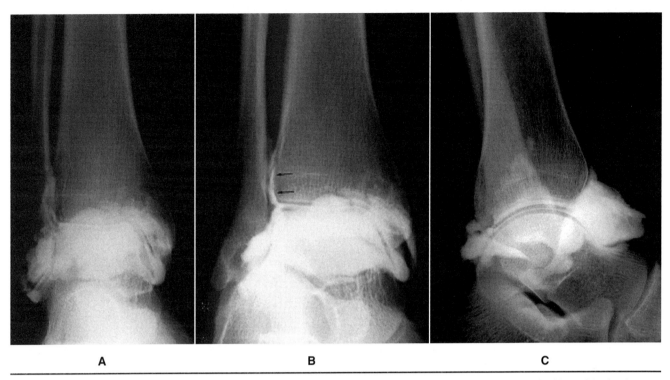

Figure 16-3    Normal ankle arthrogram. **A**, AP view. Note the medial and lateral pouches. **B**, Oblique (mortise) view. Note the filling of the distal tibiofibular joint. **C**, Lateral view. Note the anterior and posterior pouches.

extravasation of dye superior to the distal tibiofibular synovial recess, and filling of the peroneal tendon sheath.[26]

Arthrography has been performed with cross-sectional imaging studies. For example, talar osteochondritis dissecans has been assessed with CT arthrography.[27] Recently, it has been suggested that MRI arthrography would serve as a useful adjunct for evaluation of ankle pathology.[15,16] With MRI, gadolinium compounds are used as contrast-enhancing agents.

## Tenography

Tenography is also performed with an iodinated, radiopaque contrast agent. It is performed on the tendon and tendon sheath structures about the ankle joint, primarily the peroneal tendons (Figure 16-5), although it can also be used on the medial and anterior compartment tendons (Figures 16-6 and 16-7).

The injection site is selected proximal to the point of maximal tendon tenderness. After sterile preparation, the technique is performed in the following manner[28]: A needle and syringe with local anesthetic is inserted into the tendon until firm resistance is encountered. The technician inserts gentle pressure on the plunger while slowly withdrawing it from the tendon. (The needle is within the sheath when the anesthetic flows easily.) While the needle remains in place,

the syringe is removed and replaced with a second syringe containing the contrast agent. Contrast is injected until it fails to fill distally and extravasates proximally. Standard lateral foot and ankle, AP ankle, and dorsoplantar foot views are obtained following injection. Variations of this technique have also been described.[29]

Indications for tenography include tendon and tendon sheath damage, impingement, dislocation, and tenosynovitis.[28,30] Peroneal tenography can also be used to assess calcaneofibular ligament ruptures. Subsequent filling of the ankle joint with contrast indicates rupture of the calcaneofibular ligament.[31,32]

## Sinography

Sinography is used to determine whether or not a sinus or cavity in the soft tissues communicates with an underlying bone or joint.[33] This type of study can be useful for evaluating infection.[34] Radiopaque contrast material is injected into a small catheter that has been placed deeply into the sinus. Plain films are then obtained, delineating the extent and complexity of the sinus from the retrograde or gravitational filling of the contrast material[35] (Figure 16-8). It has also been used in combination with 1% methylene blue to evaluate a chronic plantar ulceration and to visibly outline its sinus tract before an operation.[36]

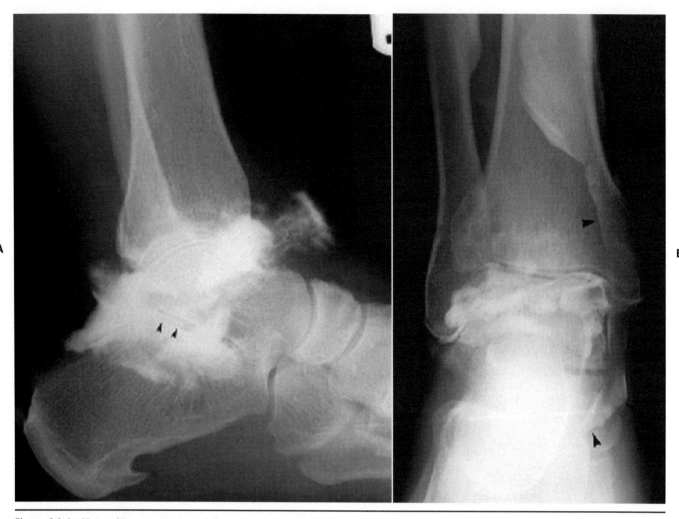

Figure 16-4    Variant filling presentations. **A**, Posterior subtalar joint. **B**, Flexor tendons.

## Bursography

Bursography of the retrocalcaneal bursa can be performed after fluid aspiration.[37] It is used to evaluate irregularity and nodularity of the synovial lining in patients with rheumatoid arthritis.[38] Frey and associates advocate bursography for evaluating and differentiating hindfoot pathology.[39]

## Gangliography

Ganglion cysts on the dorsum of the foot are not uncommon. Gangliography performed before surgery can help the surgeon understand the clinical extent of the cyst (Figure 16-9). In 1982 Reinherz published a report of one case.[40] Ly and McCarty recently outlined the technique and complications of gangliography.[41]

## Angiography

Angiography is primarily used to assess the patency of blood vessels in the foot. Arteriography evaluates arteries and venography (or phlebography), veins. It can be used to evaluate conditions exhibiting dilated, constricted, or blocked vessels. A thrombus, for example, can be clearly demonstrated by venography.[42] Arteriograms are advocated for most penetrating and violent extremity injuries with blunt instrument[43] and are useful for evaluating arteriovenous fistula.[44] Examples of musculoskeletal disorders in the foot evaluated with angiography include reflex sympathetic dystrophy, frostbite, and vascular malformations (hemangioma).[45]

Lower-extremity arteriography (Figure 16-10) is not used solely as a diagnostic study; it also serves as a

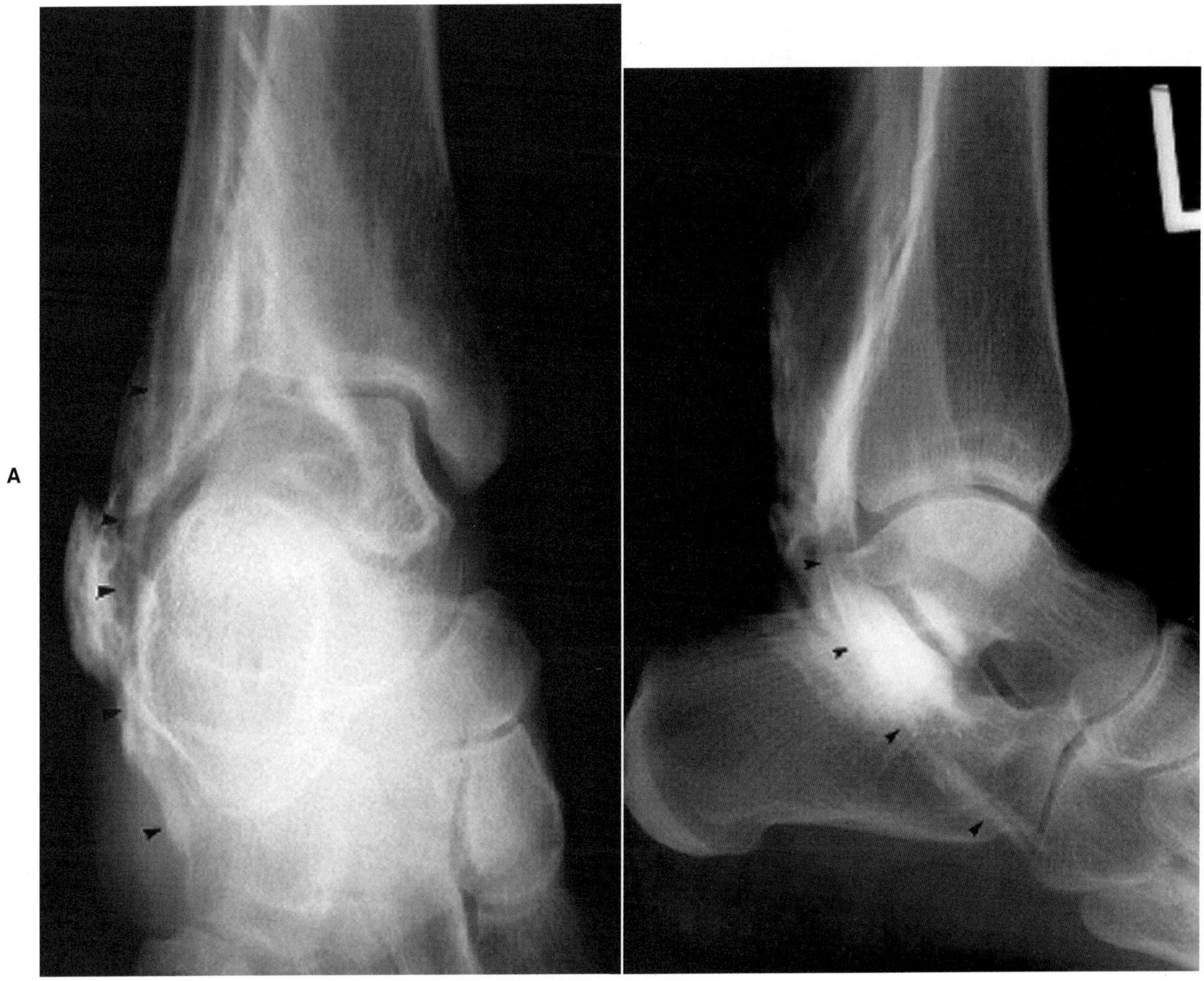

Figure 16-5   Tenography (peroneal tendon). **A**, AP view. **B**, Lateral view.

preparatory procedure for nonsurgical endovascular therapy.[46] Contrast agent is injected at the aortic bifurcation or more distally for conventional arteriography of the lower extremities. Plain films are then obtained.

Another method for evaluating the arterial vasculature is by digital subtraction angiography (DSA). Contrast material is injected intravenously, and images are obtained by computed fluoroscopy.[47] It is simpler, less invasive, and less costly than arteriography; it subjects the patient to decreased discomfort and can be performed on an outpatient basis.[48] Disadvantages include higher contrast-medium loads and decreased spatial resolution (therefore poorer-quality images).[49]

Currently, magnetic resonance angiography (Figure 16-11) is being studied and used for imaging the lower extremity.[50,51] It is believed to have excellent prospects for routine clinical use in the peripheral vessels.[52]

Venography is best performed using fluoroscopic guidance and can be performed as either an ascending (the procedure of choice) or descending study. The ascending study venogram is performed in the following manner: A radiopaque contrast medium is injected into a distal superficial vein with or without a tourniquet; the procedure is monitored by fluoroscopy, and multiple-spot plain films are obtained.[53] Descending venography is performed by injecting the iodinated contrast agent more proximally; the

Figure 16-6    Tenography (tibialis posterior tendon). *A*, AP view. **B**, Lateral view.

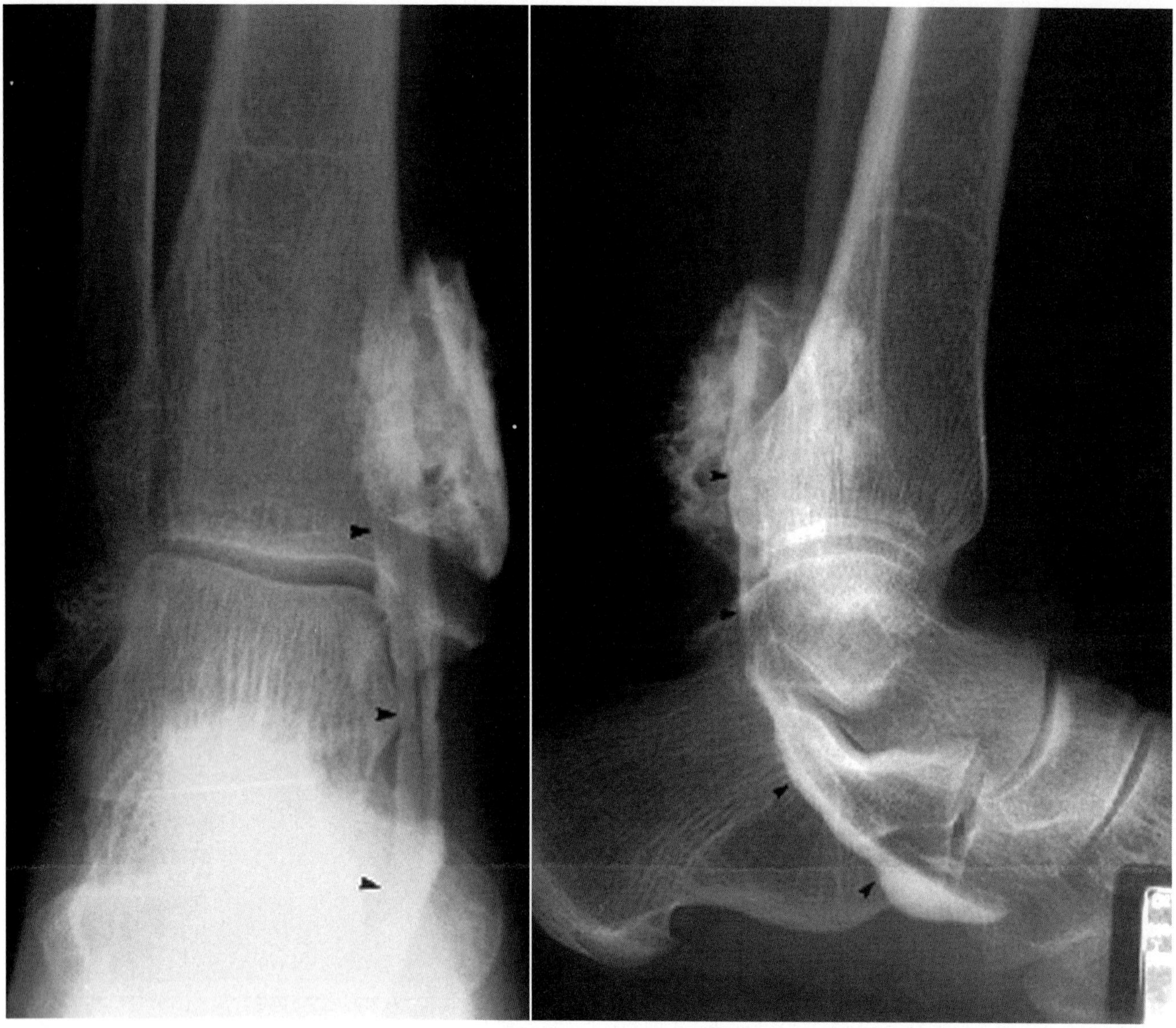

patient performs a Valsalva maneuver (forced expiration against the closed glottis), and the degree of competency is determined based on reflux.[54] Because of potential reaction to the contrast agent and significant discomfort from the procedure, noninvasive techniques for diagnosing lower-extremity deep venous thrombosis are being investigated.[55]

### ■ NUCLEAR MEDICINE STUDIES

Nuclear medicine is that branch of diagnostic radiology that uses radioactive nucleotides (or radioisotopes) to image the body. This type of study is called scintigraphy. Scintigraphy evaluates physiologic activity, in contrast to the plain film assessment of morphology and tissue densities. In the lower extremity, scintigraphy is used to evaluate the musculoskeletal system.

The performance of a radioisotope study is quite different from plain film radiography. First, a radioisotope is injected into the body; for lower-extremity studies, an antecubital intravenous site is typical. The radiopharmaceutical is distributed throughout the body and gives off gamma radiation. (Gamma rays are a form of ionizing radiation similar to x rays except for their origin: Gamma rays are produced inside the nucleus of a radioactive atom, and x rays are artificially produced outside the nucleus.[56]) A

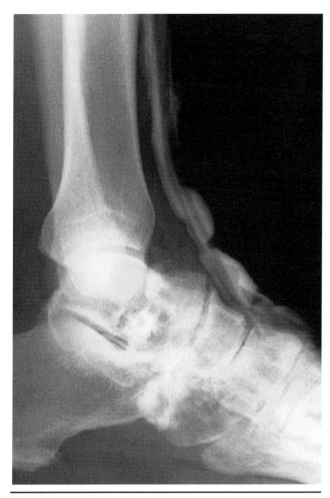

Figure 16-7   Tenography (tibialis anterior tendon) (lateral view).

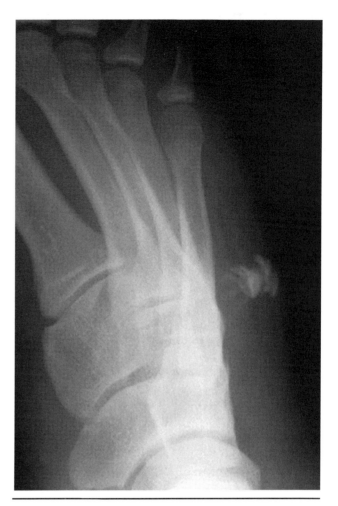

Figure 16-8   Sinography. The extent of this sinus is demonstrated clearly in the lateral oblique view.

gamma (or scintillation) camera is positioned over the body part in question and detects ionizing radiation being emitted (scintillating) from the patient. Scintillation detectors in the camera measure the radiation, which can then be recorded onto transparent film. The final image is known as a scintiscan or scintigram. In contrast to plain film radiography, in scintigraphy x rays are not transmitted through the patient.

Different aspects of the foot and ankle can be imaged. The name of the view is based on that surface of the extremity nearest to the gamma camera. For example, if the dorsum of the foot were closest to the camera, the resultant image would be a dorsal view of the foot. Plantar, medial, and lateral views of the foot and anterior, posterior, medial, and lateral ankle views can also be obtained. Occasionally you may hear the term "pinhole collimation" in reference to scintigraphy. This technique magnifies or increases the number of counts (or information density) available when recording the resulting image.[57]

The resultant image does not demonstrate the resolution seen in the plain film. In fact, it may even be difficult to recognize the foot (Figure 16-12). Small black dots are seen on a transparent film (white dots on a black background if Polaroid film is used); their overall contribution resembles the form of the foot and ankle. Individual toes may be identifiable in the dorsal and plantar views. The black dots reflect the detection of the radioisotope by the camera. A focal, increased accumulation of dots on the scintigram is called a "hot spot" and corresponds to the accumulation of radiopharmaceutical in tissue; absent accumulation (or an area of photopenia) is known as a "cold spot."

The radioisotopes used to image foot and ankle pathology are technetium, gallium, and indium. They frequently are used individually or in combination to assess musculoskeletal infection in the foot. Keep in mind that scintigraphy does not detect the presence of infection but reflects the reaction of bone (or inflammatory process) possibly associated with infection.[58]

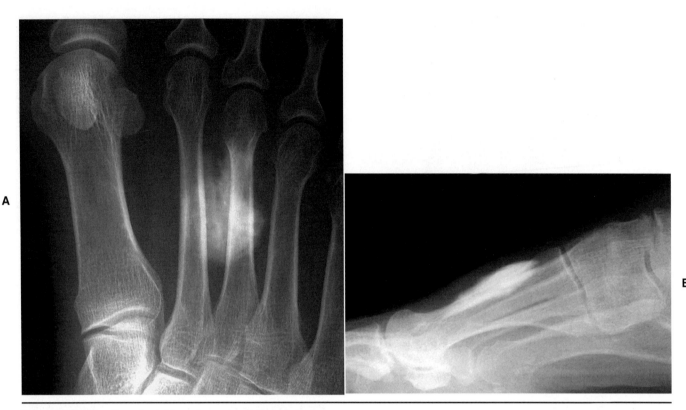

Figure 16-9    Gangliography. **A,** Dorsoplantar view. **B,** Lateral view.

## Technetium

Technetium is the most widely used of the three radioisotopes. The procedure that uses Tc-99m methylene diphosphonate (MDP) is known as the three-phase bone scan or bone scintigraphy. The technetium-phosphate complex is incorporated into bone that has increased osteoblastic activity. Its distribution is highly dependent on patent vascularity.

Bone scintigraphy is a valuable adjunct to plain film radiography. Before it may be seen on a plain film, 30% to 50% of bone must be resorbed or destroyed,[59] whereas bone scintigraphy readily detects pathology with accompanying osteoblastic activity. Although bone scintigraphy is an extremely sensitive technique for detecting increased (or decreased) bone activity, it is not highly specific. Many pathologic conditions have increased bone activity that shows increased skeletal uptake of radioisotope. To increase specificity, the results must be associated with history, clinical, and plain film findings.

Bone scintigraphy is typically performed in three phases[60]: dynamic flow, blood pool, and delayed. The dynamic flow phase (see Figure 16-12) is actually an angiogram of the part being imaged, performed promptly after antecubital injection of the radioisotope. The blood

pool phase (Figure 16-13) is performed a few minutes after injection of the radiopharmaceutical. Localized accumulation of the radioisotope is seen in areas of hyperemia. The delayed or bone scan phase (Figure 16-14) is performed two to four hours after the injection. By this time the technetium-phosphate complex has been incorporated into bone with increased osteoblastic/metabolic activity. A fourth phase, performed 24 hours after the injection, has been advocated for patients with compromised vascularity to the part in question.[61] Israel and associates[62] noted that although the uptake of Tc-99m MDP stops at approximately 4 hours in normal bone, it continues at 24 hours in abnormal bone. Indications for triple-phase bone scintigraphy[63] include trauma (stress fracture, occult fracture,[64] reflex sympathetic dystrophy, osteonecrosis, myositis ossificans, frostbite, bone graft, pseudoarthrosis), bone tumors[65] (primary and metastatic), osteomyelitis, and arthritis.[66] Bone scintigraphy is especially useful for evaluating undiagnosed bone pain in the presence of normal plain film radiographs.

A newer agent, Tc-99m hexamethylpropyleneamine oxime (HMPAO), has been used to image inflammatory processes, in particular osteomyelitis.[67] Tc-99m HMPAO selectively labels leukocytes (granulocytes) and is prepared in

a

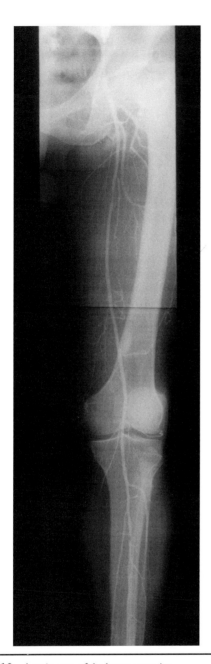

Figure 16-10    Arteriogram of the lower extremity.

manner similar to indium-111 (see following discussion). Compared with In-111, Tc-99m HMPAO has been reported to offer similar accuracy, be more convenient to use, require lower radiation dose, and be capable of imaging low-level inflammation more readily.[68]

## Gallium and Indium

The radiopharmaceuticals gallium-67 and indium-111 are frequently used with Tc-99m MDP for evaluating

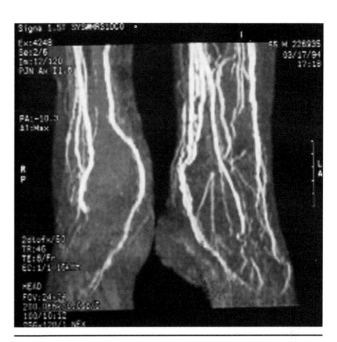

Figure 16-11    Magnetic resonance angiography.

osteomyelitis (Figure 16-15). This is especially the case if another underlying skeletal disorder (osteoarthritis, neuroarthropathy, fracture, and postoperative healing, for example) presents at the same location on plain radiographs. Although bone scintigraphy may be sensitive for bone infection, adding these studies improves specificity.

During the 1970s and early 1980s, gallium was used concomitantly with bone scintigraphy for assessing osteo-myelitis. It has been shown to be very sensitive for detecting inflammatory foot lesions[69] and useful for following the efficacy of treatment, because it doesn't localize in healing bone.[70] Images for the gallium-67 citrate scan are typically acquired 24 hours following injection. Gallium depends less on blood flow and accumulates in areas of infection. The intensity of gallium uptake at the suspected site of infection must be equal to or greater than that seen in the bone scan.[71] However, in current practice the indium-111–labeled leukocyte scan, when available, is preferable to gallium for diagnosing osteomyelitis,[72] except in children.[73]

Indium is probably superior to gallium for imaging most musculoskeletal infections,[74] although some argue that the gallium technique is still useful, given its proven clinical efficacy and practical advantages (less expensive, readily available, easier to perform, and less problematic).[75] It is felt that the results of indium in combination with technetium is more sensitive and specific for osteomyelitis, especially in the foot demonstrating neuropathic osteoarthropathy, than technetium alone or technetium in combination with gallium.[76,77] Indium scanning was shown to be valuable in

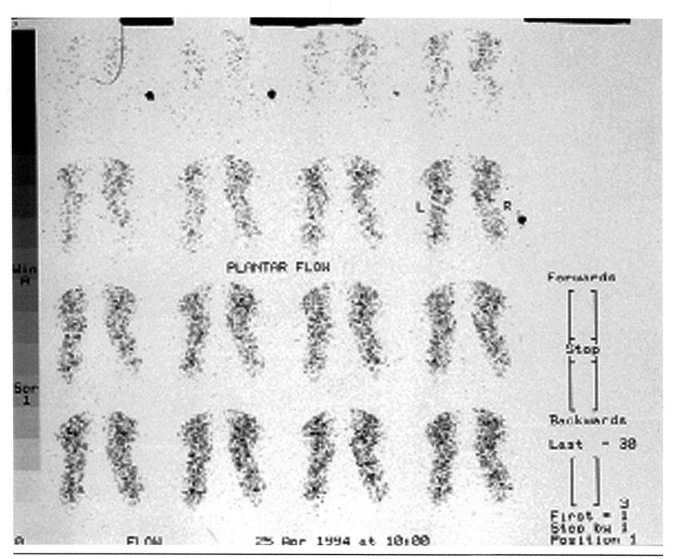

Figure 16-12   Bone scintigraphy: Phase 1 (flow study or arteriogram).

assessing diabetic foot ulcers; many of these patients have an underlying osteomyelitis that is unsuspected clinically.[78] Unfortunately, indium is not widely available and requires technical expertise in its prolonged preparation.[79] Blood is drawn from the patient; the white blood cells are separated and tagged to indium, then injected into the patient. Images are obtained 24 hours after injection. Other disadvantages include its poor resolution, the high radiation dose, and the fact that In-111 imaging alone does not consistently differentiate from infection disorders that alter bone marrow activity.[80] Tc-99m sulfur colloid marrow imaging has been used with In-111 to improve the sensitivity, specificity, and accuracy in the latter instance.[81] Another preparation, indium-111-polyclonal IgG, is thought to be useful for

evaluating infection and is safer and easier to prepare than labeled leukocytes.[82]

## ■ CROSS-SECTIONAL IMAGING STUDIES

Complex skeletal areas, especially where irregular bones are superimposed on other bones, are difficult to assess with standard plain film techniques. This is especially true in the tarsus and ankle regions. Cross-sectional imaging studies allow a single plane of interest to be examined while differentially blurring or eliminating all other structures that normally would be superimposed and impair visualization. Conventional tomography, CT, and MRI are modalities

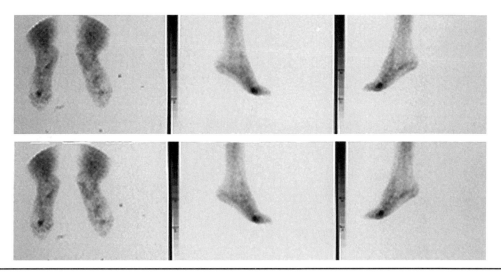

Figure 16-13    Bone scintigraphy: Phase 2 (blood pool study).

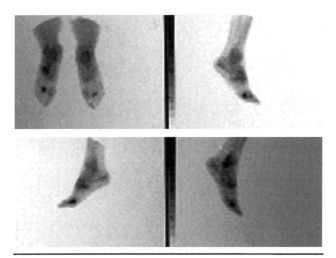

Figure 16-14    Bone scintigraphy: Phase 3 (the bone scan).

used for evaluating complex skeletal regions of the foot and ankle. In addition, CT and, more importantly, MRI provide images of soft tissue structures that cannot be visualized by plain film radiography.

## Conventional Tomography

Although the least expensive of the three cross-sectional modalities, conventional tomography yields an image that is far inferior to the remaining two types of studies. It is a variation of the simple plain film method. The x-ray tube head and film move in opposite directions about a fulcrum but in parallel planes; the fulcrum corresponds to the plane of the focal area of interest.[83] Structures above and below or to the sides of the plane of interest are blurred. Foot sections are typically obtained at 0.5-cm intervals. Osseous structures

that are not clearly identified with plain films (such as the tarsal bones) may be more clearly seen with tomography (Figures 16-16 and 16-17). Applications where this study may be useful include tarsal coalition, tarsal fracture, subtalar arthritis, osteocartilaginous lesions, loose bodies, and fracture healing.[84] A major disadvantage is the increased radiation dose compared to CT and standard radiography.[85]

## Computed Tomography

Computed tomography has the advantage of high-contrast resolution; that is, it can distinguish between two tissue types that have only slightly different attenuation characteristics.[86] Overlying tissue blurring found with conventional tomography is not seen in the CT image. The patient's extremity is placed inside the gantry of the unit. An x-ray tube rotates 360 degrees around the extremity.[87] Detectors measure the x-ray beam after it is transmitted through the patient. Attenuation values (also known as CT numbers) can be determined for all tissues and are expressed as Hounsfield units (HU). In addition, the image can be computer adjusted so that either soft tissue or bone is more visible. These are referred to as either soft tissue or bone windows, respectively (Figure 16-18). Images can be obtained in axial and coronal planes; reformatted computer images in the sagittal plane and three-dimensional images can also be obtained.[88] Slice thicknesses can be obtained between 1.5 and 12 mm; 1.5- to 2.0-mm slices are recommended for foot pathology.[89] Indications include all indications mentioned for conventional tomography; in fact, CT may very well have eliminated the need for conventional tomographic imaging of foot and ankle pathology.[89] It is useful for evaluating subtalar joint pathology[90] and is valuable for the assessment of calcaneal fractures,[91,92] even

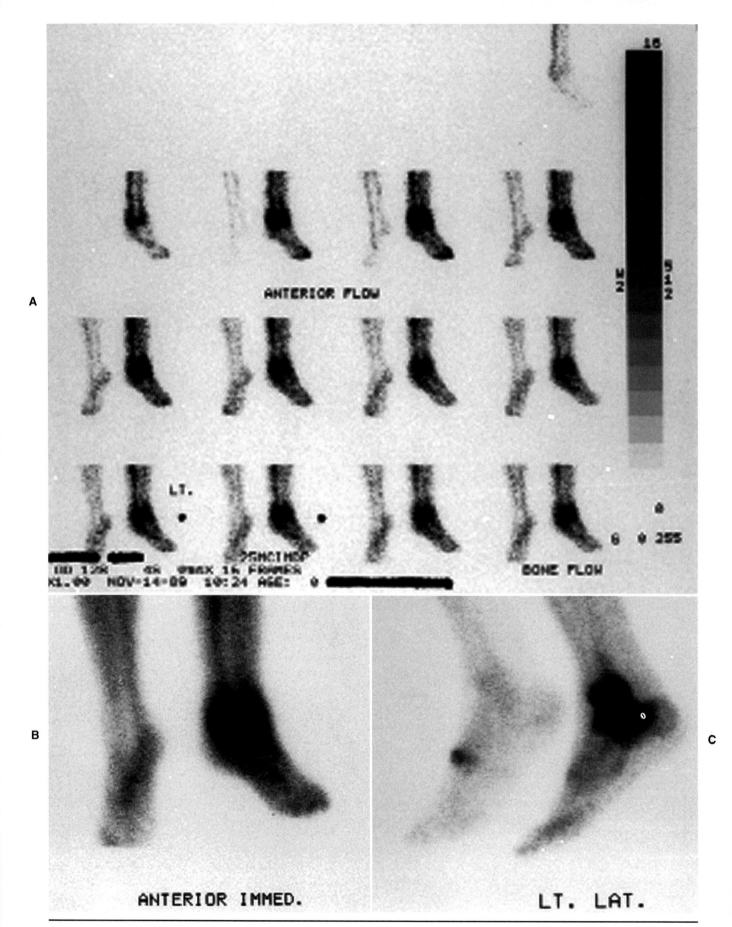

Figure 16-15 Combination of technetium, gallium, and indium scans for assessment of possible ankle infection. **A**, Bone scintigraphy, dynamic flow phase. **B**, Bone scintigraphy, blood pool phase. **C**, Bone scan (third phase).

*Continued*

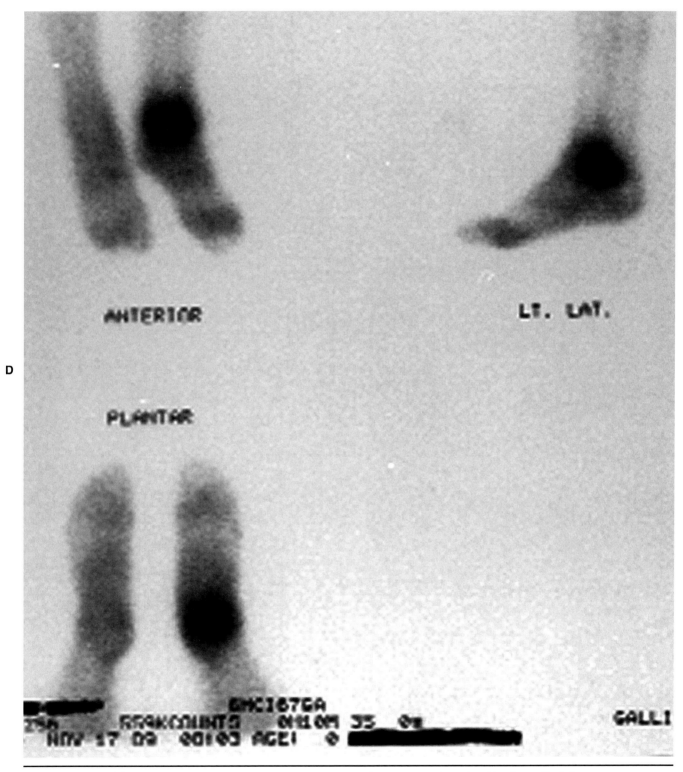

Figure 16-15, cont'd   Combination of technetium, gallium, and indium scans for assessment of possible ankle infection. **D,** Gallium scan.

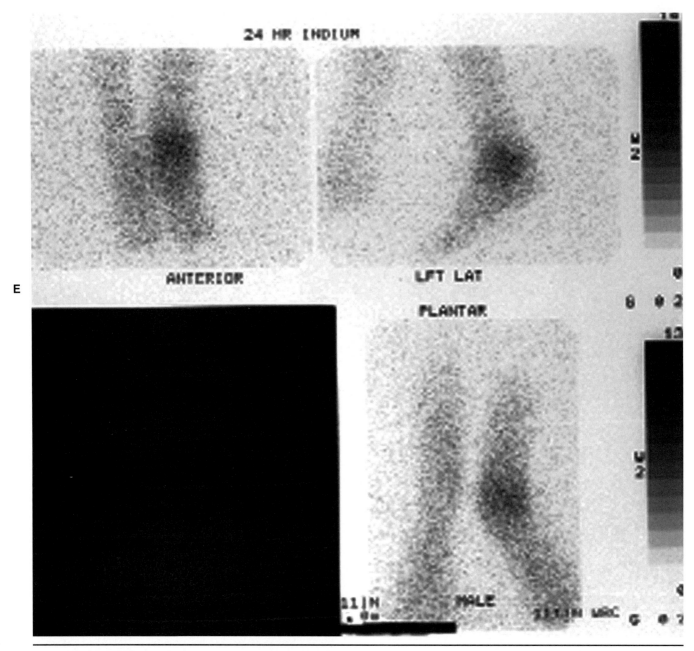

Figure 16-15, cont'd   Combination of technetium, gallium, and indium scans for assessment of possible ankle infection. **E,** Indium scan.

with three-dimensional reconstruction.[93] Although CT can be used to evaluate soft tissue pathology, MRI is usually reserved for this purpose.

## Magnetic Resonance Imaging

Unlike conventional and computed tomography, magnetic resonance imaging does not use ionizing radiation. High-quality images are obtained as radio frequency pulses are absorbed and then re-emitted by the extremity lying inside a magnetic field.[94] Cross-sectional images can be obtained in any plane, unlike the limitations placed on CT images. Furthermore, soft tissue contrast is superior to that provided by CT, making MRI the choice for soft tissue pathology.[95] Typically, two images of each section are obtained, referred to as T1- and T2-weighted images (Figure 16-19). Simply

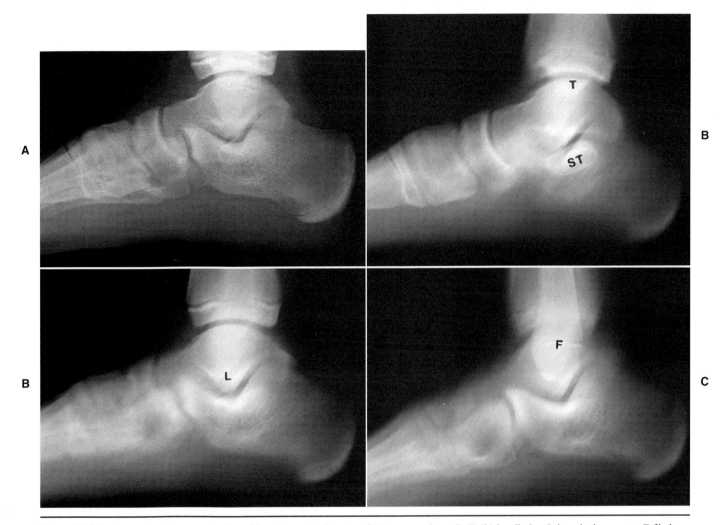

Figure 16-16   Conventional tomography, lateral foot view, sagittal sections (*ST*, sustentaculum tali; *T*, tibial malleolus; *L*, lateral talar process; *F*, fibular malleolus). **A,** Plain film. **B,** Section at 7.5 cm (from lateral side of foot). **C,** Section at 6 cm. **D,** Section at 4 cm.

speaking, the T1-weighted image represents an anatomic image; fat demonstrates the highest signal intensity. Water has the strongest signal intensity in the T2-weighted image and reflects areas of inflammation. This latter image therefore is used to assess pathology.

Indications for performing MRI of the foot or ankle include both soft tissue and osseous abnormalities. Tendon and ligament injuries receive the most attention.[96-102] Much attention has been directed recently toward the assessment of osteomyelitis, especially in the diabetic foot.[103-110] MRI also has been used to assess neuroma,[111,112] pigmented villonodular synovitis,[113,114] bone bruise,[115,116] stress fracture,[117,118] physeal fracture,[119] osteonecrosis,[120] tarsal tunnel syndrome,[121,122] and plantar fasciitis.[123] Chapter 17 provides examples of the many applications for this special imaging technique.

## MISCELLANEOUS STUDIES

Imaging procedures that are not frequently used but have limited application for foot or ankle pathology include magnification radiography, ultrasonography, xeroradiography, fluoroscopy, and low-kilovoltage radiography. Each of these procedures requires special equipment and, with the exception of magnification radiography, cannot be performed with lower extremity–specific radiographic units.

### Magnification Radiography

The purpose of magnification radiography is to obtain enlargement of the part in question while minimizing geometric blurring of the image. This can be performed by

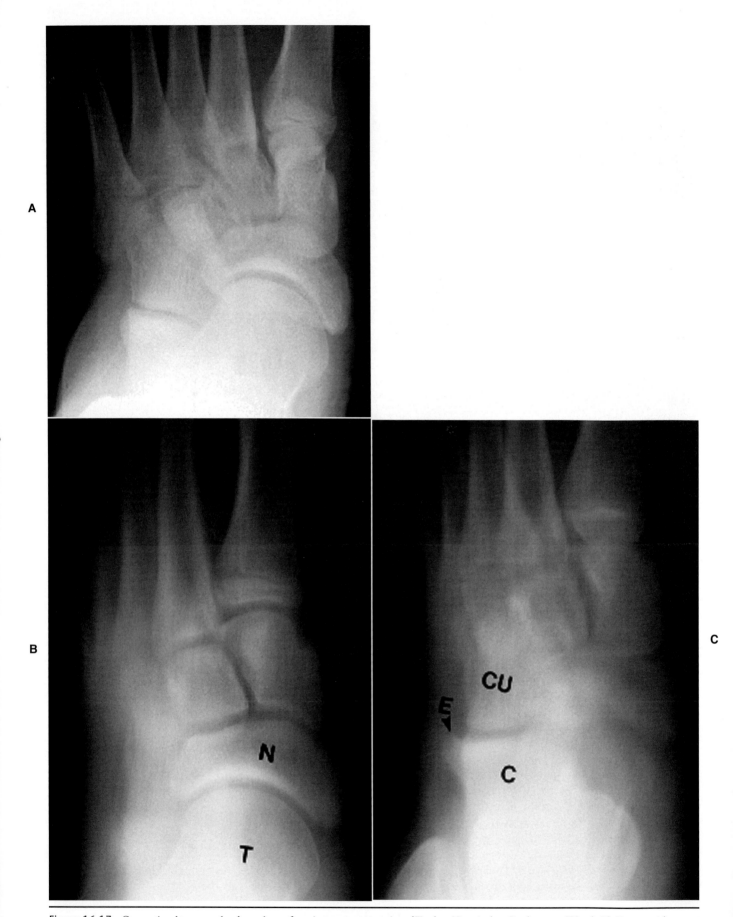

**Figure 16-17** Conventional tomography, dorsoplantar foot view, transverse sections (*T*, talus; *N*, navicular; *C*, calcaneus; *CU*, cuboid; *E*, exostosis). **A**, Plain film. **B**, Section at 7.5 cm (from sole of foot). **C**, Section at 5.5 cm.

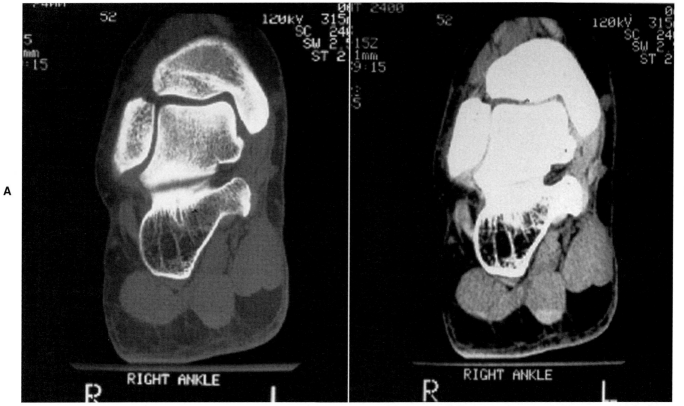

Figure 16-18    Computed tomography, ankle/rearfoot (coronal plane). **A**, Bone window. **B**, Soft tissue window.

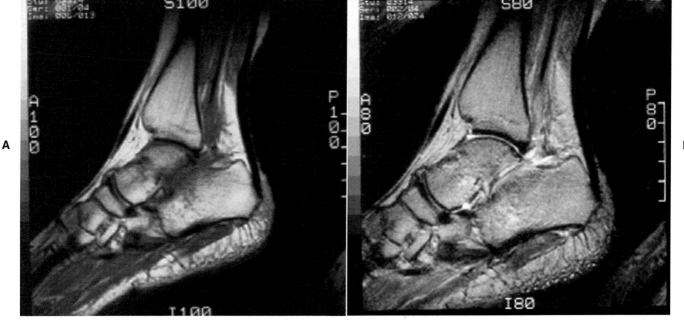

Figure 16-19    Magnetic resonance imaging, ankle/rearfoot (sagittal plane). **A**, T1-weighted image. **B**, T2-weighted image.

either of two methods: optical magnification or radiographic magnification.[124]

Optical magnification uses industrial x-ray film (such as Kodak Type M film) with a standard x-ray tube and high milliamperage. The object (the foot, in this case) is placed against the film as with standard positioning techniques. Industrial x-ray film has an extremely fine grain and sharpness; the final image is examined with the aid of a magnifying glass. However, the tradeoff is the amount of radiation or mAs required to expose this type of film. Because lower extremity–specific x-ray units are equipped with low mA settings (between 10 and 30 mA), the exposure time must be increased considerably to achieve adequate film blackening. (For example, a 100-cm source-to-image distance and 15 mA requires approximately 17 seconds exposure time with this type of film!) It is likely that patient movement, causing image blurring, will accompany high exposure time, defeating the purpose of using industrial x-ray film.

Radiographic magnification is performed with an x-ray tube that has an extremely small focal spot (100 μm). (The focal spot size of lower extremity–specific x-ray units is approximately 1 mm.) Because the object is placed at a distance from the film, a smaller focal spot results in less geometric blurring of the image than does the focal spot of standard size. Standard detail film is used with this technique. The object can be placed at any distance from the film, depending on the amount of magnification desired. The magnification factor is determined by dividing the source-to-image distance (SID) by the source-to-object distance (SOD).[125] For example, to obtain 3 times magnification of a phalanx with a 100-cm SID, the SOD must be 33 cm. The obvious disadvantage of this technique is the high skin exposure to ionizing radiation.

Radiographic magnification using a lower-extremity x-ray unit is not recommended. As noted, the focal spot size is too large (1 mm), which results in increased geometric blurring of the resultant image (Figure 16-20). Also, if

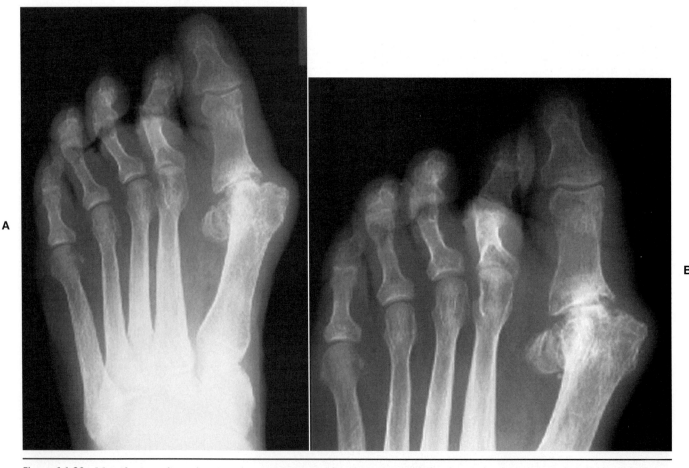

**A**

**B**

Figure 16-20  Magnification radiography using a lower extremity–specific radiographic unit (SID, 28 inches) and a 7-inch platform (SOD, 21 inches). **A,** Standard radiography. **B,** Radiographic magnification (magnification factor, 1.33). The resultant image using this equipment is less sharp than the standard study shown in **A.**

a magniposer[126] is used that raises the foot approximately 7 inches from the film, the magnification factor (MF) is not that significant (28-inch SID/21-inch SOD, 1.33 MF).

Indications for magnification radiography include the early stages of osteomyelitis[127] and rheumatoid arthritis.[124]

## Ultrasonography

Ultrasound uses inaudible high-frequency sound waves to produce an image; it is a form of non-ionizing radiation. A transducer transmits ultrasounds into the tissue; some are absorbed, others are reflected back to the transducer.[128] The procedure is inexpensive compared to MRI and can be performed more quickly.

Sonography can be used to examine any accessible soft tissues. Examples of pathologic conditions include soft tissue tumors, inflammatory changes, and trauma.[129] In fact, it appears to be becoming the initial method of choice for deep venous thrombosis of the lower leg.[130-132] However, tendons and muscle have only recently been investigated.[133] Ultrasound has been used to evaluate Achilles tendon pathology,[134-137] including complete and partial rupture (Figure 16-21), tendonitis/tenosynovitis, nodules, xanthomas, calcifications, and postoperative changes. It has even been recommended as a useful first-line imaging technique for evaluating Achilles tendon symptomatology.[138] Sonographic diagnosis of posterior tibial tenosynovitis has also been reported.[139] Recent pedal investigations include evaluation of Morton's neuroma,[140,141] plantarflexed metatarsal head position,[142] metatarsophalangeal and talocrural joint inflammation,[143] ankle ligaments,[144,145] and nonradiopaque foreign bodies.[146] It has even been used to assess leg length

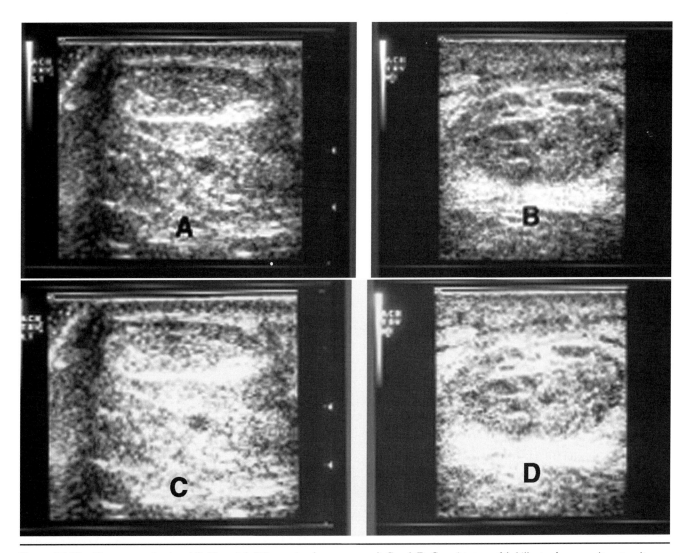

**Figure 16-21**    Ultrasonography. **A** and **B**, Normal Achilles tendon (transverse scan). **C** and **D**, Complete tear of Achilles tendon, opposite extremity. (Study courtesy Dr. L. N. Nazarian, Philadelphia.)

discrepancy[147,148] and tibial torsion.[149,150] Abiri and associates have found that the sonographic finding of fluid directly adjacent to bone is pathognomonic of bone infection in an animal model.[151]

The recent attention paid in the literature to ultrasonography of the extremities is exciting. As applications continue to be defined, its use may increase accordingly. Advantages include its use of non-ionizing radiation, widespread availability, time efficiency, and cost (especially when compared to MRI).

## Xeroradiography

Xeroradiography, although it uses x rays, is quite different from plain film radiography. The image receptor is an aluminum plate that is coated with selenium, a photoconductor.[152] It is then placed in a light-tight cassette. The extremity is positioned on the cassette the same as it would be for a plain film examination, and exposed to x rays to produce the latent image. The latent image is then transformed onto a piece of paper by a dry processing technique. The final image, compared with the plain film, has greater latitude, accentuates soft tissue and bone with similar emphasis, and enhances the edges of tissue structures (called edge enhancement)[153] (Figure 16-22).

Xeroradiography is primarily used for mammography. Although applications have been suggested for foot and ankle imaging,[154,155] it has not been widely used. In comparison to the plain film, applications for the foot and ankle may include soft tissue masses, subtle fractures, foreign objects, and early joint diseases. It also is useful for imaging an extremity through a cast. Disadvantages include its greater radiation dosage (compared with plain film radiography) and limited availability. The improvement and advent of CT and MRI studies, respectively, appear to have further assured its limited musculoskeletal usage.

## Fluoroscopy

Plain film radiography obtains static images of the skeleton. The primary function of fluoroscopy is to obtain dynamic

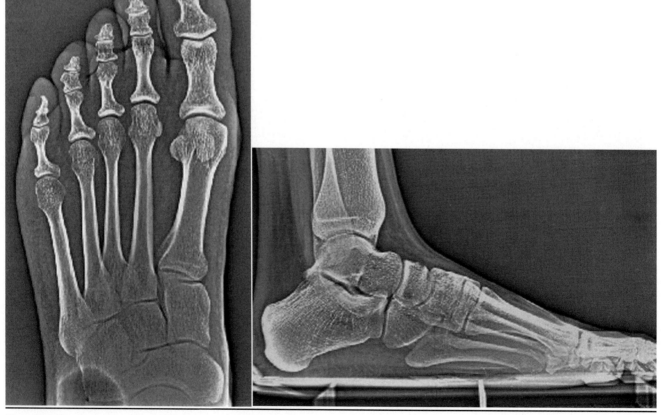

**Figure 16-22** Xeroradiography. **A,** Dorsoplantar view. **B,** Lateral view.

images, such as during angiography. It is especially useful in musculoskeletal applications for guidance of needle placement during arthrography, tenography, and bursography. Subtle fractures—those not seen with plain film radiography—may be picked up with fluoroscopy while the bone or joint in question is placed in different positions.[156] Fluoroscopy has also been used during surgical excision of radiopaque foreign bodies[157] and to evaluate sesamoid fracture/partite sesamoid disruption.[158]

## Low-Kilovoltage Radiography

Low-kilovolt radiography uses voltage in the range between 28 and 35 kilovolts. The tendons, tendon sheaths and joint capsules of the toes, and the Achilles tendon and retrocalcaneal bursa can be imaged with this mammography technique. Possible applications include periarticular edema and capsular distension associated with rheumatoid and seronegative arthritis, Achilles peritenonitis, and retrocalcaneal bursitis.[159]

## References

1. Simon RR, Hoffman JR: Radiographic comparison of plain films in second- and third-degree ankle sprains, *Am J Emerg Med* 4(5):387, 1986.
2. Smith RW, Reischl SF: Treatment of ankle sprains in young athletes, *Journal of Sports Medicine* 14(6):465, 1986.
3. Christensen JC, Dockery GL, Schuberth JM: Evaluation of ankle ligamentous insufficiency using the Telos ankle stress device, *J Am Podiatr Med Assoc* 76(9):527, 1986.
4. Sauser DD, Nelson RC, Lavine MH et al: Acute injuries of the lateral ligaments of the ankle: comparison of stress radiography and arthrography, *Radiology* 148:653, 1983.
5. Rijke AM, Jones B, Vierhout PAM: Stress examination of traumatized lateral ligaments of the ankle, *Clin Orthop* 210:143, 1986.
6. Seligson D, Gassman J, Pope M: Ankle instability: evaluation of the lateral ligaments, *Am J Sports Med* 8(1):39, 1980.
7. Rubin G, Witten M: The talar-tilt angle and the fibular collateral ligaments, *J Bone Joint Surg* 42A(2):311, 1960.
8. Cox JS, Hewes TF: "Normal" talar tilt, *Clin Orthop* 140:37, 1979.
9. Chrisman OD, Snook GA: Reconstruction of lateral ligament tears of the ankle, *J Bone Joint Surg* 51A(5):904, 1969.
10. Cass J, Morrey BF: Ankle instability: current concepts, diagnosis, and treatment, *Mayo Clin Proc* 59:165, 1984.
11. Weissman BNW, Sledge CB: *Orthopedic radiology,* Philadelphia, 1986, Saunders.
12. Grace DL: Lateral ankle ligament injuries, *Clin Orthop* 183:153, 1984.
13. Schoenberg NY, Beltran J: Contrast enhancement in musculoskeletal imaging, *Radiol Clin North Am* 32(2):337, 1994.
14. Kramer J, Stiglbauer R, Engel A et al: MR contrast arthrography (MRA) in osteochondrosis dissecans, *J Comput Assist Tomogr* 16(2):254, 1992.
15. Chandnani VP, Harper MT, Ficke JR et al: Chronic ankle instability: evaluation with MR arthrography, MR imaging, and stress radiography, *Radiology* 192:189, 1994.
16. Mayer DP, Jay RM, Schoenhaus H et al: Magnetic resonance arthrography of the ankle, *JFS* 31(6):584, 1992
17. Perlman MD: Usage of radiopaque contrast media in the foot and ankle, *JFS* 27(1):3, 1988.
18. Goldman AB: Arthrography for rheumatic disease, *Rheum Dis Clin North Am* 17(3):505, 1991.
19. Haller J, Resnick D, Sartoris D et al: Arthrography, tenography, and bursography of the ankle and foot, *Clin Podiatr Med Surg* 5(4):893, 1988.
20. Vogler HW, Bauer GR: Contrast studies of the foot and ankle. In Weissman SD, editor: *Radiology of the foot,* p 439, Baltimore, 1989, Williams & Wilkins.
21. Karpman RR, MacCollum MS: Arthrography of the metatarsophalangeal joint, *Foot & Ankle* 9(3):125, 1988.
22. Resnick D: *Bone and joint imaging,* Philadelphia, 1989, Saunders.
23. Gordon RB: Arthrography of the ankle joint, *J Bone Joint Surg* 52A(8):1623, 1970.
24. Freiberger RH, Kaye JJ: *Arthrography,* New York, 1979, Appleton-Century-Crofts.
25. Brostrom L, Liljedahl SO, Lindvall N: Sprained ankles. II. Arthrographic diagnosis of recent ligament ruptures, *Acta Chirurgica Scandinavica* 129:485, 1965.
26. Olson RW: Ankle arthrography, *Radiol Clin North Am* 19(2):255, 1981.
27. Heare MM, Gillespy T, Bittar ES: Direct coronal computed tomography arthrography of osteochondritis dissecans of the talus, *Skeletal Radiol* 17:187, 1988.
28. Destouet JM, Monsees B, Gilula LZ: Ankle tenography. In Goldman AB, editor: *Procedures in skeletal radiology,* p 679, Orlando, Fla, 1984, Grune & Stratton.
29. Reinherz RP, Zawada SJ, Sheldon DP: Tenography around the ankle and introduction of a new technique, *JFS* 25(5):357, 1986.
30. Reinus WR, Gilula LA, Lesiak LF et al: Tenography in unresolved ankle tenosynovitis, *Orthopedics* 10:497, 1987.
31. Black HM, Brand RL, Eichelberger MR: An improved technique for the evaluation of ligamentous injury in severe ankle sprains, *Am J Sports Med* 6(5):276, 1978.

32. Eichelberger RP, Lichtenstein P, Brogdan BG: Peroneal tenography, *JAMA* 247:2587, 1982.

33. Resnick D, Niwayama G: *Diagnosis of bone and joint disorders*, ed 2, p 2525, Philadelphia, 1988, Saunders.

34. Goldman F, Manzi J, Carver A et al: Sinography in the diagnosis of foot infections, *J Am Podiatry Assoc* 71:497, 1981.

35. Berquist TH, Hall BB: Interventional orthopedic radiology. In Berquist TH, editor: *Imaging of orthopedic trauma and surgery*, p 767, Philadelphia, 1986, Saunders.

36. Ayres M, Kanat IO, Joshi K: Sinography and methylene blue, *J Am Podiatr Med Assoc* 77(7):343, 1987.

37. Haller J, Resnick, D, Sartoris D et al: Arthrography, tenography, and bursography of the foot and ankle, *Clin Podiatr Med Surg* 5(4):893, 1988.

38. Resnick D, Niwayama G, editors: *Diagnosis of bone and joint disorders*, ed 2, p 303, Philadelphia, 1988, Saunders.

39. Frey C, Rosenberg Z, Shereff MJ et al: The retrocalcaneal bursa: anatomy and bursography, *Foot & Ankle* 13:203, 1992.

40. Reinherz RP: Contrast media in the foot, *J Am Podiatr Assoc* 72(11):569, 1982.

41. Ly PN, McCarty JM: Gangliography, *JFS* 31(1):52, 1992.

42. Settlemire WE, Beneson DE: Deep venous thrombosis and pulmonary embolism, *J Am Podiatr Med Assoc* 74:268, 1984.

43. Ben-Menachem Y: Vascular injuries of the extremities: hazards of unnecessary delays in diagnosis, *Orthopaedics* 9:333, 1986.

44. Mauro G, Yudkoff N, Resnick M et al: Arteriovenous fistula of the lower extremity, *J Am Podiatr Assoc* 70(12):614, 1980.

45. Bookstein JJ: Angiography. In Resnick D, Niwayama G, editors: *Diagnosis of bone and joint disorders*, ed 2, p 441, Philadelphia, 1988, Saunders.

46. Darcy MD: Lower extremity arteriography: current approach and techniques, *Radiology* 178:615, 1991.

47. Silver K, Sollitto RJ, Jamil Z: Digital subtraction angiography versus noninvasive testing in the vascular assessment of the ischemic foot, *J Am Podiatr Med Assoc* 26:217, 1987.

48. Wayrynen RE, Schwenker RP: Intravenous subtraction angiography, *Imaging Management* 3:1, 1981.

49. Sibbitt RR, Palmaz JC, Garcia F, Reuter SR: Trauma of the extremities: prospective comparison of digital and conventional angiography, *Radiology* 160:179, 1986.

50. Owen RS, Baum RA, Carpenter JP et al: Symptomatic peripheral vascular disease: selection of imaging parameters and clinical evaluation with MR angiography, *Radiology* 187:627, 1993.

51. Yucel EK, Kaufman JA, Geller SC et al: Atherosclerotic occlusive disease of the lower extremity: prospective evaluation with two-dimensional time-of-flight MR angiography, *Radiology* 187:637, 1993.

52. Dumoulin CL: Magnetic resonance imaging: today and tomorrow, *Nucl Med Biol* 21(5):683, 1994.

53. Settlemire WE, Beneson DE: Deep venous thrombosis and pulmonary embolism, *J Am Podiatr Assoc* 74:268, 1984.

54. Jacobson HG, Edeiken J: Radiological evaluation of the chronic venous stasis syndrome, *JAMA* 258:941, 1987.

55. Richlie DG: Noninvasive imaging of the lower extremity for deep venous thrombosis, *J Gen Intern Med* 8:271, 1993.

56. Bushong SC: *Radiologic science for technologists*, ed 4, St. Louis, 1988, Mosby-Year Book.

57. Brown ML, O'Connor MK, Hung JC et al: Technical aspects of bone scintigraphy, *Radiol Clin North Am* 31(4):721, 1993.

58. Wegener WA, Alavi A: Diagnostic imaging of musculoskeletal infection, *Orthop Clin North Am* 22(3):401, 1991.

59. Bonakdarpour A, Gaines VD: The radiology of osteomyelitis, *Orthop Clin North Am* 14:21, 1983.

60. Hughes J: Techniques of bone imaging. In Silberstein EB, editor: *Bone scintigraphy*, p 39, Mt. Kisco, NY, 1984, Futura.

61. Alazraki N, Dries D, Datz F et al: Value of a 24-hour image (four phase bone scan) in assessing osteomyelitis in patients with peripheral vascular disease, *J Nucl Med* 26:711, 1985.

62. Israel O, Gips S, Jerushalmi J et al: Osteomyelitis and soft tissue infection: differential diagnosis with 24 hour/4 hour ratio of Tc99m MDP uptake, *Radiology* 163:725, 1985.

63. Silberstein EB, editor: *Bone scintigraphy*, Mt. Kisco, NY, 1984, Futura.

64. Moss EH, Carty H: Scintigraphy in the diagnosis of occult fractures of the calcaneus, *Skeletal Radiol* 19:575, 1990.

65. Brown ML: Bone scintigraphy in benign and malignant tumors, *Radiol Clin North Am* 31(4):731, 1993.

66. Rosenthall L: Nuclear medicine techniques in arthritis, *Rheum Dis Clin North Am* 17(3):585, 1991.

67. Peters AM, Lavender JP: Uses of labeled white cells, *Br J Hosp Med* 48:40, 1992.

68. Roddie ME, Peters AM, Danpure HJ et al: Inflammation: imaging with Tc-99m HMPAO-labeled leukocytes, *Radiology* 166:767, 1988.

69. Karl RD, Hammes CS: Nuclear medicine imaging in podiatric disorders, *Clin Podiatr Med Surg* 5(4):909, 1988.

70. Alazraki NP, Fierer J, Resnick D: The role of gallium and bone scanning in monitoring response to therapy in chronic osteomyelitis, *J Nucl Med* 19:696, 1978.

71. Rosenthall L, Kloiber R, Damtew B et al: Sequential use

of radiophosphate and radiogallium imaging in the differential diagnosis of bone, joint, and soft tissue infection: quantitative analysis, *Diagn Imaging* 51:249, 1982.

72. Schauwecker DS: The scintigraphic diagnosis of osteomyelitis, *AJR* 158:9, 1992.

73. Alazraki NP: Radionuclide imaging in the evaluation of infections and inflammatory disease, *Radiol Clin North Am* 31(4):783, 1993.

74. Palestro CJ: The current role of gallium imaging in infection, *Sem Nucl Med* 24(2):128, 1994.

75. Sorsdahl OA, Goodhart GL, Williams HT et al: Quantitative bone gallium scintigraphy in osteomyelitis, *Skeletal Radiol* 22:239, 1993.

76. Larcos G, Brown ML, Sutton RT: Diagnosis of osteomyelitis of the foot in diabetic patients: value of [111]In-leukocyte scintigraphy, *AJR* 157:527, 1991.

77. Zeiger LS, Fox IM: Use of indium-111-labeled white blood cells in the diagnosis of diabetic foot infections, *JFS* 29(1):46, 1990.

78. Newman LG, Waller J, Palestro CJ et al: Unsuspected osteomyelitis in diabetic foot ulcers, *JAMA* 266(9):1246, 1991.

79. Rosenthall L: Radionuclide investigation of osteomyelitis, *Current Opinion in Radiology* 4:62, 1992.

80. Seabold JE, Justin EP, Marsh JL et al: Altered bone marrow activity: potential cause for false-positive indium-111-labeled leukocyte patterns in complicated cases of suspected osteomyelitis, *Abstract Radiology* 177:160, 1990.

81. Palestro CJ, Roumanas P, Swyer AJ et al: Diagnosis of musculoskeletal infection using combined In-111 labeled leukocyte and Tc-99m SC marrow imaging, *Clin Nucl Med* 17(4):269, 1992.

82. Datz FL, Anderson CE, Ahluwalia R et al: The efficacy of indium-111-polyclonal IgG for the detection of infection and inflammation, *J Nucl Med* 35(1):74, 1994.

83. Schlefman BS, Katz FN: Tomographic interpretation of the subtalar joint, *J Am Podiatr Assoc* 73(2):65, 1983.

84. Resnick D: Conventional tomography. In Resnick D, editor: *Bone and joint imaging*, p 98, Philadelphia, 1989, Saunders.

85. Sartoris DJ, Resnick D: Computed tomography of podiatric disorders: a review, *JFS* 25(5):394, 1986.

86. Adams JE: Computed tomography—applications to musculoskeletal disease. In Murray RO, Jacobsen HG, Stoker DJ, editors: *The radiology of skeletal disorders*, ed 3, p 1943, New York, 1990, Churchill-Livingstone.

87. Christensen EE, Curry TS, Dowdey JE: *An introduction to the physics of diagnostic radiology*, ed 2, Philadelphia, 1978, Lea & Febiger.

88. Andre M, Resnick D: Computed tomography. In Resnick D, Niwayama G, editors: *Diagnosis of bone and joint disorders*, ed 2, p 143, Saunders, Philadelphia, 1988.

89. Oloff-Solomon J, Solomon MA: Computed tomographic scanning of the foot and ankle, *Clin Podiatr Med Surg* 5(4):931, 1988.

90. Winalski CS, Shapiro AW: Computed tomography in the evaluation of arthritis, *Rheum Dis Clin North Am* 17(3):543, 1991.

91. Kerr PS, James A, Cole AS et al: The use of the axial CT scan in intra-articular fractures of the calcaneum, *Injury* 25:359, 1994

92. Bradley SA, Davies AM: Computed tomographic assessment of old calcaneal fractures, *Br J Radiol* 63(756):926, 1990.

93. Vannier MW, Hildebolt CF, Gilula LA et al: Calcaneal and pelvic fractures: diagnostic evaluation by three-dimensional computed tomography scans, *J Digit Imaging* 4(3):143, 1991.

94. Worthington BS: Magnetic resonance imaging of the musculoskeletal system. In Murray RO, Jacobsen HG, Stoker DJ, editors: *The radiology of skeletal disorders*, ed 3, p 1991, New York, 1990, Churchill-Livingstone.

95. Solomon MA, Oloff-Solomon J: Magnetic resonance imaging in the foot and ankle, *Clin Podiatr Med Surg* 5(4):945, 1988.

96. Tehranzedah J, Ker R, Amster J: MRI of trauma and sports-related injuries of tendons and ligaments. II. Pelvis and lower extremities, *Crit Rev Diagn Imaging* 35(2):131, 1994.

97. Klein MA: MR imaging of the ankle: normal and abnormal findings in the medial collateral ligament, *AJR* 162:377, 1994.

98. Kabbani YM, Mayer DP: Magnetic resonance imaging of tendon pathology about the foot and ankle. I. Achilles tendon, *J Am Podiatr Med Assoc* 83(7):418, 1993.

99. Kabbani YM, Mayer DP: Magnetic resonance imaging of tendon pathology about the foot and ankle. II. Tendon ruptures, *J Am Podiatr Med Assoc* 83(8):466, 1993.

100. Rijke AM, Goitz HT, McCue FC et al: Magnetic resonance imaging of injury to the lateral collateral ligaments, *Am J Sports Med* 21(4):528, 1993.

101. Schweitzer ME, Caccese R, Karasick D et al: Posterior tibial tendon tears: utility of secondary signs for MR imaging diagnosis, *Radiology* 188:655, 1993.

102. Oloff LM, Sullivan BT, Heard GS et al: Magnetic resonance imaging of traumatized ligaments of the ankle, *J Am Podiatr Med Assoc* 82(1):25, 1992.

103. Moore TE, Yuh WTC, Kathol MH et al: Abnormalities of the foot in patients with diabetes mellitus: findings on MR imaging, *AJR* 157:813, 1991.

104. Durham JR, Lukens ML, Campanini DS et al: Impact of magnetic resonance imaging on the management of diabetic foot infections, *Am J Surg* 162:150, 1991.

105. Beltran J, Campanini DS, Knight C et al: The diabetic foot: magnetic resonance imaging evaluation, *Skeletal Radiol* 19:37, 1990.

106. Sartoris DJ, Resnick D: Magnetic resonance imaging of the diabetic foot, *JFS* 28(5):485, 1989.

107. O'Hanlon JM, Keating SE: Osteomyelitis of the foot in diabetic patients: evaluation with magnetic resonance imaging, *JFS* 30(2):137, 1991.

108. Morrison WB, Schweitzer ME, Bock GW et al: Diagnosis of osteomyelitis: utility of fat-suppressed contrast-enhanced MR imaging, *Radiology* 189:251, 1993.

109. Wang A, Weinstein D, Greenfield L et al: MRI and diabetic foot infections, *Magn Reson Imaging* 8(6):805, 1990.

110. Nigro ND, Bartynski WS, Grossman SJ et al: Clinical impact of magnetic resonance imaging in foot osteomyelitis, *J Am Podiatr Med Assoc* 82(12):603, 1992.

111. Terk MR, Kwong PK, Suthar M et al: Morton neuroma: evaluation with MR imaging performed with contrast enhancement and fat suppression, *Radiology* 189:239, 1993.

112. Hoskins CL, Sartoris DJ, Resnick D: Magnetic resonance imaging of foot neuromas, *JFS* 31(1):10, 1992.

113. Ugai K, Morimoto K: Magnetic resonance imaging of pigmented villonodular synovitis in subtalar joint, *Clin Orthop* 283:281, 1992.

114. Konrath GA, Shifrin LZ, Nahigian K: Magnetic resonance imaging in the diagnosis of localized pigmented villonodular synovitis of the ankle: a case report, *Foot & Ankle* 15(2):84, 1994.

115. Terk MR, Kwong K: Magnetic resonance imaging of the foot and ankle, *Clin Sports Med* 13(4):883, 1994.

116. Schweitzer ME: Magnetic resonance imaging of the foot and ankle, *Magn Reson Q* 9(4):214, 1993.

117. Steinbronn DJ, Bennett GL, Kay DB: The use of magnetic resonance imaging in the diagnosis of stress fractures of the foot and ankle: four case reports, *Foot & Ankle* 15(2):80, 1994.

118. Santi M, Sartoris DJ, Resnick D: Magnetic resonance imaging in the diagnosis of metatarsal stress fracture, *JFS* 27(2):172, 1988.

119. Smith BG, Rand F, Jaramillo D et al: Early MR imaging of lower-extremity physeal fracture-separations: a preliminary report, *J Pediatr Orthop* 14:526, 1994.

120. Kabbani YM, Mayer DP, Downey MS: Avascular necrosis imaging with magnetic resonance imaging, *J Am Podiatr Med Assoc* 84(3): 1994.

121. Kerr R, Frey C: MR imaging in tarsal tunnel syndrome, *J Comput Assist Tomogr* 15:280, 1991.

122. Frey C, Kerr R: Magnetic resonance imaging and the evaluation of tarsal tunnel syndrome, *Foot & Ankle* 14(3):159, 1993.

123. Berkowitz JF, Kier R, Rudicel S: Plantar fasciitis: MR imaging, *Radiology* 179:665, 1991.

124. Genant HK, Resnick D: Magnification radiography. In Resnick D, editor: *Bone and joint imaging*, p 85, Philadelphia, 1989, Saunders.

125. Bushong SC: *Radiologic science for technologists*, ed 5, St. Louis, 1993, Mosby-Year Book.

126. Weissman SD: X-ray techniques. In Weissman SD, editor: *Radiology of the foot*, ed 2, Baltimore, 1989, Williams & Wilkins.

127. Lee SM, Lee RGL, Wilinsky J et al: Magnification radiography in osteomyelitis, *Skeletal Radiol* 15:625, 1986.

128. Dewbury KC: Ultrasonography in musculoskeletal disorders. In Murray RO, Jacobsen HG, Stoker DJ: *The radiology of skeletal disorders*, ed 3, p 2015, New York, 1990, Churchill-Livingstone.

129. Chhem RK, Beauregard G, Schmutz GR et al: Ultrasonography of the ankle and hindfoot, *Can Assoc Radiol J* 44(5):337, 1993.

130. Appleman PT, DeJong TE, Lampmann LE: Deep venous thrombosis of the leg: US findings, *Radiology* 163:743, 1987.

131. Gaitini D, Torem S, Pery M et al: Image-directed Doppler ultrasound in the diagnosis of lower-limb venous insufficiency, *J Clin Ultrasound* 22:291, 1994.

132. Derner R, Brantigan CO: Diagnosis of deep vein thrombosis using real-time B-mode ultrasound imaging, *J Am Podiatr Med Assoc* 80(10):531, 1990.

133. Fornage BD, Rifkin MD: Ultrasound examination of tendons, *Radiol Clin North Am* 26(1):87, 1988.

134. Blei CL, Nirschl RP, Grant EG: Achilles tendon: Ultrasound diagnosis of pathologic conditions, *Radiology* 159:765, 1986.

135. Fornage BD: Achilles tendon: ultrasound examination, *Radiology* 159:759, 1986.

136. Kälebo P, Allenmark C, Peterson L et al: Diagnostic value of ultrasonography in partial ruptures of the Achilles tendon, *Am J Sports Med* 20:378, 1992.

137. Koivunen-Niemela T, Alanen A, Viikari J: Sonography of the Achilles tendon in hypercholesterolaemia, *J Intern Med* 234:401, 1993.

138. O'Reilly MAR, Massouh H: Pictorial review: the sonographic diagnosis of pathology in the Achilles tendon, *Clin Radiol* 48:202, 1993.

139. Stephenson CA, Seibert JJ, McAndrew MP et al: Sonographic diagnosis of tenosynovitis of the posterior tibial tendon, *J Clin Ultrasound* 18:114, 1990.

140. Redd RA, Peters VJ, Emery SF et al: Morton's neuroma: sonographic evaluation, *Radiology* 171:415, 1989.

141. Pollak RA, Bellacosa RA, Dornbluth NC et al: Sonographic analysis of Morton's neuroma, *JFS* 31(6):534, 1992.

142. Graf PM, Farac K, Stess RM, Gooding GAW: High-resolution ultrasound in the preoperative and postoperative assessment of distal metatarsal osteotomy, *Invest Radiol* 23(11):827, 1988.

143. Koski JM: Ultrasonography of the metatarsophalangeal and talocrural joints, *Clin Exp Rheumatol* 8:347, 1990.

144. Friedrich JM, Schnarkowski P, Rubenacker S et al: Ultrasonography of capsular morphology in normal and traumatic ankle joints, *J Clin Ultrasound* 21:179, 1993.

145. Brasseur JL, Lazennec JY, Guerin-Surville H et al: Ultrasono-anatomy of the ankle ligaments, *Surg Radiol Anat* 16:87, 1994.

146. Gilbert FJ, Campbell RSD, Bayliss AP: The role of ultrasound in the detection of non-radiopaque foreign bodies, *Clin Radiol* 41:109, 1990.

147. Terjesen T, Benum P, Rossvoll I et al: Leg-length discrepancy measured by ultrasonography, *Acta Orthop Scand* 62:121, 1991.

148. Junk S, Terjesen T, Rossvoll I et al: Leg length inequality measured by ultrasound and clinical methods, *Eur J Radiol* 14:185, 1992.

149. Butler-Manuel PA, Guy RL, Heatley FW: Measurement of tibial torsion: a new technique applicable to ultrasound and computed tomography, *BJR* 65:119, 1992.

150. Joseph B, Carver RA, Bell MJ et al: Measurement of tibial torsion by ultrasound, *J Pediatr Orthop* 7:317, 1987.

151. Abiri MM, DeAngelis GA, Kirpekar M et al: Ultrasonic detection of osteomyelitis, *Invest Radiol* 27(2):111, 1992.

152. Bushong SC: *Radiologic science for technologists*, ed 5, p 336, St. Louis, 1993, Mosby-Year Book.

153. Genant HK, Andre M: Xeroradiography. In Resnick D, Niwayama G, editors: *Diagnosis of bone and joint disorders*, ed 2, p 125, Philadelphia, 1988, Saunders.

154. Winiecki DG, Biggs EW: Xeroradiography and its application in podiatry, *J Am Podiatr Assoc* 67(6):393, 1977.

155. Pagliano JD, Wexler CE: Xeroradiography for detection of neuromas in podiatry, *J Am Podiatr Assoc* 68(1):393, 1978.

156. Resnick D: Fluoroscopy. In Resnick D, editor: *Bone and joint imaging*, p 82, Philadelphia, 1989, Saunders.

157. Puhl RW, Altman MI, Seto JE et al: The use of fluoroscopy in the detection and excision of foreign bodies in the foot, *J Am Podiatr Assoc* 73(10):514, 1983.

158. Ward WG, Bergfeld JA: Fluoroscopic demonstration of acute disruption of the fifth metatarsophalangeal sesamoid bones, *Am J Sports Med* 21(6):895, 1993.

159. Fischer E: Low kilovolt radiography. In Resnick D, Niwayama G, editors: *Diagnosis of bone and joint disorders*, ed 2, p 108, Philadelphia, 1988, Saunders.

## Suggested Readings

Alazraki N: Radionuclide techniques. In Resnick D, Niwayama G, editors: *Diagnosis of bone and joint disorders*, ed 2, p 460, Philadelphia, 1988, Saunders.

Meschan I, Ott DJ: *Introduction to diagnostic imaging*, p 343, Philadelphia, 1984, Saunders.

Murray ICP: Skeletal scintigraphy in the investigation of disorders of bone. In Murray RO, Jacobsen HG, Stoker DJ, editors: *The radiology of skeletal disorders*, ed 3, p 1859, New York, 1990, Churchill-Livingstone.

# CHAPTER 17

# MRI/Cross-Sectional Imaging

DAVID P. MAYER • YOUSSEF M. KABBANI

The figures in the beginning of this chapter are normal cross-sectional MRI images selected from *Foot and Ankle: A Sectional Imaging Atlas*, by Mayer, Hirsch, and Simon (1993), reprinted with permission from W.B. Saunders, Philadelphia. Figures 17-1 through 17-6 are coronal views, Figures 17-7 through 17-12 are transverse views, and Figures 17-13 through 17-18 are sagittal views. Box 17-1 provides the label identification key. Immediately after the normal cross-sectional images are descriptions of the three diagnostic techniques, conventional tomography, computed tomography (CT), and magnetic resonance imaging (MRI). Following these descriptions is an overview of foot and ankle pathologies evaluated with cross-sectional imaging, including descriptions of characteristic MRI findings.

## ■ DIAGNOSTIC TECHNIQUES

### Conventional Tomography

Tomography is the technique whereby a predetermined plane of the body is demonstrated in focus on a radiograph.[1] Conventional tomography is a technique that produces differential blurring of tissues above and below the plane of section within the body. Hence conventional tomography is sometimes referred to as "motion-blurring tomography."[2]

In fact, conventional tomography doesn't truly visualize the layer of tissue of interest: It merely blurs out details above and below the plane of interest more than it blurs the plane of interest itself.[3] Thus the image formed by conventional tomography is less sharp than standard radiography. Its advantage is that the image is less obscured by structures that are located above and below the plane of interest. The further a structure is located from the plane of interest, the greater is the relative degree of blurring.[3]

Conventional tomography has three main components: the x-ray source, the object under study, and the recording medium (such as film). This process requires synchronous

motion of the x-ray source and the recording medium. Under ideal conditions, the structure under study should remain motionless.

Tomography takes two main forms: narrow-angle or thick-section tomography, which is also known as "zonography," and wide-angle tomography, which acquires thin-section images. Zonography is typically defined as between 1 and 2.5 cm in thickness, and wide-angle tomography lies in the range of 1 to 5 mm in thickness. High-contrast tissues (such as bone) are better imaged by conventional tomography than are soft tissues. The thinnest slices are acquired by use of complex-angle tomography, which is also known as "pluridirectional," and thicker slices are typically acquired by the more conventionally available "linear" tomography. Although the slices are thinnest with wide-angle tomography, the contrast is greatest with zonography (narrow angle). Pluridirectional tomography (thin-section, complex-motion tomography) produces in general less artifact than narrow angle, or zonography. A variant of tomography is "plesiotomography," which uses a book cassette, allowing multiple slices to be obtained in a single pass. This latter technique has some unfortunate tradeoffs in image quality.[2]

Newer techniques using digital acquisition and digital processing hold the promise of lower dose and improved contrast, and they may eventually create more indications for this technique. This new technique has been termed "tomosynthesis."

The indications for conventional tomography include

1. Scanning patients who are contraindicated for CT or MRI (for example, patients on life support and those with aneurysm clips or metallic fixation devices).
2. Localizing occult fractures, including stress fractures.
3. Defining the extent of known fractures.
4. Following the healing of fractures.
5. Diagnosing osteochondral fractures.

## BOX 17-1    Label Key for Figures 17-1 to 17-18

| | | | |
|---|---|---|---|
| ABH | Abductor hallucis | LTA | Lateral tarsal artery |
| ABM | Abductor digit minimi | M1 | First metatarsal |
| AHO | Adductor hallucis, oblique head | M2 | Second metatarsal |
| AHT | Adductor hallucis, transverse head | M3 | Third metatarsal |
| AJ | Ankle joint | M4 | Fourth metatarsal |
| AO | Accessory ossicle | M5 | Fifth metatarsal |
| ATF | Anterior talofibular ligament | MC | Medial cuneiform |
| BL | Bifurcate ligament | MMV | Medial marginal vein |
| CA | Calcaneus | MPA | Medial plantar artery |
| CCJ | Calcaneocuboid joint | MPN | Medial plantar nerve |
| CFL | Calcaneofibular ligament | MT | Medial tubercle of talus |
| CL | Cervical ligament | NA | Navicular |
| CU | Cuboid | OT | Os trigonum |
| D2 | Second dorsal interosseous muscle | P3 | Third plantar interosseous |
| D3 | Third dorsal interosseous muscle | PA | Plantar aponeurosis |
| D4 | Fourth dorsal interosseous muscle | PAC | Plantar aponeurosis, central part |
| DPA | Dorsalis pedis artery | PAL | Plantar aponeurosis, lateral part |
| DPN | Deep peroneal nerve | PB | Peroneus brevis |
| DPP | Deep plantar branch vessel | PCC | Plantar calcaneocuboid ligament |
| DS | Deep transverse intermuscular septum | PCN | Plantar calcaneonavicular ligament |
| EDB | Extensor digitorum brevis | PL | Peroneus longus |
| EDL | Extensor digitorum longus | PP | Proximal phalanx |
| EHL | Extensor hallucis longus | PT | Peroneus tertius |
| FDB | Flexor digitorum brevis | PTA | Posterior tibial artery |
| FDL | Flexor digitorum longus | PTC | Posterior talocalcaneal ligament |
| FDM | Flexor digiti minimi brevis | PTF | Posterior talofibular ligament |
| FHB | Flexor hallucis brevis | PTN | Posterior tibial neurovascular bundle |
| FHL | Flexor hallucis longus | PTT | Posterior tibiotalar ligament |
| FI | Fibula | QP | Quadratus plantae |
| FR | Flexor retinaculum | S | Soleus |
| HS | Heel spur | SNT | Sinus tarsi |
| IC | Intermediate cuneiform | ST | Sustentaculum tali of calcaneus |
| IER | Inferior extensor retinaculum | STJ | Subtalar joint |
| INT | Interossei | T | Talus |
| IPR | Inferior peroneal retinaculum | TA | Tibialis anterior |
| ITC | Interosseous talocalcaneal ligament | TC | Calcaneal tendon |
| L1 | First lumbrical muscle | TCL | Tibiocalcaneal ligament |
| L3 | Third lumbrical muscle | TCM | Talocalcaneonavicular joint, middle facets |
| L4 | Fourth lumbrical muscle | TCN | Talocalcaneonavicular joint, talonavicular part |
| LC | Lateral cuneiform | TI | Tibia |
| LPA | Lateral plantar artery | TIN | Tibionavicular ligament |
| LPL | Long plantar ligament | TN | Tibial nerve |
| LPN | Lateral plantar nerve | TNL | Talonavicular ligament |
| LPV | Lateral plantar vein | TP | Tibialis posterior |
| LT | Lateral tubercle of talus | | |

6. Localizing intra-articular osseous loose bodies. Intra-articular cartilaginous loose bodies are best diagnosed following intra-articular placement of contrast with arthrotomography.

7. Visualizing cortical disruption in lesions such as osteomyelitis.[4]

In routine practice, conventional tomography is commonly used for renal imaging with intravenous urography.

In general, when high-resolution multiplanar computed tomography (CT) can image the structure under study, the image quality for soft tissue and bone lesions is superior to that of conventional tomography. MRI of course adds the advantages of excellent resolution, multiplanar acquisition, no x-radiation, and superb soft tissue contrast. Among the disadvantages of MRI, and to some extent of CT as well, is their limited availability and cost. However, with the increasing clinical utility of MRI and CT the expertise and

*Text continued on p. 355*

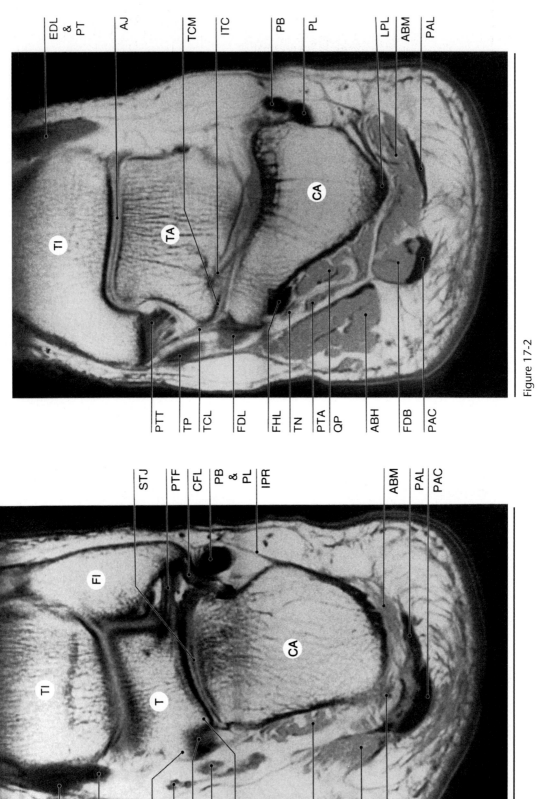

Figure 17-2

Figure 17-1

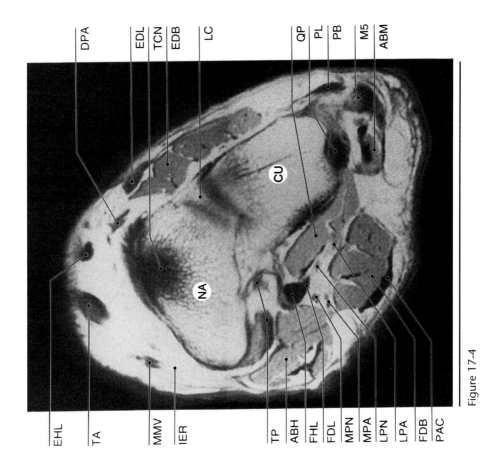

Figure 17-4

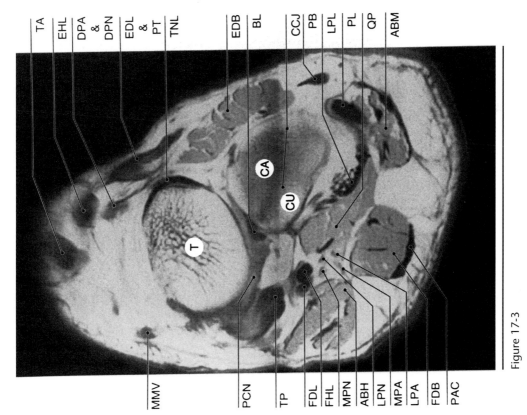

Figure 17-3

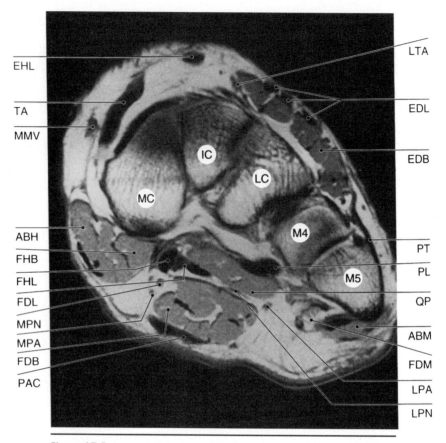

Figure 17-5

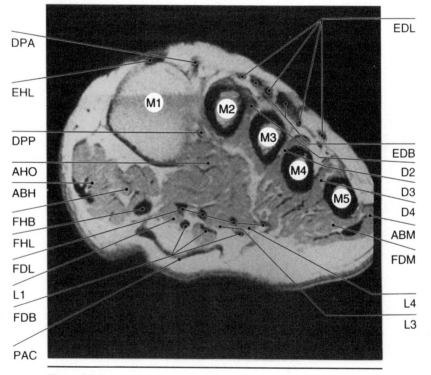

Figure 17-6

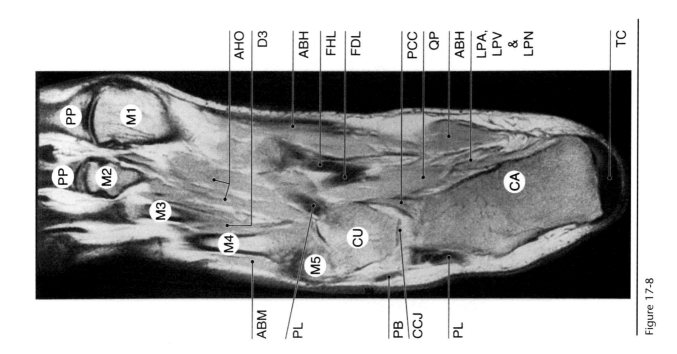

Figure 17-8

Figure 17-7

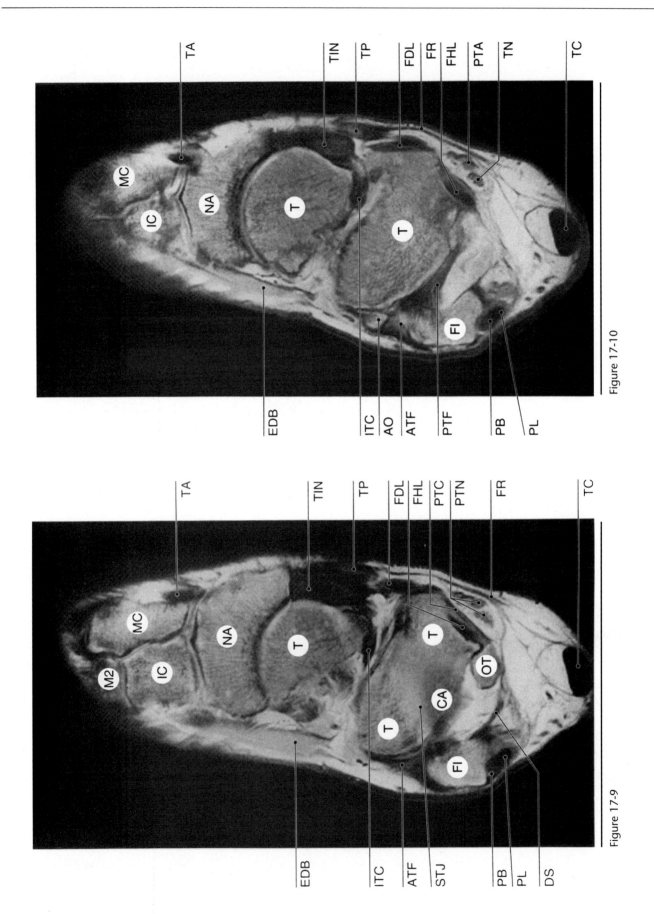

Figure 17-10

Figure 17-9

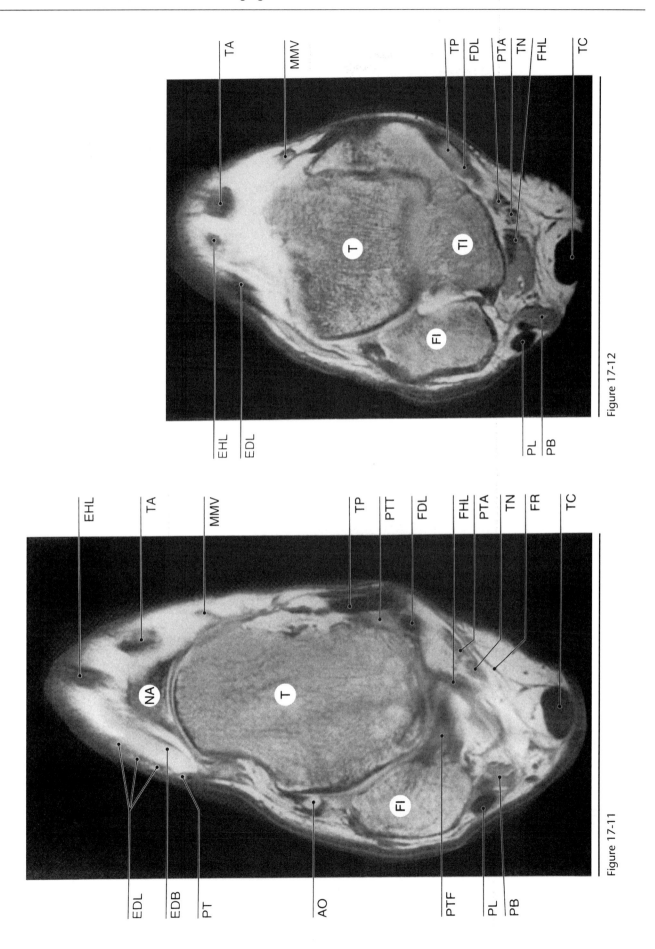

Figure 17-12

Figure 17-11

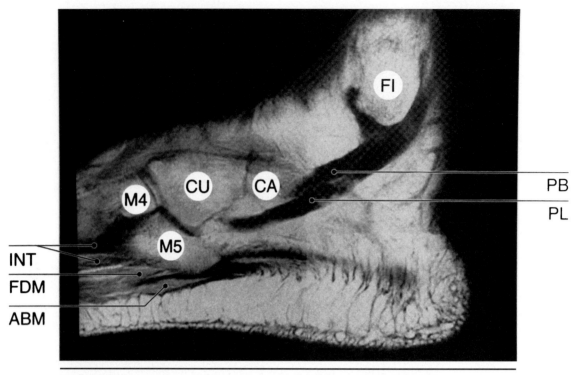

Figure 17-13

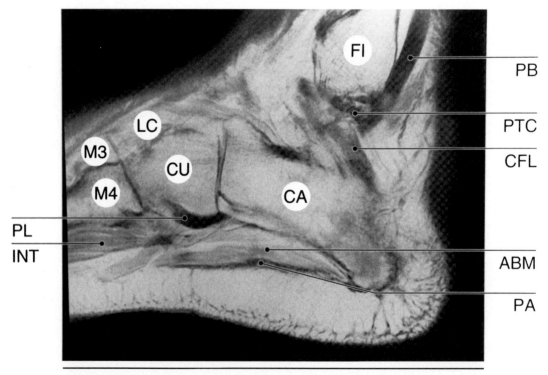

Figure 17-14

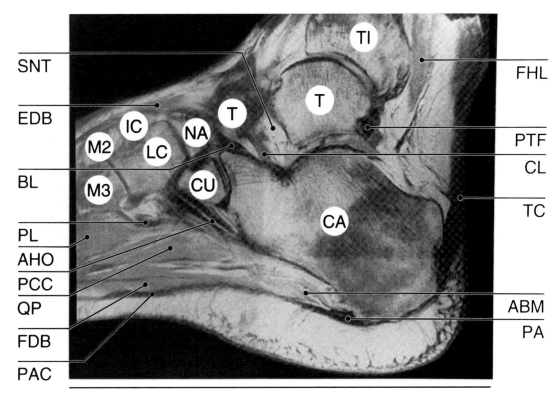

Figure 17-15

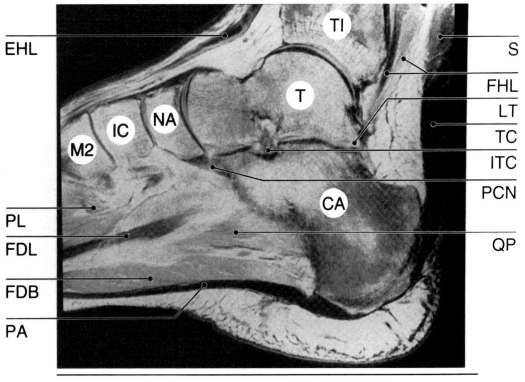

Figure 17-16

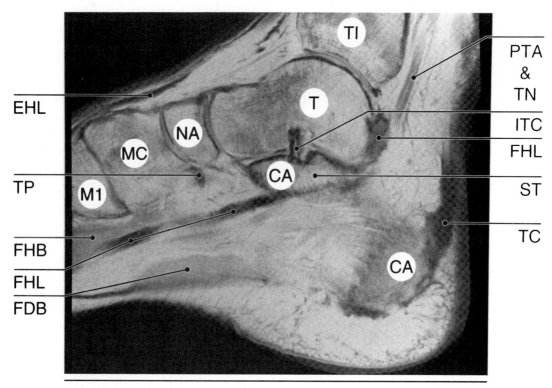

Figure 17-17

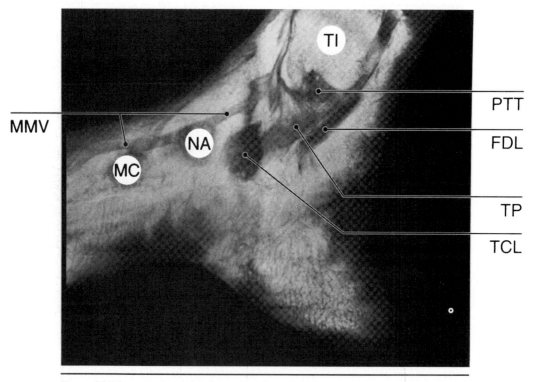

Figure 17-18

equipment necessary to perform conventional tomography is less available than previously.

Typical conventional tomography techniques for the foot and ankle include slice thicknesses in the 5-mm range with acquisition in the anteroposterior (AP) and lateral planes. The extremity position is optimized to demonstrate the lesion.

## Computed Tomography

Computed tomography (CT) of the foot and ankle uses direct multiplanar image acquisition with an ultra–high-resolution bone algorithm. The original raw data are then re-reconstructed, using the CT computer, with a soft tissue algorithm. A slice thickness of 2.5 mm is used routinely with an increment of 3 mm. Hence a 0.5-mm gap is not scanned between each CT slice and the next slice. Contiguous or overlapping slices can be acquired when computer-generated off-axis reconstructions are required. Images are routinely obtained in a minimum of two planes, such as sagittal and coronal, or coronal and axial. On occasion all three orthogonal planes may be required to define a lesion completely. Box 17-2 describes the views we currently use to image the anatomic regions of interest.

The patient is positioned as comfortably as possible, and then the foot/ankle is immobilized with cushions and tape. In our experience, the majority of patients (60% to 70%, unpublished data) are capable of being positioned for direct sagittal (parasagittal) as well as for more conventional axial and direct coronal images. A high–heat-unit x-ray tube with rapid computer reconstruction allows the data to be acquired quickly before patient discomfort causes loss of positioning and causes motion artifacts. The axial and coronal images are obtained following acquisition of a localizer image (computed radiograph). The direct sagittal images are obtained without a localizer. The typical x-ray factors are 240 to 315 mA and 140 kVp, with a scan time of 2 seconds.

---

**BOX 17-2**

| AREA OF INTEREST | VIEWS USED TO BEST DEMONSTRATE |
|---|---|
| Ankle (subtalar joint) | Sagittal, coronal |
| Calcaneus | Sagittal, axial |
| Metatarsals | Sagittal, axial* |
| Lisfranc joint | Sagittal, axial* |
| Foot | Sagittal, axial |
| Glass/foreign body | Sagittal, coronal (overlaps of one view) |
| Specific toe(s) scan 2.5 × 2.0 | Sagittal, axial* |

*In this view the gantry is tilted with regard to the foot and the bed is swiveled with regard to the arch.

---

## Magnetic Resonance Imaging

MRI is the best diagnostic radiology modality to image non-bony abnormalities because of its multiplanar imaging capability, superior soft tissue contrast, and noninvasiveness. Some facilities believe it is good practice to image both ankles simultaneously, because abnormalities are better seen as asymmetric patterns. However, imaging both extremities simultaneously inherently decreases image quality. Hence in most facilities only a single limb is imaged at a time. Bony changes such as osteoarthritis or fractures are visible on MRI or CT, but the capability to evaluate soft tissue changes associated with bone changes makes MRI superior to CT. With its excellent soft tissue contrast resolution and multi-planar imaging capabilities as well as lack of ionizing radia-tion, MRI has become the method most used in evaluating musculoskeletal disorders of the foot and ankle. MRI of the foot and ankle is typically performed on a GE 1.5 T Signa scanner with the send/ receive linearly polarized extremity coil with conven-tional and fast spin echo and volumetric gradient echo techniques.

Images may be acquired using a matrix of 192 × 256 to 256 × 256, and in some cases a matrix of 256 × 512 or even 512 × 512 can be used. Increasing matrix size causes diminution in signal to noise and also may require an increase in time of acquisition. Decreasing the matrix and increasing the field of view yields a faster scan with less noise but diminished resolution.

For typical ankle or midfoot study, a 12- to 14-cm field of view with a 192 × 256 or 256 × 256 matrix is employed. Slice thickness is 3 mm or less throughout. T1-weighted spin echo pulse sequences using TE = 20 ms, TR = 600 ms, and conventional T2-weighted spin echo pulse sequences of TE = 30 to 80 ms and TR = 2000 ms are typically em-ployed. Typically, fast spin echo (FSE) techniques include TE = 40/100 ms, TR = 4000 ms, flip angle 90 degrees, echo train length 8. The matrix is 256 × 256 with 1 nex. Images should be obtained in the optimal planes for the specific structures under study. The optimal plane of section should be chosen interactively on a localizer imager.

Additional three-dimensional volumetric acquisition using gradient echo techniques and with the following parameters are also used routinely. These techniques include TE = 10 ms, TR = 26 ms, flip angle 30 degrees, field of view 13 cm, and slice thickness 2 mm. These data can be placed into an off-line independent console and re-reconstructed in any desired plane.

## ■ TRAUMA

### Ligamentous Injuries

Ligaments are bands of fibrous tissue that connect two or more bones. The ten major ligaments of the ankle are the anterior and posterior (AP) tibiofibular, AP talofibular, calcaneofibular, calcaneonavicular, interosseous talocalcaneal, tibiotalar, tibionavicular, and tibiocalcaneal. However, the AP talofibular ligaments and the calcaneofibular ligament, which make up the lateral collateral ligament, are the ones most commonly injured.

Ankle sprains are the most common types of injuries to the ankle. Ankle sprains are injuries resulting from direct trauma to the ankle where ligaments sustain forceful flexion or stretching injuries. These ankle injuries are classified according to grades: Grade 1 represents mild stretching without ligament disruption or instability: grade 2 is marked by incomplete ligament tear, associated with pain, swelling, and ecchymosis, and grade 3 represents complete ligament tear.[5] Such injuries usually result from inversion and external rotation forces with the ankle plantarflexed.

The lateral collateral ligament is responsible for preventing inversion of the foot. Despite this strong ligamentous complex, the common mode of injury involving this ligament is inversion where the anterior talofibular ligament (ATFL) is injured. Of the three ligaments previously mentioned, the anterior talofibular ligament is most commonly injured. This ligament arises from the anterior surface of the distal fibula and inserts on the talar neck. On MR images the ATFL is 2 to 3 mm in thickness, of low signal intensity, extending obliquely in an anteriomedial course from the fibula to the talus.

The posterior talofibular ligament supports the calcaneus. Injury to the posterior talofibular ligament is rare; when it occurs, it is usually associated with anterior talofibular and calcaneofibular ligamentous injury. The calcaneofibular ligament is the strongest lateral ligament. In addition, these ligamentous tears frequently coexist with ATFL tears. Major injuries that involve these ligaments include complete ligament rupture or severe sprain from an inversion episode with associated hematoma and edema of the surrounding soft tissues.

CT has a limited role in the evaluation of ligaments with the exception of its ability to detect avulsion fragments and effusions and situations when arthrographic contrast (iodinated) has been placed into the joint space.

Because of their paucicellular fibrous composition, normal ligaments demonstrate low signal on T1- and T2-weighted images. On MRI most normal ligaments appear black, like tendons, as a result of their low water content. However, whereas most normal ligaments, including the normal talofibular ligament, display a homogeneously hypointense signal on all MR pulse sequences, the posterior talofibular ligament portrays a signal that is not homogeneous.[6] Size and orientation is an important consideration when MR is used in visualizing ligaments and similar structures. It is therefore essential to scan in the coronal, sagittal, and axial planes for optimal visualization of the ligaments and their associated structures.[7] The angle that the tendon makes with respect to the main magnetic field of the MR scanner can possibly produce variability in the signal intensity pattern of the ligament. This is the so-called "Fullerton" or "magic angle" effect.

Acute ligamentous tears (Figure 17-19) present as thickened or retracted structures with increased signal on T2-weighted images secondary to hemorrhage and edema.[8] However, the use of MRI has not become widespread in evaluating ligamentous injuries of the foot and ankle, because the anatomic complexity and small size of these body parts make it difficult to visualize small defects in their structural components. Such lesions are usually clinically diagnosed through physical examination and stress views using conventional x-rays studies. Therefore it has been recommended that ligamentous injuries such as partial and complete tears not demonstrated by MRI be visualized by arthrography and tenography.[9] In these cases MR arthro-

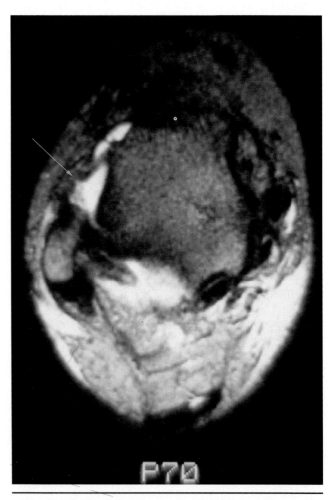

Figure 17-19    Axial T2-weighted image showing the complete absence of the anterior talofibular ligament secondary to a tear with joint effusion distending the capsule.

graphy (MRA) using a dilute gadolinium-diethylenetriamine-pantaacetic acid (Gd-DTPA) solution with saline (1:250 solution) may prove helpful as a substitute imaging modality for conventional x-ray or CT arthrography. Vicarious excretion of Gd-DTPA into joint spaces after intravenous injection has also been reported.[10] This may also prove helpful in diagnosing these injuries.

Contrast-enhanced MR imaging with intravenous Gd-DTPA is used when specific questions are raised concerning inflammatory and/or neoplastic process. In this case, 0.1 mg per kilogram is administered intravenously and images are obtained before and after contrast. T1-weighted postcontrast imaging with gadolinium is best performed using fat saturation techniques. This is because the gadolinium enhances the signal intensity of lesions that are already surrounded by the (enhancing) high-signal-intensity fat. Hence the net contrast is frequently diminished. By lowering the signal intensity of the surrounding fat, the enhanced tissue becomes easier to visualize compared with the relatively lower-signal (grayer) fat. MRI can thus define complete and incomplete disruptions or tears as well as inflammatory changes.

Minor ligamentous disruptions such as incomplete tears or inflammatory changes are usually successfully treated through conservative treatment; more serious ligamentous injuries usually require surgical intervention. Reruptures are common, especially in patients whose initial ruptures were treated conservatively. Follow-up evaluation may usually be successfully accomplished by MRI.

## Tendonous Injuries

Tendons are fibrous cords or bands that connect muscle to bone. Tendons consist of fascicles of very dense, nearly parallel collagenous fibers, elongated tendon cells, and a minimal amount of ground substance. As a reflection of their basic composition and low intrinsic water content, normal tendons demonstrate very low signal intensity on all MRI pulse sequences.[11]

The various types of tendon injuries include acute traumatic disruptions yielding partial or complete tendon tears, acute inflammation (tenosynovitis), chronic tendonitis and postsurgical abnormalities.[11] The most common type of injury is a traumatic defect that occurs in people engaged in physical activity. These injuries have become more common in the general population as participation in sports increases.[12] Tendon rupture may occur as an isolated traumatic event, or may be associated with a fracture with degenerative joint disease. Inflammation of the substance of the tendon is called *tendonitis*. As the condition progressively worsens, and the tendon sheath shows inflammatory irritation, it is classified as *tenosynovitis*. Certain types of tendon injuries may occur secondary to predisposing factors, such as infection, bone and tendon anomalies, altered foot mechanics, and neoplastic processes.[12] Clinically, there is restricted motion associated with pain, tenderness, and swelling.

**Achilles Tendon.**    Thirteen tendons cross the ankle. The tendons most commonly injured in decreasing order of frequency are the Achilles, posterior tibial, peroneus longus, peroneus brevis, and anterior tibial. With the exception of the Achilles, all tendons are enclosed in sheaths.[5]

The Achilles tendon, which functions to support dorsiflexion activity of the foot, is the largest and strongest tendon in the foot and ankle. This tendon is formed by the gastrocnemius and soleus muscles and inserts on the posterior calcaneus. The normal shape of the Achilles tendon on cross-sectional (axial) images is crescentic in shape with the convex surface posteriorly. Although it is the strongest tendon, it is the one most commonly torn in the foot and ankle.

Injury to this tendon results from athletic activity that involves forceful stretching with high-impact loading with the foot dorsiflexed.[8,13] Falling or landing on the forefoot, resulting in forceful dorsiflexion of the foot, may also result in Achilles tendon rupture. The typical location of the injury is between 2 and 6 cm proximal to its insertion. This site is said to be a vascular watershed, and the fibers from the gastrocnemius and soleus muscles are here obliquely oriented.[11]

Injury to the Achilles tendon is particularly common in people of 30 to 50 years of age who are not athletes and in cases where predisposing factors contribute to the injury. These factors include gout, systemic lupus erythematosus, rheumatoid arthritis, hyperparathyroidism, chronic renal failure, diabetes, and steroid treatment.[5,14] Males typically experience 80% of Achilles injuries.[11] Rupture of this tendon is not common in elderly people, because they do not engage in vigorous physical activity.

Patients with Achilles tears present with significant pain, occasionally with a palpable gap indicating a complete disruption. An accessory soleus muscle may sometimes be present, mimicking a mass or injury of the Achilles tendon. Patients with this anomaly may experience pain after exercising.[5] In some cases the tendon may be enlarged, with mucoid degeneration within the substance of the tendon.[11] However, as a result of soft tissue swelling even a complete defect may be difficult to diagnose by physical examination. Researchers report that as many as 20% to 30% of significant Achilles tears are missed clinically.[8,15,16] It has been well documented that MRI has proven effective in evaluating Achilles tendon disruptions.

**Posterior Tibial Tendon.**    Anatomically, the posterior tibial tendon passes through the flexor retinaculum and most commonly inserts on the tuberosity of the navicular bone and the first-metatarsal bone. Occasionally the posterior tibial tendon may insert along the undersurface of the bones of the hindfoot and midfoot. Functionally, the posterior tibial tendon stabilizes the hindfoot, supports the long arch of the foot, and aids in inversion. Rupture of this tendon yields progressive flatfoot deformity.[17]

The most common site of injury is posterior to the medial malleolus. Injuries occur at this site because of relative avascularity of the tendon at this site and the recurrent stress of the tendon against the bone of the medial malleolus with inversion and eversion motions. Of all posterior tendon injuries, 25% represent avulsion of the tendon from its insertion on the navicular. However, note that approximately 50% of normal posterior tibial tendons flare out in their distal aspect, thus increasing their diameter and displaying variable increase in signal intensity at their insertion on the navicular.[8,17,18]

Posterior tibial tendon injuries are generally classified into three types. Type I represents incomplete tear with fusiform enlargement (the defect is usually a longitudinal split).[17] This injury is usually associated with intrasubstance tendon fiber discontinuity. The inhomogeneous signal intensity pattern on MR images is frequently associated with peritendoneous fluid, which shows increased signal on the more T2-weighted images. A type II injury is characterized as a worsened, incomplete tear with decreased tendon caliber. A complete tear of the posterior tibial tendon is classified as a type III injury resulting in flatfoot deformity, weakness, and inversion of the foot. Associated with this complete rupture is pain, tenderness, swelling, and (usually) the presence of a tendon gap on palpation.[8,19,20]

Also note that although MRI is the study of choice to diagnose posterior tibial tendon tears, it has been reported that MRI may underestimate the extent of the tendon tear.[11,21] This limitation in part may well be related to technique.

### Peroneus Brevis and Peroneus Longus Tendons.
Anatomically, the peroneus brevis and peroneus longus tendons pass through the peroneal retinaculum and the retrofibular sulcus.[8,13,16,22] Injuries to these tendons typically occur posterior to the lateral malleolus. Minor injuries of the peroneus brevis and peroneus longus tendons usually include dislocations and inflammatory changes. Such minor injuries may occur through falls or may result from sports-related injuries. The mechanism of injury is similar to that of the posterior tibial tendon. Sports-related injuries are the most common source of trauma. These injuries are said to be secondary to violent reflex contraction of the peroneal muscles. If the injury is severe enough, it may also tear the peroneal retinaculum overlying these tendons. This allows lateral subluxation of the tendons.[8] Complete rupture of the peroneus brevis and peroneus longus tendons is uncommon.

However, when such rupture occurs the patient cannot evert the foot.

CT may be helpful in evaluating the peroneal notch, which is located along the posterior aspect of the distal fibula. Inadequate depth of this notch predisposes to lateral subluxation. CT can be helpful in evaluating this notch as well as disruption of the os perineum.[5]

### Anterior Tibial Tendon.
The anterior tibial tendon passes through the extensor retinaculum and inserts onto the medial and plantar aspect of the midfoot and proximal forefoot. This tendon helps dorsiflex the foot. Injuries of the anterior tibial tendon as well as that of the extensor hallucis longus and extensor digitorum longus tendons are usually associated with predisposing factors. These predisposing factors include previous fractures, degenerative joint disease, and running. Such injuries usually occur just distal to the extensor retinaculum.[5] Acute rupture of this tendon is usually rare, because ruptures normally occur through a chronic mechanism.[12] Chronic tendonitis and tenosynovitis, which have been known to occur secondary to downhill running and hiking, may contribute to rupture of this tendon. A complete rupture of this tendon clinically presents with a drop foot. This appearance can mimic the symptoms of an L4, 5 herniated disc. The typical patient is usually a middle-aged nonathletic individual.[8]

### Imaging of Tendon Pathology.
Computed tomography demonstrates tendons as round areas of increased density (relative to muscle) at the ends of their muscles, areas that are surrounded by fat and connective tissue when they are imaged distal to the muscle.[12] Although CT can accurately depict tendons, the surrounding fat and edema may obscure the site of injury. On the average, normal tendons measure about 75 to 95 Hounsfield units (HU), whereas ruptured or degenerated tendons should measure about 30 to 50 HU. CT has played a major role in the examination of bony ankle injuries; however, it provides limited information about the pathologic conditions of associated soft tissues. In addition, CT has not been reported to scan tendons consistently in the direct coronal and sagittal planes. However, with appropriate technology, equipment, and well-trained staff it is possible to acquire excellent direct sagittal and coronal images in most patients.[12] Although CT has been well documented to be excellent for depicting bony detail,[5] subtle injuries as well as total tendon disruptions are generally much better demonstrated on MRI.

MRI allows direct multiplanar imaging of tendons, ligaments, and associated structures.[18] MRI studies demonstrate normal tendons as black or very low in signal intensity. The higher the signal intensity, the brighter will be the pixel (picture) element on the scanner display screen or film. The low signal of normal tendons is due to their high collagen content and low water content. These normal tendons, with their low signal, are well contrasted against the surrounding high signal intensity of fat. A normal tendon in its sheath is surrounded by a very small amount of synovial fluid. On MRI this is demonstrated as a centrally located region of hypointensity with increased signal intensity material in the periphery secondary to fluid on the T2-weighted images. A tendon tear is demonstrated as an area of increased signal intensity internally on T2-weighted images within the substance of the tendon.

Injury to tendons is sometimes associated with increased accumulation of fluid and blood in the affected region. This is displayed as material of high signal intensity on T2-weighted sequences. Injured tendons are also well contrasted against adjacent edema by high signal intensity on T2-weighted images. Abnormal or disrupted tendons, in contrast, display higher signal intensity on all pulse sequences.

Partial tears (Figure 17-20) usually present as fusiform thickening and less frequently as focal, incomplete disruptions. Imaging in the axial, sagittal, coronal, and off-axis oblique planes is useful in detecting complete, partial, or old tendon tears.[5] A focus of increased signal within a tendon on all images, including the T2-weighted images, is more likely to represent a frank tear than is a focus of increased signal seen on only the T1 or proton density images. Partial and complete acute or subacute tendon tears exhibit increased signal intensity on MRI because of edema, fluid, or blood in the tendon substance.[5] Old tears usually appear thickened with areas of intermediate intensity within the substance of the tendons on MRI and have associated fluid accumulation in the tendon sheath.

Gradient echo techniques have been helpful in imaging slightly displaced tendons. Gradient echo techniques can be also used with volume acquisition techniques. Volume

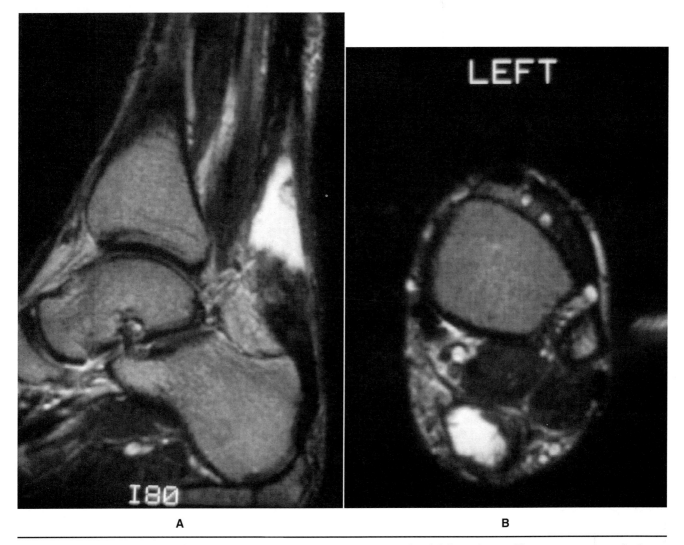

**A**                                        **B**

Figure 17-20   Sagittal **(A)** and axial **(B)** T2-weighted images in a patient with a near complete Achilles tendon tear. The paratenon appears to be the only part of the native Achilles tendon that maintains continuity.

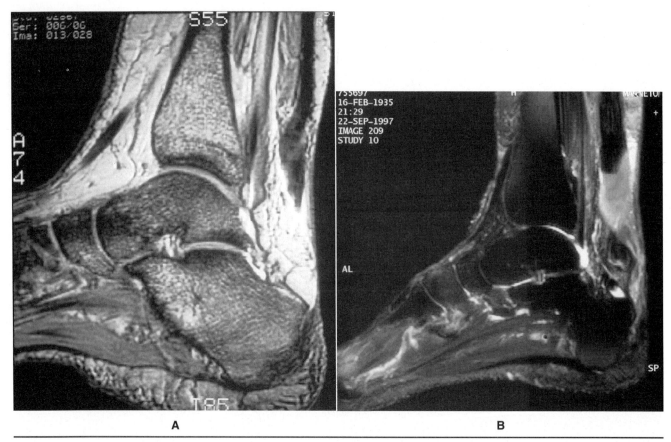

**A**                                                          **B**

Figure 17-21    **A** and **B**, Sagittal scans through the Achilles tendon in two patients showing the effects of complete tears and retraction of the proximal tendon.

acquisition techniques allow thin contiguous slices. These slices can even be less than a millimeter in thickness. These data can also be reconstructed in multiple planes on an off-line computer system.[5] Contrast enhancement for isolated tendon injuries is rarely required.

Tendon abnormalities on MR images are seen as areas of increased signal. Complete tears (Figure 17-21) present with increased signal on T2-weighted images as well as discontinuity of tendon fibers with widening of the tendon diameter and retraction of the tendons on the muscle side of the tear into the calf.

Tendonitis (Figure 17-22) usually yields a focal increase in signal within the tendon without a gap in the fibers, as well as an increase in tendon diameter. Further developments in coil technology may allow enhancement of signal-to-noise ratio, thus increasing the visualization of structures that may be difficult to see with existing technology.

## Fractures

Any bone in the foot may be susceptible to fracture; however, the metatarsals are the most commonly fractured bones. Metatarsal fractures commonly result from a direct blow to the foot. Inversion injuries generally lead to avulsion fractures involving the tuberosity of the fifth metatarsal. Phalangeal fractures are the most common types of injuries of the forefoot, usually occurring through toe stubbing. The other bones are less frequently injured. The tarsal bones are also fractured; the most commonly injured are the calcaneus and talus.

Fractures of the calcaneus are broken down into two broad categories, intra-articular and extra-articular. Intra-articular fractures of the body of the calcaneus account for about 75% of all calcaneal fractures, whereas extra-articular fractures account for about only 25%.[23]

Most fractures of the foot and ankle may be detected using plain radiography; however, the intricate anatomy of the talus and calcaneus, where most injuries occur, does not allow proper examination of multicurved cortical surfaces and overlapping structures. It is thus necessary to use a tomographic technique that allows evaluation of such bony structures and visualization of associated soft tissue. Thus direct multiplanar CT has proven beneficial in assessing fractures, because it can depict the bony anatomy of complex articular structures.

CT examination of calcaneal fractures may be accomplished in the axial, sagittal, and coronal planes. Coronal

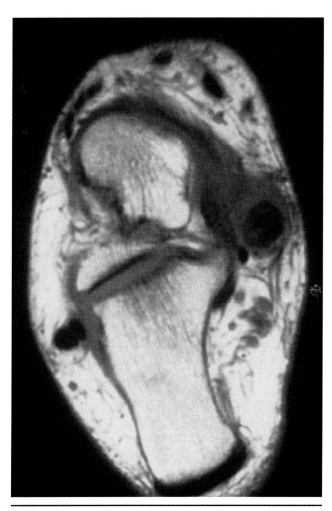

**Figure 17-22**  Axial proton density image through the ankle showing high-grade tendinosis (tendonitis) of the posterior tibial tendon with minor partial tear.

images are particularly useful for detecting disruptions of the posterior facet as well as widening or loss of height of the calcaneus. With proper technique, direct sagittal CT images can be accomplished in most patients. Such imaging adds additional information in evaluating the initial traumatic event as well as sequelae of the injury. It is important to select the appropriate scanning plane, because the information obtained may be of benefit in operative planning; however, patient discomfort and physical factors that may restrict movement may impose positioning limitations. Talar fractures have also been successfully detected with CT, because it shows intra-articular involvement and provides information on the extent of displacement. Whereas CT may adequately depict bony pathologies, MRI is particularly helpful in evaluating occult abnormalities that may be misdiagnosed or even missed entirely using conventional radiographic or CT techniques.

Subtle pathologic conditions such as occult cortical fractures, stress fractures, and osteochondral fractures have been reported to be successfully detected on MRI.[8] Fracture lines typically show decreased signal intensity that involves medullary space and cortex. The fracture line may be discontinuous. Usually signal intensity is increased next to fracture lines secondary to associated marrow edema and/or hemorrhage on T2-weighted images.[8] High-resolution MR images of the foot and ankle are usually obtained using T1-weighted (SE 600/20) and conventional or FSE T2-weighted (conventional SE 2000/30–80) spin-echo sequences in the axial plane using a small field of view and large matrix with thin sections. FSE techniques allow faster image acquisition with higher matrixes.[8] It is important to realize that although these are basic imaging techniques, the selection of other techniques in different planes depends on the specific clinical problems.

**Occult Cortical Fractures.**  In assessing occult cortical fractures, T1-weighted images in the axial, coronal, and sagittal planes demonstrate fractures of the talus and calcaneus well. The fracture lines are usually well defined and appear as linear areas of decreased signal intensity coursing through the medullary spaces and extending to the cortical surfaces on T1-weighted images.[8] These lines are well described on T1-weighted images because of the high contrast between the fracture line and the marrow fat. Soft tissue changes such as edema as well as bone bruises are well demonstrated on T2-weighted images.

**Stress Fractures.**  Stress fractures (Figure 17-23) occur as a result of repeated cyclic loading on bone. It has been reported that stress fractures account for about 30% to 40% of ankle injuries.[8] These types of fractures include fatigue fractures and insufficiency fractures. Fatigue fractures result from abnormal stress on normal bone, whereas insufficiency fractures result from normal stress on abnormal bone.

Fatigue fractures are common in people who are very physically active. Clinically, the patient has pain with tenderness and sometimes swelling is evident. Anatomically, the structures most commonly affected are the talus, calcaneus, distal tibia, and fibula. Researchers define two fracture patterns: The linear pattern is a well-defined zone of decreased signal surrounded by a poorly defined, less dark band on T1-weighted images. The linear band remains dark but is surrounded by a less well-defined zone of increased signal on T2-weighted images. The amorphous pattern displays a more focal globular focus of decreased signal on T1-weighted images. On T2-weighted images this globular focus presents as a region of increased signal. This pattern may also resemble a bone bruise.[24] MRI is at least as sensitive as nuclear medicine (bone scintigraphy) for detecting occult fractures.[8,25]

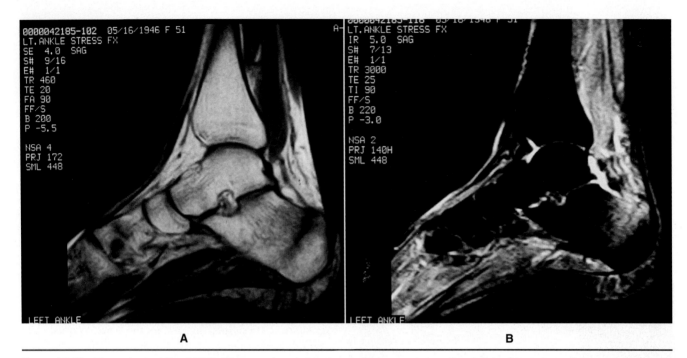

**Figure 17-23**   Proton density **(A)** and STIR **(B)** images through the calcaneus in the sagittal plane. A well-defined linear focus of abnormal signal intensity oriented perpendicular to the dorsal calcaneal cortex, almost always pathognomonic for a stress fracture, is demonstrated.

Insufficiency fracture is a specific type of stress fracture that occurs as a result of diminished bone mass, a condition termed *osteopenia*. Predisposing factors contribute to the osteopenic condition. Insufficiency fractures are common in the elderly, because these fractures are associated with osteoporotic conditions caused by disease processes that primarily affect older people. If the stress continues on the affected region, complete fracture may occur.

**Osteochondral Fractures.**   Osteochondral fractures, also termed *osteochondritis dissecans* and *transchondral fractures*, most often involve the talar dome as a result of trauma to this region.[8] Impactive loading resulting in laceration of articular cartilage and fractures of underlying bone is one of the major causative factors of osteochondral lesions.[8] Lateral osteochondral defects occur as a result of an eversion and dorsiflexion and compression on the middle third of the talar dome with impaction of the fibula, whereas in medial injuries they result from inversion, plantarflexion, and rotation forces that compress the tibia against the posterior third of the talar dome.[8] Previous trauma may cause 98% of lateral lesions and 70% of medial dome lesions.[26,27]

Osteochondral fractures are classified into four stages; stage I, localized subchondral trabecular compression; stage II, incomplete separate fragment; stage III, complete separation of cortical bone but nondisplaced fragment; and stage IV, completely separated free-floating displaced fragment.[8,27] Osteochondral lesions are also frequently associated with lateral collateral ligament injury. Lateral lesions have bone fragments displaced into the joint space more commonly than do medial transchondral fractures. Lateral lesions tend to be thinner (more waferlike), whereas medial transchondral fractures tend to be more spherical. Lateral lesions are more commonly associated with other foot and ankle injuries than are medial transchondral fractures.[26] Other etiological factors that may contribute to osteochondral lesions include ischemic necrosis, ossific abnormalities, hereditary predisposition, and hormonal and constitutional factors.[26,28–34] Typical age of involvement is between 20 and 35 years.[26,35]

Plain radiographs often fail to show osteochondral lesions, delaying diagnosis. In one series of 16 patients, 43% were initially misdiagnosed as ankle sprains.[26,36] However, CT has been reported as a valuable tool in detecting these lesions.[37,38] CT can demonstrate the full size and the extent of the lesion. Also, CT was helpful in determining the healing status of these lesions postoperatively[37] and excellent in demonstrating the complications of intra-articular free fragments.[39]

CT evaluation of talar dome fractures may be enhanced by injecting free air into the ankle joint prior to CT examination.[40] Nevertheless, stage I lesions are difficult to detect by CT, because this modality cannot readily demonstrate marrow changes. Detection at this stage is readily enabled by MRI, and, although nonspecific, by scintigraphy.

Osteochondral fractures of the talar dome (Figure 17-24) are best appreciated on coronal and sagittal MR images using T1- and T2-weighted imaging techniques. On T1-weighted images, stage I lesions reveal a decreased signal intensity, suggestive of trabecular compression. T2-weighted images may show an increase in the signal intensity secondary to bone edema. On both images the articular surface is intact.[38]

Stage II osteochondral lesions are best revealed on T2-weighted images and are characterized by the presence of a thin, irregular high-signal line at the talar interface with the fragment.[41] On T1-weighted images, the osteochondral junction appears as low signal intensity with an underlying low-signal region because of sclerotic bone.

Stage III lesions demonstrate a smooth high-signal line encircling the fragment, which represents joint fluid at the osteochondral junction.[42] This aids in differentiating between stage II and III lesions. The articular cartilage is seen as an abnormal contour thickening with an increased signal intensity.

Stage IV osteochondral fractures are best detected within the joint with gradient echo techniques. CT is superior to MR in detecting and localizing these free-floating fragments.[38]

MRI's high sensitivity permits one to predict fragment stability[26,43] as well as osteonecrosis, cartilage loss, and sometimes loose body formation.[8,31,34,44] Axial images do not demonstrate these lesions as well.

**Lisfranc Injuries.** The Lisfranc joint, also called the tarsometatarsal joint complex, is formed by the articulation of the five metatarsals with the three cuneiforms and the

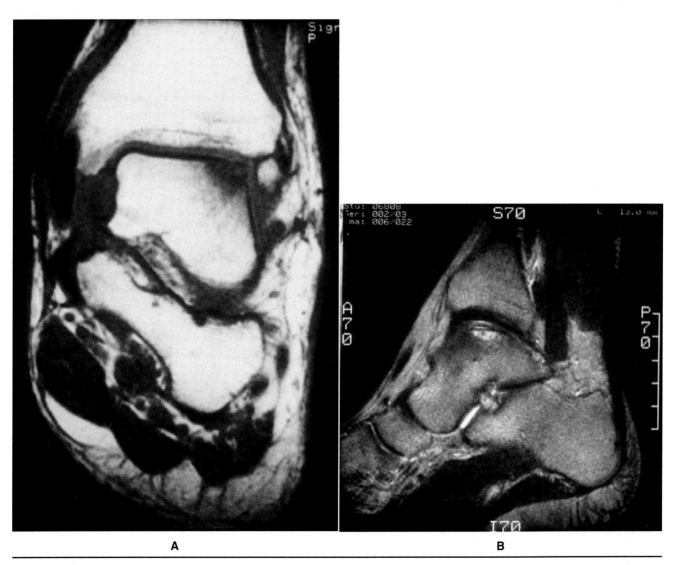

**A**    **B**

Figure 17-24    Coronal (A) and sagittal (B) T2-weighted images through the talar dome. A well-defined lesion in the subchondral bone of the talar dome secondary to a prior transchondral injury is demonstrated. A is suggestive of osteochondral defect, and B suggests a more common variety of posttraumatic transchondral injury.

cuboid bone. Injuries involving this joint are referred to as either Lisfranc fracture or Lisfranc dislocation. These injuries are named after the French surgeon Jacques Lisfranc, who first described amputation through this joint complex.[45]

Injuries involving the Lisfranc joint are rare, a number of studies have reported an incidence of 1 case per 55,000 per year.[46–49] Such injury may occur as a result of direct or indirect trauma. A heavy object striking the forefoot, often occurring as an industrial accident, is a classic example of direct trauma. Indirect injuries include a fall from a height or a fall down a flight of stairs.

The patient with a Lisfranc injury may present with pain, edema, and hematoma of the forefoot. There may be anterior and posterior shortening of the foot and transversal broadening of the foot.[46] In addition, the Lisfranc joint area shows a pathological range of motion.

The original system for classifying Lisfranc injuries presented by Quenu and Kuss in 1909 has been for the most part accepted, and it is simple to apply. A modification to this classification system, described by Hardcastle and associates, has been most commonly used.[50]

This currently used classification scheme divides Lisfranc injuries into three types:

*Type A:* Incongruity of the entire tarsometatarsal joint complex with segment displacement in one plane
*Type B:* Partial incongruity of the joint complex with medial or lateral displacement of the segment
*Type C:* Partial or total incongruity where the first metatarsal is displaced medially and the lateral four metatarsals are displaced laterally

Identifying abnormalities in the Lisfranc area depends on a thorough understanding of the normal anatomy of the joint complex. Evaluation includes radiographically observing the alignment of the metatarsals with the tarsal bones.

Reports indicate that Lisfranc injuries are overlooked on initial radiographs in as many as 20% of the cases.[46,51] The most constant and reliable radiographic sign is separation between the bases of the first and second metatarsals. Routine dorsoplantar, oblique, and lateral views are usually adequate to visualize pathologic conditions involving the tarsometatarsal joint complex. Careful observation of plain radiographs allows detection of misalignment of the metatarsal and tarsal bones that suggests subluxation and hypermobility of the Lisfranc joint. In general, radiographic evaluation of Lisfranc joint injuries include dorsoplantar views for detecting large metatarsal subluxations, oblique, and lateral views for visualizing tarsal dislocations and fractures of the cuboid bone, and lateral views for depicting cuneiform and navicular dislocation.

CT evaluation allows detection of overlapping between the metatarsals and tarsal bones. CT allows assessment of the definition of cortical margins of the tarsal bones.[52]

Congruity of the articular surfaces may also be assessed. Axial CT scans can show dorsolateral dislocations of the metatarsal bases in a type C injury. Axial scans can also detect fractures of the cuneiforms and cuboid bones. Sagittal or coronal CT scans allow evaluation of any vertical displacement about the Lisfranc joint that may not be adequately detected on axial scans.

**Ankle Fractures.**    Ankle fractures are those fractures occurring about the distal tibia and fibula. Most ankle fractures occur as a result of inversion or eversion forces that in turn occur as a result of falling with the foot firmly planted. Patients may present with pain, swelling, and ecchymosis. Weight bearing may not be possible with unstable fractures.

A number of classification schemes have been used in categorizing ankle fractures.[53–56] The more commonly used scheme is that proposed by Lauge-Hansen.[53] The Lauge-Hansen system is a two-word scheme in which the first word indicates the first position of the foot at the time of injury and the second indicates the direction of the injuring force. Based on this system, the ankle injuries are categorized into four major categories. Within each category are different levels of injury. The Lauge-Hansen classification scheme is as follows:

**Pronation-Abduction:**
*Stage 1:* Transverse fracture of the medial malleolus or rupture of the deltoid ligament
*Stage 2:* Disruption of anteroposterior tibiofibular ligaments with fracture of the posterior tibia
*Stage 3:* Oblique fibular fracture at the joint level

**Pronation-Lateral Rotation:**
*Stage 1:* Rupture of deltoid ligament with fracture of the medial malleolus
*Stage 2:* Disruption of the anterior tibiofibular ligament and interosseous membrane
*Stage 3:* Spiral fracture of the fibula (usually 6 cm above the ankle joint)
*Stage 4:* Fracture of the posterior tibia or rupture of the posterior tibiofibular ligament

**Supination-Adduction:**
*Stage 1:* Lateral ligament injury or lateral malleolus fracture
*Stage 2:* Near-vertical oblique fracture of the medial malleolus

**Supination-Lateral Rotation:**
*Stage 1:* Rupture of the anterior tibiofibular ligament
*Stage 2:* Spiral fracture of the lateral malleolus
*Stage 3:* Rupture of posterior tibiofibular ligament
*Stage 4:* Fracture of the medial malleolus

In terms of incidence, the supination-lateral injuries account for about 55% to 58% of ankle fractures followed by a supination-adduction injuries, occurring in 18% to 21% of ankle fractures, and the pronation injuries, which account for 20% of ankle fractures.[57]

Plain radiographs are sufficient for evaluating most ankle fractures. The AP, lateral, mortise, and external oblique views provide information regarding the degree of bony involvement.[54,58] The fibula is of paramount importance in classification, because injury to the fibula may indicate the direction of force.[59] The lateral view is useful in detecting anteroposterior tibial avulsion fractures as well as fibular fractures. The mortise view is helpful in evaluating talar asymmetry. In the AP view oblique fibular fracture and avulsion fractures of the tibia and fibula may be visualized. The external oblique view is useful in detecting posterior tibial fractures.

CT evaluation includes axial, coronal, and sagittal scanning where the CT images can characterize fibular articulations. CT images may help in assessing talofibular joint congruity, owing to CT's multiplanar imaging capability. Widening of the tibiofibular space in external rotation injuries may also be demonstrated on the CT images. Assessment of the overall asymmetry of the ankle joint may be achieved via coronal CT imaging with comparison to the contralateral ankle.

## Nonunions

Failure of a fracture or osteotomy to heal or show no propensity toward healing is called a nonunion. The time lapse in diagnosing this entity varies in the literature[60–63]; between 6 and 9 months is more or less indicative of a nonunion. The text *Campbell's Operative Orthopedics* places an arbitrary time for nonunion of 6 months.[64]

Nonunions result from various causes, which include disruption of blood supply, infections, excess motion, soft tissue interposition, comminution, and devitalization of the tissues surrounding the fracture.[65] Systemic factors have also been implicated, including diabetes mellitus, anemia, and growth hormones.[66–68]

Nonunions are divided into two groups: avascular and hypervascular.[69] Each group possesses certain pathologic and radiographic characteristics (see Chapter 18).

Standard radiographs are the initial means of diagnosing a nonunion. The absence of sclerotic borders across the osteotomy or the evidence of a void is pathognomonic of a diagnosis of nonunion. Diagnostic studies used to assess nonunion include fluoroscopy, scintigraphy,[70,71] and more recently CT and MRI.

## Bone Bruises

Bone bruises were first described in the knee.[17] By definition bone bruises are confined to the medullary bone, whereas the cortex and articular cartilage are intact. Bone bruises are believed to be self-limiting and typically benign.[72] Bone bruises of the foot and ankle are not as common as traumatic knee injuries that result in bone bruises.[17,72,73]

Pathologically, the trabeculae are disrupted, with edema and hemorrhage. Although little is known of bone bruises in terms of specific causative factors, it has been assumed that the major cause of this lesion is acute trauma.

The lesion may be seen as an area of decreased signal intensity that is poorly defined on T1-weighted images. On T2-weighted images, these lesions demonstrate regions of nonhomogeneously increased signal. The epiphyseal region is primarily affected, and the metaphyseal zone is secondarily affected.

## Foreign Bodies

Glass and wood are the two most common foreign objects found in the feet. To aid surgical removal, it is important to visualize foreign objects and precisely localize them. Foreign bodies are frequently visible with plain radiography; however, many objects are not easily detected by conventional means.

CT and MR have been used to detect foreign objects. CT provides excellent contrast between the foreign bodies and the soft tissues and thus is well suited for localizing foreign objects. For imaging foreign bodies, CT depends on differences of attenuation and MR relies on differences in proton density and T1 and T2 relaxation values. In acute cases, wooden objects on CT images appear as areas of low attenuation whereas chronically retained wooden objects are seen as areas of high attenuation. Glass objects are easily seen on CT images, because CT is roughly 10 times more sensitive for differences in density (linear attenuation) than conventional x-rays radiology. Thus foreign bodies should be studied by CT if plain films fail to adequately localize them. With multiplanar imaging and excellent soft tissue contrast, MR may also be able to localize foreign objects as well as visualize adjacent structures such as neurovascular bundles and assess soft tissue changes caused by these foreign bodies. Glass objects are demonstrated as signal voids on MR. In acute cases, wooden objects are also demonstrated as signal voids.

## ■ PLANTAR FASCIAL DISEASES

### Plantar Fasciitis and Heel Pain Syndrome

Plantar fasciitis is inflammation of the plantar fascia. This condition usually results from repetitive stresses on the plantar fascia, that result in microtears and subsequent fascial and perifascial inflammation.[74–77] True plantar fasciitis clinically presents with pain of the plantar fascia along its entire course, especially over the mid-foot area.[78]

Unlike heel pain syndrome, plantar fasciitis pain is exacerbated on dorsiflexion of the digits and pain on palpation along the course of the fascia.[79] This contrasts to heel pain syndrome, where fatigue fractures or periostitis of the medial calcaneal tuberosity occur at the attachment site of the plantar fascia.

For evaluating the plantar fascia and its afflictions, plain films aid in diagnosing heel spurs or fatigue fractures of the calcaneus. Bone scans may aid in the diagnosis.[80]

Recently Berkowitz and associates[81] reported on the imaging of plantar fasciitis. On MRI, normal plantar fascia appeared as a homogeneous low-signal-intensity band with uniform thickness. Flaring of the fascia was noted at its attachment. The normal plantar fascia had a thickness of 3.22 mm ±0.44 mm on sagittal images and 3.44 mm ±0.53 mm in the coronal plane.

In the symptomatic feet, the plantar fascia was significantly thickened (Figure 17-25). The mean thickness was noted to be 7.40 mm ±1.17 mm on sagittal images and 7.56 mm ±1.01 mm in the coronal plane. On proton density and T2-weighted images, areas of increased signal intensity were noted in the regions of fascial thickening. This finding was also associated with plantar subcutaneous edema, which appears as high signal intensity on T2-weighted images.

## Plantar Fascial Tears and Ruptures

Unlike plantar fasciitis, plantar fascial ruptures and partial tears are considered uncommon. Few cases have been reported in the literature.[82]

Plantar fascial rupture occurs more commonly among athletes, especially runners. The patient usually describes pain and tenderness that limits his or her activity. Physical examination of the plantar aspect of the foot reveals a palpable mass at the site of the rupture. The mass is tender to palpation and is usually localized to the medial band of the plantar fascia. Local signs of inflammation are usually present. Dorsiflexion of the digits exacerbates the symptoms.

Chronic repetitive stresses and minor repetitive trauma contribute to the etiology of these tears. Steroid injections have also been implicated.[13] Steroids have been shown to cause focal necrosis of the collagenous tissues. Cases of tendon ruptures as a result of systemic and localized steroid use and inflammatory conditions have been reported.[83]

## Plantar Fibromatosis

Plantar fibromatosis (Figure 17-26) is a soft tissue lesion that belongs to a diverse group of tumors collectively called the fibromatoses. Considered a superficial lesion, plantar fibromatosis (also known as Ledderhose's disease) usually involves the medial aspect of the plantar aponeurosis. Most lesions are unilateral and can be bilateral in up to 25% of the cases.[84]

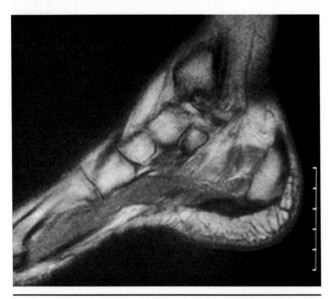

**Figure 17-25**  Sagittal T1-weighted image through the proximal plantar fascia showing the typical signs of plantar fasciitis: thickening and increase in signal intensity of the proximal plantar fascia.

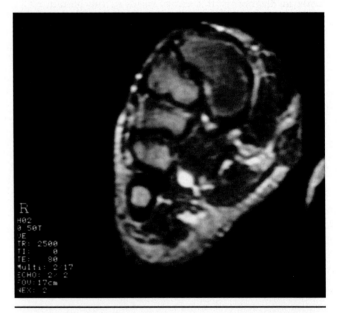

**Figure 17-26**  Coronal T2-weighted image of the midfoot. The lesion arising from the plantar fascia represents a typical plantar fibroma. It is relatively low in signal intensity due to its fibrous content. Note the absence of adjacent edema and local infiltration. The lesion is well defined, which is typical of a benign mass.

Clinically, plantar fibromatosis presents as a nodular growth on the plantar medial aspect of the foot. The lesion is firm to palpation and varies in size. Except for pressure from weight bearing, the tumor is painless and commonly recurs after local excision.

Aggressive fibromatosis or extra-abdominal dermoid is considered a deep counterpart of the superficial plantar fibromatosis. This lesion can also occur in the foot,[85] is considered rare,[86] and is highly aggressive. Unlike the superficial lesion, aggressive fibromatosis invades the local musculature and erodes the neighboring bone, causing significant destruction and deformity.

On T1-weighted MRI the superficial fibromatosis lesions appear as low-intensity nodular thickening on the medial aspect of the plantar aponeurosis. This decreased signal has been attributed to the relative acellularity and abundant collagen of this lesion.[87] On T2-weighted images the lesion demonstrates low to medium signal intensity.[88]

T2-weighted images of aggressive plantar fibromatosis demonstrates high- and low-intensity areas within the mass. Poor margination, nonhomogeneity, and bone invasion are usually seen. These MRI characteristics make it difficult to distinguish an aggressive fibromatosis from a malignant process.

## ■ INFECTION

### Cellulitis and Soft Tissue Abscess

Cellulitis is a deep infection of the skin resulting in a localized area of erythema.[89] In adults, cellulitis most frequently affects the lower legs and is a frequent finding among diabetic patients.[90,91] Although considered a clinical diagnosis, cellulitis of the foot and ankle can easily disguise an underlying abscess and/or osteomyelitis. In addition, because cellulitis is managed with antibiotics and local modalities, differentiating it from a deeper abscess is crucial, especially when the diagnosis is complicated by vascular and neurologic compromise.

Commonly employed imaging techniques employed for detecting soft tissue infections include plain x-ray studies, scintigraphy, CT, and more recently MRI.

A primary drawback of plain film radiography in evaluating soft tissue infection is the lack of early findings and limited soft tissue contrast resolution. Radionuclide scanning lacks resolution and is subject to high numbers of false positive and negative results.[92] The literature is lacking on the utility of CT scans in evaluating diabetic foot infections.[93] Gas and water attenuation material (abscess) can be detected. However, distinguishing abscesses or cellulitis from the surrounding issues is frequently difficult.

The unique ability of MRI to demonstrate soft tissue inflammatory conditions, and its high spatial and excellent contrast resolution, makes MRI an ideal tool for evaluating soft tissue infections.[94-98]

MR techniques for imaging soft tissue infections of the foot include the use of T1, T2, and STIR pulse sequences acquired with high resolution, and small fields of view.[99] Post-Gd-DPTA T1-weighted images with fat saturation are also quite helpful. Cellulitis is demonstrated as diffuse increased signal intensity in the subcutaneous tissues on T2 and STIR sequences. On T1-weighted images, cellulitis appears as a diffuse region of decreased signal replacing and infiltrating the normal high-signal subcutaneous fat.[99] The use of MRI contrast material may allow for enhancement and further delineation of the process.[94] Although both noninflammatory edema and cellulitis exhibit increased signal intensity on T2-weighted images, distortion of the soft tissues seen in cellulitis may be a distinguishing factor.[100] In addition, as a result of susceptibility effect, gas is best imaged on gradient echo images.

In the evaluation of abscesses (Figure 17-27), MRI has proven superior to CT and scintigraphy in both clinical and experimental models.[101-103] On T2 and STIR sequences, abscesses appear as well-marginated, well-localized, homogeneous high-signal-intensity collections. A peripheral rim around the abscess may be noted. This finding may be useful in differentiating abscesses from cellulitis.[94] Finally, gas within the abscess is noted by MRI and appears as focal

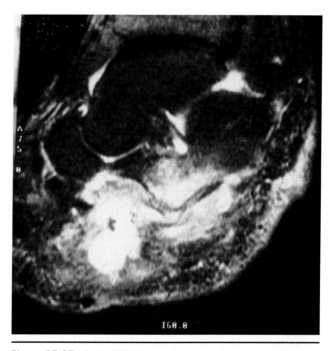

**Figure 17-27**  Sagittal T2 fat saturation image through the ankle shows marked abnormality in signal intensity. The adjacent soft tissue in the plantar aspect represents abscess and cellulitis in a diabetic patient who presented with skin ulceration.

areas of very low signal intensity on T1, T2, and STIR pulse sequences.[99]

## Osteomyelitis

Osteomyelitis, by definition, is the inflammation with infection of the marrow space of bone. Osteomyelitis may be divided into pyogenic and nonpyogenic forms. The most commonly encountered type of osteomyelitis cases are those classified as pyogenic.

Osteomyelitis is associated with up to one third of diabetic foot infections.[104] Most of the cases are a result of a contiguous spread of soft tissue infection or direct puncture wounds. About one fourth of diabetic osteomyelitis is secondary to vascular insufficiency.[105]

Osteomyelitis is extremely difficult to differentiate from diabetic osteoarthropathy. This is especially true in the later stages of arthropathy, where bone fragmentation, sclerosis, and new bone formation mimic the findings of osteomyelitis. This difficulty is complicated by the fact that the clinical picture of both conditions can be identical, presenting a diagnostic problem to the physician.

Within the broad category of osteomyelitis are three other major subdivisions: acute, subacute and chronic osteomyelitis.

**Acute.**   Clinically, acute osteomyelitis has been shown to be associated with temperature increase, local pain, soft tissue swelling, and tenderness on palpation.[106] The infective agent most commonly implicated is *Staphylococcus aureus*. The inflammatory process involves the marrow space, where subsequent edema is followed by decreased blood supply. Previous reports have suggested that acute osteomyelitis of long bones is more common in children than in adults.[106] In adults, this pyogenic form of infection usually targets the bones of the hands and feet and is usually secondary to trauma. Infection of such areas does not usually occur through hematogenic means. Rather, dissemination commonly occurs via tendon sheaths and lymphatic structures associated with the infected bone. Although acute osteomyelitis seems to occur predominantly in long bones, other skeletal structures such as the vertebrae, ilium, and the calcaneus can also be infected.[106]

CT evaluation of acute osteomyelitis may reveal increased attenuation in the medullary cavity as a result of bone marrow edema.[106] Following injection of iodinated contrast, abscess appears as a relatively low-density mass (less dense than the surrounding muscle) that is surrounded by a contrast-enhancing rim.[103] Gas, if present, appears as dark focal areas.[107] Compared with MRI, CT has been shown to be 66% sensitive and 97% specific in excluding osteomyelitis.[103]

MR imaging of acute osteomyelitis (Figures 17-28 and 17-29) cases generally exhibits decreased signal on T1-weighted images and increased signal on T2-weighted images. The decreased and increased signal intensities on T1- and T2-weighted images respectively have been attributed to a decrease in fat of the bone marrow and an increase in water content within the bone marrow.[108] STIR sequences, which suppress the signal from fat, display a markedly increased signal in osteomyelitis, indicating an increase in water content within the bone marrow secondary to edema and hyperemia.[108] Beltran[93] also reported that increased signal on T2-weighted images is a reliable means of detecting osteomyelitis. In contrast to the low signal intensities seen in neuropathic processes, increased signal intensities of osteomyelitis on conventional and fat-saturated T2-weighted images allow MR to differentiate bony infection from arthropathic changes.[108,102] Evaluating the surrounding soft tissues as well as cortical changes helps confirm the diagnosis of osteomyelitis.

**Subacute.**   Subacute osteomyelitis or Brodie's abscess is a low-grade, quiescent infection of bone. This lesion typically occurs in the younger age group (less than 25 years of age) and more frequently in males.[109] The most commonly involved bone is the femur, followed by the tibia in its metadiaphyseal regions.[106]

Clinically, Brodie's abscess presents with intermittent pain, local swelling, and tenderness. Laboratory findings are usually normal, and the sedimentation rate may not be elevated.[105] *S. aureus* is the most frequently organism isolated on culture.[110] In children, Brodie's abscess can cross the growth plate and cause septic arthritis.[106]

CT of Brodie's abscess reveals an eccentrically located lucent lesion, well circumscribed with sclerotic margins, typical of benign, slowly growing processes. Small osseous densities within the lesion representing sequestra are occasionally seen. Rarely, fluid levels within Brodie's abscess have been reported.[106] If present, periosteal changes or sinus tracts are well demonstrated by CT.

MRI of subacute osteomyelitis or Brodie's abscess reveal a low to intermediate signal on T1-weighed images and very high on T2-weighed images in the center. A thick low-signal-intensity rim outlines the abscess on both T1- and T2-weighted images. The signal is usually homogeneous, and soft tissue extension may be noted.[111]

**Chronic.**   Chronic osteomyelitis is a continuous infectious process that prevails over a period of time usually measured in months or years. Chronic osteomyelitis has been reported to most commonly affect middle-aged men. It is sometimes possible to localize areas having sequestra, which are regions of devitalized bony material surrounded by newly formed bone.

CT evaluation of chronic osteomyelitis reveal sequestra as bony fragments that are free or within the medullary

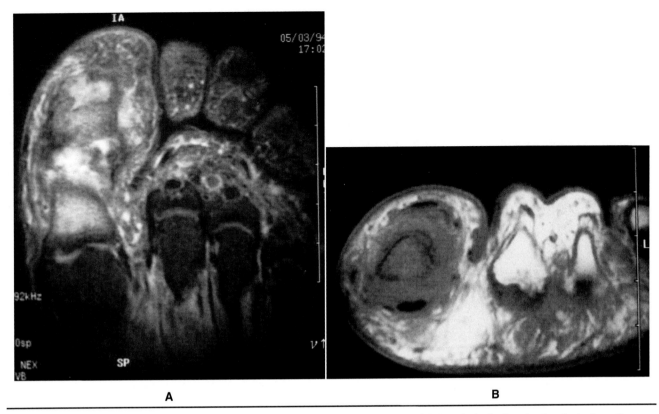

**Figure 17-28  A,** Axial T2-weighted image with fat saturation and coronal T1-weighted image **(B)** through the forefoot showing classic signs of osteomyelitis. Marrow fat signal intensity is replaced with material that is lower on the non-contrast T1-weighted image and increased on the T2 fat-saturated image. While this pattern is typical, it is not pathognomonic for osteomyelitis. Correlation with gadolinium enhancement and clinical signs and symptoms is also essential to establish the diagnosis.

cavity. Their relationship to the cortex is also well demonstrated by CT.[106] Unlike radiography, CT can distinguish between single and multiple adjacent sequestra.

Cortical defects as a result of chronic osteomyelitis appear as radiolucent gaps radiating from the medullary cavity through the cortex. A sinus tract is demonstrated as a low area of attenuation and may be filled with pus and/or sequestra.

Chronic osteomyelitis and associated pathologies are also well demonstrated by MRI. On T2-weighted images, sinus tracts appear as linear areas of increased signal intensity extending from the skin surface. Cortical disruption if present, is also well demonstrated. Sequestra appear as areas of low signal intensity against the background of a high-signal-intensity infection and edema on T2-weighted images.[111] The peripheral rim that surrounds a focus of chronic osteomyelitis appears as a band of low signal intensity on T2-weighted images.

## Deep Plantar Space Infection

Deep plantar space infections in diabetics are potentially life threatening. The complex anatomy of the plantar spaces allows bacteria to fester and infection to spread beyond the confines of the plantar vault. This fact, coupled with neuropathy and the propensity of diabetics toward foot infections, clearly demonstrate the need for early diagnosis and intervention.

Central compartment infections are probably the most serious by virtue of anatomic location.[112] Infections in this space are caused by direct penetration, web space infections, and nail bed infections.[113] Clinical findings include distension of the plantar arch with loss of skin, increased dorsal edema, and systemic signs of infection.

CT has been used in delineating diabetic plantar space infections.[40,114] Compartmental abscess appears as soft tissue nonhomogeneity either isolated to one compartment or pancompartmental. Infected interseptal fat planes appear obliterated, and transitional zones between infected and noninfected areas are well demonstrated.[40] The proximal extent of the disease process seen on CT correlates well with surgical findings.[114]

Some limitations of CT in evaluating soft tissue infection are its inability to show distinctions among edema, fibrosis, and reactive granulation tissue[40] and its relatively fair image contrast and spatial resolution.

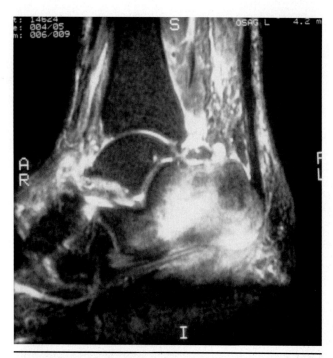

Figure 17-29    Sagittal T1 fat saturation after contrast shows an extensive lesion that begins in the soft tissues of the heel pad and extensively involves the calcaneus—a typical enhancement pattern for osteomyelitis in a diabetic patient whose disease started with a skin ulcer in the heel.

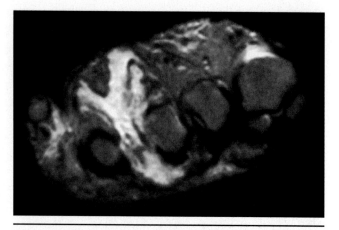

Figure 17-30    Coronal T2-weighted image from the midfoot of a diabetic patient. The Y-shaped lesion represents an abscess that spans the third intermetatarsal space.

On MRI, deep space infections (Figure 17-30) appear as homogeneous high-intensity collections on T2 and STIR images. The abscess is well outlined and delineated from the surrounding soft tissue and bony structures. On T1-weighted images that have not been contrast enhanced, abscess appears hypo- to isointense with muscle. Frank pus appears as a high signal intensity on T2-weighted images and may be distinguishable from collections of inflammatory fluid. Small focal, rounded very-low-signal foci within the abscess represent gas.[111]

## ARTICULAR DISORDERS

### Degenerative Joint Disease

Degenerative joint disease (DJD), also called *osteoarthrosis*, is a common pathologic condition occurring in the foot and ankle. It is characterized by osteophytes, asymmetric joint space narrowing, subchondral cysts, and osteocartilaginous loose bodies.[115] The condition has been speculated to be related to aging of articular structures; however, its exact etiology is unknown. It may occur as a primary osteoarthritic condition as in the hands of postmenopausal women[115] or as secondary osteoarthritis in joints with previous disease. The most common site of involvement in the foot and ankle is the metatarsophalangeal joint of the great toe.[115]

CT is useful in assessing both soft tissue and bone changes of DJD. However, MRI has proven more useful for such purposes, because it provides superior soft tissue contrast than CT. MR is also useful in assessing the extent of disease. Cartilage thinning is appreciated on images acquired orthogonal to the joint under examination. Joint effusions are seen as low-signal-intensity regions on T1-weighted images and are of high signal intensity on T2-weighted images.

On T2-weighted images irregularity and narrowing of the articular cartilage can be discerned. Loose bodies may be demonstrated on T2-weighted images as low-signal-intensity foci distinguished from the surrounding synovial fluid that is of high signal intensity on T2-weighted scans.

Subchondral cysts are well demonstrated by both CT and MR because of their tomographic nature. However, subchondral cysts are best imaged on MR using T2-weighted spin echo or gradient echo sequences, because the increased signal of the fluid within the cyst yields increased signal versus the medium to low signal intensity of the adjacent bone marrow, and hence yields improved contrast. Specifically, with T2-weighted spin echo pulse sequences, subchondral cysts are appreciated as high signal intensity, differentiating them from normal marrow and subchondral bone, which are discerned as areas of medium to low signal intensity. Osteophytes are very common in osteoarthrosis. They may be depicted on both MR and CT.

### Vacuum Joint Phenomenon

Vacuum joint phenomenon is a collection of gas within a joint not related to infection. The gas is said to be composed of 90% to 92% nitrogen gathered from the surrounding tissues.[116] Reports indicate that the vacuum phenomenon can be observed in any joint under mechanical traction.[117]

Gas in joints may also result iatrogenically from arthrographic studies or joint aspiration. Because it is associated with degenerative disease, it is common among the elderly, who are more susceptible to such processes. It has also been reported to occur in athletes after rapid distension of joints.[116]

On T1-weighted spin echo images, gas in the joint space may produce a signal void simulating ligamentous injury. On gradient echo images, magnetic susceptibility artifact may simulate cartilaginous disease.[118] CT scans easily confirms the presence of gas within joint of the foot and ankle.

## Inflammatory Arthritis

**Rheumatoid Arthritis.**    Rheumatoid arthritis is a systemic inflammatory disease of unknown origin. Radiographically, rheumatoid arthritis is characterized by periarticular swelling, joint space narrowing, osteoporosis, and subchondral cysts. Other pathologic conditions include synovial hypertrophy, joint effusion, and edema of the soft tissue structures. Osteoporosis almost always occurs in patients with rheumatoid arthritis. Rheumatoid arthritis is more common in women than men by a ratio of 3 to 1. The foot is a most common site of involvement. Soft tissue swelling is more common in the foot than in the ankle. Cortical erosions and rheumatoid cysts commonly appear throughout the foot. The articular cartilage is destroyed, narrowing the joint space symmetrically. Periosteal reactions, including the formation of new bone, are rare. Typically, inflammatory changes in the articular structures eventually result in misalignment and subluxation deformities.

The diagnosis of rheumatoid arthritis has traditionally been made using laboratory tests and conventional radiographic findings with clinical correlation. Routine radiographs may demonstrate bony changes directly. However, the articular cartilage, synovium, and other related structures are not depicted by such conventional means.

Soft tissue swelling, alignment abnormalities, erosions, and joint space narrowing are all well demonstrated on CT. In one series, coronally oriented CT images were able to depict subtalar erosions and associated structural abnormalities.[119]

MRI has been quite useful in assessing this inflammatory process. MRI evaluation of rheumatoid arthritis provides superior soft tissue contrast and multiplanar imaging demonstration of joint abnormalities. MRI can also provide valuable information concerning the extent of soft tissue and cartilaginous destruction. Cortical bony erosions are also better demonstrated by MRI than by radiography.[120] However, some researchers have reported that synovial fluid and joint effusions emit similar signal patterns on both T1- and T2-weighted pulse sequences, making it difficult to differentiate between the two.[121]

Contrast enhancement with Gd-DTPA is used when inadequate contrast between the synovium and the joint effusion makes differentiation difficult. Contrast enhancement not only allows differentiation of the synovium and joint effusions but also separates normal and inflammatory synovium. Contrast may be administered by direct arthrographic techniques. It has been reported that intravenous Gd-DTPA can enhance the joint effusion within the joint space by vicarious excretion.[121]

## Metabolic Deposition Disease

**Gouty Arthritis.**    Gout is the best understood of the metabolic diseases. It occurs in hyperuricemic individuals where a buildup of uric acid in the serum is then deposited as crystals in and around joints. Gout is common in adult men in their 50s; only 5% of cases occur in women.[122,123] Gout may be divided into three types: primary, secondary, and idiopathic. The primary form of gout is the most common. Patients with primary gout show urate overproduction and enzyme defects.[122] Secondary gout occurs as a consequence of other underlying disorders such as renal insufficiency, excessive alcohol consumption, and drug therapy, which disturb uric acid metabolism.[124,125] The designation of idiopathic gout is assigned to cases that cannot otherwise a precisely categorized.[122]

Clinically, the four stages of gout are asymptomatic hyperuricemia, acute gout, intercritical gout, and chronic gout.[126] Asymptomatic hyperuricemia may be present throughout life and precedes the first attack of acute gout. Serum uric acid levels are raised in this category of gout. Acute gout shows an abrupt onset of painful monoarticular arthritis. The typical first site of involvement is the first metatarsophalangeal joint. The initial attack of gout may be mild or severe, lasting several days. Intercritical gout is defined as gout in that period between attack. This period may be as long as years. The chronic phase of gout is characterized by a collection of urate crystals around an amorphous protein matrix with a rim of fibroblasts, histiocytes, and multinucleated giant cells.

**Calcium Pyrophosphate Dihydrate (CPPD) Deposition Disease.**    The metabolic disorder called calcium pyrophosphate dihydrate deposition disease occurs because pyrophosphate builds up excessively, resulting in CPPD deposition in the joints, which in turn results in synovitis and arthritis. Clinically, patients usually present with pain and goutlike symptoms.[127] Most patients are middle aged or elderly. Articular and periarticular structures show calcification, as may the joint capsule. This type of deposition disease causes cartilage loss, osteophytosis, and subchondral cysts. The foot and ankle are not frequently affected. However, when the foot and ankle are involved the disorder commonly affects the tarsal and metatarsophalangeal joints. CT is much better than MRI for identifying calcium deposits in joints.

**Hemochromatosis.** Hemochromatosis is a disease process in which iron is excessively deposited in various tissues. It may arise as a primary disorder or secondary to cirrhosis, anemia, or excessive iron ingestion, including multiple transfusions. The disorder affects men more commonly than females. Patients with this syndrome are typically over 40 years of age. Metacarpal and intercarpal joints are most commonly affected. However, the foot and ankle may sometimes be involved. Associated with this disorder is symmetric joint space narrowing.

## Neuropathic Arthropathy

Neuropathic arthropathy is a condition in which neural function is diminished, leading to an underlying bone and joint abnormality. This condition was first described by Charcot in 1868. It is estimated that 5% to 10% of diabetics develop Charcot joint disease during the course of their diabetes.[128]

Charcot joint disease is thought to have both neuro-vascular and neurotraumatic contributions factors.[129,130] The sympathetic control of bone blood flow is altered, leading to hyperemia and active bone resorption. This—coupled with lack of proprioception—leads to joint subluxation, fractures, and deformity.

Cofield and associates[131] in a study of 116 neuropathic extremities found the first metatarsophalangeal joint to be the most affected by this process. Lisfranc and the midtarsal joints were the next most frequently involved.

On initial presentation, the foot or ankle is usually edematous, erythematous, and warm to palpation. Pulses are usually intact and accompanied by sensory loss and absent deep tendon reflexes. About one third of these patients present with a painful foot.

CT evaluation of a Charcot joint reveals articular fracture displacement and fragmentation. All demonstrate sclerosis and shard formation, which appears as multiple minute fragments suspended within the soft tissues. Joint effusion is demonstrated as areas of relatively increased attenuation. Subchondral bone fragmentation as well as fracture orientation are well depicted, making CT ideal in preoperative planning for the surgical reconstruction of Charcot joints.

MRI findings of acute neuropathic fractures show decreased signal in the marrow on T1-weighted images.[93,94] Fracture callus appears as low signal intensity on both T1- and T2-weighted images. Effusions appear as high signal intensity on T2. Also evident is subchondral bone destruction accompanied by low signal intensity of underlying trabecular bone. Chronic neuroarthropathy may show a decreased signal intensity on all imaging sequences.

## ■ NEOPLASM

### Skeletal Neoplasms

#### Benign Neoplasms

##### Cysts

*Unicameral bone cyst.* Unicameral bone cyst, also known as solitary or simple bone cyst, is a benign lesion typically occurring in young adults. The etiology of these cysts is controversial, and many theories have been put forth.[132–134] More recent studies emphasize the importance of venous obstruction with resultant accumulation of interstitial fluid as a possible cause.[135,136]

Unicameral bone cysts most commonly affect patients below the age of 20 and more frequently involve long tubular bones.[137,138] The lesion occurs more frequently in males than in females. After age of 20 it tends to occur in flat bones and in the calcaneus.[139]

Clinically, the unicameral bone cyst is usually asymptomatic. When symptoms occur, they are usually associated with pathologic fractures. These pathologic fractures are clinically significant, because they can result in growth disturbances and angulation deformities, especially the lesions occurring near the growth plate.[140]

CT evaluation of unicameral bone cyst reveals the attenuation pattern (density) of the bone cyst to be homogeneous and of water density. The cortical margins are well defined and frequently scalloped and sclerotic. Fractures are particularly well demonstrated by CT.

On T1-weighted images MRI reveals low signal intensity, and reveals high signal intensity on T2-weighted images. The wall of cyst appears as a dark rim around the lesion on T2-weighted images. T2 signal images are consistent with the fluid composition of these cysts. If there has been prior hemorrhage, usually secondary to trauma, a fluid level with low-signal hemorrhage elements may appear in a dependent location.

*Aneurysmal bone cyst.* Aneurysmal bone cyst (ABC) is a solitary expansile lytic lesion of bone first described by Jaffe in 1921.[141] It is a non-neoplastic lesion that tends to behave aggressively, mimicking a malignancy. These lesions usually occur in patients younger than 20 years old, in the dorsal elements of the spine and the metaphysis of long bones.[137] The gender distribution appears about equal. In the lower extremity, ABCs occur most frequently in the distal tibia and fibula. In the foot, the calcaneus is the most frequently involved tarsal bone, whereas metatarsal and phalangeal involvement occurs with lessened frequency.[142]

The clinical presentation is that of a slowly growing mass over a period of months. Pain and swelling may or may not be present. Calcaneal involvement may mimic symptoms of heel spur syndrome. Metatarsal or phalangeal involvement are usually detected early, because of the lack of soft tissue in the foot.

The exact etiology of ABC cysts is not clearly understood. The most accepted theory to date suggests that the cyst forms in response to increased intraosseous venous pressure.[143] Some reports indicate that this lesion may result from traumatic fracture in certain cases.[137] Grossly, the tumor is composed of spaces filled with blood. Microscopically, the lesion contains cavernous spaces consisting of fibrous walls and giant cells, and lacks features of normal blood vessels.[144]

CT is far superior to plain radiography in defining ABC lesions.[144] CT shows an expansile lytic mass with thinning cortical margins. The outer limits of the mass is surrounded by a thin cortical shell. Multiple fluid levels in an ABC are characteristic of these lesions, on CT scans these lesions present as layers of different densities.[145] Although CT can demonstrate the expansile nature of the tumor and detect the calcified rims surrounding the lesion, it does not depict soft tissue involvement as well as MRI can. The well-defined cystic spaces with varying range of signal intensities and multiple fluid levels are even better demonstrated on MRI.

T1-weighted MR images reveal a mass of generally intermediate signal intensity with foci of both high and low signal intensity. The mass is sharply marginated by a low-signal-intensity rim consistent with fibrocartilage or bone,[146] a characteristic that is typical of most benign processes.

T2-weighted images reveal the multilocular appearance of these lesions. Multiple fluid levels appear as low to intermediate signal intensity in the dependent collection, with the nondependent collection demonstrating high signal intensity. The low-signal-intensity material represents red blood cells with plasma being located in an nondependent location. Although multiple fluid levels are characteristics of ABCs on CT and MRI, this phenomenon also occurs in telangiectatic osteosarcoma, chondroblastoma, giant cell tumor, and intraosseous lipoma.[147]

### Cartilaginous Tumors

*Osteochondroma.* Osteochondroma, also known as osteocartilaginous exostosis, represents approximately 50% of benign bone lesions, making it the most common benign bone tumor.[137] This lesion is thought to be hyperplastic displaced or aberrant growth plate cartilage.[148] Classically, the lesion consists of a bony protrusion with a cartilaginous cap, perichondrium, and a bony stalk. It is possible for this lesion to undergo sarcomatous degeneration, thus becoming a chondrosarcoma. However, such degeneration does not commonly occur in the foot and ankle. Osteochondromas typically occur in patients under 20 years of age. It seems to occur in twice as many males as in females, commonly in the distal metaphyseal region of the femur. Other locations include the distal tibia and fibula, humerus, proximal femur, and scapula.[149]

Clinically no pain is usually associated with this lesion per se, and thus osteochondroma is asymptomatic until accidental radiologic examination discovers the lesion. Symptoms may result from impingement on adjacent neurovascular structures, bursitis, or from fracture of the tumor that is associated with pain. Pain associated with rapid growth suggests malignancy, especially after age 30.[150]

The cartilaginous mass may sometimes contain calcified material that is detectable on plain radiographs as areas of increased density. Although radiographically the tumor's morphology is diagnostic, the cartilage cap and its thickness cannot be determined on plain films.

CT evaluation reveals a continuity of cortex and spongiosa of the tumor with the parent bone. The cortical structure shows an organized pattern with a center of cancellous bone. Usually no soft tissue mass or bony destruction is associated. CT can demonstrate the thickness of the cartilaginous cap.[151]

Although CT is useful in differentiating the lesion from a chondrosarcoma, lesion size is sometimes difficult to assess with CT. The problem lies with the similarity in attenuation values of cartilage and muscle and difficulty in obtaining the optimal plane of imaging.

MRI clearly demonstrates the continuity of the exostotic cortex and medullary cavity with that of the parent bone. On T2-weighted images, the perichondrium is demonstrated as a smooth, low-signal-intensity region adjacent to a high-intensity area of cartilage. The cartilaginous cap is of low to intermediate signal intensity on T1-weighted images, and on T2-weighted images the cap appears as an area of intense signal. MR imaging can precisely measure the thickening of the cartilage cap. The cap normally measures between 2 and 2.5 mm in thickness. MR is capable of detecting mass lesions as small as 3 mm and can accurately estimate the cartilage thickness. These kinds of morphometric measurements are usually accomplished using T2-weighted pulse sequences. When present, cartilage calcification can be detected by MR as a focus of low signal intensity. This calcification correlates with malignant degeneration of the lesion. The benign osteochondromas are usually nonsurgically treated unless the lesion is so large that it causes pain and derangement, in which case surgery is required.

*Chondroblastoma.* Chondroblastoma is a rare lesion of immature cartilage. Chondroblastoma normally occurs in the epiphysis of long bones, with 70% involving the distal femur, proximal tibia, proximal humerus, and tarsal bones, in descending order of frequency.[152] About 60% of the patients are in the second decade of life, with an age range of 2 to 73 and with a predilection for males over females by a ratio of 2:1.[137]

Originally confused with giant cell tumor of bone, the lesion does not produce mature cartilage and hence has the name chondroblastoma.[153] Approximately 700 lesions in the world literature have been reported, giving chondroblastoma an incidence of about 1.4% of all benign bone tumors.[154]

Over 60 lesions have been reported in the foot, most of which were in the tarsal bones.[155–158]

Clinically, pain and sometimes swelling are the most common symptoms, usually found locally. Because of their location in the epiphysis, joint symptoms such as impaired range of motion, pain and tenderness, limping, muscle atrophy, and synovial effusion accompany chondroblastomas.[152]

CT findings of chondroblastoma demonstrate a lytic lesion with calcifications within the tumor.[159] CT may also demonstrate cortical destruction, extraosseous component, and soft tissue extension. Fluid–fluid levels in cystic chondroblastomas are also well demonstrated by CT.[158] In addition, the thick periosteal response is well depicted with CT. Marrow changes, edema, and synovial effusions are all better demonstrated by MRI.

MRI signal intensity depends on the degree of calcification within the lesion.[160,161] A heavily calcified tumor demonstrates a low signal intensity on T1- and T2-weighted images. The uncalcified chondroid portion of the tumor demonstrates a high signal intensity on T2-weighted images. Joint effusion is revealed as low signal intensity on T1 and high on T2. Medullary involvement is better demonstrated by MRI because of its multiplanar capability and superior contrast resolution.

*Enchondroma.*    Enchondromas are cartilaginous tumors arising with the medullary cavity of long tubular bones. These tumors make up about 10% of all benign tumors of bone and 19% of benign cartilaginous tumors in Dahlin's series of almost 5000 primary tumors of bone.[162]

Most enchondromas occur in the third and fourth decade of life and about equally in men and women.[163] Approximately half of these lesions involve hands and feet. Most lesions are usually discovered incidentally on radiographs and are asymptomatic. The occurrence of pain should arouse suspicion of malignant transformation.[163]

CT evaluation reveals cortical expansion with thinning and endosteal scalloping. The punctate, flocculent calcification within the lesion is clear. Pathologic fractures as well as intra-articular extension are particularly well demonstrated by CT.

T1-weighted images of MR reveal a low-signal-intensity mass that may contain some high-signal bands. The tumor is usually isointense with muscle. T2-weighted images demonstrate a high-intensity-signal lesion that is usually heterogeneous. On T1-weighted images, enhancing endochondromas with Gd-DTPA reveals a pattern comprised of arcs and rings.[164]

**Synovial Chondromatosis.**    Synovial osteochondromatosis is an articular disorder in which osteocartilaginous bodies are produced as a result of synovial metaplasia or neoplasia.[165] This monoarticular condition usually affects the knee and, less frequently, the hip and shoulder. Other joint involvements have been reported.[166–170]

Synovial osteochondromatosis occurs in the third to fifth decade of life and is more common in men. Clinically, joint pain and limitation of motion are common. Joint instability can also occur, resulting in pain.[170] Adjacent bony erosions with synovial osteochondromatosis as well as subsequent degenerative joint change may occur.[171]

Early radiographic evaluation of synovial osteochondromatosis may show synovial thickening. The loose bodies calcify or ossify and cluster within the joint. The lesions can form plaques within the synovium or become attached to the synovium by a pedicle.[172] These lesions, which can number in the hundreds, frequently measure less than 10 mm in diameter.

CT evaluation of synovial chondromatosis[173] reveals multiple calcifications enclosed within the joint capsule. These calcifications appear confluent and stippled, forming a conglomerated mass.[173] The joint capsule may also be distended. Osseous erosions occurred in up to 30% of cases in one review.[171] CT clearly shows these erosions at the articular ends of the involved bone, which may allow differentiation between this entity and malignant synovial tumors.

MRI has been shown to define the exophytic extent of synovial chondromatosis with more clarity than CT.[174] In addition, MRI is useful in ruling out medullary involvement, which aids in differentiation from a malignant lesion. On T1-weighted images, the lesion appears as a low-signal-intensity mass containing dark foci. Adjacent cortical erosions or scalloping is well noted by MRI. On T2-weighted images, the lesion appears as a high-signal-intensity mass with low-signal foci within the tumor, consistent with osteocartilaginous bodies.

**Bony Tumors**

*Osteoblastoma.*    Like chondroblastomas, osteoblastomas are also considered rare tumors. Osteoblastomas (occasionally referred to as giant osteoid osteomas) are highly vascular tumors with an abundance of osteoblasts. The tumor has an unlimited growth potential and is larger than an osteoid osteoma, with an average size of 3.5 cm.[175] Histopathologically, the tumor is similar to osteoid osteomas, occasionally making histological distinction between the two difficult.[175]

Osteoblastoma occurs most commonly in adolescents and in young adults in the second and third decades of life.[175] The lesion occurs most frequently in males, at a ratio of 3 males to 1 female. Most osteoblastomas are found in the spine and in long tubular bones. In the foot, the talus is the most frequently involved bone. When in the metatarsals, the lesion is usually diaphyseal, with a glass bubble appearance on radiographs.

Clinically, the pain with osteoblastoma is mild, with limited response to salicylates. The pain is worse at night in only 13% of the cases.[176] Soft tissue swelling and osteoporosis are frequently seen with osteoblastomas that affect the talus. Muscle wasting and limping are often advanced symptoms.

CT findings reveal an expansive lytic lesion with matrix mineralization surrounded by a thin rim bone.[177-179] Soft tissue swelling and related periosteal reaction is well demonstrated by CT. A pseudocapsule surrounding the tumor may also be shown by CT. Unlike plain radiography, CT demonstrates the exact origin of the tumor as well as its intra- or extraosseous involvement.

T1-weighted MR images show the lesion to be of low signal intensity. The tumor is of high signal intensity on T2-weighted images. MRI easily demonstrates the surrounding soft tissue edema and marrow involvement. The pseudocapsule of the tumor is also well demonstrated by MRI. The nature of the changes surrounding the tumor are best demonstrated by MRI, whereas CT is superior in demonstrating the tumor's cortical shell and subtle calcifications or ossifications within the tumor.

*Osteoid osteoma.*    Osteoid osteoma is considered among the most frequently reported primary tumors of bone. Since its description by Jaffe in 1935, over 1000 cases have been reported.[180] Initially of debatable origin, osteoid osteoma is now generally accepted as an osteoblastic bone tumor consisting of variably calcified osteoid in a stroma of loose connective tissue surrounded by a zone of sclerotic bone.[181]

Osteoid osteoma occurs most frequently in the second and third decade of life. It occurs three times as often in males as in females.[175] The long tubular bones are involved about 71% of the time, most of which are in the tibia and the femur.[175] The foot is a relatively common site for osteoid osteomas (20%), with the talus and calcaneus being most commonly involved.[177] In the foot, most lesions are localized in the subperiosteal region or in cancellous bone and can be (rarely) intra-articular, associated with synovitis and other manifestations of joint disease.[182,183]

The clinical presentation alone may be diagnostic of osteoid osteoma. The pain is typically greatest at night and is relieved by salicylates. Local sensory stimulation from unmyelinated nerve fibers within the nidus and prostoglandins released by tumor tissue have been implicated as causative factors for these symptoms.[184] In advanced stages, local tenderness and swelling may be present.

CT findings include a well-localized, lucent nidus within the involved bone. Areas of calcification within the nidus are usually present. Sclerosis is frequently seen surrounding the nidus. CT clearly demonstrates subperiosteal lesions that evoke little subperiosteal reaction.

On T1-weighted images of MRI, the nidus of osteoid osteomas has a low signal intensity. T2-weighted images may also have a low signal intensity secondary to the calcification of the osteoid matrix and rapid blood flow within the nidus.[185,186] Surrounding inflammation and hyperemia present as high signal intensity on T2-weighted images and may involve a large area surrounding the lesion. MRI is an excellent modality for demonstrating joint inflammation and effusions secondary to intra-articular lesions.

*Giant cell tumor.*    Giant cell tumor (GCT), also referred as osteoclastoma, is a common and a locally aggressive lesion of unknown origin. Considered a transitional tumor, it possesses characteristics of both benign and malignant lesions.[187]

Giant cell tumors occur in the third and fourth decades of life, most commonly in males. The long tubular bones especially the distal femur and the proximal tibia, are most frequently involved.[187] Other bony involvement includes the distal radius, proximal humerus, distal tibia, and sacrum. Approximately 5% of GCT localize in the bones of the hands and less commonly in the feet.[188,189]

Clinically, pain is the most common complaint, followed by local swelling and limitation of motion in the adjacent joint.[190] The lesion is tender to palpation, and muscle atrophy and pathologic fractures are advanced clinical presentations.

CT reveals thinning of the involved cortex and cortical destruction by the tumor. Penetration of subarticular cortical bone as well as joint invasion may also be seen. Areas of low attenuation within the lesion may be noted secondary to fluid levels, hemorrhage, or necrosis.[191]

On MRI, GCT demonstrates low signal intensity on T1-weighted images and a higher signal on T2-weighted images.[192] Also on T2-weighted images, the lesion may demonstrate intermediate signal intensity and may show foci of higher signal intensity that correspond to cyst formation, hemorrhage, or necrosis.[192]

MRI is far superior to CT for demonstrating the extraosseous extension of the tumor. However, CT remains superior for demonstrating subtle cortical destruction and small bone fragments. This is because (1) MRI generally provides poorer spatial resolution (especially in older scanners), (2) MRI fundamentally cannot demonstrate calcified structures, and (3) MR images may suffer from occasional increased motion artifact because of prolonged acquisition time, especially on conventional T2-weighed images.[193]

*Nonossifying fibroma.*    Nonossifying fibroma, also known as fibrous cortical defect, is a common bone tumor. Despite the name, the lesion is mostly intramedullary, and cortical involvement is not always present.[194]

Nonossifying fibromas occur most frequently in childhood and adolescence (in the second decade of life). Most lesions are asymptomatic and incidentally discovered on radiographs.

The long tubular bones are usually affected in 90% of cases.[195] The tibia is involved 43% of the time, the femur in 38%, and the fibula in about 8% of the cases.[195] Upper extremity as well as foot involvement is rare.

Nonossifying fibroma is more common in boys and is usually asymptomatic. Symptoms result from pathologic fractures.[196] Otherwise most lesions ossify after closure of epiphysis without incident.

Both MRI and CT reveal the precise location of these lesions. Usually images show scalloping and expansion of the cortex. Thin trabeculae are usually noted within the lesion and described as showing a "honeycomb" appearance. Very subtle pathologic fractures are well demonstrated by CT.

MRI shows these lesions as having a low signal periphery with variably increased signal within the lesion on T2-weighted images.

*Intraosseous lipoma.* Compared to the common soft tissue lipomas, intraosseous lipomas are considered among the rarest of tumors. To date, approximately 70 intraosseous lipomas have been reported.[197] These lesions are usually metaphyseal in location, occurring most frequently in the proximal portions of the fibula and the femur. In the foot, intraosseous lipomas have a predilection for involving the calcaneus, making up 14% of the reported lesions.[198]

Intraosseous lipoma occurs equally in both males and females. The typical patient is about age 40. Patients are usually asymptomatic, with most lesions discovered accidentally on routine radiographs. However, intraosseous lipomas can be painful, and potential complications include pathologic and stress fractures.[199]

Several hypotheses about the origin of intraosseous lipoma have been proposed.[200] Those include, trauma, infection, and infraction. However, these lesions are increasingly becoming more accepted as primary bone tumors.[201] Histologically, the tumor is characterized by mature lipocytes in a background of fibroblasts and occasional foci of necrosis.[200]

CT findings reveal a well-delineated medullary lytic lesion.[197,202] The lesion has a thin sclerotic margin and a central calcific body. With a CT value of fat, the lesion is almost always histologically identifiable. However, lesions containing histiocyte laden with fat vacuoles may yield comparable low CT attenuation values. Also, fluid levels may be demonstrated within these lesions as in aneurysmal bone cysts.

On MRI, intraosseous lipomas demonstrate a high signal intensity on T1-weighted images and medium to low signal on T2-weighted images. The central calcified necrotic matter within the lipomas appears as a dark focus. MR is superior to plain radiography in determining the extent of these tumors. Furthermore, nonhomogeneous tissue is readily depicted by MR, making it superior to CT in the differential diagnosis of these lesions. Fat saturation techniques significantly increase specificity in diagnosing fatty lesions.

## Malignant Skeletal Neoplasms

**Osteosarcoma.** Osteogenic sarcoma is the second most common malignant primary bone tumor, with about 15% incidence, second only to multiple myeloma.[203] Of reported cases, 85% involve patients under 30 years of age, most

between the ages of 15 and 25. The ratio of its incidence in males versus females is about 1.5 to 1.0.[203]

Osteogenic sarcoma occurs most commonly in the distal femur/proximal tibial region.[204] The pelvis, skull, and the jaw are the next most frequently affected sites, respectively. Its occurrence in the foot is very uncommon, and only a limited number of cases have been reported.[205,206] A recent review of the literature indicated that the frequency of foot involvement ranged from 0.17% to 2.08%, with an average of 0.83%.[207]

In the foot, the tarsal bones are usually involved. The metatarsals or the phalanges are rarely if ever involved. In long bones, the lesion is usually 90% metaphyseal and about 9% diaphyseal.[204] About 85% of patients with OGS develop micrometastasis to the lungs.[204] When osteosarcoma affects the tarsus, the recommended conventional treatment is amputation below the knee.

CT evaluation may show sclerosis of bone with a surrounding soft tissue mass.[208–213] The involved bone may show lytic changes and fragmentation. There is usually soft tissue thickening and generalized osteopenia. Thus, bony involvement is well demonstrated by CT.

MRI may show scattered areas of higher or lower signal intensity typical of malignancy secondary to hemorrhage, necrosis, or calcifications.[208,209,211–215] Cortical involvement may be indistinct, suggesting cortical invasion. A soft tissue mass is clearly outlined, differentiating it well from the surrounding normal musculature. Often a pseudocapsule surrounds the mass. Surrounding vessel displacement, physeal, medullary, as well as articular involvement are all well demonstrated by MRI. Uncalcified lesions involving the bone marrow demonstrates increased signal on inversion recovery and T1-weighted pulse sequences. Uncalcified marrow lesions on T2-weighted spin echo sequences also give an increased signal intensity pattern. Surrounding edema frequently appears adjacent to the extraosseous component of these tumors. This extraosseous edema generally resolves after chemotherapy.

**Ewing sarcoma.** Ewing sarcoma was first described as a separate entity in 1921. It's a relatively common, highly malignant tumor of uncertain origin. About 5% of all tumor biopsies are diagnosed as Ewing sarcoma.[216] Of the patients presenting with Ewing sarcoma, 75% are between the ages of 10 and 25.[216] Patients as young as 18 months and as old as 61 years of age have been reported.[216]

The most frequent sites of Ewing sarcoma are the femur, ilium, humerus, fibula, and ribs.[217] Involvement of the foot bones have been reported about four times more often than that of the hand.[217] Any bones of the foot may be involved, including the phalanges.

Radiographically, osteosclerosis and ill-defined osteolysis along with cortical permeation dominate the picture. In diagnosing and staging, CT findings, which basically augment plain films, include permeative osteolysis, cortical erosions, and increased attenuation of bone. Poorly defined margins and a soft tissue mass are common.[218,219] Soft tissue extension can occur in the absence of significant bony destruction.[220] The tumor is usually homogeneous unless necrosis is present. CT scans have been used in preoperative surgical planning and in assessing postoperative response of the tumor to radiation therapy.

T1-weighted images using MRI usually show the lesion as a low-signal-intensity mass. The lesion emits a high and/or an intermediate signal on T2-weighted images. Intramedullary extension on T1 shows a low signal against a background of high signal intensity produced by the normal fatty marrow.[221] MRI is also very useful in evaluating postchemotherapy behavior.

**Chondrosarcoma.** Chondrosarcoma is a destructive low-grade malignancy occurring in the fourth to sixth decades of life. It is relatively rare in the bones distal to the ankle joint.[222]

Wu and Guise reviewed 19 cases of chondrosarcomas of the foot and reported an age range of 14 to 71.[223] In their series, the ratio of incidence in males to females was 3:2. Frequent sites were the tarsus, phalanges, and metatarsals respectively, with the calcaneus being the most frequently involved.

Chondrosarcomas are divided into central and peripheral lesions.[224] The peripheral lesions are further subdivided into exostotic (arising from osteochondromas), juxtacortical, and periosteal chondrosarcomas.[224]

Clinically, pain is the most characteristic presenting symptom of chondrosarcoma. Usually a mass is associated with erythema and tenderness.

CT findings include sclerosis of the bone involved, along with calcifications or ossifications of the adjacent soft tissues. Cortical as well as periosteal involvement may present as punctate calcifications.[225] Dense rings or spicules of calcifications, absence of necrosis, and eccentric lobular growths correlate with a low-grade malignancy.[226] High-grade lesions are characterized as having faint amorphous calcifications, concentric patterns of growth, a large component of soft tissue density, and necrotic areas of even lower density.[226]

T1-weighted MRI shows a generally homogeneous mass with low-signal-intensity medullary involvement. The lobulated nature of the tumor matrix, typical of chondrosarcomas, is well revealed by MRI. Low-intensity septa within the tumor matrix are also well appreciated. Periosteal, articular, and physeal and soft tissue involvement, including involvement of neurovascular structures, are also well demonstrated by MRI.

**Fibrosarcoma.** Fibrosarcoma is a malignant fibroblastic tumor of bone and is considered a rare malignancy.[227,228] This tumor can either be a primary lesion or a secondary one arising in an area of osteonecrosis, chronic osteomyelitis,

giant cell tumor, or Paget's disease, or appear following irradiation.[194] Histologically, fibrosarcomas can be well or poorly differentiated.[229] Fibrosarcoma can occur at any age; however, it is most frequent in the fourth to sixth decade of life.[230] The femur is the most frequently involved bone, followed by the tibia and the pelvis.[230] In Dahlin and Unni's series, 4.4% of fibrosarcomas arose in the ankle.[222]

Clinically, pain, swelling, and limitation of motion are the initial complaints. The clinical presentation is usually within the first 6 months of occurrence. About a third of the patients present initially with a pathologic fracture of the involved bone.[230]

CT of fibrosarcoma reveals extensive cortical destruction, poor margination, soft tissue extension, and lack of sclerosis.[210] Osteoporosis may also be noted with fibrosarcoma on CT, because of tumor-related hyperemia.

T1- and T2-weighted images on MRI usually reveal a nonhomogeneous mass of low or intermediate density.[231] Osseous soft tissue and as intra-articular involvement are well demonstrated by MRI. Relationship of the tumor to nearby neurovascular bundle is well demonstrated on MRI studies.

**Adamantinoma.** Adamantinoma is a locally aggressive, rare, malignant tumor originally described by Fischer in 1913.[232] Although the tumor was initially of controversial origin, researchers now generally accept that the tumor originates from epithelial cells.[233] However, some lesions are histologically variable and have been found to contain cells that resemble those of Ewing sarcoma, as well as tissue resembling fibrous dysplasia and ossifying fibroma.[233]

Most adamantinomas occur in the third decade of life and are more common in males. Rare cases in children and in elderly patients have been reported.[234] Of the lesions, 90% arise in the tibia, and approximately 17.5% occur in the ankle region, in either the tibia or fibula.[222,235]

Clinically, patients presents with local swelling and erythema with or without pain of the involved extremity. A history of trauma to the area is not infrequent. Radiographically, adamantinomas resemble fibrous dysplasia, and it is very difficult to distinguish between the two lesions.[236]

On CT, cortical involvement is well demonstrated. This includes cortical destruction as well as medullary space involvement. The appearance of adamantinomas on MRI mimics those of fibrous dysplasia.[237] These include low signal intensity on T1-weighted images and variable signal intensity on T2-weighted images. Soft tissue involvement as well as articular and adjacent bony invasion is also well demonstrated by MRI.

## Soft Tissue Neoplasms
### Benign Tumors

**Neuroma.** The most common neuroma in the foot is Morton's interdigital neuroma. Morton's neuroma commonly involves the third plantar common digital nerve. This lesion represents perineural fibrosis of the involved nerve with associated vascular and perivascular proliferation.[238] A frequent location of Morton's neuroma is the third interspace. This has been reported in the second interspace; adjacent neuromas in both interspaces have also been reported.[239]

The etiology of Morton's neuromas has been attributed to faulty biomechanics.[240] Compression of the nerve against the intermetatarsal ligament causes inflammation and reactive perineural fibrosis. The marked female predominance is generally attributed to the wearing of high-heeled shoes.[239]

Clinically, symptoms include pain and numbness in the forefoot and sometimes the feeling of electricity radiating either proximally or distally into the foot. Firm compression in the involved interspace usually reproduces the symptoms.

Plain radiography and CT have little to offer in evaluating interdigital neuromas. Sonography has been reported to successfully localize these lesions.[241] MRI is by far the method of choice in localizing as well as delineating this lesion from adjacent soft tissue structures such as bursae and fat (Figure 17-31).

MRI using T1-weighted images frequently shows a low-signal-intensity mass well demarcated from adjacent fatty tissue.[242] The low signal intensity is attributed to the fibrous composition of these tumors. The mass is usually localized plantar to the third-metatarsal interspace. It may extend and become prominent between the metatarsal heads up to the phalangeal bases. Neuromas maintain close apposition to adjacent osseous structures, and no bony abnormality is usually seen.

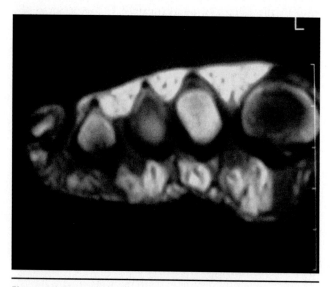

**Figure 17-31**  Coronal T1-weighted image through the metatarsophalangeal joints demonstrates a typical Morton's neuroma. The neuroma is teardrop shaped and originates from the third distal intermetatarsal space.

In one series reviewed, Morton's neuromas were frequently associated with proximal high-signal-intensity foci on the T2-weighted image.[243] These foci were attributed to fluid-filled intermetatarsal bursae located dorsal to the deep transverse intermetatarsal ligament. The Morton's neuromas have been demonstrated to enhance on post-Gd-DTPA scans. The use of fat saturation techniques increases contrast on post-Gd-DTPA T1-weighted images and hence increases lesion conspicuity. In addition, high-resolution techniques are quite helpful in localizing small neuromas.

**Neurofibroma.**  Neurofibromas are benign peripheral nerve-sheath tumors that arise from sensory or motor nerves. They can be either multiple, as seen in von Recklinghausen's disease, or the more frequent solitary type.[244]

Solitary neurofibromas affect both males and females in equal frequency. They occurs in persons between the ages of 20 and 30.[244] The superficial variety of neurofibromas occur as solitary nodules, are usually painless, and are removed by marginal excision. Grossly, these lesions appear as white-gray well-encapsulated masses occurring within the subcutaneous tissues.[245]

The deeper neurofibromas involving major nerves permeate between nerve fibers and cause fusiform swelling of the involved nerve. When confined to the epineurium, they possess a true capsule.[245] Frequently the value of surgically excising these tumors must be weighed against loss of neurologic function.

**Lipoma.**  Lipomas are abnormal accumulations of fat and are found in areas of abundant fatty tissues. They usually occur in the thighs, shoulders, and back. Lipomas involving the feet have been reported.[246–248]

Lipomas are usually painless; however, they do cause discomfort when exerting pressure on adjacent structures. They occur frequently in the fifth and sixth decades of life. Females are affected more than males.

Lipomas can either be simple or multilobed. The thin capsular covering surrounding lipomas delineate these lesions from surrounding soft tissue structures and is characteristic of their benign nature. Thickening of dividing septa and poor margination are signs of malignancy, as seen in liposarcoma.

CT evaluation shows a sharply marginated, smoothly bordered homogeneous mass of fatty attenuation. Lipomas may contain thin, linear streaks representing fibrous septa. They have a low linear attenuation (density) on CT studies between −80 and −160 Hounsfield units. They are uniform in density and lack significant contrast enhancement.[249]

T1-weighted MR images show a homogeneous high-signal-intensity mass that is isointense with subcutaneous fat. Lower-signal-intensity streaks on T1-weighted images represent septa within the lesion. These streaks must be differentiated from necrosis and the soft tissue component seen in liposarcomas.[250] Because of the specificity of the low linear attenuation coefficient (density) of fat, CT is more specific than MRI in diagnosing lipomas[250] unless fat saturation techniques are employed.

**Hemangioma.** Hemangiomas are vascular malformations that are usually benign.[251] Histologically, they are characterized by increased number of vascular channels and overgrowth of endothelial lining. Hemangiomas may be composed of adipose or fibrous tissue, smooth muscle, and—rarely—bone.

Hemangiomas occur most often in Caucasian infants and occur twice as frequently in females as in males.[252] Berlin reported 33 cases involving the foot and found the majority of hemangiomas involving muscle and connective tissue.[253]

Despite their nonmalignant nature, hemangiomas can produce devastating deformities. In the extremities, bone and cartilage involvement may lead to fracture and regional giantism. In the foot, hemangiomas have been reported on the plantar surface, involving the plantar musculature and the plantar aponeurosis[254-256] and resulting in gross abnormality.

Surgical resection of hemangiomas and argon laser therapy are the most widely used and effective forms of treatment.[257] Knowing the full extent of the lesion prior to surgery is essential, because recurrence usually follows inadequate removal.[258]

X-rays studies may reveal soft tissue swelling, and phleboliths may be demonstrated. Erosions and periosteal reaction may also be seen. Angiography has been used to demonstrate the feeding vessels. However, angiography fails to demonstrate the full extent of the lesion and its relationship to muscle and neurovascular bundles.[259]

Dynamic CT scanning with administration of contrast material has been used with some success to demonstrate these lesions.[260] However, CT may be limited in available imaging planes and is hampered by beam hardening artifact from bone and requires contrast material that has potential for morbidity and mortality.

In the foot, MRI may show a well-defined mass occupying the plantar aspect.[261-264] Involvement of flexor muscles and plantar aponeurosis involvement have both been reported. Usually no bones are involved, and little or no calcification is present.

The typical signal characteristic of this lesion is one of high signal intensity on the T2-weighted images. This signal reflects the cystic nature of these lesions. Also on T2-weighted images of hemangiomas may show a homogeneous or inhomogeneous pattern of signal intensity. In addition, phleboliths may be demonstrated in some lesions as low-signal-intensity foci on T2-weighted images. A feeding artery and a draining vein are demonstrated as serpiginous channels of low signal intensity (flow void). MR angiography (MRA) can be quite helpful in demonstrating the hemangiomas and their associated vascular channels. On MRA studies, the vessels can be demonstrated as high or low in signal intensity.

**Pigmented Villinodular Synovitis.** Pigmented villinodular synovitis (PVNS) is thought to be a proliferative disorder of the synovium arising from the synovial lining of joints, tendons, and ligaments.[265] The exact etiology of PVNS remains unknown. Both sides of the joint space are frequently involved. Proposed causes include hemorrhage into the joint, neoplasia, lipid deposition disorders, and minor trauma.[266]

PVNS occurs in young adults between ages 20 and 50 and is slightly more common in men. The knee joint is most frequently involved, with the hip, wrist, shoulder, and ankle being also involved, in descending order of frequency.[267] Lesions involving the small joints of the hands and feet have also been reported.[268]

Clinically, the lesion appears as a nonpainful soft tissue mass. Minimal to mild joint swelling and tenderness are the most common presenting complaints. The lesions are primarily monoarticular; however, rare cases of polyarticular involvement have been reported.[269] In the foot and ankle the lesions appear as lobulated soft tissue masses. Radiographically one sees multiple bony erosions and subchondral lucencies of the involved bones.

CT findings may reveal erosions of the involved articulations with a soft tissue mass. The lesion may have mixed attenuation, with foci of density higher than the surrounding muscle tissue.[270] The high attenuation of these masses correlates with hemosiderin deposits within the lesion. PVNS containing coarse calcifications is well depicted by CT.[271]

MR signal intensities are related to the histological components of PVNS. The signal changes depend on the amount of hemosiderin present.[272] The region is usually hypointense signal on T1- and T2-weighted images. Cystic components of the lesion are characterized by higher signal intensity on T2-weighted image and low signal intensity on T1-weighted images.[273]

**Ganglion Cyst.** Ganglion cysts are superficially located myxoid lesions resulting from connective tissue degeneration secondary to trauma. They commonly present as spheroid cystic cavities occurring on the dorsum of the wrist in young people between the ages of 25 and 45.[274] Less often, they are found on the volar surface of wrist or finger and dorsum of foot and toes.[275] Nine percent of the reported ganglion cysts are said to occur around the foot and ankle.[276]

Ganglion cysts measure about 1 to 3 inches in diameter and are movable within the surrounding tissue. They are loosely attached to the tendon sheaths. It is not clear whether ganglia arise from tendon sheaths and other synovial structures. Usually there is no communication between the ganglion cyst and the joint space.[274]

Clinically, ganglion cysts about the foot and ankle are more painful than the corresponding lesions around the wrist.[276] The symptoms usually depend on the size of the cyst and its relationship to neighboring structures.[277] Pressure on nearby nerves can cause paresthesia and even impair function.

CT evaluation of a ganglion cyst reveals a well-defined periarticular mass with attenuation values that are within the range of water.[278] It appears smoothly bordered, with a thin, capsular rim.

On T1-weighted images of MRI, ganglion cysts demonstrate low-intensity signal and on T2-weighted images, a very-high-intensity signal.[264,174] The lesion is demonstrated to be homogeneous and smooth bordered. The relationship to tendons and neurovascular structures is particularly well demonstrated by MRI using its multiplanar capability (Figures 17-32 and 17-33).

## Malignant Tumors

**Synovial Cell Sarcoma.**    Synovial cell sarcoma is an uncommon tumor with a predilection for the foot. Despite its name, synovial cell sarcomas do not originate from synovial tissue or from joints.[279] Mesenchymal tissue adjacent to joints and synovial lined tissues gives origin to these tumors.

Synovial cell sarcoma usually occurs between the ages of 20 and 40 but can appear at any age. Clinical presentation is that of a slowly growing, painful mass associated with erythema and edema. Slow growth is characteristic of synovial cell sarcoma.[280] Considered highly aggressive, local recurrence after surgery is common and is associated with poor prognosis. Identifying the entire extent of the tumor is crucial when considering surgical intervention of a synovial cell sarcoma.

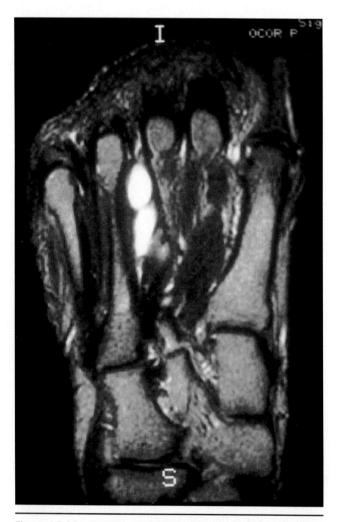

**Figure 17-32**    Axial T2-weighted image shows a lobulated high signal intensity lesion in the third intermetatarsal space that represents a ganglion cyst.

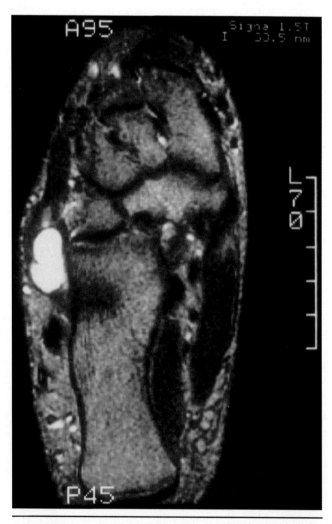

**Figure 17-33**    Axial T2-weighted image through the midfoot shows a rounded high-signal-intensity lesion with very thin walls and no adjacent edema or bony abnormality—a typical pattern for a benign ganglion cyst.

CT may show a soft tissue thickening with a mass. The extent of the mass, with involvement of adjacent normal soft tissues, is also visualized, as are intralesional calcifications. Calcifications have been associated with a more favorable prognosis. Contrast enhancement may or may not aid in delineating the mass.

T1-weighted MR images show a low-signal-intensity mass and demonstrate its extent along with any adjacent bony and soft tissue involvement.[96,264,281,282] The lesion may be of high and/or intermediate signal intensity on T2-weighted images. High signal intensity on T2-weighted images represents areas of necrosis within the tumor. Focal calcifications or hemorrhage may also be seen as dark foci (low signal intensity) within the lesion.[281]

**Malignant Fibrous Histiocytoma.** Malignant fibrous histiocytoma (MFH) is evident in adult life.[283] It occurs in the extremities, especially in the legs. Occurrence in the foot has been reported.[284–286] MFH occurs primarily in middle-aged Caucasian males (ages 50 to 70) and is considered rare in children and in those below age 20.[283]

Clinical presentation of MFH is that of a slowly enlarging, painless mass. Usually no systemic signs appear unless the tumor occurs in the retroperitoneum. MFH has variable histological presentations and a high recurrence rate.[284] Although considered infrequent, metastasis does occur.[284,285]

CT shows a dense, multilobed, mixed-density soft tissue mass with or without underlying bony involvement. The exact relationship of the tumor to muscle and even bone may not be clearly demonstrated by CT.[287] Inflammatory response and surrounding edema cannot be discerned from muscle. Calcifications within the mass may or may not be present.[288] In addition, the evaluation is limited in the axial plane.

On T1-weighted images, MFH presents with a low to moderate signal intensity, lower than that of fat but higher than that of muscle. T2-weighted images demonstrate a high signal intensity that representing hemorrhage, necrosis, and an occasional low-signal-intensity focus representing hemosiderin deposits or fibrosis. Resolution of peritumoral edema following chemotherapy is also well documented by MRI.

Unlike CT, MRI shows the exact relationships among the tumor, surrounding muscle, fascia, and vessels. In addition, edema is well differentiated from muscle in MR evaluation of MFH.[211]

**Liposarcoma.** Liposarcoma is a common soft tissue sarcoma. It is commonly found in the thigh, gluteal region, the leg, and the retroperitoneum. Rarely does it occur in the foot or arise from a pre-existing lipoma.

Liposarcomas are divided into five different categories: embryonal, myxoid, pleomorphic, well differentiated, and round cell.[289] Histologically, they vary in the amounts of fat and soft tissue components.

Radiographically, liposarcoma appears as an ill-defined mass with both water and fat densities. Calcifications, ossifications, and increased density correlates with the aggressiveness of the tumor.

CT evaluation usually reveals a fatty mass that contains linear areas of low attenuation.[290] The mass is nonhomogeneous, and internal calcifications may be present. The borders of the tumor may not be well demonstrated by CT. Contrast-enhanced CT has been used to better evaluate liposarcomas.[287]

Histologically, different liposarcomas have different MR characteristics.[291,292] Depending on the relative amount of fatty tissue within the liposarcoma, they may be of a higher signal intensity on T1-weighted images.[250] They can thus have a higher signal intensity than surrounding muscle. However, if little fatty tissue is present (very common in liposarcomas), they may well have a lower signal intensity than a lipoma or subcutaneous fat.

In myxoid liposarcomas the relative water content causes the lesion to emit a low signal intensity on T1-weighted images. Overall, MR is superior to CT in delineating these lesions from surrounding soft tissue structures. Low-grade liposarcoma may be difficult to distinguish from benign lipoma.

## Metastatic Disease

One of the most deadly aspects of cancer is metastasis. The skeletal system is the third most common site of metastasis in terms of both frequency and clinical effects.[293] Up to 30% of all patients with primary tumors demonstrate microscopic evidence of osseous metastasis at autopsy.[294] The term *acrometastasis* refers to metastatic lesions of the hand and foot. Between 0.007% and 0.3% of all metastatic lesions are in this category.[294]

Although rare, acrometastases are important for several reasons:

1. They may be the first manifestation of an occult cancer.
2. They may herald the presence of other more widespread metastasis.
3. They mimic other disease processes and if misdiagnosed may delay diagnosis and treatment.[295]

The first reported case of acrometastasis was in the bones of the hand, in 1906. Bloodgood in 1920 reported the first case of metastatic disease involving bones of the foot.[296] Since then, sporadic cases of foot metastasis have been reported. In his paper, Gall reviewed 2800 osseous tumors and found only 11 involving the foot.[297] In 1980, Bunkis reviewed and presented 27 cases of osseous metastasis to the foot.[298] Zindrich and associates reported on 72 cases of metastatic tumors to the bones of the foot, in a world literature review.[299] Recently Libson and associates reported on 22 new cases,[300] for a combined reported case total of 94 metastatic tumors to the foot.

The specific mechanism of osseous metastasis to the peripheral skeleton are not well understood. Anatomic aspects of the vasculature, special characteristics of the osseous, and differential properties of the tumor cells all have been implicated.[301] Trauma, thermal differences, hormonal influence, local hemodynamic factors, and host immune response have all been implicated in affecting the chances of tumor emboli implanting at a particular site.[301]

Radiographically, these lesions are predominantly osteo-lytic, although osteoblastic lesions have been reported. Initial radiographic findings may be very subtle and can be easily missed. Because the calcaneus is predominantly cancellous in substance, lytic lesions are not readily recognizable. At least a 2-week lag delays detecting density changes in cancellous bone on conventional radiography, making ancillary studies a necessity in early diagnosis. As it enlarges, the neoplasm may cause ballooning of the thinned cortical shell of the calcaneus. Once the neoplasm has broken through the cortical shell, it usually involves the contiguous soft tissues.

CT has also completely replaced conventional tomography in delineating metastatic lesions. The contrast resolution of computed tomography is 10 times greater than that of conventional radiography, and it better discloses trabecular and cortical bone destruction, replacement of marrow fat by neoplastic tissue, extension into the surrounding soft tissue, and involvement of neurovascular structures.[302] CT is especially useful when percutaneous biopsy is being considered.[303] CT has demonstrated metastasis to the spine where conventional radiography has failed to do so.[304]

MRI is superior to CT for detecting metastasis involving the marrow space. However, CT is superior in demonstrating cortical involvement of bony fragmentation or calcification associated with the tumor. MRI is excellent in revealing soft tissue involvement as well as extent of the lesion. Osseous metastases typically demonstrate decreased signal intensity on T1-weighted images.[305] The occasional exception is tumor in which there has been recent hemorrhage. T2-weighted images of metastases vary according to the nature of the tissue, (including degree of cellularity and water content) but in general appear as increased in signal intensity.[305]

In conclusion, CT and MRI are excellent modalities in evaluating metastatic disease, especially when surgery or radiotherapy are being considered. Both modalities have proved effective in early detection of spinal metastasis and play an increasing role in the detection and evaluation of metastatic disease. MRI is more sensitive for detecting metastasis.

# ■ CONGENITAL ANOMALIES

## Tarsal Coalition

Tarsal coalition is a congenital anomaly in which two or more tarsal bone are fused. The tarsal bones may be fused together by fibrous, cartilaginous, or bony tissue. Coalitions are usually present at birth and are rarely of the bony type. Physical examination usually shows limited subtalar motion associated with pes planus and spasm of the peroneal muscles,[306] with routine radiographic studies, diagnosis of coalitions may sometimes be missed. Nuclear medicine, although it shows radioactive tracer uptake that indicates abnormalities, is usually nonspecific. Overlapping structures are not easily detected by conventional radiography; thus a tomographic technique is often necessary for evaluating the tarsal bones and their articulations in these lesions. MRI and CT are quite useful for evaluating overlapping structures that are often found in coalitions. Tarsal coalitions may be evaluated using T1- and T2-weighted spin echo, and volumetric gradient echo MR pulse sequence. These techniques are useful for detecting bony, cartilaginous, and fibrous fusions as well as any soft tissue or marrow space changes that may be associated with these foot deformities.

Coronal and sagittal CT sections through the talus and calcaneus are quite helpful as well. CT can distinguish between osseous and nonosseous coalition. It can provide information regarding other articulations throughout the foot. CT not only detects the coalition, but it can also assess the extent of the coalition, as is important for preoperative planning. Moreover, it can provide a three-dimensional assessment of height, width, and depth of the coalition.[307] CT is also quite useful in evaluating degenerative changes within a joint complex. Because CT only allows limited soft tissue evaluation, MRI with its superior soft tissue contrast can better assess soft tissue involvement and other related changes.

**Calcaneonavicular Coalition.**  Occurring in more than 50% of the cases, calcaneonavicular coalition is the most frequent type of tarsal coalition.[308] In this type of coalition, the calcaneus is fused with the navicular bones. Although the condition is relatively asymptomatic, patients may present with pain, persistent discomfort in the subtalar region, and spastic flatfoot deformity. These signs and symptoms usually develop in the second or third decades of life. Males predominate.

This type of coalition may sometimes be detected on plain radiography; however, routine anterior, posterior, and lateral views of the foot may not clearly demonstrate such a deformity.[309] Bony fusions per se are usually seen in routine radiographic studies, whereas bony sclerosis and irregularity of the cortices of the calcaneus and navicular are signs suggestive of fibrous and cartilaginous fusion. The actual cartilaginous and fibrous fusions themselves, in contrast, are not detected on radiography.

### Talocalcaneal Coalition.

In talocalcaneal coalition (Figure 17-34), the middle facet of the talus are fused with the calcaneus. Talocalcaneal coalition is the second most common coalition, occurring in 35% of the cases diagnosed with congenital coalitions.[308] Patients present with vague pain, discomfort, and flatfoot deformity. Talocalcaneal coalition limits any inversion and eversion of the ankle.[310] Again, as in calcaneonavicular coalition, males predominate.

Owing to the complexity of the talocalcaneal joint, it is difficult for routine radiography to visualize coalition in its entirety. Thus, secondary signs are used to diagnose the fusions. These signs include talar beak, rounding of the

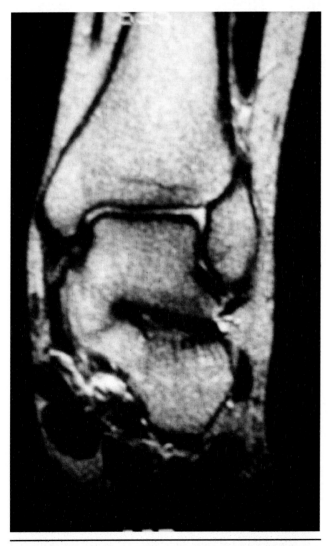

**Figure 17-34** Coronal T2-weighted image through the hind foot demonstrating a bony coalition between the talus and the calcaneus. The marrow space is continuous between the two bones.

lateral process of the talus, talocalcaneal joint space narrowing, and asymmetry of the anterior subtalar joints as seen on lateral oblique views. However, these signs are only suggestive of talocalcaneal coalition and thus not diagnostic. Here too, MRI and CT can be extremely helpful in diagnosing these lesions and guiding the surgeon toward the appropriate therapy.

### Other Types of Coalition.

Other extremely rare forms of coalition include talonavicular coalition and calcaneocuboid coalition. Talonavicular coalition is a fusion between the talus and the navicular. The bridges can be osseous, cartilaginous, or fibrous. Diagnosis is usually made by conventional radiography. The calcaneocuboid coalition may also be osseous, fibrous, or cartilaginous. Frequently these entities can be adequately assessed by conventional radiography. However, high-resolution multiplanar CT or even MRI can be used to diagnose occult lesions and/or help guide preoperative planning.

## Other Congenital Anomalies

*Talipes equinovarus* (also termed clubfoot) is a serious congenital anomaly. The anomaly usually occurs in isolation; however, it may be seen with other abnormalities. The talocalcaneal angle is markedly reduced, often seen with the long axes of a talus and calcaneus superimposed.[308] The long axes of the first and fifth metatarsal converge laterally to the calcaneus.

*Metatarsus adductus* is a deformity that is present at birth. However, this anomaly is not typically diagnosed until 3 to 4 months later.[308] All metatarsals are adducted at the tarsometatarsal joints while the calcaneus is in normal position.

*Calcaneovalgus* is usually bilateral and uncommon. In this deformity, the foot is dorsiflexed and against the lower leg. While the heel is in calcaneovalgus, the forefoot has an abduction planus.

## ■ NEURAL IMPINGEMENT SYNDROME

### Tarsal Tunnel Syndrome

Tarsal tunnel syndrome is a neuropathic condition involving the impingement or compression of the posterior tibial nerve and branches as it passes through the tunnel under the flexor retinaculum. Tarsal tunnel syndrome was first described by Keck.[311] The tunnel is a fibro-osseous canal containing the long toe flexors, flexor digitorum longus tendon, flexor hallux longus, posterior tibial tendon, and the neurovascular bundle that contains the posterior tibial nerve.[312, 313]

A number of factors contributing to the impingement have been reported. These include thickening of the flexor retinaculum, distension of tendon sheaths caused by tenosynovitis, neoplastic processes, and variscosities.[312,314] The clinical presentation includes pain along the plantar surface of the foot, soft tissue edema, and tenderness about the medial aspect of the ankle. As the condition progressively worsens, sensory impairment may develop. The diagnosis of tarsal tunnel syndrome requires adequate anatomic delineation. Depiction of the structures within the tunnel and other associated anatomic structures proximal and distal to the overlying flexor retinaculum are demonstrated using T1- and T2-weighted MR imaging. On axial MR scans, the nerve may be seen as a tiny, round, gray (low signal intensity) structure closely associated with the flexor hallux longus tendon; adjacent to the nerve is the posterior tibial tendon, which is characterized as a low-signal ovoid structure.[315] In addition, all tunnel boundaries may also be identified on MRI studies.[315]

Sagittal MR images can show the bifurcating nerve within the tunnel. However, sagittal images do not depict all the boundaries of the tunnel. MR images in the axial and sagittal planes are best for depiction of the tunnel, because these orientations provide visualization of posterior tibial nerve, the tunnel's boundaries, and other structures within the tunnel.

The use of MRA vascular flow techniques with/without selective saturation bands allows selective delineation of the vascular structures within the tarsal tunnel. In addition, T1-weighted MR pulse sequences provide high-resolution images depicting the tunnel with great anatomic detail. Neoplastic processes, ganglions cysts, edema, hemorrhage, and other soft tissue changes may also be demonstrated by MRI using T2 pulse sequences.

The diagnosis of tarsal tunnel syndrome is confirmed by abnormal nerve conduction studies.[316] As conservative forms of treatment, anti-inflammatory agents and corticosteroid injections may provide only transient relief. Surgical decompression, in contrast, has proven successful in providing long-term relief in some patients.[312,317]

## ■ MARROW SPACE DISORDERS

### Ischemic Necrosis

**Osteonecrosis of the Bone.** The general term *ischemia* is used to describe pathologic changes associated with deficient blood supply and its sequelae in tissues. The term *ischemic necrosis of bone (osteonecrosis)* refers to death of bone and its marrow secondary to ischemia. Other terms frequently used to describe osteonecrosis include *aseptic necrosis, avascular necrosis,* and *osteochondritis.*[318]

Ischemia to bone can be a result of a whole host of conditions. Extraosseous causes include trauma, vasculitis, vasospasms, baronecrosis or decompression sickness, and elevated extraosseous venous pressure. Intraosseous causes of bone ischemia include sinusoidal obstruction, sickle cell

disease, thrombosis, tumors, hypertrophy of lipid cells, and idiopathic causes.[319]

Systemic conditions that have been associated with osteonecrosis include pancreatitis, systemic lupus erythematosus, rheumatoid arthritis, Cushing's disease, hemophilia, Gaucher's disease, alcoholic fatty liver disease, and chronic steroid use.[320]

**Pathophysiology.** The pathophysiology and sequelae of ischemic necrosis of bone depend on (1) location of the ischemic insult and (2) the nature and composition of the bone marrow at the site of infarct.[321]

Infarcts in metaphyseal and diaphyseal regions lend themselves to significant collateralization and are fairly well protected against ischemic necrosis. Epiphyseal regions are predominantly cartilaginous and therefore lack direct blood supply and are more susceptible to necrosis.

The composition of the involved bone marrow is also relevant in ischemic necrosis.[322] Hematopoietic marrow (red marrow) is highly vascular and is less vulnerable to ischemia. Red marrow is found in the axial skeleton, skull, proximal humeri, and proximal femoral. The blood supply in yellow (fatty) marrow is relatively sparse, compared with red marrow, and hence is more susceptible to osteonecrosis.[321]

Zizic and associates postulated that an increase in bone marrow pressure either directly or as a result of ischemia, causes resistance to blood flow, and thus congestion, with eventual ischemia, edema, and eventually cell damage or death.[319]

**Histology.** Histologically the ischemic insult eventually results in cell death.[318,323] Although red marrow is highly vascular, the hematopietic cells are most vulnerable to ischemia and die within the first 6 to 12 hours. A host response is initiated, resulting in inflammation and hyperemia that cause edema. Fat cells are more resistant to ischemia and survive 2 to 5 days after the ischemic insult. Next, within 48 hours, the bone cells die. These include osteoblasts, osteoclasts, and osteocytes.

A reactive interface results at the periphery of the ischemic focus, which is characterized by inflammation, increased vascularity, granulation, and fibroblastic tissue. Continued hyperemia and edema can eventually cause significant bony resorption, allowing articular collapse and subsequent degenerative joint disease on continued weight bearing.

### Osteonecrosis Involving the Bones of the Foot

**Osteonecrosis of the Metatarsals—Freiberg Disease.** Avascular necrosis of the metatarsals was described first by Freiberg in 1914. Since then numerous authors have described the condition and proposed various etiologies.[324–326] It is now accepted that repetitive trauma is responsible for Freiberg's infarct.[318,327] The second metatarsal is most frequently involved. The third and fourth metatarsals are less frequently involved. The first and fifth metatarsals are also affected.[328]

Smilie and Helal described in detail the pathologic staging of Freiberg disease.[327,329] Essentially, a fracture of the subchondral bone plate occurs, with subsequent resorption of the metatarsal head as it flattens. This description correlates with the radiographic findings of this entity.

Clinically, the condition is more common in females than males by a ratio of 4:1. The teenage years are most commonly affected. A "variant" of Freiberg's disease also has been reported in older age groups.[330] Pain and swelling are the initial findings, subsequently progressing to degenerative joint disease with limitation of motion and deformity.

**Osteonecrosis of the Talus.**    A significant complication of talar fractures is avascular necrosis. The complication usually follows talar neck and talar body fractures and arthrodesis involving the subtalar joint complex.

Avascular necrosis involving the talar body can be suspected as early as 6 to 8 weeks after injury. The extent of necrosis depends on the degree of displacement of the fracture(s). Evidence of bone resorption, revealed as subchondral bony demineralization in the dome of the talus, is evidence of an intact blood supply.[331] The talar body is relatively dense if the blood supply is interrupted secondary to avascular necrosis.

**Osteonecrosis of the Navicular—Köhler Disease.**    Köhler's disease, or osteonecrosis of the tarsal navicular, in children is thought to result from repetitive compression forces on the navicular during weight bearing.[332] This disease was first described by Köhler in 1908.

Köhler's disease is about four to six times more frequent in males than in females, and the involvement is usually unilateral in 80% of the cases. Clinically, the child presents with a limp with pain and swelling overlying the navicular.

Radiographically, the navicular appears narrowed on a lateral view in the foot. To confirm the diagnosis of avascular necrosis of the tarsal navicular, comparative views of the appropriate foot are mandatory.

**Imaging of Osteonecrosis.**    Radionuclide imaging has been traditionally used for early detection of avascular necrosis (AVN). Radionuclide scintigraphy has been shown to be on average 85% sensitive and specific in diagnosing ischemic necrosis of bone.[333]

Scintigraphy, however, is not without pitfalls. Positive scans may also indicate fracture healing or early revascularization of bone, limiting the utility of bone scans in early detection and followup of AVN. False negative results can be as high as 49%.[319] In addition, patients with systemic causes of AVN may have multiple sites of bony involvement. This makes bone scans more difficult to interpret. In early bilateral symptomatic involvement, both bones may be interpreted as negative. In asymmetric bilateral AVN, the less affected side is frequently overlooked.[319]

CT evaluation of AVN offers helpful information concerning the extent of the process. In the presence of AVN, the normal arrangement of trabecular bone becomes altered. CT allows detection of subtle cortical, subchondral, and cancellous fractures resulting from the ischemic process.[334] Thus CT can be important in surgical planning for treatment of AVN.

Among the modalities used in detecting AVN, MRI has proved the most effective.[334-337] This is because MRI is very sensitive for detection of abnormal bone marrow.[321] Because marrow necrosis is an early part of AVN, MRI is generally considered somewhat superior to scintigraphy and much better than CT for detecting avascular necrosis (Figure 17-35).

The MRI finding in AVN corresponds to the pathologic staging of the disease.[321] T1-weighted images of early AVN reveal the lesion to be lower in signal intensity than is fat. This lowered signal represents areas of edema and increased cellularity. Thus the area is usually irregular, with low signal intensity on T1- and high on T2-weighted images. This is consistent with the acute inflammatory stage, marked by increased hyperperfusion and edema. In the later stages, replacement of the fatty marrow by cellular debris, granulation tissue, fibrosis, and necrosis result in decreased signal intensity on *both* T1- and T2-weighted images.

The interface between the necrotic focus and the healthy bone in AVN is well demonstrated by MRI. The interface is depicted as a low-signal-intensity rim on T1-weighted images and a raised signal intensity on T2-weighted images. When present, this double-line sign is thought to be characteristic of ischemic necrosis.[334]

## Reflex Sympathetic Dystrophy

Reflex sympathetic dystrophy (RSD) is a sympathetically maintained pain disorder with a wide range of a clinical manifestations mediated by the sympathetic nerves. Numerous names have been used to describe RSD, including *Sudek's atrophy, causalgia, post-traumatic dystrophy,* and many others.[338,339]

The exact etiology of RSD is unknown. RSD can be described as an abnormal physiologic response or an exaggerated negative response of an extremity to trauma. The condition results from microtrauma, surgical procedures, tendon or ligament sprains, infections, and neoplasms.[340,341]

The clinical manifestation of reflex sympathetic dystrophy always includes pain that is out of proportion to the visible injury and is intractable. The clinical spectrum occurs in three stages. Stage 1 is characterized by diffuse pain, inflammation, edema, hypothermia, or hyperthermia. Stage 2, also known as the dystrophic stage, occurs 2 to 6 months after the onset of RSD. This stage is characterized by brawny edema, hyperhydrosis, muscle atrophy, and spotty osteoporosis. Stage 3 is the atrophic stage and is characterized by irreversible atrophic changes. This includes pale, cool, dry skin, generalized osteoporosis, and complete joint stiffness.

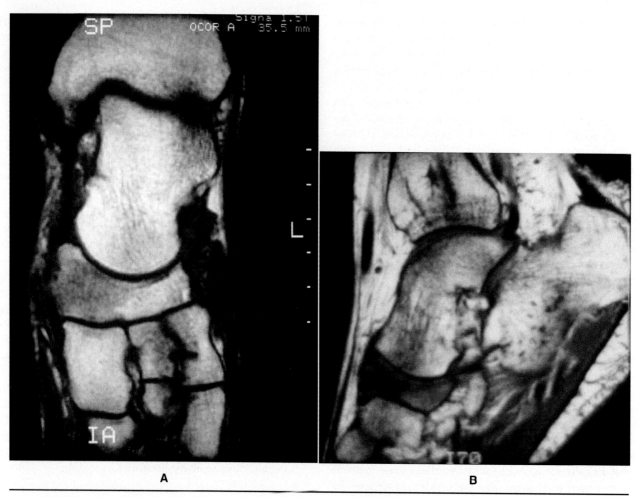

**Figure 17-35**    Axial (A) and sagittal (B) T1-weighted images through the midfoot show diminished signal intensity in the navicular bone secondary to early avascular necrosis.

Hartley described the types of radiographic changes related to RSD.[342]

*Type A:* Consists of the discrete mottling throughout a large portion of the involved bone. These findings are particularly prominent in the tarsal bones and the cancellous portion of long bones of the extremities.

*Type B:* Manifested by deossification in metaphyseal ends of the toes, producing a rarefaction band. These bands were also found in the metatarsals and the distal ends of the tibia and fibula.

*Type C:* Characterized by subchondral deossification.

*Type D:* Characterized by diffuse mottling of all portions of the involved bones.

Radionuclide bone scintigraphy and thermography have been successfully used as aids in the diagnosis of RSD. However, neither of these modalities are specific. Bone scans usually reveal diffuse increased uptake in the area involved. This is caused by the associated hyperemia resulting from an abnormal sympathetic reflex.[339,343]

MRI findings in RSD are also not specific. T1-weighted images may show a diffuse signal intensity decrease or a complete loss of signal of the involved bone. However, the bone marrow may be normal and only changes in the local musculature may be seen. T2-weighted images may show mottled nonhomogeneity of the involved bone. However, here too bone marrow may be completely normal. Although muscle atrophy and joint effusion may be present, these findings are not specific for RSD. In this study of 25 patients with RSD, Koch and associates concluded that MRI may improve the diagnostic specificity of RSD when used in conjunction with scintigraphy.[344]

## ■ COLLAGEN DISORDERS

### Marfan's Syndrome

Marfan's syndrome is a connective tissue disorder that is inherited as an autosomal dominant trait.[345,346] It affects males and females equally. Clinical manifestations most commonly involve three organ systems: skeletal, ocular, and cardiovascular.

Skeletal manifestations include arachnodactyly, dolichostenomelia, hyperextensibility in joints, deformity involving the chest wall, and asymmetric bone growth in childhood. The foot may present with arachnodactyly, pronation, pes planus, and clubfoot.

The major ocular manifestation is the ectopic lens. This abnormality may be severe, resulting in blindness, or it may not affect visual acuity at all.

Numerous cardiovascular complications have been identified throughout the literature. These include mitral valve prolapse and aortic root dilation as the most common abnormalities encountered.[346,347]

## Ehlers-Danlos Syndrome

Ehlers-Danlos syndrome is a connective tissue disorder that is inherited as an autosomal dominant trait. It is characterized by hyperextensibility in joints, fragility of blood vessels, and ligamentous and capsular laxity.

## References

1. Brooks JA: Tomography. In Ballinger PW, editor: *Radiographic positions and radiologic procedures,* ed 6, vol 3, p 22, St. Louis, 1986, Mosby.

2. Stanton L: Conventional tomography. In Taveras J, Ferrucci J, editors: *Radiology: diagnosis-imaging-intervention,* chap 12, p 1, Philadelphia, 1991, Lippincott.

3. Ho C, Sartoris DJ, Resnick D: Conventional tomography in musculoskeletal trauma, *Radiol Clin North Am* 27(5):929, 1989.

4. Resnick D: Conventional tomography. In Resnick, D, Niwayama G, editors: *Diagnosis of bone and joint disorders,* vol 1, p 313, Philadelphia, 1981, Sanders.

5. Cass JR, Morrey BF: Ankle instability: current concepts, diagnosis, and treatment, *Mayo Clin Proc* 59: 165, 1984.

6. Erickson SJ, Smith JW, Ruiz ME et al: MR imaging of the collateral ligament of the ankle, *AJR* 156:131, 1991.

7. Kier R, Dietz MJ, McCarthy SM, Rudicel SA: MR imaging of the normal ligaments and tendons of the ankle, *J Comput Assist Tomogr* 15(3):477, 1991.

8. Liou J, Totty WG, Magnetic resonance imaging of ankle injuries, *Top Magn Reson Imaging* 3(4):1, 1991.

9. Berquist TH: Magnetic resonance imaging of the foot and ankle, *Semin Ultrasound CT MR* 11(4):327, 1990.

10. Hajek PC, Baker LL, Sartoris DJ et al: MR arthrography: anatomic pathologic investigation, *Radiology* 163:141, 1987.

11. Deutsche AL, Mink JH: Musculoskeletal trauma, *Top Magn Reson Imaging* 1(4):53, 1989.

12. Rosenberg ZS, Feldman F, Singson RD, Kane R: Ankle tendons: evaluation with CT, *Radiology* 166:221, 1988.

13. Frey CC, Shereff MJ: Tendon injuries about the ankle in athletes, *Clin Sports Med* 7:103, 1988.

14. Marcus DS, Reicher MA, Kellerhouse LE: Achilles tendon injuries: the role of MR imaging, *J Comput Assist Tomogr* 13(3):480, 1989.

15. Scheller AD, Kasser JR, Quigley TB: Tendon injuries about the ankle, *Orthop Clin North Am* 11:801, 1980.

16. Inglis AE, Scott WN, Sculco TP: Rupture of the tendo Achille: an objective assessment of surgical and nonsurgical treatment, *J Bone Joint Surg* 58A:990, 1976.

17. Deutsch AL, Mink JH: Magnetic resonance imaging of musculoskeletal injuries, *Radiol Clin North Am* 27(5):983, 1989.

18. Noto AM, Cheung Y, Rosenberg ZS et al: MR imaging of the ankle: normal variants, *Radiology* 170:121, 1989.

19. Rosenberg ZS, Cheung Y, Jahss MH: Computed tomography scan and magnetic resonance imaging of ankle tendons: an overview, *Foot & Ankle* 8:297, 1988.

20. Rosenberg ZS, Cheung Y, Jahss MH et al: Rupture of posterior tibial tendon: CT and MR imaging with surgical correlation, *Radiology* 169:229, 1988.

21. Kieft GJ, Bloem JL, Rozing PM et al: MR imaging of recurrent anterior dislocation of the shoulder: comparison with CT arthrography, *AJR* 150:1083, 1988.

22. Zeiss J, Saddemi SR, Ebraheim NA: MR imaging of the peroneal tunnel, *J Comput Assist Tomogr* 13(5):840-844, 1989.

23. Kerr R, Computed tomography. In Forrester DM, Kricun ME, Kerr R, editors: *Imaging of the foot and ankle,* Rockville, Md, 1988, Aspen.

24. Deutsch AL, Mink JH, Shellock FG: Magnetic resonance imaging of injuries to bone and articular cartilage: emphasis on radiographically occult abnormalities, *Orthop Rev* 19(1):66, 1990.

25. Stafford SA, Rosenthal DI, Gebhardt MC, Brady TJ, Scott JA: MRI in stress fracture, *AJR* 147:553, 1986.

26. Folik AB, Gould N: Osteochondritis dissecans of the talus (transchondral fractures of the talus): review of the literature and new surgical approach for the medial dome lesions, *Foot & Ankle* 5(4):165, 1985.

27. Berndt AL, Harty M: Transchondral fractures (osteochondritis dissecans)of the talus, *J Bone Joint Surg* 41A:988, 1959.

28. Mesgarzadeh M, Sapega AA, Bonakdarpour A et al: Osteochondritis dissecans: analysis of mechanical stability with radiography, scintigraphy, and MR imaging, *Radiology* 165:775, 1987.

29. Aichroth P: Osteochondritis dissecans of the knee: a clinical survey, *J Bone Joint Surg* 53B:440, 1971.

30. Caffey J, Madell SH, Royer C et al: Ossification of the distal femoral epiphysis, *J Bone Joint Surg* 40A:647, 1958.

31. Silverman FN, *Caffey's pediatric x-ray diagnosis,* ed 8, Chicago, 1985, Mosby-Year Book.

32. Smilie IS, *Injuries of knee joint,* ed 4, Edinburgh, 1970, Livingstone.

33. Langer F, Percy EC: Osteochondritis dissecans and anomalous centers of ossification: a review of 80 lesions in 61 patients, *Can J Surg* 14:208-215, 1971.

34. Ribbing S: Hereditary multiple epiphyseal disturbance and its consequences for osteogenesis of local malacias particularly osteochondritis dissecans, *Acta Orthop Scan* 24:286, 1955.

35. Paul GR: Transchondral fractures of the talus. In Yablon IG, Segal D, Leach RE, editors: *Ankle injuries,* p 113, New York, 1983, Churchill-Livingstone.

36. Bosien WR, Staples OS, Russell SW: Residual disability following acute ankle sprains, *J Bone Joint Surg* 37A: 1237, 1955.

37. Zinman C, Wolison N, Reis D: Osteochondritis dissecans of the dome of the talus: computed tomography scanning in diagnosis and follow-up, *J Bone Joint Surg* 70A(7):1017, 1988.

38. Anderson I, Crighton K, Grattan-Smith T et al: Osteochondral fractures of the dome of the talus, *J Bone Joint Surg* 71A(8):1143, 1989.

39. Zinam C, Reis N: Osteochondritis dissecans of the talus: use of the high resolution computed tomography scanner, *Acta Orthop Scand* 53:697, 1982.

40. Sartoris D, Resnick D: Computed tomography of podiatric disorders: review, *JFS* 25(5):394, 1986.

41. DeSmet A, Fisher D, Burstein M et al: Value of MR imaging in staging osteochondral lesions of the talus (osteochondritis dissecans) in 14 patients, *AJR* 154:555, 1990.

42. Yulish B, Mulopulos G, Goodfellow D et al: MR imaging of osteochondral lesions of the talus, *J Comput Assist Tomogr* 11(2):296, 1987.

43. Alexander AH, Lichtman DM: Surgical treatment of transchondral talar-dome fracture (osteochondritis dissecans), long-term follow-up, *J Bone Joint Surg* 62A:646, 1980.

44. Linden B: Osteochondritis dissecans of the femoral condyles, *J Bone Joint Surg* 95A:95:769, 1977.

45. Cassebaum WH: Lisfranc fracture-dislocations, *Clin Orthop* 30:116, 1963.

46. Goosens M, De Stoop N: Lisfranc's fracture-dislocations: etiology, radiology, and results of treatment, *Clin Orthop* 176:154, 1983.

47. Aitken AP, Poulson D: Dislocations of the tarso-metatarsal joint, *J Bone Joint Surg* 45A:246, 1963.

48. Geckeler EO: Dislocations and fracture-dislocations of the foot: transfixion and Kirschner wires, *Surgery* 25:730, 1949.

49. Faciszewski T, Burks RT, Manaster BJ: Subtle injuries of the Lisfranc joint, *J Bone Joint Surg* 72A:1519, 1990.

50. Hardcastle PH, Reschauer R, Kutscha-Lissberg E, Schoffmann W: Injuries to the tarsometatarsal joint: incidence, classification, and treatment, *J Bone Joint Surg* 64B:349, 1982.

51. Foster SC, Foster RR: Lisfranc's tarsometatarsal fracture-dislocations, *Radiology* 120:798, 1976.

52. Goiney RC, Connell DG, Nichols DM: CT evaluation of tarsometatarsal fracture-dislocation injuries, *AJR* 144:985, 1985.

53. Lauge-Hansen N: Fractures of the ankle. II. Combined experimental-surgical and experimental-roentgenologic investigations, *Arch Surg* 60:957, 1950.

54. Morrey BF, Cass JR, Johnson KA, Berquist TH: Imaging of orthopedic trauma and surgery. In Berquist TH, editor: *Foot and ankle,* p 407, Philadelphia, 1986, Saunders.

55. Yablon IG, Heller FG, Shouse L: The key role of the lateral malleolus in displaced fractures of the ankle, *J Bone Joint Surg* 59A:169, 1977.

56. Yablon IG, Wasilewski S: Management of unstable ankle fractures, *Foot & Ankle* 1:11, 1980.

57. Yde J, Kristensen KD: Ankle fractures: supination eversion fractures stage II: primary and late operative and non-operative treatment, *Acta Orthop Scand* 51:695, 1980.

58. Edeiken J, Cotler JM, Ankle trauma, *Semin Roentgenol* 13:145, 1978.

59. Arimoto HK, Forrester DM: Classification of ankle fractures: an algorithm, *AJR* 135:1057, 1980.

60. Boyd HH: Causes and treatment of nonunion of the shafts of the long bones with a review of 741 patients, *AAOS Instructional Course Lecture,* vol 17, p 165, St. Louis, 1960, Mosby.

61. Boyd HB, Lipinski SW, Wiley JH: Observations on nonunion of the shafts of long bones with a statistical analysis of 842 patients, *J Bone Joint Surg* 43A:159, 1961.

62. Vogler H, Randolph T: Nonunions and delayed unions, *JFS* 24(1):62, 1984.

63. Costa A: Delayed union in metatarsal osteotomies, *J Am Podiatr Assoc* 16(4):127, 1977.

64. Crenshaw AH: Nonunions. In Crenshaw AH, editor: *Campbell's operative orthopedics,* vol 1, p 761, St Louis, 1974, Mosby.

65. Gudas CJ, Cann JE: Nonunions and related disorders, *Clin Podiatr Med Surg* 8(2):321-339, 1991.

66. Cozens L: Does diabetes delay fracture healing? *Clin Orthop* 82:134, 1972.

67. Rothman R: The effect of iron deficiency anemia on fracture healing, *Clin Orthop* 77:276, 1971.

68. Misol S: Growth hormone in delayed fracture union, *Clin Orthop* 74:206, 1971.

69. Weber GB, Cech O: *Pseudoarthritis,* pp 40-44, New York, 1976, Grune & Stratton.

70. Lund BG, Lund JO: Evaluation of fracture healing in

man by serial 99m Tc-Sn-pyrophosphate scintimetry, *Acta Orthop Scand* 49:435, 1978.

71. Esterhal JL Jr, Brighton CT, Heppenstall RB et al: Detection of synovial pseudoarthritis by 99m-Tc scintigraphy, *Clin Orthop* 96:15, 1981.

72. Mink JH, Deutsch AL: Occult cartilage and bone injuries of the knee: detection, classification, and assessment with MR imaging, *Radiology* 167:749-751, 1988.

73. Yao L, Lee JK: Occult intraosseous fracture: detection with MR imaging, *Radiology* 167:749-751, 1988.

74. Leach RE, Seavey MS, Salter DK: Results of surgery in athletes with plantar fasciitis, *Foot & Ankle* 7:156, 1986.

75. Hill JJ Jr, Cutting PJ: Heel pain and body weight, *Foot & Ankle* 9:254, 1989.

76. Kwong PK, Kay D, Vower RT, White MW: Plantar fasciitis: mechanics and pathomechanics of treatment, *Clin Sports Med* 11:215, 1983.

77. Snider MP, Clancy WG, McBath AA: Plantar fascia release for chronic plantar fasciitis in runners, *Am J Sports Med* 14:481, 1986.

78. Campbell JW, Inman VT: Treatment of plantar fasciitis and calcaneal spurs with the UCBL shoe insert, *Clin Orthop* 103:57, 1974.

79. Jahss M: Surgery of the adult heel. In Jahss M, editor: *Disorders of the foot and ankle: medical and surgical management*, vol 2, p 1396, Philadelphia, 1991, Saunders.

80. Williams PL, Smibert JG, Cox R et al: Imaging study of the painful heel syndrome, *Foot & Ankle* 7:345, 1987.

81. Berkowitz J, Kier R, Rudicel S: Plantar fasciitis: MR imaging, *Radiology* 179:665, 1991.

82. Leach R, Jones R, Silva T: Ruptures of the plantar fascia in athletes, *J Bone Joint Surg* 60A(4):537, 1978.

83. Jahss M: *Disorders of the foot and ankle*, vol 2, Philadelphia, 1991, Saunders.

84. Enzinger FM, Weiss SW: *Soft tissue tumors*, ed 2, pp 136-163, St Louis, 1988, Mosby.

85. Wetzel LH, Levine E: Soft tissue tumors of the foot: value of MR imaging for specific diagnosis, *AJR* 155:1025-1030, 1990.

86. Reitano JJ, Hauvy P, Nykyri E et al: The desmoid tumor. I. Incidence, sex age, and anatomical distribution in the Finnish population, *Am J Clin Pathol* 7:665-685, 1982.

87. Sundaram M, McGuire MH, Schajowicz F, Soft tissue masses: histologic basis for decreased signal on T2 weighted MR image, *AJR* 148:1247-1250, 1987.

88. Totty WG, Murphy WA, Lee JKT, Soft tissue tumors: MR imaging, *Radiology* 160:135-141, 1986.

89. Looking B, Marks J: Cellulitis. In Looking B, editor: *Principles of dermatology*, p 189, Philadelphia, 1986, Saunders.

90. Lankin J, Frier B, Ireland J: Diabetes mellitus and infection, *Postgrad Med* 61:233, 1985.

91. Arensow DJ, Sherwood C, Wilson R: Neuropathy, angiopathy and sepsis in the diabetic foot. III. Sepsis. *J Am Podiatr Assoc* 72:35, 1982.

92. Sullivan DC, Rosenfield NS, Ogden J, Gotschalk A: Problems in scintigraphic detection of osteomyelitis in children, *Radiology* 135:731, 1980.

93. Beltran J, Campanini S, Knight C, McCalla M: The diabetic foot: magnetic resonance imaging evaluation, *Skeletal Radiol* 19:37, 1990.

94. Moore T, Yuh W, Kathol M et al: Abnormalities of the foot in patients with diabetes mellitus: findings on MR imaging, *AJR* 157:9813, 1991.

95. Wall S, Fisher M, Amparo E et al: Magnetic resonance imaging in the evaluation of abscess, *AJR* 144:1217, 1985.

96. Kransdorf M, Jelinek J, Moser R et al: Soft tissue masses: diagnosis using MR imaging, *AJR* 153:541, 1989.

97. Tang J, Gold R, Bassett L, Seeger L: Musculoskeletal infection of the extremities: evaluation with MR imaging, *Radiology* 166:205, 1988.

98. Modic MT, Pflanze W, Feiglin D et al: MRI of musculo-skeletal infections, *Radiol Clin North Am* 24:247, 1986.

99. Deutsch A: Bone and soft tissue infection. In Deutsch A, Mink J, Kerr R, editors: *MRI of the foot and ankle*, p 199, New York, 1992, Raven Press.

100. Mason M, Zlatkin M, Esterhal J et al: Chronic complicated osteomyelitis of the lower extremity: evaluation with MR imaging, *Radiology* 173:355, 1989.

101. Beltran J, McGhee RB, Shaffer PB et al: Experimental infections of the musculoskeletal system: evaluation MR imaging and Tc-99m MDP and GA 67 scintography, *Radiology* 167:167, 1988.

102. Yuh W, Corson J, Baraniewski H et al: Osteomyelitis of the foot in diabetic patients: evaluation with plain film, 99m Tc MDP bone scintigraphy and MR imaging, *AJR* 152(4):795, 1989.

103. Chandnani VP, Beltran J, Morris CS et al: Acute experimental osteomyelitis and abscess: detection with MR imaging versus CT, *Radiology* 174:233, 1990.

104. Waldvogel FA, Medoof G, Swartz MN: Osteomyelitis: a review of clinical features, therapeutic considerations and unusual aspects, *N Engl J Med* 282:198, 260, 316, 1970.

105. Bamberger DM, Daus GP, Gerding DM: Osteomyelitis in the feet of diabetic patients: long term results, prognostic factors and the role of antimicrobial and surgical therapy, *Am J Med* 83:653, 1987.

106. David R, Barron BJ, Madewell JE: Osteomyelitis, acute and chronic, *Radiol Clin North Am* 25(6):1171, 1987.

107. Golimbu C, Firooznia H, Rafii M: CT of osteomyelitis of the spine, *AJR* 142:159, 1984.

108. Unger E, Moldofsky P, Gatenby R, Hartz W, Broder G: Diagnosis of osteomyelitis by MR imaging, *AJR* 150:605, 1988.

109. Miller WB, Murphy WA, Gilula LA: Brodie's abscess: reappraisal, *Radiology* 132:15, 1979.

110. Brailsford JF: Brodie's abscess and its differential diagnosis, *BMJ* 120:119, 1938.

111. Erdman WA, Tamburro F, Jayson HT et al: Osteomyelitis: characteristics and pitfalls of diagnosis with MR imaging, *Radiology* 180:533, 1991.

112. Tan J, Flanagan P, Donovan D, File T: Team approach in the management of diabetic foot infections, *JFS* (suppl) 23(1):12, 1987.

113. Bose K: A surgical approach for the infected diabetic foot, *Int Orthop* 3:177, 1979.

114. Sartoris D, Devine S, Resnick D et al: Plantar compartmental infection in the diabetic foot: the role of computed tomography, *Invest Radiol* 20:772, 1980.

115. McLeod RA: Arthritis. In Berquist TH, editor: *Radiology of the foot and ankle,* pp 213-246, New York, 1989, Raven Press.

116. Hertzanu Y, Bar-Ziv J: Case report 606, *Skeletal Radiol* 19:225-226, 1990.

117. Ehara S, Kattapuram SV, Khurana JS: Case report 551, *Skeletal Radiol* 18:329-330, 1989.

118. Shogry MEC, Pope TL Jr: Vacuum phenomenon simulating meniscal or cartilaginous injury of the knee at MR imaging, *Radiology* 180:513-515, 1991.

119. Seltzer SE, Weissman BN, Braunstein EM et al: Computed tomography of the hindfoot, *J Comput Assist Tomogr* 8(3):488, 1984.

120. Beltran J, Caudill JL, Herman LA et al: Rheumatoid arthritis: MR imaging manifestations, *Radiology* 165:153-157, 1987.

121. Adam G, Dammer M, Bohndorf K et al: Rheumatoid arthritis of the knee: value of gaodopentetate dimeglumine-enhanced MR imaging, *AJR* 156:125-129, 1991.

122. Rubenstein J, Pritzker KPH: Crystal-associated arthropathies, *AJR* 152:685, 1989.

123. Grahame R, Scott JT: Clinical survey of 354 patients with gout, *Ann Rheum Dis* 29:461, 1970.

124. Cornelius R, Schneider HJ: Gouty arthritis in the adult, *Radiol Clin North Am* 26:1267, 1988.

125. Boss GR, Seegmiller JE: Hyperuricemia and gout: classification, complications and management, *N Engl J Med* 300:1459, 1985.

126. Wyngaarden JB, Kelley WN: *Gout and hyperuricemia,* New York, 1976, Grune & Stratton.

127. Jensen PS, Putman CE: Current concepts with respect to chondrocalcinosis and the pseudogout syndrome, *AJR* 123:531-539, 1975.

128. Brower A, Allman RM: Pathogenesis of the neurotrophic joint: neurotraumatic vs. neurovascular, *Radiology* 139:349, 1981.

129. Brower A, Allman RM: The neurotrophic joint: a neurovascular bone disorders, *Radiol Clin North Am* 19:571, 1981.

130. Troman NM, Kelly WD: The effect of sympathectomy on blood flow to bone, *JAMA* 183:121, 1963.

131. Cofield RH, Morrison MJ, Beabout JW: Diabetic neuropathy in the foot: patient characteristics and patterns of radiographic change, *Foot & Ankle* 4(1):16, 1983.

132. Jaffe HL, Lichtenstein L: Solitary unicameral bone cyst with emphasis on roentgen picture: The pathologic appearance and pathogenesis, *Arch Surg* 44:1004, 1942.

133. Cohen J: Simple bone cyst: studies of cyst fluid in six cases with a theory on pathogenesis, *J Bone Joint Surg* 42A:609, 1960.

134. Cohen J: Etiology of bone cyst, *J Bone Joint Surg* 52A:1493, 1970.

135. Cohen J: Unicameral bone cysts: a current synthesis of reported cases, *Orthop Clin North Am* 8:715, 1977.

136. Chigira M, Mae H, Arita S, Udagawa E: The etiology and treatment of simple bone cyst, *J Bone Joint Surg* 65B:633, 1983.

137. Huvos AG: *Bone tumors: diagnosis, treatment, and prognosis,* ed 2, Philadelphia, 1991, Saunders.

138. Neer CS, Francis KC, Johnson AD, Kieran HA: The etiology and treatment of simple bone cysts: current concepts on the treatment of solitary unicameral bone cysts, *Clin Orthop North Am* 997:40, 1973.

139. Resnick D, Niwayama G: Simple bone cyst. In Resnick D, Niwayama G, editors: *Diagnosis of bone and joint disorders,* ed 2, vol 6, p 3820, Philadelphia, 1988, Saunders.

140. Capanna R, Van Horn J, Ruggieri P, Biagini R: Epiphyseal involvement of unicameral bone cysts, *Skeletal Radiol* 15:428, 1988.

141. Jaffe HL: *Tumors and tumorous conditions of the bone and joints,* pp 54-62, Philadelphia, 1958, Lea & Febiger.

142. Resnick D, Niwayama G: Aneurysmal bone cyst. In Resnick D, Niwayama G, editors: *Diagnosis of bone and joint disorders,* ed 2, vol 6, p 3831, Philadelphia, 1988, Saunders.

143. Jaffe HL, Aneurysmal bone cyst, *Bull Hosp Jt Dis,* 11:3, 1950.

144. Banakdapour A, Levy WN, Aegerter E: Primary and secondary aneurysmal bone cysts: a radiological study of 75 cases, *Radiology* 126:75-83, 1978.

145. Hudson TM: Fluid levels of aneurysmal bone cysts: a CT feature, *AJR* 141:1001-1004, 1984.

146. Zimmer W, Berquist TH et al: Magnetic resonance imaging of aneurysmal bone cyst, *Mayo Clin Proc* 59:633-636, 1984.

147. Tsai J, Dalinka M, Fallon M, Zlatkin M, Kressel H: Fluid-fluid level: a nonspecific finding in tumors of bone and soft tissue, *Radiology* 175:779-782, 1980.

148. Langenskiold A: Normal and pathological bone growth in the light of the development of cartilaginous foci in chondrodysplasia, *Acta Chir Scand* 95:367, 1947.

149. Resnick D, Niwayama G: Osteochondroma. In Resnick D, Niwayama G, editors: *Diagnosis of bone and joint disorders,* ed 2, vol 6, p 3701, Philadelphia, 1988, Saunders.

150. Huvos AG: *Bone tumors: diagnosis, treatment, and prognosis,* Philadelphia, 1979, Saunders.

151. Hudson TM, Springfield DS, Spanier SS et al: Benign exostoses and exostotic chondrosarcomas: evaluation of cartilage thickness by CT, *Radiology* 152:595, 1984.

152. Resnick D, Niwayama G: Chondroblastoma. In Resnick D, Niwayama G, editors: *Diagnosis of bone and joint disorders,* ed 2, vol 6, pp 3688-3697, Philadelphia, 1988, Saunders.

153. Jaffe H, Lichtenstein L: Benign chondroblastoma of bone: reinterpretation of so-called calcifying or chondromatous giant cell tumor, *Am J Pathol* 18:969, 1942.

154. Feldman F: Chondroblastoma and chondromyxoid fibroma. In Taveras J, Ferrucci JC, editors: *Radiology: diagnosis-imaging-intervention,* chap 79, pp 1-14, Philadelphia, 1984, Lippincott.

155. Kricun ME, Kricun R, Haskin ME: Chondroblastoma of the calcaneus: radiographic features with emphasis on location, *AJR* 128:613, 1977.

156. Moore TM, Roe JB, Harvey JP, Chondroblastoma of the talus: case report, *J Bone Joint Surg* 59A:830, 1977.

157. Ohno T, Kadoya H, Park P et al: Case report 382, *Skeletal Radiol* 15:478, 1986.

158. Kahmann R, Gold RH, Eckhart JT, Mirra JM: Case report 337, *Skeletal Radiol* 14:301, 1985.

159. Quint L, Gross B, Glazer G, Bramstein E, White S: CT evaluation of chondroblastoma, *J Comput Assist Tomogr* 8(5):907-910, 1984.

160. Fobben ES, Dalinka MK, Schiebler ML: The magnetic resonance imaging appearance at 1.5 tesla of cartilaginous tumors involving the epiphysis, *Skeletal Radiol* 16:647, 1987.

161. Moss AA, Gamsu G, Genant HK: Chondroblastoma. In *Computed tomography of the body with magnetic resonance imaging,* ed 2, p 574, Philadelphia, 1992, Saunders.

162. Dahlin DC: *Bone tumors,* ed 2, pp 28-37, Springfield, III, Charles C Thomas, 1967.

163. Resnick D, Niwayama G: Enchondroma. In Resnick D, Niwayama G, editors: *Diagnosis of bone and joint disorders,* ed 2, vol 6, p 3679, Philadelphia, 1988, Saunders.

164. Aoki J et al: MR of enchondroma and chondrosarcoma rings and arcs of Gd-DTPA enhancement, *J Comput Assist Tomogr* 15(6):1011-1016, 1991.

165. Milgram JW: Synovial osteochondromatosis: a histopathological study of thirty cases, *J Bone Joint Surg* 59A:792, 1977.

166. Giustra PE, Furman RS, Roberts L, Killoran PJ: Synovial chondromatosis of the elbow, *AJR* 127:347, 1976.

167. Lyritis G: Synovial chondromatosis of the inferior ulnar joint, *Acta Orthop Scand* 47:373, 1971.

168. Ronald JB, Keller EE, Veiland LH: Synovial chondromatosis of the temporomandibular joint, *J Oral Surg* 36:13, 1978.

169. Szepesi J: Synovial chondromatosis of the metacarpophalangeal joint, *Acta Orthop Scand* 46:426, 1975.

170. Weiss C, Averbuch PF, Steiner GC, Rusoff JH: Synovial chondromatosis and instability of the proximal tibiofibular joint, *Clin Orthop* 108:187, 19795.

171. Norman A, Steiner G: Bone erosion in synovial chondromatosis, *Radiology* 161:749, 1986.

172. Kleiger B: Osteochondral bodies in the ankle joint. In Taveras J, Ferrucci J, editors: *Radiology: diagnosis-imaging-intervention,* chap 27, pp 1-7, Philadelphia, 1991, Lippincott.

173. Ginaldi S: Computed tomography feature of synovial chondromatosis, *Skeletal Radiol* 5:219, 1980.

174. Sundaram M, McGuire M, Fletcher J et al: Magnetic resonance imaging of lesions of synovial origin, *Skeletal Radiol* 15:110, 1986.

175. Norman A: Benign osteoblastic lesions. In Taveras J, Ferrucci J, editors: *Radiology: diagnosis-imaging-intervention,* chap 76, pp 1-9, Philadelphia, 1991, Lippincott.

176. McLeod RA, Dahlin DC, Beabout JW, The spectrum of osteoblastoma, *AJR* 126:321, 1976.

177. Farmlett EJ, Magid D, Fishman EK: Osteoblastoma of the tibia: CT demonstration, *J Comput Assist Tomogr* 9:577-579, 1985.

178. Torricelli P, Martinelli C, Boriani S, Ferraro A: Computerized tomography in spinal osteoblastoma: observations in 10 cases, *Radiat Med* 72:267-271, 1986.

179. Sundaram M, McGuire MH: Computed tomography or magnetic resonance for evaluating the solitary tumor with tumorlike lesions of bone? *Skeletal Radiol* 117:393-401, 1988.

180. Resnick D, Niwayama G: Osteoid osteoma. In Resnick D, Niwayama G, editors: *Diagnosis of bone and joint disorders,* ed 2, vol 6, p 3621, Philadelphia, 1988, Saunders.

181. Swee R, McLeod R, Beabout J: Osteoid osteoma: detection, diagnosis, and location, *Radiology* 130:117-123, 1979.

182. Gould N: Articular osteoid osteoma of the talus: a case report, *Foot & Ankle* 1(5):284-285, 1981.

183. Simon WH, Beller ML: Intracapsular epiphyseal osteoid osteoma of the ankle joint: a case report, *Clin Orthop* 108:200-203, 1975.

184. Sherman MS, McFarland G Jr: Mechanism of pain in osteoid osteomas, *South Med J* 58:163-166, 1965.

185. Glass RBJ, Poznanski AIC, Fisher MR et al: MR imaging of osteoid osteoma, *J Comput Assist Tomogr* 10:1065-1067, 1986.

186. Yeager BA, Schiehler ML, Wertheim SB et al: MR imaging of osteoid osteoma of the talus, *J Comput Assist Tomogr* 11:916-917, 1986.

187. Norman A: Giant cell tumor (osteoclastoma). In Taveras J, Ferrucci J, editors: *Radiology: diagnosis-imaging-intervention,* p 1, Philadelphia, 1991, Lippincott.

188. World LE, Swee RG: Giant cell tumor of the small bones of the hands and feet, *Semin Diag Pathol* 1:173, 1984.

189. Mechlin MB, Kricun ME, Stead J, Schwamm HA: giant cell tumor of the tarsal bones: report of three cases and review of the literature, *Skeletal Radiol* 11:266, 1984.

190. Resnick D, Niwayama G, editors: *Diagnosis of bone and joint disorders,* ed 2, Philadelphia, 1988, Saunders.

191. Tehranzadeh J, Murphy B, Mwaymneh W: Giant cell tumor of the proximal tibia: MR and CT appearance, *J Comput Assist Tomogr* 13(2):282, 1989.

192. Herman, Mezgarzadeh M, Bonakdarpour A, Dalinka M: The role of magnetic resonance imaging in giant cell tumor of bone, *Skeletal Radiol* 16:635-643, 1987.

193. Kerr R: Magnetic resonance imaging. In Forrester D, Kricun M, Kerr R, editors: *Imaging of the foot and ankle,* p 283, Rockville, Md, 1988, Aspen.

194. Kumar R, Madeweel JE, Lindell MM, Swischuk LE: Fibrous lesions of bones, *Radiographics* 10(2):237, 1990.

195. Resnick D, Niwayama G: Nonossifying fibroma. In Resnick D, Niwayama G, editors: *Diagnosis of bone and joint disorders,* ed 2, vol 6, p 3739, Philadelphia, 1988, Saunders.

196. Renan DB, Maylahn DJ, Fahey JJ: Fracture through large ossifying fibromas, *Clin Orthop* 103:82, 1974.

197. Ramos et al: Osseous lipoma: CT appearance, *Radiology* 157:617-619, 1985.

198. Resnick D, Niwayama G: Lipoma. In Resnick D, Niwayama G, editors: *Diagnosis of bone and joint disorders,* ed 2, vol 6, p 3782, Philadelphia, 1988, Saunders.

199. Freiberg R, Gordon W, Gueck C, Ishikawe T, Abrams N: Multiple intraosseous lipomas with type IV hyperlipoproteinemia: a case report, *J Bone Joint Surg* 56A(8):1729-1732, 1974.

200. Hart JA, Intraosseous lipoma, *J Bone Joint Surg* 55B(3):624-631, 1973.

201. Lesson M, Kay D, Smith B: Intraosseous lipoma, *Clin Orthop* 181:186-190, 19983.

202. Reig-Box V, Guinot-Turmo J, Risent-Martinez F, Aparis-Rodriguez F, Ferrer-Jimenez R: Computed tomography of intraosseous lipoma of os calcis, *Clin Orthop* 221:286-291, 1987.

203. Mirra JM: Osteogenic sarcoma. In Mirra JM, editor: *Bone tumors: clinical, radiologic, and pathologic correlations,* vol 1, p 225, Philadelphia, 1989, Lea & Febiger.

204. Resnick D, Niwayama G: Osteogenic sarcoma. In Resnick D, Niwayama G, editors: *Diagnosis of bone and joint disorders,* ed 2, vol 6, p 3648, Philadelphia, 1988, Saunders.

205. Sneppen O, Dissing I, Schiodt T: Osteosarcoma of the metatarsal bones: review of the literature and case report, *Acta Orthop* 49:220, 1978.

206. Amini M, Colacecchi C: An unusual case of primary osteosarcoma of the talus, *Clin Orthop* 150:217, 1980.

207. Wu KK: Tumor review: osteogenic sarcoma of the foot, *JFS* 26(3):269-271, 1987.

208. Wetzel L, Levine E, Murphy M: A comparison of MR imaging and CT in the evaluation of musculoskeletal masses, *Radiographics* 7(5):851-874, 1987.

209. Aisen A, Martel W, Braunstein E, McMillin R, Philips W, Kling T: MRI and CT evaluation of primary bone and soft tissue tumors, *AJR* 146:749-756, 1988.

210. Lukens J, McLeod R, Sims F, CT evaluation of primary osseous malignant neoplasms, *AJR* 139:45-48, 1982.

211. Zimmer W et al: Bone tumors: MRI versus CT, *Radiology* 155:709-718, 1985.

212. Hudson TM, Hamlin DJ, Enneking WF, Petterson H: Magnetic resonance imaging of bone and soft tissue tumors: early experience in 31 patients compared with computed tomography, *Skeletal Radiol* 13:134-146, 1985.

213. Tehranzadeh J, Mnaymneh W, Cyrus G, Gaston M, Murphy B: Comparison of CT and MR imaging in musculoskeletal neoplasms, *J Comput Assist Tomogr* 13(3):446-472, 1989.

214. Sundaram M, McLeod R: MR imaging of tumor and tumor-like lesions of bone and soft tissue, *AJR* 155:817-824, 1990.

215. Bloem JL, Blueman RG, Taminian AHM, Oosterom AT, Stolk J, Doornbos J: MRI of primary malignant bone tumors, *Radiographics* 7(3):425-445, 1987.

216. Mirra JM: Ewing sarcoma. In Mirra JM, editor: *Bone tumors: clinical, radiologic, and pathologic correlations,* vol 2, p 1087, Philadelphia, 1989, Lea & Febiger.

217. Resnick D, Niwayama G: Ewing sarcoma. In Resnick D, Niwayama G, editors: *Diagnosis of bone and joint disorders,* ed 2, p 3845, Philadelphia, 1988, Saunders.

218. Reinus WR, Gilula LA, Slinly SK: Radiographic appearance of Ewing sarcoma of the hands and feet: report from the intergroup Ewing's sarcoma study, *AJR* 144:331, 1985.

219. Vanel D, Contesso G, Couanet D et al: Computed tomography in the evaluation of 41 cases of Ewing sarcoma, *Skeletal Radiol* 9:8, 1982.

220. Reinus WR, Gilula LA, Radiology of Ewing's sarcoma: intergroup Ewing's sarcoma study, *Radiographics* 4:929, 1984.

221. Daffner R, Luretin A, Dash N et al: MRI in the detection of malignant infiltration of bone marrow, *AJR* 146:353, 1986.

222. Dahlin DC, Unni KK: *Bone tumors: general aspects and data on 8542 cases,* Springfield, Ill, 1986, Charles C Thomas.

223. Wu K: Chondrosarcoma of the foot, *JFS* 25(5):449,1 1987.

224. Resnick D, Niwayama G: Chondrosarcoma. In Resnick D, Niwayama G, editors: *Diagnosis of bone and joint disorders,* ed 2, vol 6, p 3720, Philadelphia, 1988, Saunders.

225. McLeod RA: Bone and soft tissue neoplasms. In Berquist TH, editor: *Radiology of the foot and ankle,* p 247, New York, 1989, Raven Press.

226. Rosenthal D, Schiller A, Mankin H: Chondrosarcoma: correlation of radiological and histological grade, *Radiology* 150:21, 1984.

227. Pritchard DJ, Sim FH, Ivins JC et al: Fibrosarcoma of bone and soft tissue of the trunk and extremities, *Orthop Clin North Am* 8:869, 1977.

228. Huvos AG, Higginbotham NL: Primary fibrosarcoma of bone: a clinicopathologic study of 130 patients, *Cancer* 35:837, 1975.

229. Taconis WK, Mulder JD: Fibrosarcoma and malignant fibrous histiocytoma of long bones: radiographic features and grading, *Skeletal Radiol* 11:237, 1984.

230. Resnick D, Niwayama G: Fibrosarcoma. In Resnick D, Niwayama G, editors: *Diagnosis of bone and joint disorders,* ed 2, vol 6, p 3750, Philadelphia, 1988, Saunders.

231. Bloem JL, Falke THM, Tamianiau AHM et al: Magnetic resonance imaging of primary malignant bone tumors, *Radiographics* 5(6):853, 1985.

232. Fischer B: Uber ein primares adamantinom der tibia, *Frankf Zfuer Pathol* 12:422, 1913.

233. Mori H, Mamnoto S, Hiramatsu K, Miura T, Moum NF: Adamantinoma of the tibia: ultrasound & immunohisto-chemical study with ref to histogenesis, *Clin Orthop* 190:299, 1984.

234. Resnick D, Niwayama G: Adamantinoma. In Resnick D, Niwayama G, editors: *Diagnosis of bone and joint disorders,* ed 2, vol 6, p 3842, Philadelphia, 1988, Saunders.

235. Unni KK, Dahlin DC, Beaoujt JW, Irvins J: Adamantinoma of long bones, *Cancer* 34:1796, 1974.

236. Bloem JL, Heul R, Schutevear H, Kuipers D: Fibrous dysplasia vs. adamantinoma of the tibia: differentiation based on discriminant analysis of clinical & plain film findings, *AJR* 156:1017-1023, 1991.

237. Utz JA, Kransdorf MJ, Jelink JS, Moser RP, Berrey BH: MR appearance of fibrous dysplasia, *J Comput Assist Tomogr* 13(5):845-851, 1989.

238. Reed R, Bliss B: Morton's neuroma, Arch Pathol 95:123, 1973.

239. Jahss MH: Disorders of the foot and ankle: medical surgical management. Philadelphia, 1991, Saunders.

240. Mulder JD: The causative mechanism of Morton's metatarsalgia, *J Bone Joint Surg* 33B:94, 1951.

241. Sartoris DJ, Brozinsky S, Resnick D, MR images: interdigital or Morton's neuroma, *JFS* 28:78-82, 1989.

242. Sartoris DJ, Brozinsky S, Resnick D: MR images: interdigital or Morton's neuroma, J Foot Surg 28:78-82, 1989.

243. Erickson S, Canale P, Carrera G, Johnson J et al: Interdigital Morton's neuroma: high resolution MR imaging with a solenoid coil, *Radiology* 181:833-836, 1991.

244. Geschickter CF: Tumors of the peripheral nerves, *Am J Cancer* 25:377, 1935.

245. Enzinger FM, Weiss SW: Benign tumors of the peripheral nerves. In Enzinger FM, Weiss SW, editors: *Soft tissue tumors,* ed 2, p 7191, St. Louis, 1988, Mosby.

246. Booker RJ: Lipoblastic tumors of the hands and feet: review of the literature and report of 33 cases, *J Bone Joint Surg* 47A:727-740, 1965.

247. Lisch M, Mittleman M, Albin R: Digital lipoma of the foot: an extraordinary case, *JFS* 21:330-334, 1982.

248. Kerman B, Foster L: Lipoma of the foot: a large and unusual case, *JFS* 24(5):345-348, 1985.

249. Moss AA, Gamsu G, Genant H: *Computed tomography of the body with MRI,* ed 2, p 582, Philadelphia, 1992, Saunders.

250. Dooms GC, Hricak H, Sollito RA et al: Lipomatous tumors and tumors of fatty components: MR imaging potential and comparison of MR & CT results, *Radiology* 157:479, 1985.

251. Pack TT, Miller TR: Hemangiomas: classification, diagnosis, and treatment, *Angiology* 1:405, 1950.

252. Berlin SJ: Vascular tumors of the foot. In *Soft somatic tumors of the foot: diagnosis and surgical management,* Mount Kisco, NY, 1976, Futura.

253. Berlin SJ: Hemangioma of the foot: report of four cases and review of the literature, *J Am Assoc Podiatr* 60:63, 1970.

254. Castillenti T: Cavernous hemangioma of the foot: case report and review of the literature, *J Am Assoc Podiatr* 79(8):406-410, 1989.

255. Tubiolo A, Jones R, Chalker D: Cavernous hemangioma of the plantar forefoot: a literature review and cases report, *J Am Assoc Podiatr* 76(3):164-167, 1986.

256. McNeill TW, Ray RD: Hemangioma of the extremities: review of 35 cases, *Clin Orthop* 101:154, 1974.

257. Apfelberg DB, Maser MR, Lash HL: Extended clinical use of the argon lasers for cutaneous lesions, *Arch Dermatol* 115:719-721, 1979.

258. Miechajev IA, Karlsson S: Vascular tumors of the hand, *Scand J Plast Reconstructive Surg* 16:67-75, 1982.

259. McNeil TW, Chan GE, Capek V, Ray RD, The value of angiography in the surgical management of deep hemangiomas, *Clin Orthop* 101:176-181, 1984.

260. Ranch RF, Silverman PM, Korbkim M et al: Computed tomography of benign angiomatous lesions of the extremities, *J Comput Assist Tomogr* 8:1143-1146, 1984.

261. Cohen J, Weinkeb J, Redman H: Arteriovenous malformations of the extremities: MR imaging, *Radiology* 158:475-479, 1986.

262. Nelson M et al: Magnetic resonance imaging of peripheral soft tissue hemangiomas, *Skeletal Radiol* 19:477-482, 1990.

263. Kaplan D, Williams S, Mucocutanous and peripheral soft tissue hemangiomas: MR imaging, *Radiology* 163: 163-166, 1987.

264. Wetzel L, Levine E: Soft tissue tumors of the foot: value of MR imaging for specific diagnosis, *AJR* 155: 1025-1030, 1990.

265. Granowitz SP, D'Antonio J, Mankin HL: The pathogenesis and long term end results of pigmented villonodular synovitis, *Clin Orthop* 114:335, 1976.

266. Docken WP: PVN: a review with illustrative case reports, *Semin Arthritis Rheum* 9:1-22, 1979.

267. Resnick D, Niwayama G: Pigmented villonodular synovitis. In Resnick D, Niwayama G, editors: *Diagnosis of bone and joint disorders,* ed 2, vol 6, p 3925, Philadelphia, 1988, Saunders.

268. Georgen TG, Resnick D, Niwayama G: Localized nodular synovitis of the knee: a report of two cases with abnormal arthrogram, *AJR* 126:647-650, 1976.

269. Leszczynski J, Huckell JR, Percy JS, Leriche JC, Lentle BC: Pigmented villonodular synovitis in multiple joints, *Ann Rheum Dis* 34:269, 1975.

270. Kottal R, Vogler J, Motanoros A, Alexander A, Cookson J: Pigmented villonodular synovitis: a report of MR imaging in two cases, *Radiology* 163:551, 1987.

271. Baker N, Klein J, Weidner N et al: Imaging of pigmented villonodular synovitis containing coarse calcifications, *AJR* 153:1228, 1989.

272. Jelinek J, Kransdorf MJ, Utz JA et al: Imaging of pigmented villonodular synovitis with emphasis on MR imaging, *AJR* 152:337, 1989.

273. Spritzer CE, Dalinka MK, Kressel HY: MRI of PVN: a report of two cases, *Skeletal Radiol* 16:316-319, 1987.

274. Enzinger F, Weiss S: Ganglion. In Enzinger F, Weiss S, editors: *Soft tissue tumors,* ed 2, p 923, St. Louis, 1988, Mosby.

275. Klimar M, Freiberg A: Ganglia of the foot and ankle, *Foot & Ankle* 3(1):45, 19082.

276. McEvedy BV: Simple ganglia, *Br J Surg* 49:585, 1962.

277. Soren A: Pathogenesis and treatment of ganglion, *Clin Orthop* 48:173, 1966.

278. Heiken J, Lee J, Smathers R et al: CT of benign soft tissue masses of the extremities, *AJR* 142:575, 1984.

279. Wright PH, Sims FH, Kelly PJ: Synovial sarcoma: an analysis of 134 tumors, *Cancer* 18:613, 1965.

280. Cadman NL, Soule EH, Kelly PJ: Synovial sarcoma: an analysis of 134 tumors. *Cancer* 18:613, 1965.

281. Moss AA, Gamsu G, Genant HK: Musculoskeletal tumors. In Moss A, Gaunsu G, editors: *Computed tomography of the whole body with MRI,* ed 2, p 597, Philadelphia, 1992, Saunders.

282. Morton M, Berquist T, McLeod R, Unni K, Sim F: MR imaging of synovial sarcoma, *AJR* 156:337, 1991.

283. Resnick D, Kyriakos M, Greenway G: Malignant fibrous histiocytoma. In Resnick D, Niwayama G, editors: *Diagnosis of bone and joint disorders,* ed 2, vol 6, p 3776, Philadelphia, 1988, Saunders.

284. Nachlas M, Ketai D: An unusual variation of malignant fibrous histiocytoma: a case report, *JFS* 19:212, 1980.

285. Weiss SW, Enzinger FM: Malignant fibrous histiocytoma: an analysis of 200 cases, *Cancer* 41:2250, 19787.

286. Kearney MM, Soule EH, Ivins JC: Malignant fibrous histiocytoma: a retrospective study of 167 cases, *Cancer* 45:167, 1980.

287. Petasnick J, Turner D, Charters et al: Soft tissue masses of the locomotor system: comparison of MR imaging with CT, *Radiology* 160:125, 1986.

288. Paling M, Hyams M: Computed tomography in malignant fibrous histiocytoma, *J Comput Assist Tomogr* 6(4):785, 1982.

289. Resnick D, Kyriakos M, Greenway G: Liposarcoma. In Resnick D, Niwayama G, editors: *Diagnosis of bone and joint disorders,* ed 2, vol 6, p 3789, Philadelphia, 1988, Saunders.

290. DeSantos LA, Ginaldi S, Wallace S: Computed tomography in liposarcoma, *Cancer* 47:46, 1981.

291. London J, Kim E, Wallace S et al: MR imaging of liposarcomas: correlation of MR features and histology, *J Comput Assist Tomogr* 13:832, 1989.

292. Sundaram M, Baran G, Memenda G, McDonald DJ: Myxoid liposarcoma: magnetic resonance imaging appearance with clinical and histological correlation, *Skeletal Radiol* 19:359, 1990.

293. Berretoni B, Carter J: Mechanism of cancer metastasis to bone: current concepts review, *J Bone Joint Surg* 68A(2):308, 1986.

294. Chung TS: Metastatic malignancy to the bones of the hand, *J Surg Oncol* 24:9, 1983.

295. Healy J, Turnbull A, Micdema B, Lanne J: Acrometastasis, *J Bone Joint Surg* 68A(5):473, 1986.

296. Bloodgood JC: Bone tumors, benign and malignant, *Am J Surg* 34:229, 1920.

297. Gall RJ, Sims F, Pritchard DJ: Metastatic tumors to the bones of the foot, *Cancer* 37:1492, 1976.

298. Bunkis J, Mehrohof A, Stayman J: Metastatic lesions of the hand and foot, *Orthop Rev* 9:97, 1980.

299. Zindrich MR, Young MP, Dailey RJ, Light TR: Metastatic tumors of the foot, *Clin Orthop* 170:219, 1982.

300. Libson E, Bloom R, Husband J, Stoker D: Metastatic tumors of bones of the hand and foot: a comparative review and report of 43 additional cases, *Skeletal Radiol* 10:387, 1987.

301. Poste G, Fidler I: The pathogenesis of cancer metastasis, *Nature* 283:139, 1980.

302. Resnick D, Niwayama G: Skeletal metastases. In Resnick D, Niwayama G, editors: *Diagnosis of bone and joint disorders,* ed 2, vol 6, p 4000, Philadelphia, 1988, Saunders.

303. Hardy D, Murphy W, Gilula L: Computed tomography in planning percutaneous biopsy, *Radiology* 134:447, 1980.

304. Harbin W: Metastatic disease and the nonspecific bone scan: value of spinal tomography, *Radiology* 145:105, 1982.

305. Gold R, Seeger L, Bassett L, Steckel R: An integrated approach to the evaluation of metastatic bone disease, *Radiol Clin North Am* 28(2):471, 1990.

306. Deutsch AL, Resnick D, Campbell G: Computed tomography and bone scintigraphy in the evaluation of tarsal coalition, *Radiology* 144:137-140, 1982.

307. Marchisello PJ: The use of computerized axial tomography for the evaluation of talocalcaneal coalition: a case report, *J Bone Joint Surg* 69A(4):609-611, 1987.

308. Kricun ME: Congenital foot deformities. In Kricun ME, editor: *Imaging of the foot and ankle,* p 47, Rockville, Md, 1988, Aspen.

309. Sarno RC, Carter BL, Bankoff MS, Semine MC: Computed tomography in tarsal coalition, *J Comput Assist Tomogr* 8(6):1155-1160, 1984.

310. Sartoris DJ, Resnick DL: Tarsal coalition, *Arthritis Rheum* 28(3):331-338, 1985.

311. Keck C: the tarsal-tunnel syndrome, *J Bone Joint Surg* 44A:180-182, 1962.

312. Erickson SJ, Quinn SF, Kneeland JB et al: MR imaging of the tarsal tunnel and related spaces: normal and abnormal findings with anatomic correlation, *AJR* 155:323-328, 1990.

313. Havel PE, Ebraheim NA, Clark SE, Jackson WT, DiDio L: Tibial nerve branching in the tarsal tunnel, *Foot & Ankle* 9(3):117-119, 1988.

314. Ricciardi-Pollini PT, Moneta MR, Falez F: The tarsal tunnel syndrome: a report of eight cases, *Foot & Ankle* 10(4):214-218, 1990.

315. Zeiss J, Fenton P, Ebraheim N, Coombs RJ: Normal magnetic resonance anatomy of the tarsal tunnel. *Foot & Ankle* 10(4):214-218, 1990.

316. Kerr R, Fey C: MR imaging in tarsal tunnel syndrome, *J Comput Assist Tomogr* 15(2):280-286, 1991.

317. Takakura Y, Kitada C, Sugimoto K, Tanaka Y, Tamai S: Tarsal tunnel syndrome, *J Bone Joint Surg* 73B(1): 125-128, 1991.

318. Sweet DE, Madewell JE: Pathogenesis of osteonecrosis. In Resnick D, Niwayama G, editors: *Diagnosis of bone and joint disorders,* vol 3, p 2780, Philadelphia, 1981, Saunders.

319. Zizic TM, Marcoux DS, Hungerford DS, Stevens MB: The early diagnosis of ischemic necrosis of bone, *Arthritis Rheum* 29(10):1177, 1986.

320. Berquist TH: Bone and soft tissue ischemia. In Berquist TH, editor: *Radiology of the foot and ankle,* p 316, New York, 1989, Raven Press.

321. Vogler J, Murphy W: Bone marrow imaging, *Radiology* 168:679, 1988.

322. Kricun ME: Red-yellow marrow conversion: Its effect on the location of some solitary bone lesions, *Skeletal Radiol* 14:10, 1985.

323. Totty WG, Murphy WA, Ganz WI et al: Magnetic resonance imaging of the normal and ischemic femoral head, *AJR* 143:1273, 1984.

324. Koehler A: A typical disease of the second metatarsal joint, *AJR* 10:705, 1923.

325. Braddock GT: Experimental epiphyseal injury and Freiberg's disease, *J Bone Joint Surg* 41B:154, 1959.

326. Levin P: Juvenile deforming metatarsophalangeal osteochondritis, *JAMA* 81:189, 1923.

327. Smilie IS: Freiberg's infraction (Köhler's second disease), *J Bone Joint Surg* 39B:580, 1957.

328. Freiberg AN: Infraction of the second metatarsal: a typical injury, *Surg Gynecol Obstet* 19:191, 1914.

329. Helal B, Gibb P: Freiberg's disease: a suggested pattern of management, *Foot & Ankle* 8(2):94,1 1987.

330. Young MC, Fornasier VL, Cameron HU: Osteochondral disruption of the second metatarsal: a variant of Freiberg's infraction? *Foot & Ankle* 8(2):103, 1987.

331. Hawkins LG: Fractures of the neck of the talus, *J Bone Joint Surg* 52A:991, 1970.

332. Karp M: Koehler's disease of the tarsal scaphoid, *J Bone Joint Surg* 19:84, 1937.

333. Beltran J, Herman CJ, Burk JM et al: Femoral head avascular necrosis: MR imaging with clinical pathologic and radionuclide correlation, *Radiology* 166:215, 1988.

334. Mitchell D, Kressel H, Arger P et al: Avascular necrosis of the femoral head: morphologic assessment by MR imaging with CT correlation, *Radiology* 161:739, 1986.

335. Glickstein M, Burk L, Schiebler M et al: Avascular necrosis versus other diseases of the hip: sensitivity of MR imaging, *Radiology* 169:213, 1988.

336. Mitchell D, Rao V, Dalkinka M et al: Hematopoietic and fatty bone marrow distribution in the normal and ischemic hip: new observations with 1.5T MR imaging, *Radiology* 161:199, 1986.

337. Thickman D, Axel L, Kressel HY et al: MRI of avascular necrosis of the femoral head, *Skeletal Radiol* 15:133, 1986.

338. Poplawski ZJ, Wiley AM, Morry JF: Postraumatic dystrophy of the extremities, *J Bone Joint Surg* 65A:642-655, 1983.

339. Genant HK, Kozin F, Beherman C, McCarthy DJ, Sims J: The reflex sympathetic dystrophy syndrome, *Radiology* 117:21-32, 1975.

340. Delorimer AA, Minear WL, Boyd HB: Reflex hyperemic deossification regional to joints of the extremities, *Radiology* 46:227, 1946.

341. Malanment I, Glick J: Sudek's atrophy: The clinical syndrome, *J Am Podiatr Med Assoc* 73(7):362-367, 1983.

342. Hartley J: Reflex hyperemic deossification, *J Mt Sinai Hosp* 22:268, 1955.

343. Resnick D, Niwayama G: Osteoporosis. In Resnick D, Niwayama G, editors: *Diagnosis of bone and joint disorders,* ed 2, vol 4, pp 2023-2085, Philadelphia, 1988, Saunders.

344. Koch E, Hofer W, Sialer G, Marincek B, Schuthess G: Failure of MR imaging to detect reflex sympathetic dystrophy of the extremities, *AJR* 156:113-115, 1991.

345. Magid D, Pyeritz RE, Fishman EK: Musculoskeletal manifestations of the Marfan syndrome: radiologic features, *AJR* 155:99-104, 1990.

346. Woerner EM, Royalty K: Marfan syndrome: what you need to know, *Postgrad Med* 87(5):229-236, 1990.

347. Pyeritz RE: The Marfan syndrome, *Am Fam Physician* 34(6):83-94, 1986.

# Bone and Joint Disorders

# CHAPTER 18

# Fractures and Related Conditions: Fundamentals

FRANK A. SPINOSA • ROBIN C. ROSS • ROBERT A. CHRISTMAN

Medical dictionaries define a fracture simply as the breaking of bone.[1] However, the physician must also know a fracture's anatomic position, its direction, and whether it is linear, comminuted, or dislocated. The biomechanics of fractures can differ, as can the rate and type of healing pattern. This chapter presents these fundamentals of fracture type and occurrence.

## ■ DIAGNOSIS

Plain film radiography is the best initial screening device to determine whether a fracture exists. At least two views, possibly three, must be taken of the area of concern. The views vary depending on skeletal location in the foot or ankle. Chapter 11 can help you select the best views to see a particular osseous site.

Radiographic examination reveals findings used to describe the type of fracture and the position of its fragments. Analysis of radiographic studies can differentiate a "hairline" fracture from obvious disruption of the normal contour of the bone.[2,3] Occult or hard-to-visualize fractures may require additional imaging studies, such as computed tomography, MRI, or radioisotope skeletal imaging.

## ■ FRACTURE TERMINOLOGY

An *open fracture* (often labeled a *compound fracture*) occurs when the overlying soft tissue has been disrupted, exposing the bone to external air.[2,4] This may be a result of the bone penetrating the skin (internal to external) or of a foreign body (such as a bullet) penetrating the bone (external to internal). According to Gustilo,[5] open fractures require immediate attention involving union of the fracture ends and prevention of wound sepsis. When the skin surface has not been breached, the fracture is considered *closed* (sometimes mislabeled as a simple fracture).

Hartman[2] describes a *comminuted fracture* as one in which multiple fracture lines exist in the same bone. In other words, the bone shows three or more fracture segments (Figure 18-1). This is in opposition to a true *simple fracture* in which one fracture line (only two fracture segments) appears in a bone (Figure 18-2). A comminuted fracture may often be found in a crush injury with extensive soft tissue damage. Harkess[4] suggests that projectiles may strike the bone, causing fragmentation, and the fragments may themselves become secondary missiles. Comminuted fractures are a common problem and must be accurately understood by the physician. In fact, Watson-Jones[6] found that the most frequent injury to the forefoot is a comminuted fracture of one or both phalanges of the hallux as the result of a crush injury. A butterfly fragment (Figure 18-3) is a portion of bone that has been sheared off by a combination of different forces acting on the bone.

The difference between a complete and incomplete fracture is best evidenced by several and varied radiographic views. A *complete fracture* line penetrates all cortices of the bone, whereas an *incomplete fracture* does not cross all cortices.[7] Examples of incomplete fractures are greenstick and torus. A *greenstick fracture*, like a torus fracture, occurs in a person (usually a child or adolescent) who has not fully matured. The greenstick fracture may result in an angulation deformity because part of the cortex has actually been breached, whereas the rest of the bone is too soft to break (Figure 18-4). A *torus fracture* is a compression fracture that may only show cortical bulging on a radiograph[2]

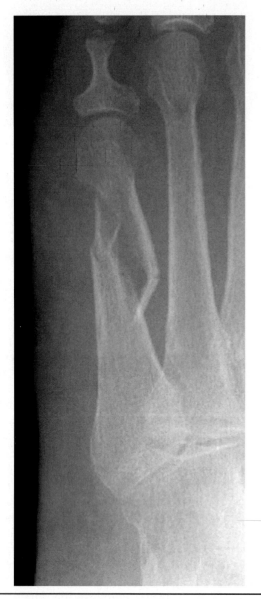

**Figure 18-1**   Comminuted fracture, fifth-metatarsal distal half diaphysis. At least four fracture fragments are present.

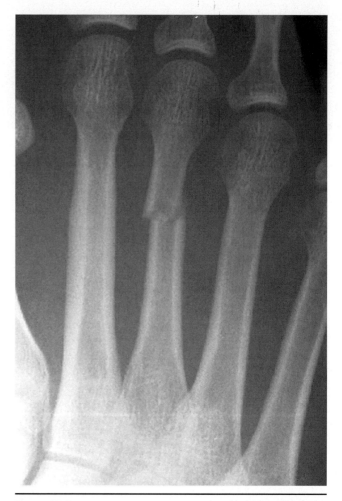

**Figure 18-2**   Simple fracture, third metatarsal, directed transversely at the junction between the middle and distal thirds of the shaft. The distal segment relative to the proximal is slightly displaced medially and angulated laterally.

(Figure 18-5). Most fractures discussed in this chapter are subcategories of complete fractures.

*Avulsion fractures* occur where muscle, tendon, or ligament insert onto bone and where an abrupt pull has been strong enough to break a portion of the bone with the attached tissue. They can occur on any bone, whether "long" or "flat" bone. An example of a ligamentous avulsion fracture is at the origin of the lateral ankle ligaments on the fibular malleolus (Figure 18-6). This point is associated with ankle injuries from abnormal pull or tension on the ligaments during severe inversion. A common tendon avulsion fracture occurs at the fifth-metatarsal tuberosity (Figure 18-7) and is

caused by an abrupt contraction or pull of the peroneus brevis at the styloid process. Take care to differentiate an avulsion fracture (often having a somewhat jagged border) from an accessory ossicle (possessing smooth cortical margins).[8-10]

Fulford[11] offers a full and complete definition of a *stress fracture* as a gradually developing fault in a bone that results from multiple repetitions of a force (or cyclic loading) that if applied only once would not cause any damage. Research has determined that the incidence of stress fractures may account for as much as 80% of all tibial, calcaneal, and metatarsal fractures.[12,13] Early diagnosis is formed on a carefully elicited history because no radiographic proof of the fracture is visible for approximately 2 weeks. The diagnosis may be confirmed before this 2-week period with the use of scintigraphy. Radiographically, the stress fracture has been described as two types. The first is the *compression*

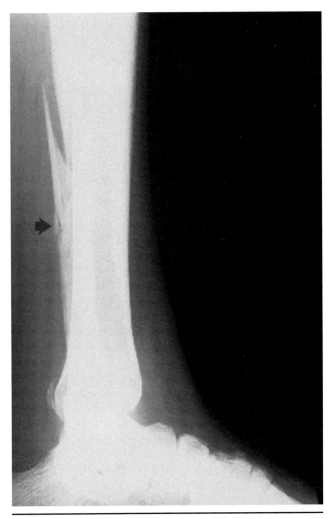

Figure 18-3   Comminuted fracture, butterfly fragment, distal fibula.

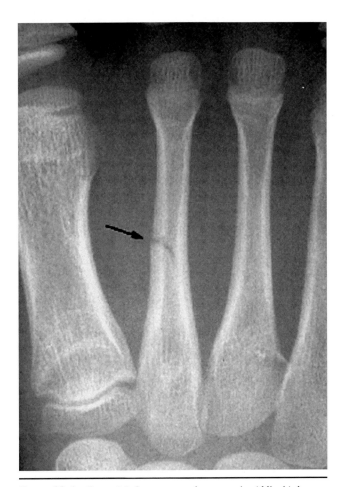

Figure 18-4   Greenstick fracture, second metatarsal, middle third diaphysis. Only the medial cortex is broken; the lateral is intact.

type, which exhibits an internal transverse callus, as is seen in cancellous bone (Figure 18-8), and the second type is the *distraction* fracture, which displays a periosteal callus as a sign of cortical disruption[12] (Figure 18-9). These types of fractures are most commonly seen in patients who have undergone rigorous and unaccustomed physical training, as, for example, dancers, athletes, and people in the armed services.

A *pathologic fracture* is one in which the bone in question is not healthy and has been weakened by pre-existing disease (Figure 18-10). In an otherwise healthy bone the amount of stress applied to this diseased area would not have been enough force to cause a fracture.[14] In fact, many osseous tumors are discovered as incidental findings on radiographs that were originally taken for what turns out to be a pathologic fracture.

Small osteocartilaginous fragments may be seen in the joints of patients with osteoarthritis (Figure 18-11). These

small chips of bone may also develop as a result of trauma. They are often referred to as "loose osseous bodies" or "joint mice." An associated condition of osteocartilaginous bodies in the ankle joint is *osteochondritis dissecans* (Figure 18-12). In this case the etiology is not arthritis but trauma or spontaneous necrosis, and such instances have only recently been classified as fractures.[15,16] The pathologic appearance of osteochondritis dissecans is that of an area of necrotic bone, covered with cartilage, that separates from the articular surface.

On diagnosing a fracture, to accurately treat the problem the physician must determine the relationship of the fracture ends, radiologically and clinically. An undisplaced fracture (Figure 18-13, *A*) reveals no change in the normal relationship of the fragment ends to each other. In a displaced fracture the distal fragment is altered from its usual relationship with the proximal fragment by at least 2 mm in distance. Fracture displacement may either be partial (Figure 18-13, *B*) or absent (0% apposition), as in the so-called bayonet fracture (Figure 18-13, *C*). According to

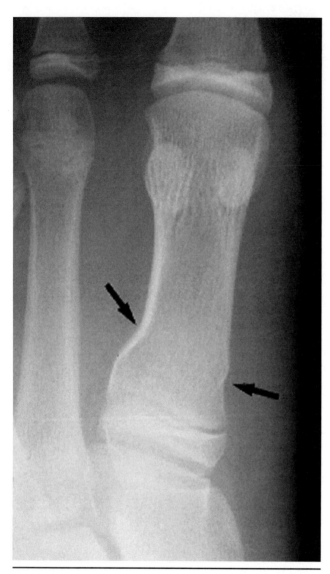

Figure 18-5   Torus fracture, first metatarsal, proximal third diaphysis. Note the "buckling" of the medial and lateral cortices; no distinct fracture line can be seen.

Hartman,[2] an angulated fracture is one in which the longitudinal axis of the displaced distal bone fragment is angled away from the proximal bone (Figure 18-14); a rotation fracture occurs with the rotation of the distal bone fragment along its longitudinal axis with respect to the proximal fragment.

## ■ DISLOCATION AND SUBLUXATION

Normally the two bony articular surfaces at a joint contact one another with 100% apposition. Less than 100%, but greater than 0%, apposition between the two bones is known as *subluxation* (Figure 18-15). Subluxation may occur as the

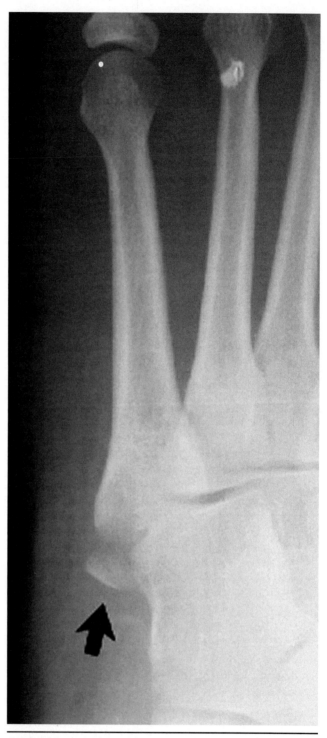

Figure 18-6   Avulsion fracture, fifth-metatarsal tuberosity. The tuberosity fragment is displaced and distracted posteriorly.

result of traumatic forces or of pathologic states where supporting structures have been weakened. Joint subluxation may or may not occur in conjunction with a fracture. Although the normal joint relationship has been altered,

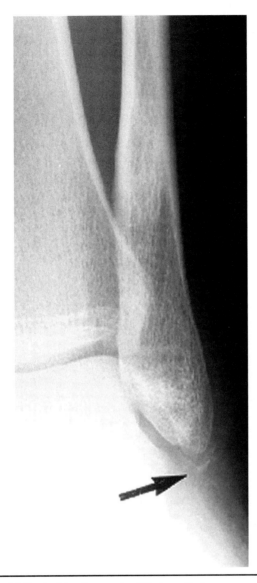

Figure 18-7    Avulsion fracture, tip of fibular malleolus.

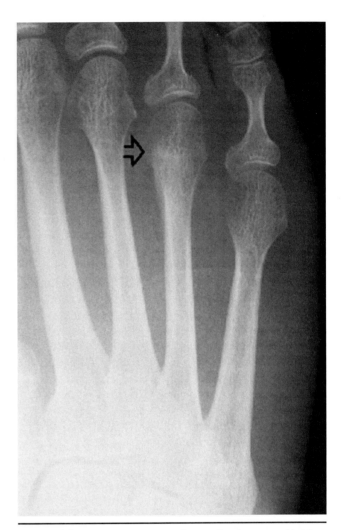

Figure 18-8    Cancellous bone stress fracture, fourth-metatarsal head. Note the ill-defined increased density directed transversely across the head/neck.

partial contact between the joint surfaces does remain. The extreme scenario of subluxation is referred to as *dislocation* where there is no contact (0% apposition) between the articular surfaces (Figure 18-16). Dislocation also may or may not be associated with fracture. Traumatic dislocations, for the most part, are not common but do occur at the metatarsophalangeal, tarsometatarsal, subtalar, and ankle joints. Clinical palpation of subluxation/dislocation is helpful in addition to radiological exam.[17,18]

Under the broad heading of dislocations, diastasis and effusion should be discussed. A *diastasis* may be any simple separation of a normally joined part. This may occur without a fracture, as in the case of a separated epiphysis in a child, or with an associated fracture as in an ankle fracture under the Lauge-Hansen category of pronation–external rotation stage 4, with separation between the tibia and fibula (Figure 18-17). An *effusion* is technically an escape of fluid from either blood or lymphatic vessels into tissues or cavities. This in itself does not cause a dislocation but may impede the reduction of a subluxation or dislocation. Joint effusion radiographically appears as an increased soft tissue density adjacent to a joint (Figure 18-18).

## BIOMECHANICS

Factors that may cause a bone to fracture may fall under one of two categories: extrinsic or intrinsic. Extrinsic factors are those comprising magnitude, duration, and direction of the forces acting on the bone as well as the rate at which the bone is loaded.[4] Extrinsic factors include stress and strain.

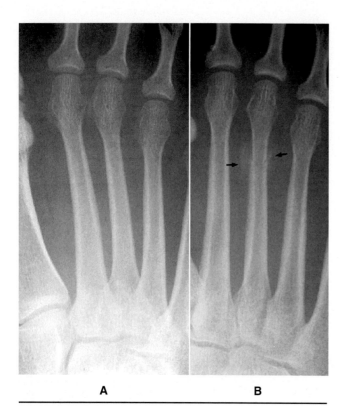

**Figure 18-9**    Cortical bone stress fracture, third-metatarsal distal third diaphysis. **A**, Initial, normal films. **B**, Two weeks later. Note the periosteal reaction along the margins of the fracture site *(arrows)*.

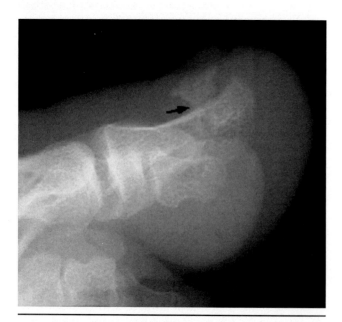

**Figure 18-10**    Pathologic fracture, hallux distal phalanx. A fracture has occurred at the junction between the phalangeal shaft and the subungual osteochondroma.

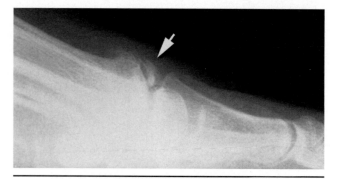

**Figure 18-11**    Loose body, first metatarsophalangeal joint. Loose bodies are frequently seen at osteoarthritic joints.

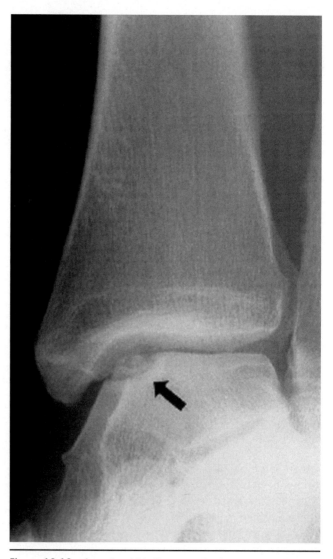

**Figure 18-12**    Osteochondritis dissecans, talar dome superomedially

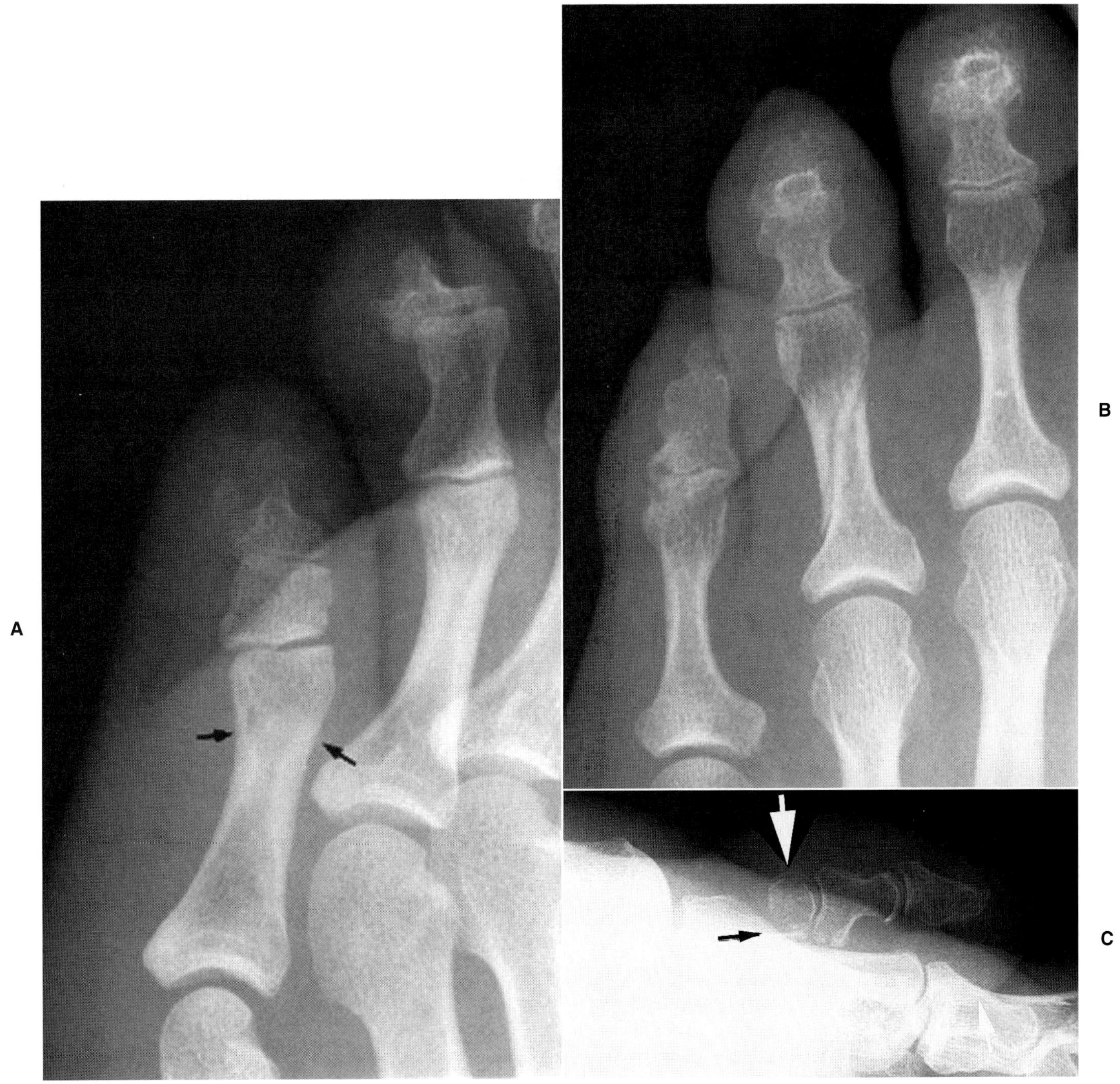

Figure 18-13   Fracture displacement: **A,** A nondisplaced (100% apposition) fracture of the fifth-toe proximal phalanx at its distal diametaphysis. **B,** Oblique fracture of the fourth-toe proximal phalanx diaphysis. The distal fragment relative to the proximal is slightly displaced laterally (partially apposed). **C,** Bayonet fracture (0% apposition), third-toe proximal phalanx. The proximal phalanx head *(large white arrow)* is resting on top of the phalanx shaft *(small black arrow).*

Stress is the resisting force set up in a body as a result of an externally applied force. Stress can be further subdivided into tension, compression, or sheer forces. Tension forces act to pull a body apart, compression forces act to squeeze a body together, and shear forces distort a body by permitting opposite parallel planes to slide over one another. Strain, in contrast, is a change in the shape of a body resulting from the application of a force or a load. Strain may be subdivided into tensile strain (increase in length), compression strain (decrease in length), or shear strain (the relative movement

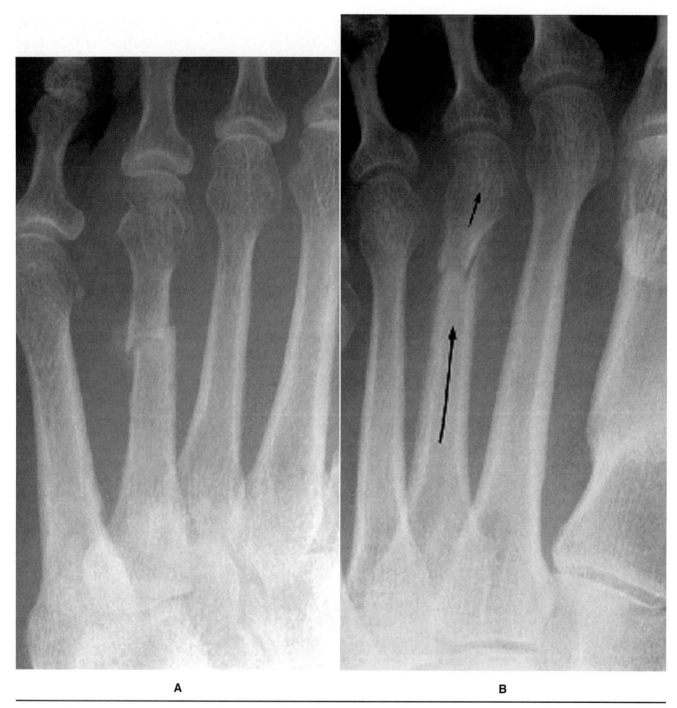

**A**                                                                                    **B**

Figure 18-14    Fracture alignment/angulation: **A,** Transverse fracture, fourth metatarsal, at the junction between the middle and proximal third diaphysis. Although the distal segment is displaced laterally relative to the proximal segment, the axes of the two fragments are parallel; this can be designated as no angulation. **B,** Transverse fracture, third-metatarsal distal third diaphysis. The distal, or capital, segment is angulated medially relative to the proximal segment. Note also the slight lateral displacement.

of any two points perpendicular to the line joining them, expressed as a fraction of the length of that line).[4]

The *intrinsic factors* include such properties as the energy-absorbing capacity, modulus of elasticity (Young's modulus), fatigue failure, and density.[4] The concept of

energy-absorbing capacity explains how fractures associated with slow loading are usually linear and not displaced, and those associated with high-energy loading are often comminuted. The faster a bone is loaded, the more rapid is the energy absorption before fracture or dislocation.

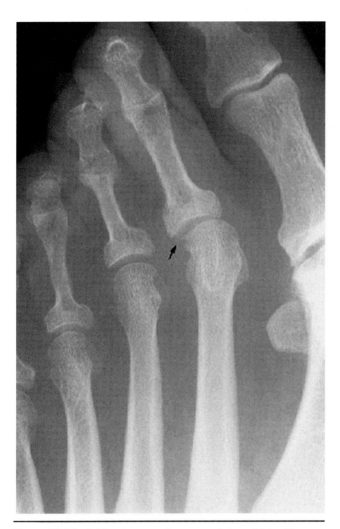

Figure 18-15  Subluxation, second metatarsophalangeal joint. The proximal phalanx base does not fully articulate (partial apposition) with the metatarsal head. It is slightly subluxated laterally.

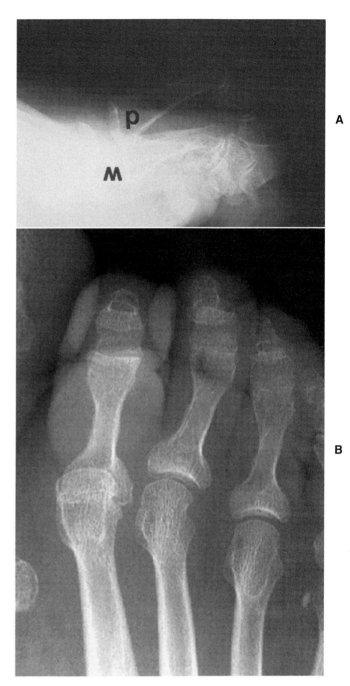

Figure 18-16  Dislocation, second metatarsophalangeal joint. **A,** Lateral view. The proximal phalanx base *(p)* does not articulate (0% apposition) with the metatarsal head *(m)* and is dislocated superiorly. **B,** Dorsoplantar view. The proximal phalanx base is superimposed on the metatarsal head. The dislocation could be missed if the lateral view were not studied closely.

Young's modulus, or the modulus of elasticity, reveals the final pathway to failure of a structure in a different light. A deforming force may be applied to a body to cause it to change shape, and when this force is removed the body returns to its normal state (elastic strain). If a greater amount of deforming force is applied and then is removed, the body may have been stressed so much that it does not revert to its normal position but is permanently deformed (plastic strain). If the deforming force increases to a greater magnitude, the body breaks and a fracture ensues (this point in the stress increase is the break point).[19]

Fatigue strength is best exemplified by a stress fracture. When a body is undergoing repeated or cyclic stresses, the body may fail, even though the forces of these individual stresses are much lower than the ultimate tensile strength of the body.

The final intrinsic factor to consider is density. Density is directly proportional to the strength of the bone and vice versa. Less stress is needed to initiate a fracture in a less dense bone than is needed in a more dense bone. Hence

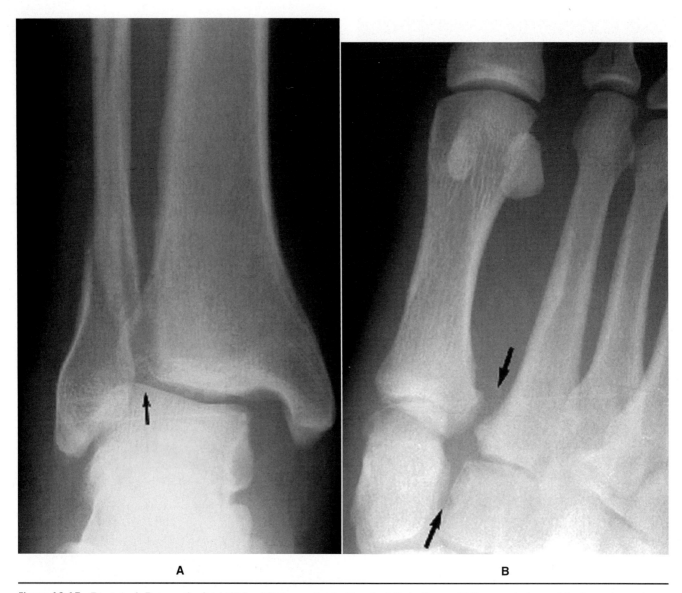

Figure 18-17   Diastasis. **A**, Between the distal tibial and fibula, associated with a distal fibular fracture. **B**, Between the bases of the first and second metatarsals, with slight subluxation of the second metatarsocuneiform joint.

individuals suffering from a condition such as osteoporosis have an increased risk of fracture.

## ■ DIRECTION AND ANATOMY OF FRACTURE

A fracture may be described in more than one fashion. Fractures have already been defined in relation to the number of fragments, associated forces such as tendons, positioning of the fracture segments relative to one another, and whether or not the fracture breached the soft tissue

casing. The fracture's anatomic position and location in relation to the bone must also be defined. The terminology used is derived from the visual picture that the fracture presents radiographically.

Fractures in tubular bones can be described based on the fracture line's direction relative to the involved bone's longitudinal axis. A *transverse fracture* is one in which the fracture line is transverse to the longitudinal axis of the bone (Figure 18-19). A fracture line that is oblique to the longitudinal axis of the bone is known as an *oblique fracture* (Figure 18-20). A *spiral fracture* is rotated around the longitudinal axis of the bone. A fracture is often considered

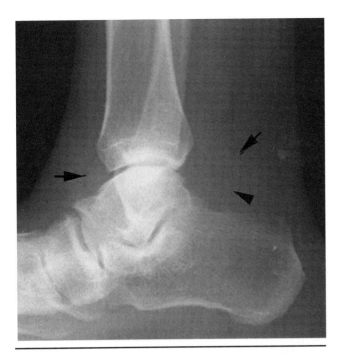

Figure 18-18   Ankle joint effusion. Note the increased soft tissue density anterior and posterior to the ankle.

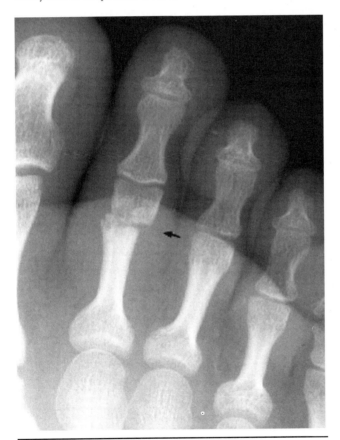

Figure 18-19   Transverse fracture, second-toe proximal phalanx distal diametaphysis. Note the slight lateral displacement of the head relative to the shaft.

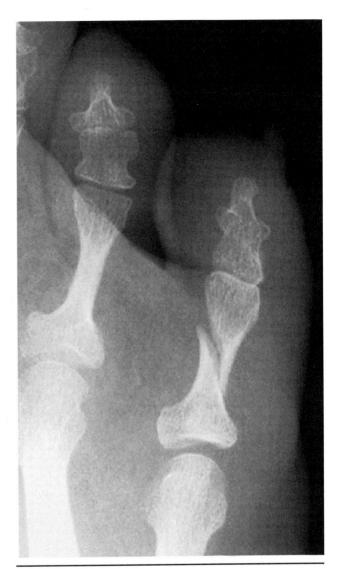

Figure 18-20   Oblique fracture, fifth-toe proximal phalangeal shaft. The distal segment is slightly displaced and angulated laterally.

spiral if its length is at least twice the distance between the medial and lateral margins of the bone (Figure 18-21).

An *impacted fracture* describes a condition of when the shaft of the long bone (usually the distal fragment) is compressed or driven into the cancellous proximal fragment (Figure 18-22). An impaction fracture often displays an inherent amount of stability. The involved bone may also be shortened.

The anatomic location of the fracture must also be included in its description. The shaft of a long bone can be divided into thirds: proximal, middle, and distal. Fractures of the shaft should include this terminology in their description: for example, "a transverse fracture of the middle third of the shaft or diaphysis" (Figure 18-23).

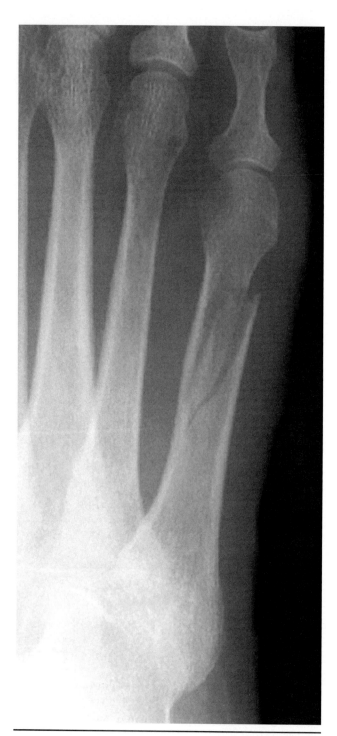

Figure 18-21   Spiral fracture, fifth-metatarsal distal half diaphysis.

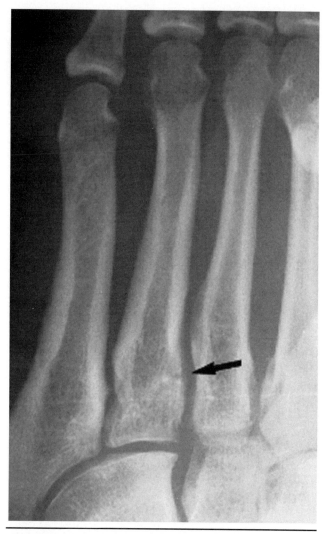

Figure 18-22   Impaction fracture, third-metatarsal proximal diametaphysis.

An *intra-articular fracture* is one that involves a joint surface (Figure 18-24). Secondary degenerative joint disease may develop at the involved joint. Fracture of a bone's anatomic process (for example, navicular tuberosity, fifth-metatarsal styloid process, calcaneal anterior process) should

be described completely, as in "fracture of the navicular tuberosity." A subcapital fracture is located just inferior to the head of a specific bone. The term *cervical fracture* may indicate a fracture of the spine but is sometimes used to describe a fracture of the neck of a particular long bone. A malleolar fracture includes the tibial and fibular processes at the level of the ankle.

## ▓ FRACTURE HEALING

Cruess and Dumont[20] suggest that fracture healing be divided into three overlapping phases: the inflammatory phase, the reparative phase, and the remodeling phase. The inflammatory phase occurs at the outset of the break: The presence of increased necrotic material elicits an immediate

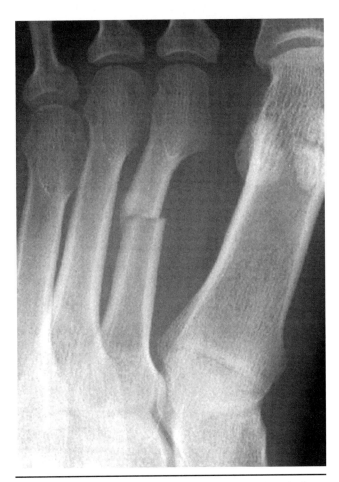

Figure 18-23  Transverse fracture, second-metatarsal, middle third diaphysis (or near its junction with the distal third diaphysis). The distal segment is slightly displaced laterally relative to the proximal segment.

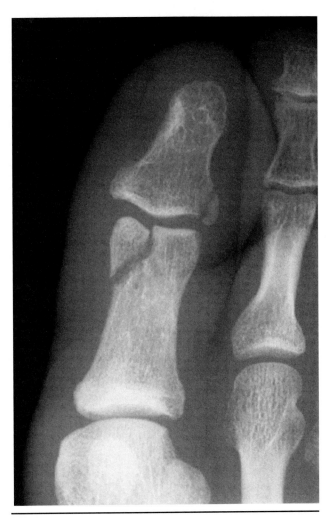

Figure 18-24  Intra-articular fracture, hallux proximal phalanx head medial aspect. (A small avulsion fracture can be seen along the lateral aspect of the distal phalangeal base, which also extends into the joint.)

and acute vasodilation and plasma exudation in the area, causing edema to develop at the break site. Other than the fracture line itself, the only other radiographic finding will be increased soft tissue density and volume (Figure 18-25, *A*). The reparative phase involves the organization of the hematoma, which primarily serves as a fibrin scaffold for the early phases of repair, with the appearance of fibrous tissue, cartilage, and immature bone commonly referred to as callus (Figure 18-25, *B*). The fracture ends become immobilized as callus and bone bridge the gap between them. Sufficient local nutrition, in the form of viable blood supply and oxygen, allows more bone to form and callus to resorb.[19] This is the remodeling phase (Figure 18-25, *C*).

Fracture healing may be affected by extrinsic and intrinsic factors that can be either beneficial or disadvantageous. Such factors may be the amount of local trauma (increased adjacent soft tissue damage slows the healing rate), bone density (bone strength is proportional to its density), the type of bone (cancellous bone has a richer

blood supply), and the degree of immobilization (increased movement of the fragment ends may cause the development of a pseudoarthrosis, "false joint" or gapping).[20] Other factors may include the presence of infection, in which case the blood supply may be diverted to fight the infection rather than for healing, or bone necrosis, which could not serve as a viable base for new bone growth. Malignancy would also affect bone healing, as would an intra-articular fracture. In the case of intra-articular fracture, synovial fluid may lyse the initial hematoma, retarding the healing rate.[21] The patient's health status may modify fracture healing with respect to age (the younger the child, the faster the rate of healing), hormones (corticosteroid inhibits fracture healing whereas growth hormone enhances it), exercise (stimulates bone formation), and electric currents (correctly applied, stimulates bone to grow).[20]

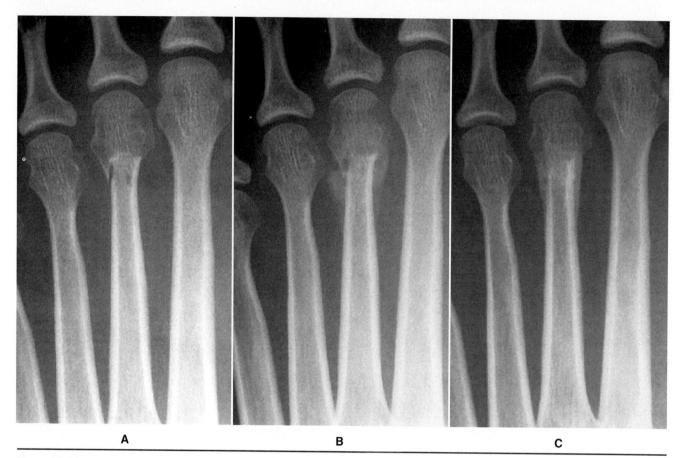

**Figure 18-25** Radiographic correlation with fracture healing, second-metatarsal distal diametaphysis. **A,** Inflammatory phase. The only findings are the fracture itself and slight increased soft tissue density. **B,** Reparative phase. Periosteal new bone formation (bone callus) surrounds the fracture site. **C,** Remodeling phase.

Despite proper treatment, some fractures may not heal as expected. Whereas Pauwells[23] and others believe that improper healing should be categorized as disturbed union or pseudoarthrosis, most modern literature describes fracture-healing complications as falling into one of three categories: delayed union, nonunion, or pseudoarthrosis. *Delayed union* indicates that fracture healing is taking longer than it should for a particular fracture type, patient age, and area of bone. Delayed union may range up to 6 months longer.[2,20-22]

A *nonunion* is a fracture site that shows no propensity toward healing, no matter how slow, at the 6-month range or later. Nonunions are subdivided into two subcategories, hypertrophic or hypotrophic.[2,21,23] The hypertrophic type has the ability to heal because of its rich blood supply but fails to do so and merely develops an overabundance of callus (Figure 18-26). Hypertrophic nonunions are further subdivided as elephant foot (having a great amount of callus), horse hoof (with a moderate amount of callus), and oligotrophic (minimal callus). These classifications are usually the result of the fracture ends not being immobilized sufficiently through the healing period. Treatment of hypertrophic nonunion does not differ from that of delayed union and includes increasing the immobilization period as well as using internal fixation.

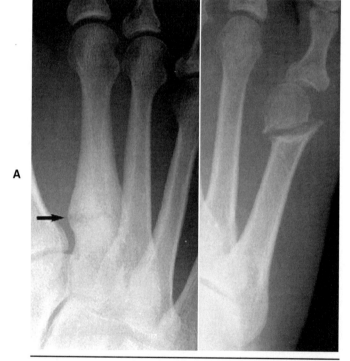

**Figure 18-26** Hypertrophic nonunion. **A,** Second-metatarsal proximal third diaphysis. Significant bone production is seen at the nonunion site. **B,** Fifth-metatarsal distal metaphysis. Some bone hypertrophy is noted at the fracture margins, but not as much as in *A*.

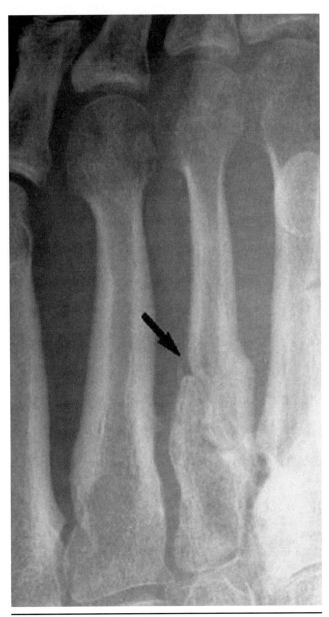

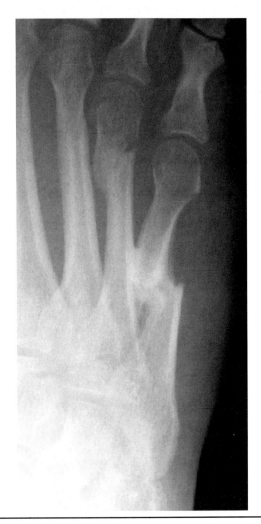

Figure 18-28   Malunion fractures, fourth-metatarsal distal third diaphysis and fifth-metatarsal, middle third diaphysis.

Figure 18-27   Hypotrophic nonunion, third-metatarsal proximal third diaphysis. Little evidence of bone production is seen at this site.

Randolph and Vogler[22] clearly described the hypotrophic or avascular group of nonunions, which were originally reported by Weber and Cech.[24] This group is subdivided into torsion wedge (in which a small bone fragment is wedged between the fracture ends causing a maligned fusion), comminution (several fracture fragments with possible necrosis), defect (a missing fracture fragment), and atrophic (which lacks total osseous integrity) (Figure 18-27). Treatment in these cases usually involves surgical intervention in the form of decortification and/or bone grafting.[22]

As stated earlier, the term pseudoarthrosis has been loosely used in association with conditions involving delayed unions and nonunions. Although *pseudoarthrosis* is a form of nonunion, it is a special type in which a fibrous joint space is formed with the presence of synovial-like fluid.[21,22]

A fracture that has healed with the relationship of its distal fragment to the proximal fragment in improper anatomic alignment is called a *malunion*[2] (Figure 18-28). A malunion causing severe disability to the patient may require surgical realignment.

## References

1. Stedman TL: *Medical dictionary*, ed 23, Baltimore, 1976, Williams & Wilkins.
2. Hartman JT: *Fracture management: a practical approach*, Philadelphia, 1978, Lea & Febiger.
3. Weissman SD: *Radiology of the foot*, 1983, Baltimore, Williams & Wilkins.
4. Harkess JW: Principles of fractures and dislocations. In Rockwood Jr CA, Green DP, editors: *Fractures*, vol 1, p 1, Philadelphia, 1975, Lippincott.
5. Gustilo RB: Management of open fractures, *Minn Med* 54:185, 1971.
6. Watson-Jones R: *Fractures and joint injuries*, ed 3, vol 2, Baltimore, 1946, Williams & Wilkins.
7. Gamble FO, Yale I: *Clinical foot roentgenology*, ed 2, Huntington, 1975, Krieger Publishing.
8. Carp L: Fracture of the fifth metatarsal bone with special reference to delayed union, *Ann Surg* 86:308, 1927.
9. Anderson L: Injuries of the forefoot, *Clin Orthop* 122:21, 1977.
10. Berquist TH: *Radiology of the foot and ankle*, New York, 1989, Raven Press.
11. Fulford P: Stress fractures, *Practitioner* 225:142, 1981.
12. Meurman KOA: Less common stress fractures in the foot, *BJR* 54:637, 1981.
13. Meurman KOA, Elfving S: Stress fracture of the cuneiform bones: case reports, *BJR* 53:626, 1980.
14. Spinosa F: Cysts and cystlike lesions. In Cole DR, DeLauro TM, editors: *Neoplasms of the foot and leg*, p 165, Baltimore, 1990, Williams & Wilkins.
15. Berndt AL, Harty M: Transchondral fractures (osteochondritis dissecans) of the talus, *J Bone Joint Surg* 41A:988, 1959.
16. Edeiken J, Hodes P: *Roentgen diagnosis of diseases of bone*, ed 2, vol 2, Baltimore, 1973, Williams & Wilkins.
17. DePalma AF: *The management of fractures and dislocations*, ed 2, vol 1, Philadelphia, 1970, Saunders.
18. Scurran BL: *Foot and ankle trauma*, New York, 1989, Churchill Livingstone.
19. Kuntscher G: *The callus problem*, St. Louis, 1974, Green.
20. Cruess RL, Dumont J: Healing of bone, tendon, and ligament. In Rockwood Jr CA, Green DP, editors: *Fractures*, vol 1, p 97, Philadelphia, 1975, Lippincott.
21. Sevitt S: *Bone repair and fracture healing in man*, New York, 1981, Churchill Livingstone.
22. Randolph TJ, Vogler H: Nonunions and delayed unions, *J Foot Surg* 24:62, 1985.
23. Pauwells F, Grunduss E: Der Biomechanic del Frakturheilung, *Verh Dtsch Ges Orthop* 34, Congress, 1940.
24. Weber GG, Cech O: *Pseudoarthrosis*, New York, 1976, Grune & Stratton.

# CHAPTER 19

# Classification of Fractures and Dislocations

FRANK A. SPINOSA

The earliest human study of fractures surely dates to the time when *Homo erectus* walked the earth and suffered wounds and injuries involving fractures and dislocations.[1] Crude attempts at treatment involved splinting with wooden branches, because immobilization was found to reduce discomfort and allow for healing. Through the centuries, war became a theater for the management of fractures and dislocations.[2]

Today the universal treatment of such trauma requires shared language and understanding of the mechanism of the injuries, so that professionals can communicate with one another with specific details about a diagnosis. The intern learns that to fixate a fracture, one must increase the deformity, separate the fragments, and replace them in normal anatomic alignment. How then does one increase a deformity, if the mechanism is not known? Clearly, this is why clinicians need fracture classification systems. Such systems outline the position, mechanism, and possible prognosis of an injury.

This chapter deals with fractures and dislocations of the foot and ankle primarily through systems of classification. The fractures of the foot presented include injuries of the first metatarsophalangeal joint, fractures of the fifth-metatarsal base, Chopart and Lisfranc joint dislocations, and navicular, talar, and calcaneal fractures. Also included are epiphyseal and ankle injuries, as well as several miscellaneous fractures.

## ■ DIGITAL AND METATARSAL FRACTURES AND DISLOCATIONS

Fractures of the phalanges are usually closed injuries caused by the toes striking on hard surfaces or heavy objects dropping on toes.[3] Digital fractures are infrequent in the distal and middle phalanges.[4] The proximal phalanges often suffer irregular transverse, oblique, or in more serious cases, comminuted fractures. Spiral fractures (Figure 19-1) are more commonly produced when the toe is jammed into an immovable object.[3]

Dorsoplantar, medial oblique, and lateral oblique radiographs are essential for proper diagnosis. Treatment usually involves immobilizing the affected digits, and open reduction is rarely indicated.[3,5,6] Displaced fractures (Figure 19-2) can usually be corrected with simple traction.[5]

Dislocations of the interphalangeal joints may remain undiagnosed because the patient does not have severe clinical symptoms. The dislocations may occur in isolation or as part of more involved trauma.[3,5]

Metatarsal fractures are most often of the oblique type, found either in diaphyseal or metaphyseal bone (Figure 19-3).[6] A higher incidence of fractures occur at the metatarsal neck (Figure 19-4), which is weaker than the shaft.[6] Spiral fractures (Figure 19-5) are commonly seen in rotational injuries such as stepping off a curb. Blunt, direct trauma causes oblique, transverse, or comminuted fractures.[3] Some metatarsal fractures occur secondary to more involved injuries such as Lisfranc's fracture-dislocation. Fracture fragments are considered displaced if they are rotated, angulated, impacted, or otherwise not in anatomic alignment.[7]

Dislocations of the metatarsophalangeal joints result most often from a forced dorsiflexion of the proximal phalanx on the metatarsal head. These injuries rarely occur without capsular rupture. Dislocations are more common at the first metatarsophalangeal joint.[6]

## ■ FIRST METATARSOPHALANGEAL JOINT FRACTURES-DISLOCATIONS

The classic injury seen at the first metatarsophalangeal joint is one of hyperextension.[8] The trauma is often caused by excessive dorsiflexion from falls or automobile accidents.[9–11] Diagnosis must be accomplished with the help of x-ray

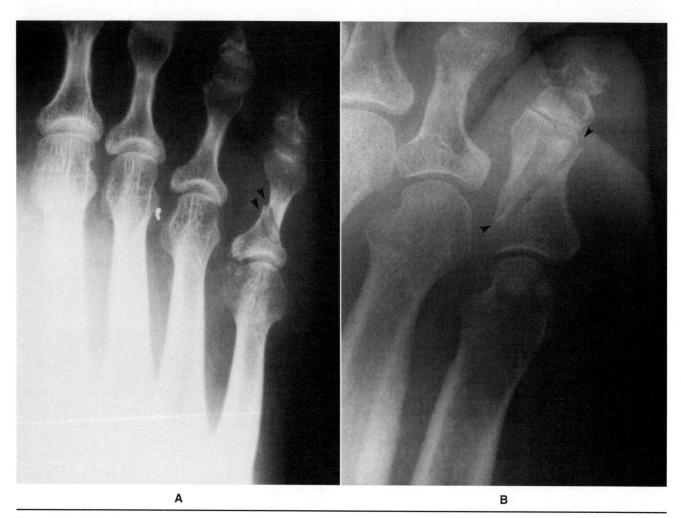

Figure 19-1    **A,** The fracture line runs from anteromedial to posterolateral in this DP view. The two arrowheads indicate superimposition of the fracture fragment edges. **B,** Medial oblique view, different patient. The fracture line extends the entire length of the phalanx.

studies, because clinical examination may not reveal the exact extent of the injury.[8,10]

The literature before 1980 reveals few articles dealing with traumatic dislocations of the first metatarsophalangeal joint. Then Jahss[12] published a classification system for these injuries (Box 19-1). According to this system, a dorsiflexion mechanism ruptures the capsule beneath the first-metatarsal neck, whereas the hallux dislocates to the dorsum of the metatarsal head, with sesamoids intact (Figure 19-6). The metatarsal head is found in a declined position in this Type I injury.[13] Such injuries are virtually always irreducible, because the metatarsal head is pushed through the plantar capsule and is tightly held between the medial and lateral tendons of the flexor hallucis brevis muscle.[9,12,14]

On increased force of dorsiflexion, the injury continues, rupturing the intersesamoidal ligament, classified by Jahss as Type II-A.[12] Thus radiograph shows a wide separation of the sesamoids. In Type II-B increased force transversely

fractures a sesamoid. If the mechanism includes an impaction injury of the first metatarsophalangeal joint, a comminuted fracture of a sesamoid may occur.[10]

As the force is relieved, the distal portion of the sesamoid remains distally displaced in the joint as a free-floating fragment.[8,10,12] In Type II injuries reduction is usually manageable.

## ■ FIFTH-METATARSAL FRACTURES

Avulsion fractures occur at the insertion of ligaments or tendons.[6] Thus injuries that involve a twisting or sudden pull by a tendon or ligament on its osseous insertion can produce a pull-off or avulsion fracture. This is often the case in fractures of the fifth-metatarsal base.

Avulsion of the proximal tuberosity is quite common (Figure 19-7) and is caused by an abrupt pull of the

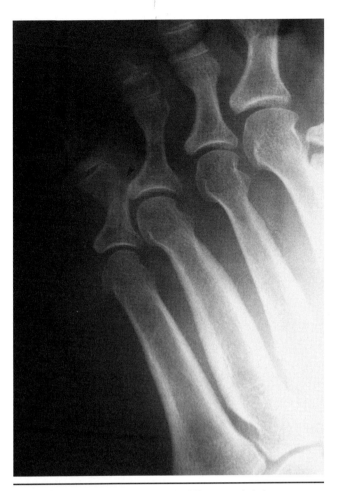

Figure 19-2    Displaced fracture of the fifth proximal phalanx.

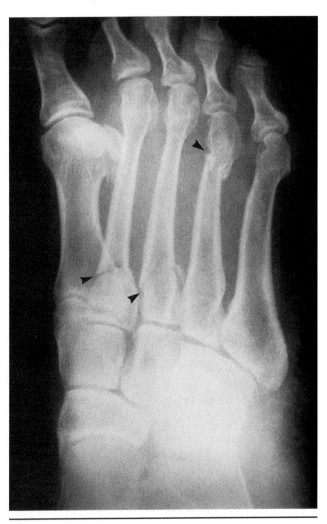

Figure 19-4    Fractures at the fourth-metatarsal neck and at second- and third-metatarsal bases.

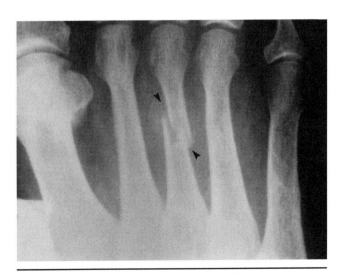

Figure 19-3    Fracture of the third-metatarsal shaft.

peroneus brevis.[6,15] Care must be taken to differentiate this fracture from a normal secondary growth center in children. Radiographically, the growth plate should appear parallel to the shaft of the fifth metatarsal, whereas a fracture lies in a more perpendicular fashion. Also consider the unlikely possibility of an avulsed epiphysis, which exhibits clinical symptoms similar to a fracture. Finally, an os vesalianum must be included in the differential diagnosis, although the edges of an accessory bone are characteristically smooth, and the bone often bilateral.[3]

Sir Robert Jones[16,17] in 1902 described a fracture of the proximal fifth metatarsal. The term today describes a fracture distal to the styloid process, involving the proximal metaphysis and diaphysis, thus differentiating it from an avulsion fracture (Box 19-2, Figure 19-8). Jones was the first to imply that the etiology of the fifth-metatarsal fracture was indirect violence rather than a direct blow. He recounts

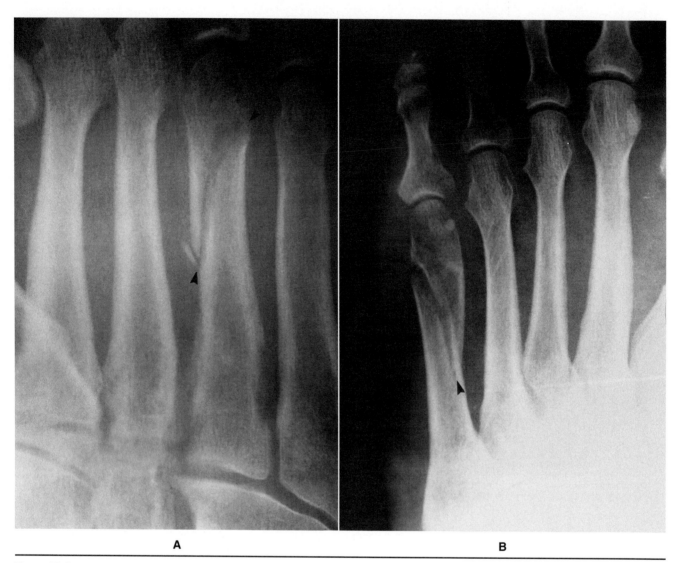

Figure 19-5  **A,** Spiral fracture of the fourth-metatarsal shaft. **B,** Spiral fracture of the fifth-metatarsal shaft.

| BOX 19-1 | First Metatarsophalangeal Joint Injury Classification |
|---|---|
| **Type** | **Classification** |
| I | Dorsal dislocation of the hallux |
| II-A | Dorsal dislocation of the hallux with rupture of the intersesamoidal ligament |
| II-B | Dorsal dislocation of the hallux with transverse fracture of one of the sesamoids |

Data from Jahss MH: *Foot & Ankle* 1:15, 1980.

his own injury, suffered while dancing. Crude roentgenograms of the day revealed a fracture "three-fourths of an inch from its base."[16] Therefore, in a Jones fracture the entire styloid process or base is separated.[18]

The mechanism of the Jones fracture appears to be a plantarflexory motion while the foot is inverted and in equinus.[3,19] This usually occurs when the person is stepping down from a curb or stairs. The anatomy of the styloid process, which overhangs the joint proximally, causes the fracture to occur distal to this site.

The anatomic attachments to the fifth-metatarsal base include the joint capsule surrounding the fifth metatarso-cuboid joint, the peroneus brevis and tertius, and fibers of the abductor digiti minimi, flexor digiti minimi, and interosseous muscles.[20] So strong are these attachments that, as Jones remarked, it is easier to fracture the bone than to cause dislocation.[16] This observation is sustained by accounts of patients with symmetric, bilateral injuries that occurred at different time intervals.[19,21]

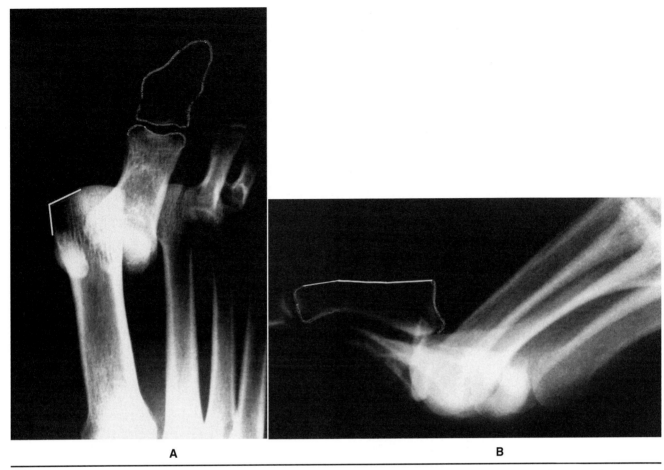

**Figure 19-6   A,** Dorsoplantar view. The hallux is displaced laterally and posteriorly. **B,** Lateral view. Superior displacement is demonstrated.

Comminution of the fifth-metatarsal base may occur when it is impacted between the ground and the cuboid and fourth-metatarsal base. Treatment of this and other fractures of the fifth-metatarsal base can occasionally be difficult, with persistent symptoms. Delayed unions or non-unions may require bone grafting.[19,22]

## ■ LISFRANC FRACTURE-DISLOCATIONS

Dislocations of the tarsometatarsal joint, commonly known as Lisfranc's joint, are rare.[3] Anatomically, the four lesser-metatarsal bases are joined to each other by the intermetatarsal ligaments. No ligament attaches the bases of the first and second metatarsals. The oblique ligament from the medial cuneiform to the base of the second metatarsal, Lisfranc's ligament, is the cause of avulsion fractures of the second-metatarsal base.[3,6,8,23] The second-metatarsal base is held snugly in a mortise formed by the first and third metatarsocuneiform joints.[24] Plantar ligaments maintain

stronger support than the weaker dorsal ligaments, thus allowing for more dorsal dislocations.[24]

Early authors as well as Bohler[18] (1935) and Gissane[25] (1951) felt that injuries to the tarsometatarsal joint may be caused by indirect forces such as falling from a low height, or stepping off a curb, invoking forced plantarflexion of the foot. Today, motor vehicle accidents where the foot violently strikes the firewall account for most of these injuries, and are often missed because other, more severe trauma has been sustained.[3,24,26–28] In its keystone position, the second metatarsal cannot move until it fractures at its base. When some or all lesser metatarsals move laterally, the cuboid is crushed.[29]

The mechanisms of injury are variable, and the literature differs as to discreet classification.[30,31] Quenu and Kuss[32] in 1909 proposed a simplified system of classification (Box 19-3) that included three types of injury. The first, *homolateral*, displayed all five metatarsals medially or laterally dislocated in the frontal plane. The second, *isolated*, takes into account either a medially displaced first metatarsal or a lateral

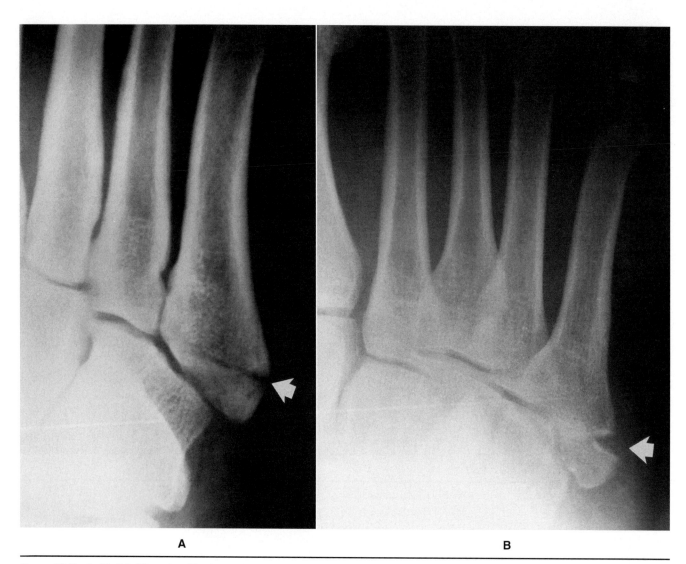

**A**    **B**

Figure 19-7    **A,** Medial oblique view. The fracture line nearly parallels the articular surface. **B,** Dorsoplantar view, different patient. The fracture line is intra-articular; the avulsed tuberosity is angulated and distracted posteriorly.

| BOX 19-2 | Classification of Fractures of Base of Fifth Metatarsal |
|---|---|

| Type | Classification |
|---|---|
| 1A | Fracture at the junction of shaft and base (Jones) |
| 1B | Comminuted fracture of shaft and base |
| 2A | Fracture of styloid process (avulsion) |
| 2B | Fracture of styloid process (avulsion) with joint involvement |

Data from Stewart IM: *Clin Orthop* 16:190, 1960.

displacement of one or more lesser metatarsals. The third type, *divergent*, involves both medial displacement of the first metatarsal as well as lateral displacement of one or more lesser metatarsals.

Wiley[29] described only two mechanisms of injury at Lisfranc's joint: abduction and plantarflexion. In abduction, the base of the second metatarsal fractures and the metatarsals displace laterally. Continued abduction causes a crush fracture of the cuboid. This injury is likened to the "nutcracker" compression fracture of the cuboid described by Hermel and Gershon-Cohen.[33] In their studies, the cuboid is caught between the bases of the fourth and fifth metatarsals as well as the calcaneus.

In Wiley's Lisfranc injury description, when the foot is in plantarflexion, longitudinal forces displace the tarso-metatarsal joints dorsally as well as either laterally or medially.

Wilson,[34] in 1972, experimented with cadaver feet and classified the types of Lisfranc dislocations according to supination or pronation injuries (Box 19-4). According to

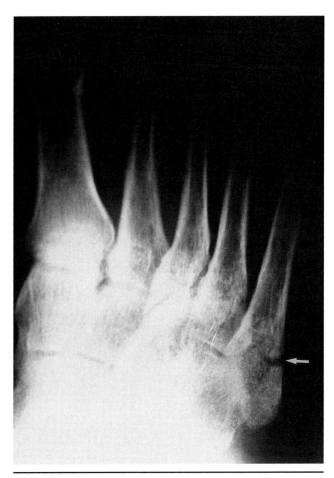

Figure 19-8  Jones's fracture of the fifth metatarsal.

BOX 19-4    Lisfranc Joint Fracture-Dislocations

| Type | Classification |
|------|----------------|
| Pronation 1 | Medial displacement of first metatarsal |
| Pronation 2 | Medial displacement of first metatarsal with dorsolateral displacement of lesser metatarsals |
| Supination 1 | Dorsolateral displacement of three or four lesser metatarsals |
| Supination 2 | Dorsolateral displacement of all five metatarsals |

Data from Wilson DW: *J Bone Joint Surg* 54B:677, 1972.

**TABLE 19-1    Lisfranc Joint Fracture-Dislocation**

| Type | Classification | Injury |
|------|----------------|--------|
| A | Total incongruity | Lateral deviation of all metatarsals<br>Medial deviation of all metatarsals |
| B | Partial incongruity<br>Medial dislocation | Medial deviation of first metatarsal in isolation or with deviation of one or more of the lesser metatarsals |
|  | Lateral dislocation | One or more of the lateral four metatarsals deviated laterally |
| C | Divergent | First metatarsal is deviated medially<br>Any combination of the lateral four metatarsals deviated laterally |

Data from Hardcastle PH, Reschaver R, Kutscha-Lissberg E, Schoffmann W: *J Bone Joint Surg* 64B:349, 1982.

**BOX 19-3    Lisfranc Joint Fracture-Dislocations**

| Type | Classification |
|------|----------------|
| Homolateral | Five metatarsals displaced in the frontal plane |
| Isolated | Medial displacement of the first metatarsal or lateral displacement of one or more lesser metatarsals |
| Divergent | Medial displacement of the first metatarsal and lateral displacement of one or more lesser metatarsals |

Data from Quenu E, Kuss 6: *Revista deChirurgie* 39:1, 1909.

this four-stage system, pronation-eversion causes an initial medial displacement of the first metatarsal.

A more severe injury further incurs dorsolateral deviation of the lesser metatarsals. In the supination-inversion stages, dorsolateral displacement of three or four lesser metatarsals occurs beginning laterally, and in a later stage the first metatarsal follows suit, displacing dorsally and laterally.

Wilson as well as Hesp, van der Werken, and Goris[35] found in their studies that forced plantarflexion was not a frequent cause of injury.

Because the Quenu and Kuss classification did not take into account all varieties of displacement, Hardcastle, Reschauer, Kutscha-Lissberg, and Schoffmann,[30] in 1982, proposed specific variations of this classification (Table 19-1, Figure 19-9). In this classification, Type A involves total incongruity of Lisfranc's joint, with lateral or medial deviation of all metatarsals, as seen in the homolateral type of Quenu and Kuss. In Type B, either medial dislocation or lateral dislocation occurs. In medial dislocation, the first metatarsal may be medially displaced in isolation, or it can occur with the additional displacement of one or more of the lesser metatarsals (Figure 19-10). In lateral dislocation, one or more of the lesser metatarsals deviates laterally. Type C is described as divergent, with the first metatarsal medially deviated and a combination of the lesser metatarsals laterally deviated (Figure 19-11).

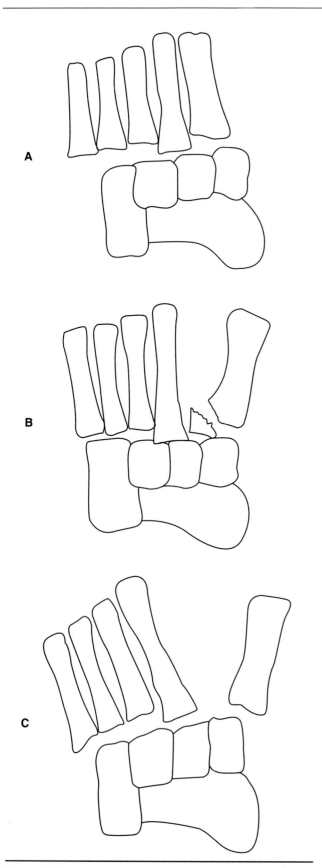

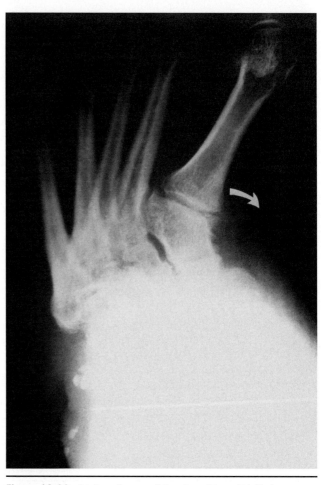

**Figure 19-10**  Lisfranc fracture-dislocation with medial displacement of the first ray.

**Figure 19-9**  A schematic representation of a Lisfranc fracture-dislocation classification. (Data from Quenu E, Kuss G: *Rev Chir* 39:1, 1909.)

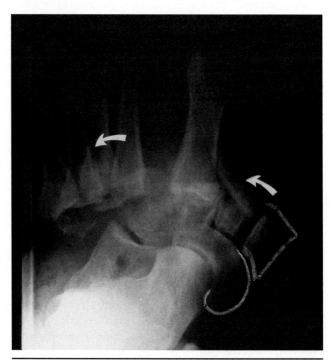

**Figure 19-11**  Divergent Lisfranc fracture-dislocation.

## ■ MIDTARSAL JOINT FRACTURE-DISLOCATIONS

The midtarsal joint, Chopart's joint, consists of the calcaneocuboid and talonavicular articulations. Injuries to this joint are not uncommon but yet often overlooked unless adequate radiographs, including dorsoplantar, oblique, and lateral views, are taken.[8,36,37] Main and Jowett[36] published a midtarsal joint injury classification system in 1975. The system arranges the injuries by mechanism and direction of the deforming force. A simplified arrangement is shown in Table 19-2.

Most midtarsal joint injuries are caused by medial forces and longitudinal forces. A force applied medially causes inversion of the foot with dorsal avulsion/chip fractures of the talus, navicular, or lateral aspects of the cuboid or calcaneus.[5] Medial subluxation or dislocation of the forefoot may also occur. The medial swivel force, as described by Main and Jowett,[36] causes dislocation at the talonavicular joint, while the calcaneocuboid joint remains intact.

Longitudinal forces with the ankle plantarflexed cause the metatarsals and cuneiforms to compress the navicular, resulting in several possible vertical lines of fracture across the body of the navicular. Note that in 1988 Rymaszewski and Robb[37] suggested that the deforming force behind vertical fractures of the navicular is forced plantarflexion rather than longitudinal compression on an already plantarflexed foot.

Lateral forces produced by falls from heights produce avulsion of the medial navicular tuberosity and/or talus. One may also encounter impaction fractures of the calcaneus or cuboid.

Plantar forces, sometimes seen in motorcycle accidents or in injuries where the foot unnaturally twists beneath the body, cause plantar dislocation of the cuboid and navicular. Avulsion fractures of the navicular, talus, or anterior process of the calcaneus are also possible.[36]

Last, injuries caused by crush forces produce severe comminution fractures of one or more bones of the midtarsal joint, in no appreciable pattern. If open fractures occur, they are most common in the crush type of injury.

## ■ NAVICULAR FRACTURES

An encounter with a navicular fracture must be accompanied by examination of the entire midtarsal joint area. Although an isolated navicular fracture is certainly possible, other evidence of midtarsal joint subluxation, dislocation, or flake fractures must be searched for.

Watson-Jones[38] described three types of navicular fractures (Box 19-5). The first, a fracture of the tuberosity,

---

**TABLE 19-2** Midtarsal Joint Fracture-Dislocation

| Deforming Force | Direction of Force | Mechanism | Injuries |
|---|---|---|---|
| Medial | Medial force on lateral side of foot | Inversion of foot | Chip fracture of talus, navicular, or lateral aspect of cuboid or calcaneus; forefoot dislocated medially |
| Medial | Medial swivel force applied to forefoot | Fall from height with rotation at talocalcaneal joint | Talonavicular joint dislocation; calcaneocuboid joint intact |
| Longitudinal | Frontal impact with ankle plantarflexion | Compression of navicular between talus and cuneiforms | Vertical fractures through navicular |
| Longitudinal | Frontal impact with little or no ankle plantarflexion | Compression of inferior aspect of navicular between talus and cuneiforms | Vertical fractures through navicular with possible crush of inferior aspect, and dorsal dislocation of superior fragments |
| Lateral | Lateral forces on medial side of foot | Fall from low height forcing forefoot into valgus | Avulsion of medial navicular tuberosity; chip fracture of talus or navicular; impaction fracture of calcaneus and/or cuboid |
| | | High fall or vehicle wheel rolls over foot | Talonavicular joint subluxates laterally; comminution of calcaneocuboid articulation |
| Lateral | Lateral swivel force to medial side of foot | Awkward landing on foot from low height | Laterally displaced talus; intact calcaneocuboid joint |
| Plantar | Plantar force on the forefoot and midfoot | Falls with foot twisted under the body | Avulsion fractures of navicular, talus, or anterior process of calcaneus; plantar dislocation of cuboid and navicular |
| Crush | Impaction force from dorsal to plantar | Impaction | Comminution and displacement, possibly open |

Data from Main BJ, Jowett RL: *J Bone Joint Surg* 57B:89, 1975.

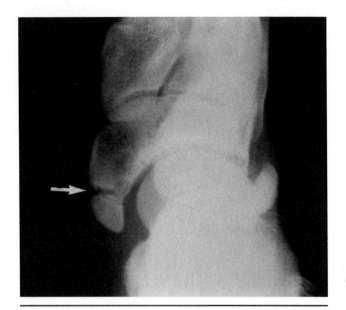

Figure 19-12    Fracture of the medial tuberosity of the navicular.

| BOX 19-5 | Classification of Navicular Fractures |
|----------|----------------------------------------|
| **Type** | **Classification** |
| 1 | Fracture of the medial tuberosity |
| 2 | Fracture of the dorsal lip |
| 3 | Transverse fracture through the body |

Data from Watson-Jones R: *Fractures and joint injuries,* ed 3, vol 2, Baltimore, 1946, Williams & Wilkins.

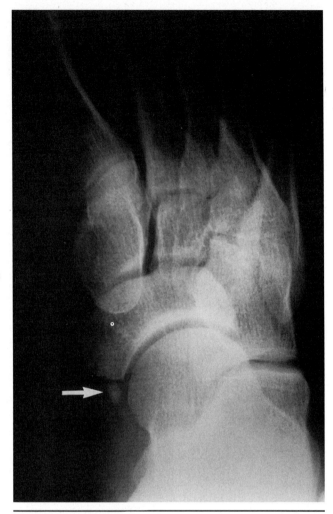

Figure 19-13    Os tibiale externum.

may be produced when an extreme pull from the tibialis posterior tendon causes an avulsion at its major insertion (Figure 19-12). The mechanism might be a twisting of the foot on a step.[39] Remember that portions of the insertion of the tibialis posterior may be found at the sustentaculum tali of the calcaneus, as well as the three cuneiforms, the cuboid, and the second-, third-, and fourth- metatarsal bases.[39]

The fracture of the tuberosity is best viewed on dorsoplantar and lateral oblique foot views. One must distinguish this fracture from the os tibiale externum, a secondary ossification center (Figure 19-13).[40] Fractures, especially when acute, routinely exhibit jagged edges and may seem to fit together like pieces of a puzzle. Accessory bones commonly are smooth, somewhat rounded, and are often bilateral.[20,38,41] A pull on the insertion of the tibialis posterior when an os tibiale externum is present can produce the same symptoms of pain and swelling as in a true fracture.

The second type of navicular fracture described by Watson-Jones[38] is a fracture of the dorsal lip. The navicular

is, in essence, a keystone for vertical stress on the arch,[39,42] so falls that produce eversion and vertical stress cause the tibionavicular ligament to avulse a chip fracture from the dorsal surface of the navicular (Figure 19-14).

Third, a transverse fracture may occur across the navicular in a horizontal plane, separating the bone into large superior and smaller inferior segments.[38] A lateral radiograph is best used for visualizing this injury. The findings often reveal a dorsal dislocation of the large superior fragment.[38]

According to Eichenholtz and Levine,[39] the Watson-Jones Type 2 chip fractures make up almost half of all navicular fractures, with the remainder separated equally into Types 1 and 3. Moreover, in their 1964 study Eichenholtz and Levine found that it was likely for the deltoid and spring ligament attachments to produce more stress than did the tibialis posterior tendon in causing a fracture of the navicular tuberosity.

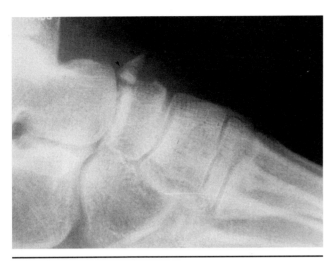

Figure 19-14   Dorsal fracture of the navicular.

## ◼ TRANSCHONDRAL FRACTURES OF THE TALAR DOME

The most common talar fracture is the talar dome fracture.[6] This injury is found most often in adults, in males twice as frequently as females. Although the etiology has been somewhat controversial, trauma is considered the most likely.[6,43]

The talar dome injury, first thought to be a pure case of osteochondritis dissecans (Figure 19-15), was described as such by Kappis[44] in 1922. A talar dome fracture, similar in description to osteochondritis dissecans, was reported in 1932 by Rendu.[45] Berndt and Harty[43] published a classic analysis of 24 cases of talar dome lesions and concluded that trauma was nearly always the cause of this fracture of an

articular surface, which appeared identical to previously described osteochondritis dissecans.

The talar dome transchondral fracture occurs through the articular layer to subchondral bone. The resultant injury ranges from a cartilaginous depression to an avulsed chip fracture (Figure 19-16).[46,47] Symptomotology in acute cases is similar to that of ankle sprains, and diagnosis is difficult if not impossible without the help of radiographs. Chronic presentations mimic arthritic conditions.[46] Anteroposterior, mortise, and medial oblique ankle views are recommended for diagnosis; the lateral view is minimally useful for diagnosis of this fracture.[6,48] If the lesion is not readily visible, these radiographic views should be repeated with the foot in mild dorsiflexion and plantarflexion, or computed tomography (Figure 19-17) should be employed. Fracture healing is evidenced by trabeculae crossing the fracture site.[43]

Many talar dome injuries cannot be directly related to trauma, because the fracture fragment is free of blood and nerve supplies.[20] Consequently, avascular necrosis is not an unlikely complication.

The basic concept of fracture involves recognizable trauma and pain, but in talar dome injuries pain is only

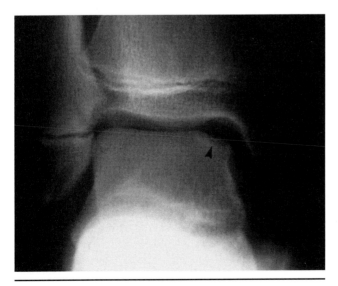

Figure 19-15   Osteochondritis dissecans at the talar dome.

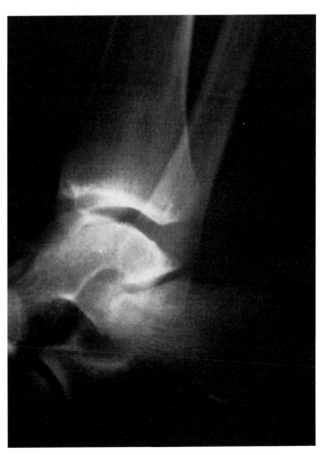

Figure 19-16   Lateral view of a large talar dome fracture with slight anterior displacement.

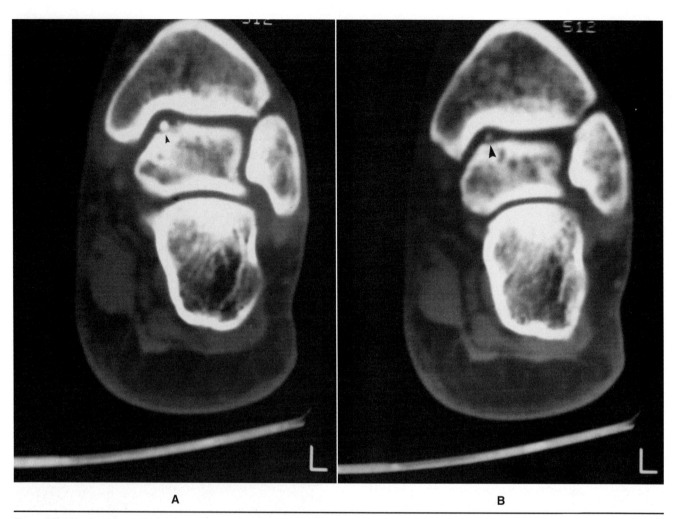

Figure 19-17   **A** and **B** are coronal plane images of slightly different anatomic slices that depict the lesion *(arrowhead).*

present when collateral ligament damage is encountered. If no history of pain is reported in mild injuries, clinical and radiographic diagnosis is often missed. A history of moderate pain in more severe injuries may mislead the examiner into diagnosing an inversion ankle sprain only. These are the reasons for the diagnostic confusion between nontraumatic osteochondritis dissecans and a true transchondral fracture.

Berndt and Harty proposed mechanisms of injury based on their case studies and cadaver experiments.[43] They described four stages of injury based on these mechanisms (Boxes 19-6 and 19-7). The injuries appear either on the lateral or medial aspect of the talar dome (Figure 19-18).

Lateral lesions are found on the anterior or middle half of the lateral talar dome. These injuries are caused by inversion of the ankle with the talus in a dorsiflexed position. As the talus dorsiflexes, the wide anterior portion of the talar dome shifts posteriorly. As an inversion force is applied, the dome rotates laterally and strikes the fibula, causing a depression in the articular surface. This injury, which Berndt and Harty

| BOX 19-6 | Talar Dome Injury Classification |
| --- | --- |

| Stage | Classification |
| --- | --- |
| I | Small compression fracture |
| II | Incomplete avulsion of a fragment |
| III | Complete avulsion without displacement |
| IV | Avulsed fragment displaced within the joint |

Data from Berndt AL, Harty M: *J Bone Joint Surg* 41A:988, 1959.

called a Stage I injury, may be painless. As the force continues, a fracture fragment from the anterior lateral talar dome is produced, causing a Stage II injury. Further force would cause complete avulsion and then displacement of the fracture fragment, Stages III and IV. Pain is encountered as the lateral collateral ligaments tear.[43,49] Eversion does not produce talar dome lesions, owing to the anatomic configuration of the medial malleolus.

BOX 19-7    Talar Dome Injury Mechanism

| Mechanism | Injury to Talar Dome |
|---|---|
| Inversion and dorsiflexion | Lateral-middle |
| | Lateral-anterior |
| Inversion and plantarflexion with lateral rotation | Medial-posterior |

Data from Berndt AL, Harty M: *J Bone Joint Surg* 41A: 988, 1959.

Medial injuries are reported with less firm evidence of trauma.[46] The mechanism of injury involves plantarflexion and inversion of the talus, with anterior and lateral rotation of the tibia.[43,47] Inversion causes the medial aspect of the talar dome to abut the articular surface of the tibia. As the tibia rotates externally, its posterior surface impacts on the talus, causing a Stage I injury of the medial posterior aspect of the talar dome (Figure 19-19).[43,47] Continued rotation partially ruptures the deltoid ligament, grinding a fragment from the articular surface of the talus.[6,46] Depending on the severity of the injury, it appears as a Stage II, III, or IV.

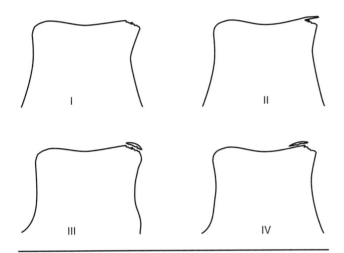

Figure 19-18    Talar dome fracture classification. (Data from Berndt AL, Harty M: *J Bone Joint Surg* 41A:988, 1959.)

## TALAR FRACTURES AND DISLOCATIONS

Fractures of the talus have had various etiologies throughout the history of modern medicine. Falls from horseback preceded airplane accidents, and today motor vehicle accidents account for the vast majority of these injuries.[50,51] In all cases, however, the mechanism is forcible dorsiflexion of the talus against the anterior-distal articular border of the tibia. In a fall from a high place, the forefoot can hit the ground first and sharply dorsiflex on the lower limb. In flying accidents, Coltart[52] described the "aviator's astragalus" as an injury caused when the forefoot dorsiflexed against the rudder pedal of an airplane. Motor vehicle accidents often

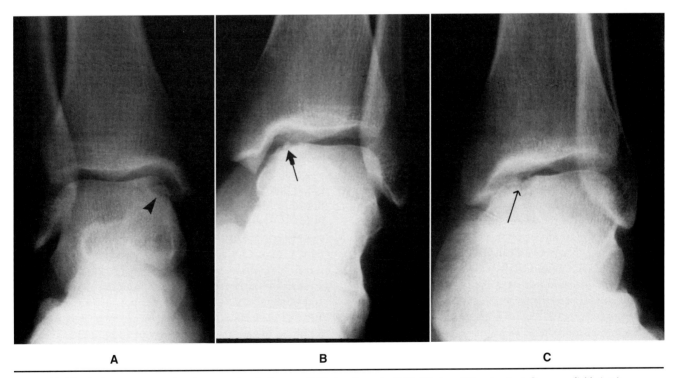

Figure 19-19    **A,** Anteroposterior view demonstrating the large medial lesion *(arrowhead).* **B,** AP view, different patient. Superomedial lesion is identified *(arrow)* with surrounding sclerosis. **C,** Lateral oblique view demonstrates a large superomedial defect and superimposed loose bodies.

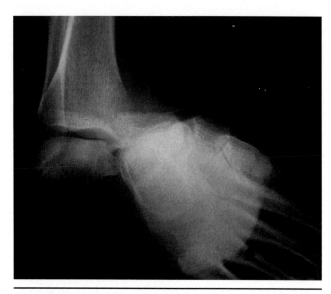

**Figure 19-20** Destructive talar fracture caused by dorsiflexion, external rotation, and adduction.

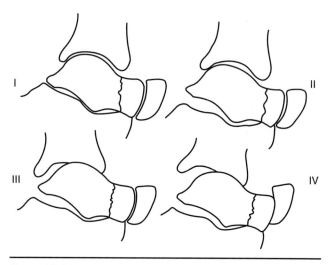

**Figure 19-21** A schematic representation of the Hawkins classification of talar neck fractures.

| **BOX 19-8** | **Talar Fractures and Dislocations Classification** |
|---|---|
| **Type** | **Classification of Injury** |
| I | Vertical fracture at talar neck, undisplaced |
| II | Vertical fracture at talar neck, displaced Subtalar joint subluxated or dislocated |
| III | Vertical fracture at talar neck, displaced Subtalar and ankle joint dislocation |
| IV | Vertical fracture at talar neck, displaced Subtalar, ankle, and talonavicular joint dislocation |

Data from Hawkins LG: *J Bone Joint Surg* 52A: 991, 1970; Canale ST, Kelly FB *J Bone Joint Surg* 60A:143, 1978.

feature a foot forced into the firewall during a collision. In addition to dorsiflexion, external rotation and adduction of the talus may occur (Figure 19-20).[53]

Hawkins[53] described a classification of three types of talar fractures (Box 19-8, Figure 19-21) with emphasis on increasing severity of injury and damage to the delicate talar blood supply. In 1978 Canale and Kelly[54] presented a long-term study that introduced a fourth type of fracture.

In a Type I injury, a vertical fracture of the neck of the talus occurs, with minimal displacement (Figure 19-22). The fracture line travels through the neck from the subtalar joint at a site between the posterior and middle facets. These injuries are usually treated by non–weight-bearing immobilization, and the prognosis is good. A low incidence of avascular necrosis is expected here.[53-55]

Type II injuries exhibit vertical fractures through the neck of the talus, with displacement of the posterior portion of the subtalar joint.[38] In addition, the subtalar joint is subluxated or dislocated. The fracture of the neck may appear somewhat more posterior than in a Type I, affecting the posterior facet of the subtalar joint.

Type III injuries include talar neck fractures with displacement, as well as dislocation at both the subtalar and ankle joints (Figure 19-23). The Type IV injury described by Canale and Kelly added a talonavicular joint dislocation to the Type III injuries. Injury Types II, III, and IV have increasing incidences of avascular necrosis and decreasing rates of successful treatment. Open reduction and internal fixation is often the treatment of choice for these injuries.[56]

Avascular necrosis is the most common and serious complication seen in talar injuries.[55] The three major blood supplies to the talus are the posterior tibial artery, the dorsalis pedis artery, and the peroneal artery. The posterior tibial artery's calcaneal branches form a network over the posterior tubercle. The artery of the tarsal canal that supplies blood to the middle third of the talus also arises from the posterior tibial artery.[20] The dorsalis pedis artery supplies blood to the sinus tarsi and gives off the medial tarsal artery branches that supply the neck and dorsal head of the talus.[6,55] Branches arise from the peroneal artery to supply the posterior region of the talus and a portion of the lateral talus. An extensive system of anastemoses supply the remaining portions of the talus.[42]

Routine radiographs of anteroposterior, mortise, lateral, and oblique views should be obtained in talar injuries. If avascular necrosis occurs, it appears approximately 2 months following injury.[53] It is evident on an x-ray study as relatively radiosclerotic dead bone and surrounding atrophic bone. Hawkins described a sign of subchondral radiolucency on radiograph in the body of the talus that seems to infer an intact blood supply and is therefore a good indication that

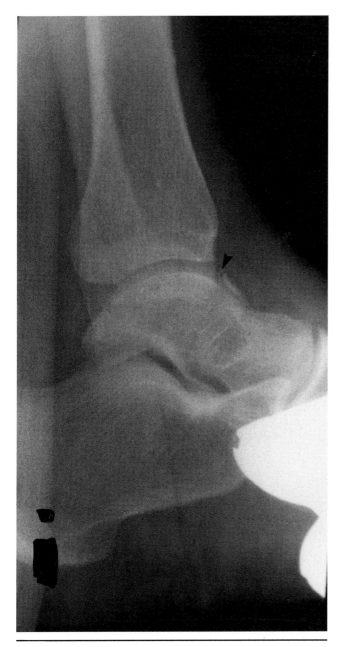

Figure 19-22    Talar neck fracture.

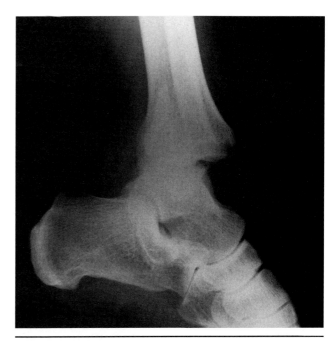

Figure 19-23    Dislocation of the ankle, subtalar, and talonavicular joints.

| BOX 19-9 | Incidence of Avascular Necrosis in Hawkins-Type Talar Fracture-Dislocations |
|---|---|

| Type | Average Incidence of Avascular Necrosis |
|---|---|
| I | 7% |
| II | 46% |
| III | 88% |

Data from Hawkins L6: *J Bone Joint Surg* 52A:991, 1970; Canale ST, Kelly FB: *J Bone Joint Surg.* 60A:143, 1978; Watson-Jones R: *Fractures and joint injuries,* ed 6, vol 2, New York, 1982, Churchill-Livingstone.

avascular necrosis will not occur.[53] The Hawkins sign is best visualized on anteroposterior and mortise ankle views.

Avascular necrosis as a result of talar injury has an extremely high incidence that increases with the severity of the injury.[50] Average occurrence, seen in Box 19-9, is 7% in Type I injuries, 46% in Type II, and 88% in Type III.[38,53,54] Type IV injuries most likely have an incidence rate of nearly 100%, although statistics on these injuries are scanty.[54]

Treatment of talar injuries must be immediate and precise. To ensure proper alignment of fracture fragments, Canale and Kelly recommend radiographs taken with the ankle in equinus, the foot pronated 15 degrees, and the x-ray beam directed toward the ankle at 75 degrees from the horizontal. If the fragments are not well visualized, computed tomography may be employed.

## ■ FRACTURE OF THE POSTERIOR PROCESS OF THE TALUS

In 1882 Francis Shepherd[57] described a previously unreported fracture of the posterior process of the talus external to the groove of the flexor hallucis longus tendon. He found some fractured portions with no attachment to the talus and others united by fibrous attachments. Shepherd rejected the possibility that these fractures could

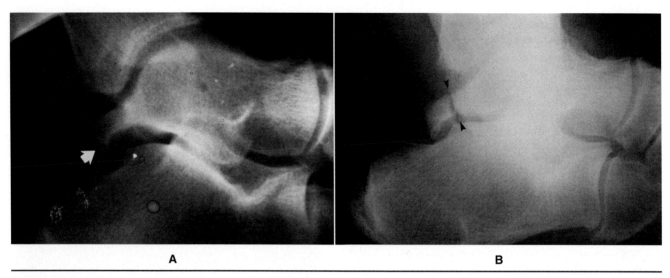

**A**                          **B**

Figure 19-24    **A,** Prominent, intact, Steida's process of talus. **B,** Shepherd's fracture of talus.

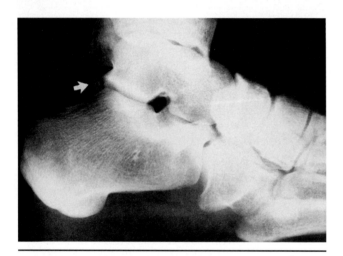

Figure 19-25    Differential diagnosis of os trigonum and Shepherd's fracture.

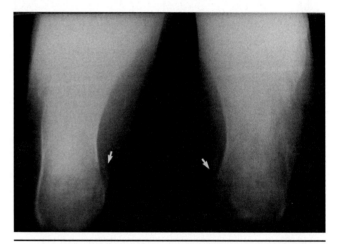

Figure 19-26    Calcaneal axial views of bilateral calcaneal fractures.

be secondary epiphyses caused by the lack of cartilage between the talus and the fractured portion (Figure 19-24).

Care must be taken during radiographic analysis not to mistake the Shepherd's fracture for an os trigonum (Figure 19-25).[38,58] As in all such cases, the fracture end is jagged and the two pieces appear to fit together. The os trigonum should appear round and smooth.

## ■ CALCANEAL FRACTURES

The calcaneus is the largest and most commonly fractured tarsal bone.[20,59,60] Calcaneal fractures occur more commonly in adults, and in children are most often extra-articular.[61] Most adult calcaneal fractures are caused by compression and displacement of the bone through high falls or motor vehicle accidents.[62,63] Extra-articular fractures may be caused by rotational injuries.[62]

Radiographic evaluation of calcaneal fractures should routinely include lateral, oblique, and calcaneal axial views (Figure 19-26).[64] Bohler's angle should be observed on lateral view, because a decrease would indicate a joint depression (Figure 19-27).[65] Computed tomography is the technique of choice if available (Figure 19-28). Radiographic examination of the spine, as well as of the tibia and fibula, is recommended.[66]

Palmer,[62] in 1948, considered different types of calcaneal fractures according to its mechanism of injury. He described three: avulsion, compression, and shearing. Palmer's intent was to simplify previous classifications. One earlier classification attempt by Bohler[65] in 1931 accurately described fractures of avulsion, the anterior process, and

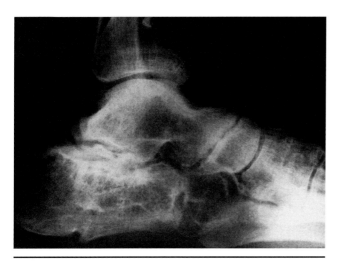

Figure 19-27    Joint depression fracture of the calcaneus.

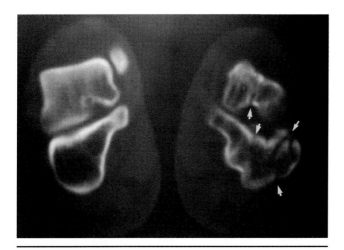

Figure 19-28    Computed tomography revealing comminuted fractures of the calcaneus and talus.

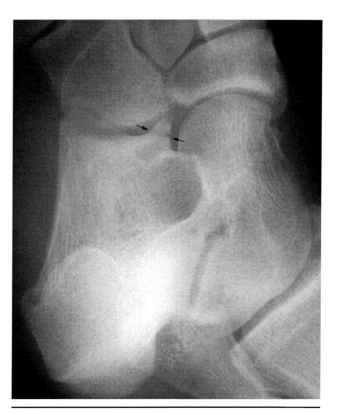

Figure 19-29    Anterior beak fracture of the calcaneus.

**BOX 19-10    Classification of Calcaneal Fractures**

| Type | Classification of Fracture |
|---|---|
| I | Extra-articular |
| A | Anterior process fracture |
| B | Fracture of the medial tuberosity |
| C | Fractures through the body (vertical or horizontal) |
| D | Fracture of the superior-lateral process |
| II | Intra-articular |
| A | Tongue type |
| B | Joint depression |

Essex-LoPresti P: *Br J Surg* 39:395, 1952.

extra-articular fractures through the body. It was on these and other works that Essex-LoPresti[67] based his classification in 1952. The Essex-LoPresti classification (Box 19-10) divides calcaneal fractures into two types, extra-articular and intra-articular. The extra-articular type represented only a quarter of his cases, and the injuries were much less severe than the intra-articular type. Type I extra-articular fractures included those of the anterior "beak" process (Figure 19-29), the medial tuberosity, vertical or horizontal fractures through the body, and fractures of the superior-lateral process (Figure 19-30).

Type II, intra-articular fractures, involve the subtalar joint. Two distinct varieties are described by Essex-LoPresti: the tongue type and joint depression. Tongue-type fractures (Figure 19-31) are caused by the talus descending into the cancellous body of the calcaneus, causing a primary vertical fracture line from the subtalar joint. A secondary fracture line runs posteriorly from the primary fracture. If force continues, the anterior portion of this tongue fracture is driven into the body of the calcaneus, and the posterior end is forced dorsally and posteriorly.

The Type II joint depression category represents a primary fracture line from the subtalar joint through the body of the calcaneus plantarly, which gaps open, thus decreasing Bohler's angle. A secondary line runs posteriorly and superiorly, displacing the subtalar joint. When the force of injury ceases, soft tissue elastic recoil allows upward displacement of the posterior aspect of the calcaneus.[62,67]

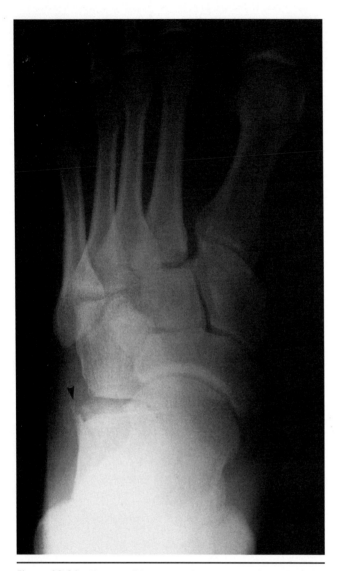

Figure 19-30  Fracture of the superior-lateral process of the calcaneus.

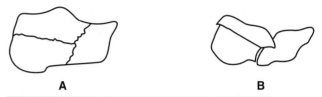

Figure 19-31   **A,** Tongue-type calcaneal fracture with slight displacement. (From Essex-LoPresti P: *Br J Surg* 39:395, 1952. With permission of the publishers, Butterworth-Heinemann Ltd.) **B,** Tongue-type calcaneal fracture with severe displacement. (From Essex-LoPresti P: *Br J Surg* 39: 395, 1952 with permission of the publishers, Butterworth-Heinemann Ltd.)

| BOX 19-11 | | Classification of Calcaneal Fractures |
|---|---|---|
| **Type** | | **Classification of Fracture** |
| I | A | Fracture of medial tuberosity |
| | B | Fracture of sustentaculum tali |
| | C | Fracture of anterior process |
| II | A | Fracture of posterior beak |
| | B | Achilles tendon avulsion fracture |
| III | A & B | Oblique fractures not involving the subtalar joint |
| IV | A & B | Intra-articular fractures involving the subtalar joint |
| V | A & B | Comminuted joint depression fractures |

Data from Rowe CR, Sakellarides HT, Freeman PA, Sorbie C: *JAMA* 184:920, 1963.

comminuted joint depression. In Rowe's study, open reduction treatment was required more often in Types II, III, and IV, whereas Type V was often manually reduced and immobilized (Figure 19-35) with variable results.

More recently, Schmidt and Weiner[61] proposed a combined classification of calcaneal fractures, using both Essex-LoPresti and Rowe classifications (Box 19-12). The Schmidt-Weiner classification was designed for use in adults and children, because it includes a posterior apophyseal fracture as Type I-A.

Small avulsion flake fractures from various areas of the body of the calcaneus are labeled as Type I-E. Schmidt and Weiner did not find Type II fractures in children. Type V fractures correspond to Essex-LoPresti intra-articular types of tongue and joint depression. In this study, Type VI fractures, a significant loss of bone and soft tissue at the area of the Achilles tendon insertion, occurred often as a result of lawnmower injuries.

## ◼ EPIPHYSEAL FRACTURES

Childhood fractures of the epiphysis or separations of the epiphyseal plate may result in arrested or deformed

These fractures are severely comminuted, and avascular necrosis is a likely complication.[40]

Lindsay,[60] in 1958, described calcaneal fractures as either moderate or severe, basing these classifications on the extent of injury. Rowe and associates[66] based their calcaneal fracture classifications (Box 19-11, Figure 19-32) on the location of the injury, modifying a Watson-Jones[38] classification.

In the Rowe classification, Type I caused mild to moderate disability and could often be treated by closed reduction and immobilization. Type I included fractures of the medial tuberosity, sustentaculum tali, and anterior process. Type II described a posterior beak fracture (Figure 19-33) as well as larger avulsion fractures that included the insertion of the Achilles tendon. Type III are oblique extra-articular fractures, and Type IV are intra-articular fractures of the subtalar joint (Figure 19-34). Type V fractures involve

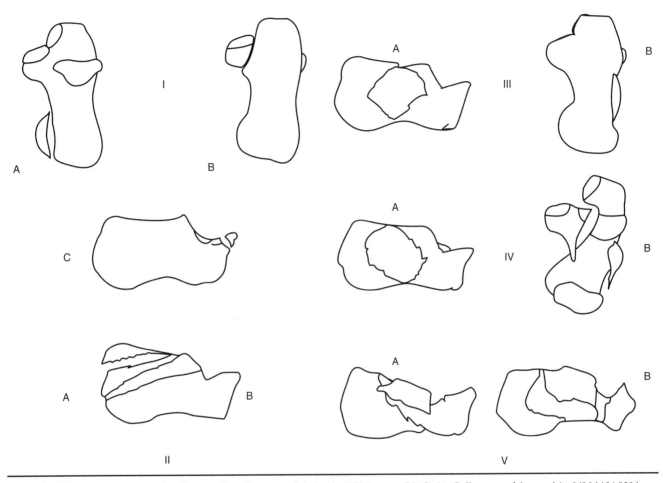

Figure 19-32    Calcaneal fracture classification. (From Rowe CR, Sakellarides HT, Freeman PA, Sorbie C: Fractures of the as calcis, *JAMA* 184:920.)

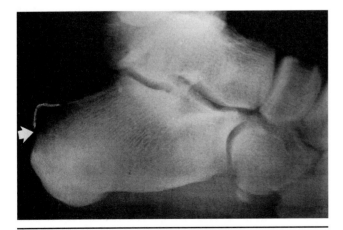

Figure 19-33    Posterior beak fracture of the calcaneus.

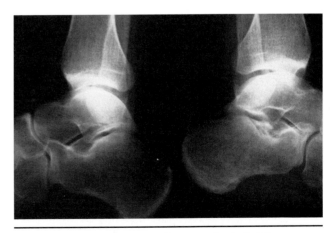

Figure 19-34    Bilateral calcaneal fractures with subtalar joint involvement.

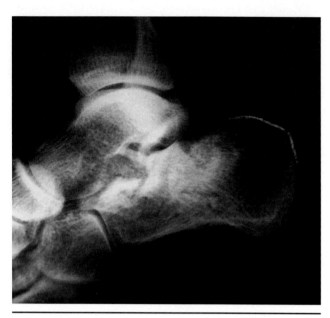

Figure 19-35    Healed calcaneal joint depression fracture.

---

**BOX 19-12    Classification of Calcaneal Fractures**

| Type | | Classification of Fracture |
|------|---|---------------------------|
| I | A | Fracture of medial tuberosity or apophysis |
| | B | Fracture of sustentaculum tali |
| | C | Fracture of anterior process |
| | D | Fracture of inferior-lateral process |
| | E | Avulsion fractures from calcaneal body |
| II | A | Fracture of posterior beak |
| | B | Achilles tendon avulsion fracture |
| III | | Extra-articular linear fracture |
| IV | | Intra-articular linear fracture into subtalar joint |
| V | A | Tongue-type fracture |
| | B | Joint depression fracture |
| VI | | Destruction of bone and soft tissue at posterior aspect with loss of Achilles tendon insertion |

Data from Schmidt TL, Weiner DS: *Clin Orthop* 171:150, 1982.

---

**TABLE 19-3    Epiphyseal Ankle Injury Classification**

| Type | Degree | Classification |
|------|--------|---------------|
| External rotation | First | Separation of epiphyseal plate of fibula with an oblique fracture into the diaphysis |
| | Second | Separation of epiphyseal plates of fibula and tibial malleolus with an oblique fracture into the disphysis of the fibula |
| | Third | Separation of fibular and tibial epiphyseal plates with an oblique fracture into the diaphysis of the fibula |
| Abduction | First | Separation of epiphyseal plate of tibial malleolus |
| | Second | Separation of epiphyseal plate of fibula and tibial malleolus |
| | Third | Separation of epiphyseal plates of fibula and tibia |
| Adduction | First | Separation of epiphyseal plate of fibula |
| | Second | Separation of epiphyseal plate of fibula and tibial malleolus with intra-articular fracture of tibial malleolus |
| | Third | Separation of epiphyseal plates of fibula and tibia with intra-articular fracture of tibial malleolus |
| Compression | | Separation of tibial epiphyseal plate with posterior fracture of diaphysis |
| Direct violence | | Epiphyseal plate separations of fibula and tibia |

Data from Bishop PA: *AJR* 28:49, 1932.

---

growth.[68] The epiphyseal growth plate is made up of four zones, from distal to proximal: the zone of calcification, zone of hypertrophic cartilage, proliferating zone, and the resting zone.[69] The hypertrophic zone contains the least collagen fibers and is therefore the weakest zone and the site of most epiphyseal separations.[70] The blood supply to the epiphysis and metaphysis of the fibula and tibia is separate, so an epiphyseal plate separation without excessive shearing may not disrupt the growth by instigating avascular necrosis.[69]

The mechanisms of fractures in children are similar to those of adults. However, before epiphyseal plates close they are weaker than ligamentous attachments. Therefore mechanisms of injury that would cause ligament rupture in adults usually result in epiphyseal injuries in children.[71]

Growth plate injuries are caused by shearing, avulsion, or crushing forces.[69,72] Throughout the years, many authors have sought to classify the injuries by mechanism and location. Several of these classifications are presented next, to give the reader a variety of etiologies and appearances of epiphyseal injuries.

Bishop,[73] in 1932, described a somewhat complicated classification of epiphyseal injuries in the ankle (Table 19-3). His classification system is based on five mechanisms of injury. The first, external rotation of the foot, separates the epiphyseal plate of the fibula and obliquely fractures the fibula proximal to the growth plate in the first-degree stage. As the injury progresses to the second degree of external rotation, the tibial epiphyseal plate separates at the medial malleolus. Continuing the force of injury separates the entire tibial epiphyseal plate.

The second mechanism of injury in Bishop's classification is abduction of the foot. In the first degree of this injury, the epiphyseal plate of the medial malleolus separates. In the second degree, the epiphyseal plate of the fibula also separates, and in the third stage the entire epiphyseal plate of the tibia separates.

In the third type of injury, adduction of the foot, the fibular epiphyseal plate separates in the first degree. If the injury progresses in adduction, additional separation of the medial malleolar epiphyseal plate and an intra-articular fracture of the medial malleolus occur. Finally, if the third degree is attained, the entire tibial epiphyseal plate separates.

The fourth mechanism is that of compression or crush injury. This force causes separation of the epiphyseal plate of the tibia with a posterior fracture of the diaphysis of that bone.

Direct violence was the fifth force described by Bishop, who claims that this injury causes separations of the tibial and fibular epiphyseal plates.

By far the most commonly used and widely accepted classification of epiphyseal injuries is that of Salter and Harris,[69] from 1963. Salter and Harris describe three main types of injury: separation of the epiphyseal plate, vertical fractures across the epiphysis, and compression injuries. Fractures of the epiphysis and crush fractures have much poorer prognoses than do separations of epiphyseal plates.

Five classifications of epiphyseal injury are described by Salter and Harris (Box 19-13, Figure 19-36). In Type I, separation of the epiphyseal plate occurs as the result of an avulsion force (Figure 19-37). Blood supply is rarely damaged, and the prognosis is excellent. In Type II, the epiphyseal plate is separated partially before exiting through the metaphysis, causing a triangular fragment (Figure 19-38) known as the Thurston Holland's sign or fragment.[74]

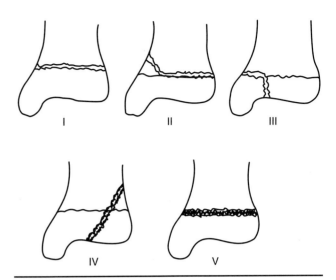

Figure 19-36   A schematic representation of the Salter-Harris classification of epiphyseal plate fractures.

A lamella sign, a detachment of a thin layer of the epiphyseal plate region, was described by Werenskiold.[75] Type II is the most common of epiphyseal plate injuries, and prognosis is also excellent.

Type III involves an intra-articular fracture extending from the articular surface to the epiphyseal growth plate, effectively fracturing the epiphysis. The fracture then extends along the weakest portion of the epiphyseal plate to the cortical margin. Because of the need for accurate realignment of the fragments, open reduction, and internal fixation may be needed.

Type IV is a vertical fracture extending from the articular surface, through both the epiphysis and growth plate, to exit through the metaphysis. Prognosis is guarded, and open reduction is often needed.

Type V is a quite uncommon and extremely destructive compression of the epiphyseal plate. Immobilization and traction are possible treatments.[69,76]

Another classification of epiphyseal injuries is one proposed by Aitken.[70] This simple classification (Box 19-14) includes three types. Type I involves an avulsion fracture-separation of the epiphyseal plate, usually with a fragment through the metaphysis. Type II is a vertical fracture through the epiphysis from the joint surface to the epiphyseal plate. In Type III, the Type II fracture extends beyond the epiphyseal plate through a portion of the metaphysis.

In 1965, Crenshaw[77] published a classification similar to Bishop's pediatric ankle injuries that were based on the direction of force of the injury (Box 19-15). In Crenshaw's classification, four forces are examined: external rotation, abduction, plantarflexion, and adduction. External rotation causes a separation through a portion of the epiphyseal plate

---

**BOX 19-13    Epiphyseal Injury Classification**

| Type | Classification of Injury |
|------|--------------------------|
| I | Separation of the epiphyseal plate |
| II | Fracture separates the epiphyseal plate along a variable distance, then exits through the metaphysis, creating a triangular fragment known as Thurston-Holland's sign |
| III | Intra-articular fracture extending from the joint surface through the epiphysis to the epiphyseal plate; the fracture extends along the epiphyseal plate to its periphery |
| IV | Intra-articular fracture extending from the joint surface through the epiphysis and the epiphyseal plate and exits in the metaphysis |
| V | Crush injury causing a compression fracture of the epiphyseal plate |

Data from Salter RB, Harris WR: *J Bone Joint Surg* 45A:587, 1963.

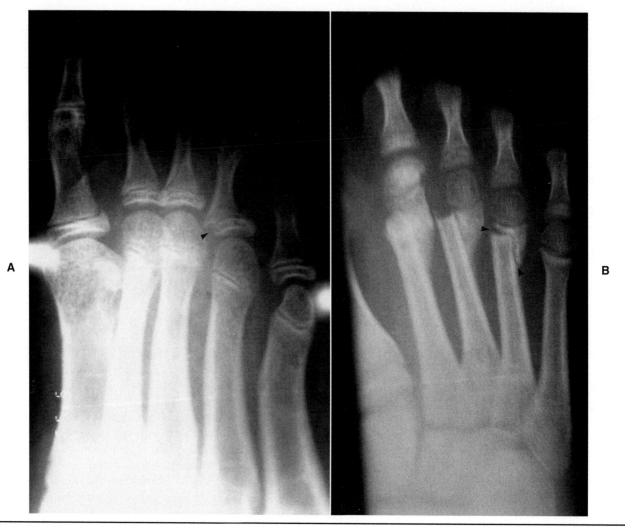

**Figure 19-37    A,** Fracture of fourth proximal phalangeal growth plate secondary to shearing force. **B,** Fractures of second, third, and fourth metatarsals, caused by blunt trauma, with no radiographic evidence of growth plate disruption.

of the tibia that exits into the posterior metaphysis. A fibular fracture above the growth plate is often seen. Abduction injuries cause a separation of the tibial epiphyseal plate with a possible fracture into the anterolateral aspect of the metaphysis. A fibular fracture may also occur. Plantarflexion injuries involve a posterior displacement of the epiphysis. If a metaphyseal fracture occurs, it will also be posteriorly displaced. Adduction force produces tension on the lateral ligaments, avulsing the fibular epiphysis. An intra-articular fracture of the medial malleolus follows if the force continues and the talus impacts on the tibia.

In 1978 Dias and Tachdjian[78] combined the Salter-Harris and Lauge-Hansen[79] classifications to develop a system of ankle injuries in children. The Dias-Tachdjian system is based on the position of the foot and direction of the injuring force (Table 19-4).

Supination-inversion involves two stages. In Stage I, a separation of the epiphyseal plate of the fibula with possible fracture into the metaphysis occurs laterally. If the injury continues to Stage II, an intra-articular fracture through the epiphysis of the tibia with possible fracture into the metaphysis is caused by the talus impacting the medial malleolus.

Supination-plantarflexion leads to a separation of the epiphyseal plate of the tibia, usually with a metaphyseal fragment.

Supination-external rotation also involves two stages of increasing severity. A Stage I injury causes separation of the epiphyseal plate of the tibia, with a spiral fracture extending into the diaphysis. As the force continues, Stage II incurs a spiral fibular fracture proximal to the epiphyseal plate.

Pronation-eversion-external rotation involves a separation of the epiphyseal plate of the tibia with an extension of

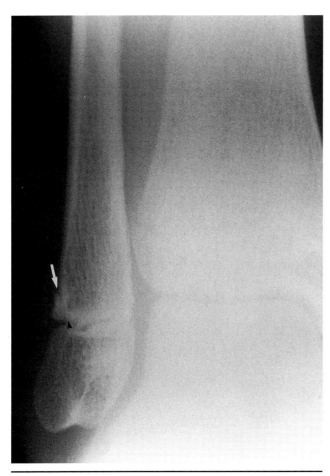

**Figure 19-38**  Epiphyseal plate and metaphyseal fractures with Thurston Holland sign.

**BOX 19-15**  Tibial Epiphyseal Injury Classification

| Type | | Classification of Injury |
|---|---|---|
| I | External rotation | Separation of the tibial epiphyseal plate along a variable distance, with fracture exiting the posterior metaphysis |
| | | A fibular fracture above the growth plate is common |
| II | Abduction | Separation of the tibial epiphyseal plate with possible fracture into the anterior lateral metaphysis |
| | | A fibular fracture is possible |
| III | Plantarflexion | Posterior displacement of epiphysis with possible metaphyseal fracture also posteriorly displaced |
| IV | Adduction | Intra-articular fracture of medial malleolus, possibly involving the metaphysis |
| | | Avulsion of fibular epiphysis precedes this fracture |

Data from Crenshaw AH: *Clin Orthop* 41:98, 1965.

**TABLE 19-4**  Epiphyseal Ankle Injury Classification

| Type | Stage | Classification of Injury |
|---|---|---|
| Supination-inversion | I | Separation of distal fibular epiphyseal plate with possible fracture into the metaphysis |
| | II | Intra-articular fracture through the tibial epiphysis with possible fracture into the metaphysis |
| Supination-plantarflexion | I | Separation of the tibial epiphyseal plate, usually with a metaphyseal fragment |
| Supination-external rotation | I | Separation of the tibial epiphyseal plate with a long spiral fracture of the distal tibia |
| | II | Separation of the tibial epiphyseal plate with a long spiral fracture of the distal tibia and a spiral fracture of the fibula above the growth plate |
| Pronation-eversion-external rotation | I | Separation of the tibial epiphyseal plate with a metaphyseal fragment and a short oblique fracture in the diaphysis of the fibula |

Data from Dias LS, Tachdjian MO: *Clin Orthop* 136:230, 1978; Dias LS, in Rockwood CA, Wilkins KE, King RE, editors: *Fractures in children*, vol 3, Philadelphia, 1984, Lippincott.

**BOX 19-14**  Epiphyseal Injury Classification

| Type | Classification of Injury |
|---|---|
| I | Transverse avulsion fracture at epiphyseal plate, usually with a fragment through the metaphysis |
| II | Vertical fracture across the epiphysis to the epiphyseal plate |
| III | Vertical fracture across the epiphysis, through the epiphyseal plate, and into the metaphysis |

Data from Aitken AP: *Clin Orthop* 41:19, 1965.

the fracture into the metaphysis. Also seen is a short oblique fracture in the diaphysis of the fibula.

Triplane fractures involve fractures of the fibular diaphysis, the anterolateral tibial epiphysis, and a tibial epiphysis-metaphysis fragment.[78] They are most likely

| BOX 19-16 | Epiphyseal Injury Classification |
|---|---|
| **Type** | **Classification of Injury** |
| 1A | Separation of epiphyseal plate |
| 1B | Separation of epiphyseal plate through the spongiosa |
| 1C | Separation of epiphyseal plate with associated injury to the germinal portion |
| 2A | Partial separation of epiphyseal plate with triangular metaphyseal fragment |
| 2B | Type 2A with displacement of the metaphyseal fragment |
| 2C | Type 2A with involvement of a significant layer of metaphyseal bone |
| 2D | Compression to a localized area of epiphyseal plate by metaphysis |
| 3A | Intra-articular fracture through the epiphysis, extending along the epiphyseal plate to its periphery |
| 3B | Type 3A with a metaphyseal layer avulsed with the epiphyseal fragment |
| 3C | Type 3A fracture through a malformed epiphysis |
| 4A | Intra-articular from articular surface through the epiphysis and epiphyseal plate into the metaphysis |
| 4B | Type 4A with an additional fracture through the epiphysis |
| 4C | Type 4A with epiphyseal plate fracture through the cartilaginous zones |
| 4D | Type 4A with multiple fractures of epiphysis, metaphysis, and epiphyseal plate |
| 5 | Compression fracture of epiphyseal plate |
| 6 | Perichondral ring abrasion or burn |
| 7A | Osteochondral fracture |
| 7B | Osteochondral fracture involving the zone of hypertrophy |
| 8 | Vascular interruption of metaphyseal growth |
| 9 | Avulsion of periosteum |

Data from Ogden JA: *Skeletal injury in the child*, Philadelphia, 1982, Lea & Febiger.

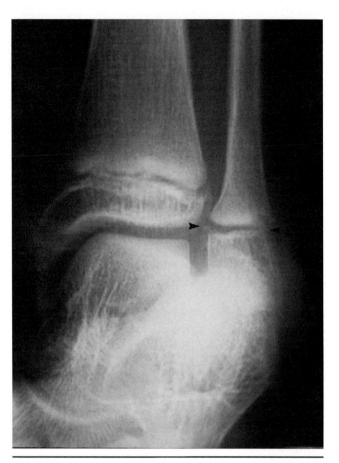

Figure 19-39    Fracture through the epiphyseal plate of the fibula.

caused by external rotation with or without plantarflexion and do not fit the Dias-Tachdjian classification.

Also not under the Dias-Tachdjian system is a Salter-Harris III injury of the tibial epiphysis known as juvenile Tillaux fracture.[77,80]

In 1982 Ogden[81] built a more extensive Salter-Harris system, with several subclassifications (Box 19-16). Type 1A injuries are more often seen in infants with limited development of the ossification center and represent separation of the epiphyseal plate. Type 1B fractures occur through the spongiosa area of the resting zone of the growth plate as opposed to the zone of hypertrophic cartilage. Diseases such as leukemia and myelomeningocele affect metaphyseal ossification and may precipitate Type 1B injuries. Type 1C is an infrequent fracture with an associated injury to the germinal portion of the epiphyseal plate.

A Type 2A injury is the most common of growth plate fractures, caused by a shearing or avulsion force (Figure 19-39). Type 2A corresponds to a Salter-Harris II, with a triangular metaphyseal fragment produced. In Type 2B the metaphyseal fracture is displaced. Type 2C involves a thin layer of metaphyseal bone, involving most of the opposing metaphysis. Type 2D occurs when an area of the metaphysis causes compression damage to a localized area.

Type 3, the intra-articular fracture, is designated with two subtypes. Type 3A represents a fracture from the articular surface through the epiphysis to the epiphyseal plate, then extending along the growth plate to the periphery as seen in a Salter-Harris III. Type 3B fractures occur through the spongiosa level, so that a layer of metaphyseal bone is avulsed along with the epiphyseal fragment. Type 3C occurs in deformed epiphyses.

Type 4A corresponds to a Salter-Harris IV, extending a fracture from the joint surface, through the epiphysis as well as the epiphyseal plate, into the metaphysis. Type 4B involves an additional fracture fragment through the epiphysis. The

Type 4C fracture passes through the cartilagenous zones. Severe trauma causes a Type 4D, with multiple fractures of the metaphysis, epiphysis, and epiphyseal growth plate.

Type 5, a compression fracture, corresponds to a Salter-Harris V. Ogden adds Type 6, an injury possibly caused by a severe burn or degloving of skin, where the perichondral area is contused. Type 7A fractures are osteochondral fractures extending from the articular surface through the epiphyseal cartilage and into the preossification region. These injuries are common at the malleoli. Type 7B fractures occur through the hypertrophic cartilaginous zone.

Type 8 injuries affect metaphyseal growth by temporarily interrupting vascular supply to the metaphysis. Type 9 injuries damage the periosteum by avulsion and affect the ability of bone to remodel.

Healing of epiphyseal injuries with no interruption of blood supply is accomplished within three weeks. If bone callus fills the growth plate, growth is partially or totally arrested. This complication is common in fractures that cross the epiphyseal plate.[69] It is therefore imperative to attain early radiographic diagnosis of epiphyseal injuries. Routine anteroposterior, lateral, and mortise ankle views that include the proximal tibia and fibula are indicated.

Salter-Harris Types I and V are difficult to view and must be differentiated from normal open or closing growth plates. Difficult injuries may require computed tomography or magnetic resonance imaging.[82]

## ■ EARLY STUDY OF ANKLE FRACTURES

To understand the complex mechanisms of ankle fractures, it is imperative to review the early studies of these injuries. Throughout the history of medicine, various diseases, conditions, lesions, symptoms, and injuries have been described by medical pioneers with such import that their names are used as eponyms. Several of these eponyms are included in the following discussion. Today's usage of these eponyms sometimes does not correlate with the original descriptions or experiments by their namesake, notably Pott,[83] Dupuytren,[84] Volkmann,[85] and Cotton[86] fractures.[79]

## Pott's Fracture

In 1768 Sir Percivall Pott[83] published a monograph on fractures that described a fibular fracture 2 to 3 inches proximal to the distal end of the bone. The injury was described as including a deltoid ligament rupture and an intact syndesmosis. This is not consistent with the more common usage of the term "Pott's fracture" as describing a bimalleolar fracture.[6,87]

## Dupuytren's Fracture

Dupuytren,[84] in 1819, described a fracture of the fibula 2½ inches proximal to its distal end. A medial injury involving a deltoid ligament tear or medial malleolar fracture preceded this injury.[87] Diastasis is always present.[79]

## Maisonneuve Fracture

In 1840 Maisonneuve[88] explained an external rotary force that fractures the medial malleolus or tears the deltoid ligament and then followed with a tibiofibular ligament tear. The force subsequently caused a torque about the proximal third of the fibula. This fibular fracture is the Maisonneuve fracture. Pankovich[89] described a classification of Maisonneuve fractures that involved five stages. Stage 1 is a tear of the anterior tibiofibular ligament or avulsion of the anterior tibial tubercle. Stage 2 involves a rupture of the posterior tibiofibular ligament or fracture of the posterior tibial tubercle. Stage 3 exhibits a rupture of the anterior medial aspect of the ankle joint capsule, and Stage 4 is the Maisonneuve fracture. Stage 5 is the medial injury, with either a medial malleolar fracture or superficial deltoid rupture.

## Chaput-Tillaux Fracture

In 1872, Tillaux[90] studied ankle trauma involving a medial injury causing a superficial deltoid tear or medial malleolar fracture, a fibular fracture approximately 2 inches above the ankle joint, and the Tillaux fracture. The Tillaux fracture occurs in the anterior lateral tibial tubercle. In 1907 Chaput[91] reproduced the avulsion fracture in laboratory specimens on radiograph and recorded several clinical injuries involving fractures of the anterior tibial tubercle.[78]

## Wagstaffe Fracture

The Wagstaffe[92] fracture, first reported in 1873, is an avulsion of the distal fibula by the anterior inferior tibiofibular ligament. This injury commonly occurs during a suppination–external rotation injury.[93]

## Von Volkmann Fracture

Von Volkman,[85] in 1875, described a fracture of the anterior lateral lip of the tibia, caused by an avulsion from the anterior tibiofibular ligament and the interosseous membrane through a force of pronation and abduction. According to Lauge-Hansen,[79] later authors erroneously classified this fracture as being on the posterolateral aspect of the tibia, as it is now known.

## LeFort Fracture

In a paper written in 1886, LeFort described yet another fibular fracture.[94] The LeFort fracture is a vertical fracture of the fibula, caused by a pull from the anterior tibiofibular ligament at the anterior medial aspect of the lateral malleolus.[6,94] This injury occurs as a result of a supination-adduction force, LeFort believed.

## Cotton Fracture

In 1915 Cotton[86] described a fracture of the posterior aspect of the tibia, the area also known as the posterior malleolus. He stated that the injury is associated with a fracture of the medial malleolus, and a fibular fracture above the joint level.[79] Thus the Cotton fracture is known as a trimalleolar fracture.

## ◼ ANKLE FRACTURES AND DISLOCATIONS

Ankle injuries are increasing in number secondary to an increase in risk factors in today's world.[95] Radiographic evaluations with anteroposterior, lateral, and mortise ankle views are routinely performed and usually sufficient for diagnosis.[96,97] If needed, computed tomography and magnetic resonance imaging readily expose occult injuries.

The early pioneers of ankle fracture research used cadavers to simulate clinical injuries. Chaput[91] was the first to use roentgenograms for studying ankle fractures. Ashhurst and Bromer[98] created one of the first comprehensive classification systems in 1922. They based their system on a study of 300 ankle fractures and classified them according to the mechanism of injury (Table 19-5).

The Ashhurst and Bromer system lists the forces of injury as external rotation, abduction, and adduction of the foot, as well as axial loading compression and direct violence. In their opinion, the spiral-oblique fracture of the fibula occurred during external rotation of the pronated foot, without diastasis. This concept is contrary to current theory. Their classification stressed osseous fractures over ligamentous tears as results of the forces of injury.[79]

Seeking to bolster the impact of the Ashhurst-Bromer classification, in 1932 Bishop[73] presented a series of more than 300 cases. These papers brought to the fore the importance of understanding mechanisms of injury to diagnose and treat them. The term *mechanism* refers not to the actual injury, such as a fall or direct trauma but rather to the position of the foot during injury and the direction of the applied force.[99] The complexity of ankle fractures is due to the fact that when the foot is planted on the ground, the body acts as a fulcrum to apply excessive torque on the ankle.[87] Because reduction of the fracture requires reversing the force of injury, understanding the mechanism is imperative.[100] Henderson[101] noted, in 1932, that it is not always possible to determine the force of injury from patient history, and he based his classification (Table 19-6) on

---

**TABLE 19-5** Ankle Fracture Classification

| Force of Injury | Degree | Classification of Injury |
|---|---|---|
| A. External rotation | First | Oblique fracture of distal fibula |
| | Second | Oblique fracture of distal fibula with medial malleolar fracture or deltoid ligament rupture and possible posterior tibial lip fracture |
| | Third | Oblique fracture of distal fibula with supramalleolar fracture of tibia |
| B. Abduction | First | Fracture of medial malleolus |
| | Second | Fracture of medial malleolus with fibular fracture at or below the tibial plafond, with or without diastasis |
| | Third | Fracture of medial malleolus and distal aspect of tibia |
| C. Adduction | First | Transverse fracture of lateral malleolus at or below the tibial plafond |
| | Second | Transverse fracture of lateral malleolus at or below the tibial plafond with fracture of the medial malleolus |
| | Third | Transverse fracture of lateral malleolus at or below the tibial plafond with a supramalleolar fracture of the tibia |
| D. Compression | | Marginal fractures of tibia; comminution of tibial plafond; T- or Y-shaped fractures of tibia into the ankle joint |
| E. Direct violence | | Supramalleolar fractures |

Data from Ashhurst APC, Bromer RS: *Arch Surg* 4:51, 1922.

**TABLE 19-6** Ankle Fracture Classification

| Fracture | Type | Classification of Injury |
|---|---|---|
| A. Fractures of the malleoli | 1. Isolated | A. Fibula fracture<br>B. Medial malleolus fracture |
| | 2. Combined | A. Low bimalleolar fractures<br>B. Bimalleolar fractures with talar displacement |
| B. Fractures of weight-bearing surface of tibia | 1. Isolated | A. Posterior tibial lip fracture<br>B. Anterior tibial tubercle fracture |
| | 2. Combined | A. Anterior tibial tubercle or posterior tibial lip fractures with trimalleolar fractures |

Data from Henderson MS: *Wisc Med J* 31:684, 1932.

**TABLE 19-7** Ankle Fracture Classification

| Force of Injury | Stage | Classification of Injury |
|---|---|---|
| Supination (adduction) | I | Fracture of lateral malleolus or ligament rupture |
| | II | Stage I plus fracture of medial malleolus |
| Pronation (abduction) | I | Fracture of medial malleolus or rupture of deltoid ligament |
| | II | Stage I plus transverse fracture of lateral malleolus below syndesmosis;<br>*Or* Stage I plus syndesmotic rupture;<br>*Or* Stage I plus syndesmotic rutpure and fibular fracture above the syndesmosis |
| Abduction and external rotation | I | Fracture of medial malleolus or rupture of deltoid ligament |
| | II | Stage I plus oblique fracture of fibula below syndesmosis |
| | III | Stage I plus syndesmotic rupture |
| | IV | Stage I plus rupture of the anterior tibiofibular ligament and fibular fracture at the syndesmotic level |
| | V | Stage I plus rupture of the anterior tibiofibular ligament and fibular fracture above the syndesmosis |

Data from Husfeldt E: *Hospitalstid* 81:717, 1938.

considerations of pathological anatomy. Thus Henderson eschewed the need for classification based on mechanical force, and questions remained as to the degree of diastasis and ligament rupture one must suspect in an accompanying ankle fractures.

In his classification, published in 1938, Husfeldt[102] sought to interpret syndesmotic damage (Table 19-7). To date, classifications lacked an all-encompassing presentation of injury force, mechanism, ligamentous rupture, as well as fracture descriptions.

By far the most used and best understood classification of ankle fractures is the one developed by Lauge-Hansen[79,102–106] in a series of five papers from 1948 through 1953. This classification (Table 19-8) is based on a dual designation in which the first word denotes the position of the foot at the moment of injury and the second word indicates the forced movement of the foot producing the injury.[104]

The Lauge-Hansen experiments classified ankle injuries on various forced motions of the foot while it is positioned in supination or pronation.[103] Supination is defined in these studies as a combination of internal rotation, adduction of the rearfoot, and inversion of the forefoot (with plantarflexion), whereas pronation is defined as a combination of external rotation, abduction of the rearfoot, and eversion of the forefoot (with dorsiflexion).[102] The term *eversion* used to describe the force of injury implies an internal rotation of the leg while the foot remains in closed chain stance. Thus lateral or external rotation is the actual force indicated.[6]

Supination-adduction injuries are designated as having two stages. The injury occurs when the foot is in a position of supination and the lower limb is moved medially over the talus.

In Stage I, a transverse fracture of the fibula occurs at the malleolar level, or ruptures of the anterior talofibular ligament, posterior talofibular ligament, and possibly the calcaneofibular ligament may occur when lateral stress is applied. If the force continues, the lateral malleolus or ligaments are released from tension, and the talus, free to swing medially and dorsally, strikes the medial malleolus, causing a vertical fracture (Figure 19-40). This fracture represents Stage 2.

The supination-external rotation injury has four stages beginning with tension on the anterior tibiofibular ligament. This ligament may remain intact,[107] or it may avulse a fragment of bone from the anterior tubercle of Chaput or from the anterior lateral aspect of the fibula, known as a Wagstaffe fracture.[91,92] Slight diastasis may appear between the tibia and fibula. As the force continues to Stage 2, the

**TABLE 19-8**  Ankle Fracture Classification

| Force of Injury | Stage | Classification of Injury |
|---|---|---|
| Supination-adduction | 1 | Transverse fracture of the lateral malleolus at the malleolar level, or ruptures of the calcaneofibular ligament or posterior talofibular ligament |
| | 2 | Vertical fracture of the medial malleolus |
| Supination-external rotation | 1 | Rupture of anterior tibiofibular ligament, with avulsion from anterior tibial tubercle or fibula |
| | 2 | Stage 1 plus a supramalleolar spiral fracture of the fibula |
| | 3 | Stage 2 plus an avulsion from the posterior tibial lip by the posterior tibiofibular ligament |
| | 4 | Stage 3 plus a horizontal fracture of the medial malleolus or rupture of the deltoid ligament |
| Supination-internal rotation | 1 | Rupture of the anterior talofibular ligament |
| | 2 | Rupture of the anterior talofibular ligament with avulsion fragments from the lateral aspect of calcaneus and cuboid |
| Pronation-abduction | 1 | Horizontal fracture of the medial malleolus or rupture of the deltoid ligament |
| | 2 | Stage 1 plus a rupture of anterior tibiofibular ligament with avulsion from anterior tibial tubercle, and a rupture of posterior tibiofibular ligament with avulsion from posterior tibial lip |
| Pronation-external rotation | 1 | Horizontal fracture of the medial malleolus or rupture of the deltoid ligament |
| | 2 | Stage 1 plus a rupture of anterior tibiofibular ligament with avulsion from anterior tibial tubercle |
| | 3 | Stage 2 plus a high spiral fracture 6–8 cm from the distal tip of the lateral malleolus |
| | 4 | Stage 3 plus a rupture of posterior tibiofibular ligament with avulsion from posterior tibial lip |
| Pronation-internal rotation | 1 | Spiral fractures of tibia and fibula |
| Pronation-dorsiflexion | 1 | Vertical fracture of medial malleolus |
| | 2 | Large avulsion from the anterior tibial tubercle |
| | 3 | Supramalleolar fracture of fibula |
| | 4 | Transverse fracture of posterior aspect of tibia |

Data from Lauge[-Hansen] N: *Arch Surg* 56:259, 1948; Lauge-Hansen N: *Arch Surg* 60:957, 1950; Lauge-Hansen N: *AJR* 71:456, 1954; Lauge-Hansen N: *Arch Surg* 64:488, 1952; Lauge-Hansen N: *Arch Surg* 67:813, 1953.

fibula twists about its longitudinal axis, and a fracture fragment from the lateral malleolus dislocates (Figure 19-41) approximately 2 to 4 mm laterally and dorsally. The anterior talofibular ligament and calcaneofibular ligament may remain intact. Increased and continued force brings Stage 3, where the lateral malleolar fragment dislocates further, and the talus subluxates dorsally and laterally. It is possible in this stage to have either a ligament tear or a fracture of the posterior tibial region.[104,107] Even greater deforming force causes increased dislocation of the talus and the fibular malleolus. The foot everts without resistance, and a medial malleolar fracture dislocates laterally and plantarly. The talus subluxates dorsally, and the foot may be at a right angle to the leg. If the medial malleolus fractures, the deltoid ligament remains intact. If the bone does not avulse and the deltoid ligament ruptures, the superficial, weaker layers, the posterior tibiotalar, tibionavicular, and tibiocalcaneal ligaments will tear, rather than the deep layer, the anterior tibiotalar ligament.[99,108]

Lauge-Hansen also described a supination-inversion injury with two stages.[104] In this internal rotation injury, rupture of the anterior talofibular ligament occurs in Stage

1, followed by avulsions from the lateral aspects of the calcaneus and cuboid in Stage 2.

Pronation-abduction injuries, caused by forced abduction of the rearfoot when the foot is in a position of pronation, begin with a medial malleolar fracture in Stage 1. The fracture fragment dislocates anteriorly and slightly laterally.[103] In Stage 2, both the medial malleolus and talus assume a valgus attitude, and tears of the anterior and posterior tibiofibular ligaments occur, with possible avulsions of the anterior and posterior tibial lips,[107] resulting in a diastasis.[109] As the injury proceeds, Stage 3 exhibits a fracture of the fibula 0.5 to 1 cm above the ankle joint, with lateral dislocation of both the lateral and medial malleolar fragments, as well as the talus (Figure 19-42).

A pronation-external rotation injury, indicated by forced external rotation of a pronated foot after the occurrence of Stage 1 in the pronation-abduction injury, causes the medial malleolar fracture fragment to dislocate anteriorly.[103] The fibula rotates externally to widen the syndesmotic space. Rupture of the anterior tibiofibular ligament with avulsion of the anterior tibial tubercle in Stage 2 initiates the syndesmotic tear and increases the widening of its space.

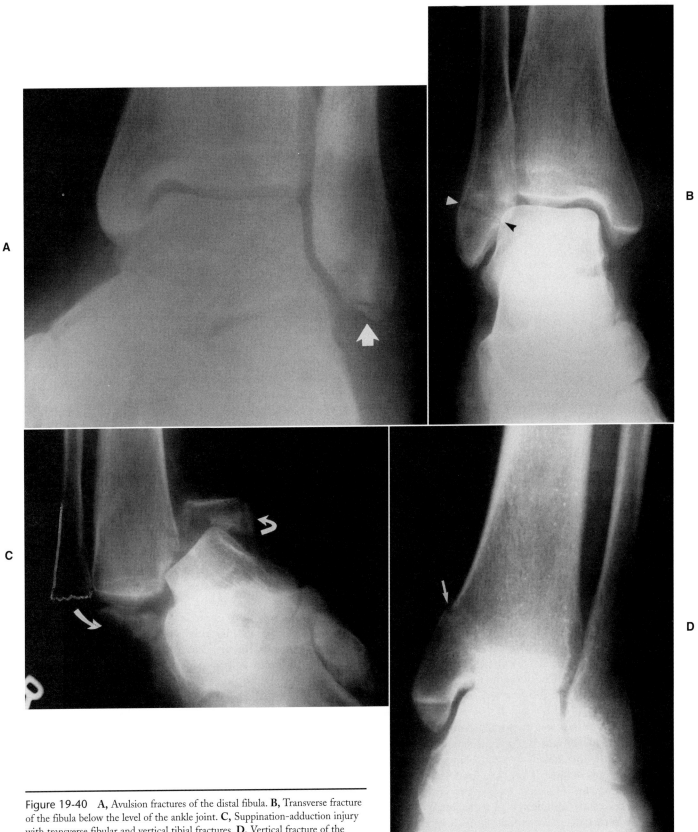

Figure 19-40   **A,** Avulsion fractures of the distal fibula. **B,** Transverse fracture of the fibula below the level of the ankle joint. **C,** Suppination-adduction injury with transverse fibular and vertical tibial fractures. **D,** Vertical fracture of the medial malleolus.

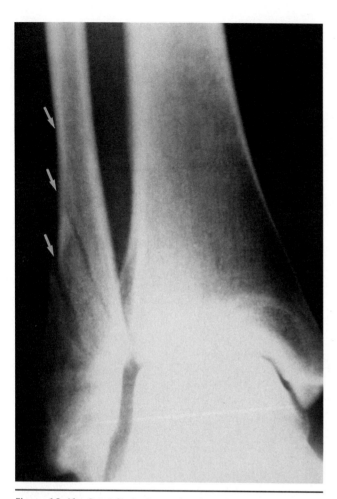

**Figure 19-41**   Spiral fibular fracture just above the joint level.

Stage 3 of pronation-external rotation causes a high spiral fracture of the fibula 6 to 8 cm from the distal tip of the lateral malleolus (Figure 19-43). This fracture occurs above the level of the syndesmotic ligaments and is secondary to extreme forces of torque. Finally, Stage 4 entails a dorsal subluxation of the talus, along with both malleolar fracture fragments. The lateral malleolus finally locates behind the tibia, and the medial malleolus rotates laterally. Rupture of the posterior tibiofibular ligament and possible avulsion fracture from the posterior tibial lip (Figure 19-44) results.[107]

A pronation-inversion (internal rotation) injury was described by Lauge-Hansen[104] as causing spiral fractures of both the tibia and fibula. Pronation-dorsiflexion causes injury in four stages. They are initiated by forced dorsiflexion of the pronated foot, often caused by axial loading during falls from heights or motor vehicle accidents. Stage 1 begins, as do all pronation injuries, with a fracture of

the medial malleolus, often a vertical fracture.[106] Stage 2 involves a large avulsion from the anterior tibial tubercle. As the injury progresses, a fracture of the fibula above the malleolar level occurs (Stage 3), and in Stage 4 a transverse fracture of the tibial plafond, also known as a pilon fracture, results.[98] These fractures may be comminuted, with spiral or oblique fractures extending into the tibial shaft (Figure 19-45).[110,111]

A classification of ankle fractures according to the level of fibular fracture, known as the Danis-Weber[112-115] classification (Box 19-17), is of great advantage to radiologists for its ease in quick visual classification on radiograph.[116,117] This classification involves three types. The first, Type A, (see Figure 19-40, *B*) is a fracture below the level of the ankle joint, usually transverse. In Type B, the fibular fracture is seen from the joint level into the syndesmosis (see Figures 19-41 and 19-42). Type C is a high fibular fracture, always associated with diastasis (see Figure 19-43). Further differentiation is described into Type C-1, which occurs at the syndesmotic level, and Type C-2, a higher fracture with greater disruption of the syndesmosis.[118]

To better understand and remember ankle fracture classifications, some authors have devised simplified systems, flowcharts, or algorithms. In 1980 Arimoto and Forrester[100] presented the Lauge-Hansen classification in an algorithm specifically to facilitate rapid radiographic identification (Table 19-9) of the mechanisms of injury and the accompanying stage. Weiss Docks, and Freedland[119] in 1983 presented a paper that described the Lauge-Hansen system in a clockwork fashion to explain the sequential sequence of injuries.

These systems were developed in part to allow for easier memorization and comprehension of ankle fracture classifications. A system of study for the Danis-Weber and the four major Lauge-Hansen categories by applying the concept of clockwork to a cross section of the right ankle has been devised (Table 19-10, Figure 19-46), as follows.

In supination-adduction Stage 1, the injury begins on the lateral (L) side and proceeds in a clockwise fashion to the Stage 2 medial (M) injury.

In supination-external rotation Stage 1, the injury begins at the anterior (A) aspect and proceeds in a clockwise fashion to the lateral (L) aspect, then to the posterior (P) ankle, and finally on to the medial (M) aspect.

Pronation-abduction Stage 1 injury begins at the medial (M) aspect and proceeds to the anterior aspect of the ankle where an anterior to posterior (A-P) syndesmotic rupture occurs. Finally, a lateral (L) injury is seen in Stage 3.

The pronation-external rotation Stage 1 injury also begins at the medial (M) aspect and proceeds to the anterior (A) aspect of the ankle, then to the lateral (L) side, and finally to the posterior (P) portion of the ankle.

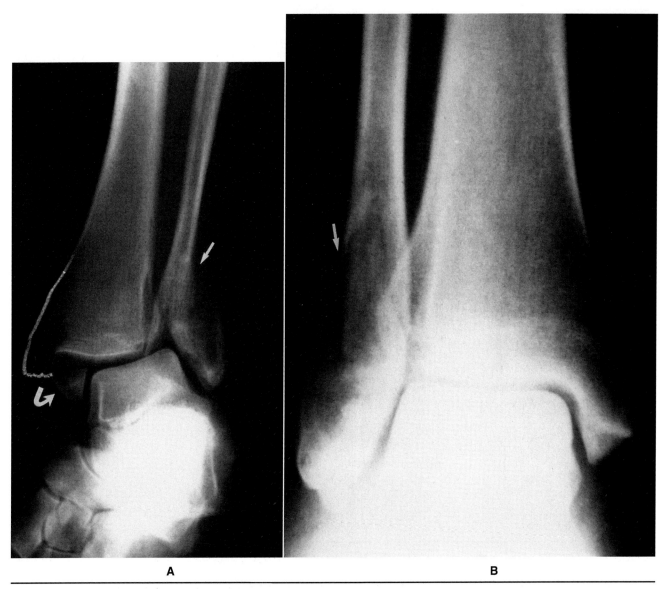

**A**                    **B**

Figure 19-42  **A,** Pronation-abduction injury exhibiting a transverse medial malleolar fracture and an oblique fibular fracture just above the level of the ankle joint. **B,** Oblique fibular fracture above the ankle joint.

The L-A-M-M designation reflects the first stages of each Lauge-Hansen injury. The T-S-O-H designation ("host" spelled backward) reflects the type of fibular fracture seen, and the V-T-T-T designation indicates the type of medial malleolar fracture encountered in Lauge-Hansen injuries.

Supination-adduction injuries classically produce a transverse (T) avulsion type of fracture from the distal portion of the fibula and a vertical (V) medial malleolar fracture. Supination-external rotation, pronation-abduction, and pronation-external rotation injuries usually cause a transverse (T) fracture of the medial malleolus.

Supination-external rotation injuries generally produce a spiral (S) type of fracture. Pronation-abduction results in oblique (O) fibular fractures just above the ankle joint level, and pronation-external rotation causes high (H) spiral fibular fractures because of the greater amount of torque involved.

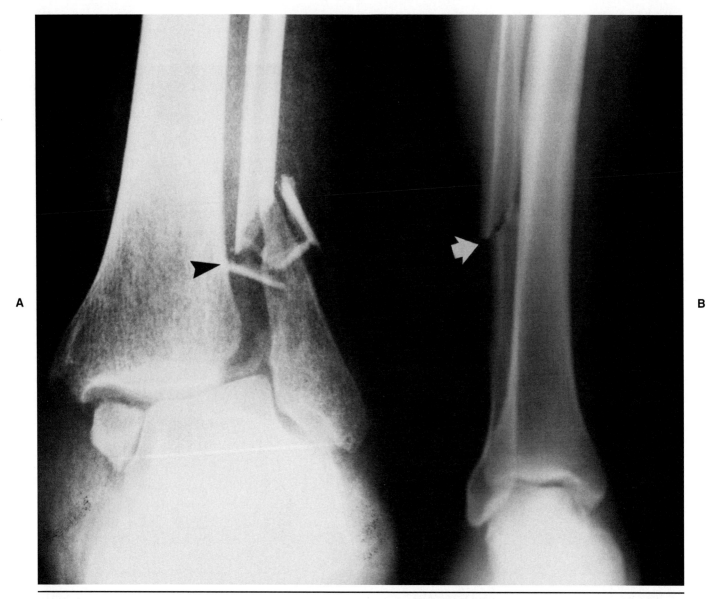

Figure 19-43    **A,** Mortise view demonstrates severe comminution and displacement/angulation of fibular fracture segments *(arrowheads)*. The talus is displaced laterally; the divulsed tibial malleolus fragment moved with the talus. **B,** AP view, different patient, Fibular fracture sight is diaphyseal *(arrow)*.

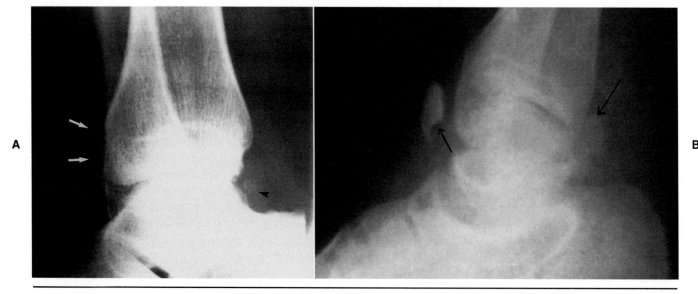

Figure 19-44    **A,** Lateral ankle view demonstrates posterior *(arrows)* and anterior *(arrowhead)* fracture features. **B,** Lateral view of different patient demonstrates large anterior and posterior fragments *(arrows)*.

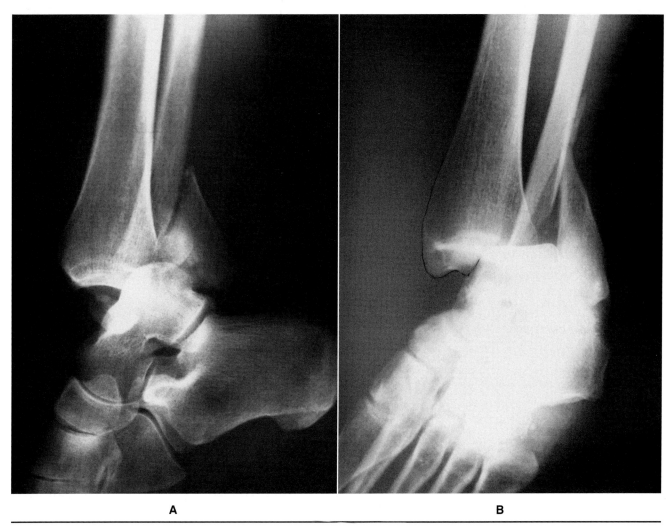

**A**                                                                                          **B**

Figure 19-45   Lateral **(A)** and AP **(B)** views demonstrate ankle dislocation and severe fracture displacement and angulation.

| BOX 19-17 | Ankle Fracture Classification |
|---|---|
| **Type** | **Classification of Injury** |
| A | Transverse fibular fracture below the level of the ankle joint |
| B | Oblique fibular fracture at the level of the ankle joint into the syndesmosis |
| C-1 | Spiral fibular fracture at or above the level of the syndesmosis |
| C-2 | High spiral fibular fracture above the level of the syndesmosis, always with diastasis |

Data from Danis R: *Theorie et pratique de l'osteosynthese,* Paris, 1949, Desoer et Masson; Weber BG: *Int Orthop* 4:789, 1981; Weber BG: *Aktuelle probleme in der chirurgie,* ed 2, Stuttgart, 1972, Haus Huber; Weber BG, Simpson LA: *Clin Orthop* 199: 61, 1985, Muller ME, Allgower M, Schneider R, Willenegger H: *Manual of internal fixation,* New York, 1979, Springer.

**TABLE 19-9** Ankle Fracture Classification

| Lauge-Hansen Type | Stage | Malleolar Fracture | Medial Malleolar Fracture | Fibular Fracture |
|---|---|---|---|---|
| Pronation-lateral rotation | IV | Posterior malleolar fracture | | High |
| Pronation-lateral rotation | III | No posterior malleolar fracture | | High |
| Supination-lateral rotation | IV | Medial malleolar fracture or deltoid tear | Spiral | Low |
| Supination-lateral rotation | III | Posterior malleolar fracture | Spiral | Low |
| Supination-lateral rotation | II | No posterior malleolar fracture | Spiral | Low |
| Pronation-abduction | III | | Oblique | Low |
| Supination-adduction | II | Medial malleolar fracture | Transverse | Low |
| Supination-adduction | I | No medial malleolar fracture | Transverse | Low |
| Pronation-lateral rotation | II | Diastasis | Oblique | Absent |
| Pronation-lateral rotation | I | No diastasis | Oblique | Absent |
| Supination-adduction | II | | Vertical | Absent |
| Pronation-abduction | II | Posterior malleolar fracture | Transverse | Absent |
| Pronation-abduction | I | No posterior malleolar fracture | Transverse | Absent |

Arimoto HK, Forrester DM: *AJR* 135: 1057, 1980.

**TABLE 19-10** Ankle Fracture Algorithm

| Classifications | | | | | |
|---|---|---|---|---|---|
| Danis-Weber | Lauge-Hansen | Number of Stages | Clockwise Rotation Begins | Fibular Fractures | Tibial Fractures |
| A | SAD | 2 | L | T | V |
| B | SEX | 4 | A | S | T |
| B | PAB | 3 | M | O | T |
| C | PEX | 4 | M | H | T |

Legend:

| *Lauge-Hansen* | *Clockwise Rotation Begins* |
|---|---|
| SAD = suppination-adduction | L  = lateral |
| SEX = suppination-external rotation | A  = anterior |
| PAB = pronation-abduction | M = medial |
| PEX = pronation-external rotation | M = medial |

| *Fibular Fractures* | *Tibial Fractures* |
|---|---|
| T  = transverse | V = vertical |
| S  = spiral | T = transverse |
| O = oblique | t = transverse |
| H = high spiral | T = transverse |

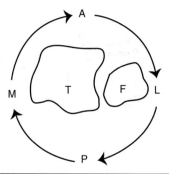

Figure 19-46  Ankle classification algorithm using a right ankle cross section. *A*, anterior; *L*, lateral; *P*, posterior; *M*, medial; *T*, tibia; *F*, fibula.

## References

1. Haeger K: *The illustrated history of surgery*, New York, 1988, Bell Publishing.
2. Gustilo RB: Management of open fractures, *Minn Med* 54:185, 1971.
3. Anderson LD: Injuries of the forefoot, *Clin Orthop* 122:185, 1977.
4. Marcinko DE, Elleby DH: Digital fractures and dislocations. In Scurran BL, editor: *Foot and ankle trauma*, p 309, New York, 1989, Churchill-Livingstone.
5. Depalma AF: *The management of fractures and dislocations*, ed 2, Philadelphia, 1970, Saunders.
6. Berquist TH, Johnson KA: Trauma. In Berquist TH, editor: *Radiology of the foot and ankle*, New York, 1989, Raven Press.
7. Kirchwhem WW, Figura MA, Binning TA, Leis SB: Fractures of internal metatarsals. In Scurran BL, editor: *Foot and ankle trauma*, p 345, New York, 1989, Churchill-Livingstone.
8. Smith TF: Pedal dislocations. *Clin Podiatr* 2(2):358, 1985.
9. Salamon PB, Gelberman RH, Huffer JM: Dorsal dislocation of the metatarsophalangeal joint of the great toe, *J Bone Joint Surg* 56A:1073, 1974.
10. Konkel KF, Muehlstein JH: Unusual fracture-dislocation of the great toe: case report, *J Trauma* 15:733, 1975.
11. Giannikas AC, Papachristou G, Papavasiliou N et al: Dorsal dislocation of the first metatarsophalangeal joint, *J Bone Joint Surg* 57B:384, 1975.
12. Jahss MH: Traumatic dislocations of the first metatarsophalangeal joint, *Foot & Ankle* 1:15, 1980.
13. Lewis AG, DeLee JC: Type I complex dislocation of the 1st metatarsophalangeal joint: open reduction through a dorsal approach, *J Bone Joint Surg* 66A:1120, 1984.
14. Daniel WL, Beck EL, Duggar GE, Bennett AJ: Traumatic dislocation of the first metatarsophalangeal joint: a case report, *Journal of the American Podiatry Association* 66:97, 1976.
15. Torg JS, Baldini FC, Zelko RR et al: Fractures of the base of the first metatarsal distal to the tuberosity, *J Bone Joint Surg* 66A:209, 1984.
16. Jones R: Fracture of the base of the fifth metatarsal bone by indirect violence, *Ann Surg* 35:6697, 1902.
17. Kavanaugh JH, Borower TD, Mann RV: The Jones' fracture revisited, *J Bone Joint Surg* 60A:776, 1978.
18. Bohler L: *The treatment of fractures*, ed 5, New York, 1958, Grune & Stratton.
19. Stewart IM: Jones fracture: fracture of the base of the fifth metatarsal, *Clin Orthop* 16:190, 1960.
20. Warwick R, Williams PL: *Gray's anatomy*, ed 35, Philadelphia, 1973, Saunders.
21. Stewart IM: Fracture of neck of femur: survival and contralateral fracture, *BMJ* 2:922, 1957.
22. Maxwell JR: Metatarsal fractures. In McGlamry ED, editor: *Comprehensive textbook of foot surgery*, vol 2, Baltimore, 1987, Williams & Wilkins.
23. Jeffreys TE: Lisfranc's fracture-dislocation, *J Bone Joint Surg* 45B:546, 1963.
24. Aitken AP, Poulson D: Dislocations of the tarso-metatarsal joint, *J Bone Joint Surg* 45A:246, 1963.
25. Gissane W: A dangerous type of fracture of the foot, *J Bone Joint Surg* 33B:535, 1951.
26. Cassebaum WH: Lisfranc's fracture dislocations, *Clin Orthop* 30:116, 1963.
27. Foster SC, Foster RR: Lisfranc's tarsometatarsal fracture dislocation, *Radiology* 120:79, 1976.
28. Goiney RC, Connell DG, Nichols DM: CT evaluation of tarsometatarsal fracture-dislocation injuries, *AJR* 144:985, 1985.
29. Wiley JJ: The mechanism of tarso-metatarsal joint injuries, *J Bone Joint Surg* 53B:474, 1971.
30. Hardcastle PH, Reschauer R, Kustcha-Lissberg E, Schoffmann W: Injuries to the tarsometatarsal joint: incidence, classification and treatment, *J Bone Joint Surg* 64B:349, 1982.
31. Perlman MD, Leveille D, Gale B: Traumatic classifications of the foot and ankle, *JFS* 28:551, 1989.
32. Quenu E, Kuss G: Etude sur les luxations du metatarse, *Revista de Chirurgie* 39:1, 1909.
33. Hermel MB, Gershon-Cohen J: The nutcracker fracture of the cuboid by indirect violence, *Radiology* 60:850, 1953.
34. Wilson DW: Injuries of the tarso-metatarsal joints, *J Bone Joint Surg* 54B:677, 1972.
35. Hesp WLEM, van der Werken C, Goris RJA: Lisfranc dislocations: fractures and/or dislocations through the tarso-metatarsal joints, *Injury* 15:261, 1984.
36. Main BJ, Jowett RL: Injuries of the midtarsal joint, *J Bone Joint Surg* 57B:89, 1975.
37. Rymasgewski LA, Robb JE: Mechanism of fracture-dislocation of the navicular: brief report, *J Bone Joint Surg* 70B:492, 1988.
38. Watson-Jones R: *Fractures and joint injuries*, ed 6, vol 2, New York, 1982, Churchill-Livingstone.
39. Eichenholtz SN, Levine DB: Fractures of the tarsal navicular bone, *Clin Orthop* 34:142, 1964.
40. Watson-Jones R: *Fractures and joint injuries*, ed 3, vol 2, New York, 1946, Churchill-Livingstone.
41. Anderson JE: *Grant's atlas of anatomy*, Baltimore, 1983, Williams & Wilkins.
42. Morton DJ: *The human foot*, New York, 1964, Hafner.
43. Berndt AL, Harty M: Transchondral fractures (osteochondritis dissecans) of the talus, *J Bone Joint Surg* 41A:988, 1959.

44. Kappis M: Weitere Beitrage zur traumatisch-mechanischen Entstehung der "spontanen" Knorpelablosungen (sogen. osteochondritis dissecans), *Deutsche Zeitschrift für Chirurgie* 171:13, 1922.

45. Rendu A: Fracture intra-articulaire parecellaire de la poulie astraglienne, *Lyon Med* 150:220, 1932.

46. Canale ST, Belding RH: Osteochondral lesions of the talus, *J Bone Joint Surg* 62A:97, 1980.

47. Naumetz VA, Schweigel, JF: Osteocartilaginous lesions of the talar dome, *J Trauma* 20:924, 1980.

48. Smith GR, Winquist RA, Allan NK, Northrop CH: Subtle transchondral fractures of the talar dome: a radiological perspective, *Radiology* 124:667, 1977.

49. Pritsch M, Horoshovski H, Farine I, Tel-hanomer IO: Arthroscopic treatment of osteochondral lesions of the talus, *J Bone Joint Surg* 68A:862, 1986.

50. Pennal GF: Fractures of the talus, *Clin Orthop* 30:53, 1963.

51. Kenwright J, Taylor RG: Major injuries of the talus, *J Bone Joint Surg* 52B:36, 1970.

52. Coltart WD: "Aviator's astragalus," *J Bone Joint Surg* 34B:545, 1952.

53. Hawkins LG: Fractures of the neck of the talus, *J Bone Joint Surg* 52A:991, 1970.

54. Canale ST, Kelly FB: Fractures of the neck of the talus, *J Bone Joint Surg* 60A:143, 1978.

55. Mulfinger GL, Trueta J: The blood supply of the talus, *J Bone Joint Surg* 52B:160, 1970.

56. Blair HC: Comminuted fractures and fracture dislocations of the body of the talus, *Am J Surg* 59:37, 1943.

57. Shepherd FJ: A hitherto undescribed fracture of the astralagus, *Journal of Anatomy and Physiology,* 17:79, 1882.

58. Cavaliere RG: Talar fractures, In McGlamry ED, editor: *Comprehensive textbook of foot surgery,* vol 2, p 904, Baltimore, 1987, Williams & Wilkins.

59. Cave EF: Fracture of the os calcis: the problem in general, *Clin Orthop* 30:64, 1963.

60. Lindsay WRN, Dewar FP: Fractures of the os calcis, *Am J Surg* 95:555, 1958.

61. Schmidt TL, Weiner DS: Calcaneal fractures in children: an evaluation of the nature of injury in 56 children, *Clin Orthop* 171:150, 1982.

62. Palmer I: The mechanism and treatment of fractures of the calcaneus, *J Bone Joint Surg* 30A:2, 1948.

63. Slatis P, Kroduoto O, Santavista S, Laasonen EM: Fractures of the calcaneus, *J Trauma* 19:939, 1979.

64. Lance EM, Corey EJ, Wade PA: Fractures of the os calcis, *J Trauma* 4:15, 1964.

65. Bohler L: Diagnosis, pathology, and treatment of fractures of the os calcis, *J Bone Joint Surg* 13:75, 1931.

66. Rowe CR, Sakellarides HT, Freeman PA, Sorbie C: Fractures of the os calcis, *JAMA* 184:920, 1963.

67. Essex-LoPresti P: The mechanism, reduction technique, and results in fractures of the os calcis, *Br J Surg* 39:395, 1952.

68. Carothers CO, Crenshaw AH: Clinical significance of a classification of epiphyseal injuries at the ankle, *Am J Surg* 89:879, 1955.

69. Salter RB, Harris WR: Injuries involving the epiphyseal plate, *J Bone Joint Surg* 45A:587, 1963.

70. Aitken AP: Fractures of the epiphyses, *Clin Orthop* 41:19, 1965.

71. Poland J: *Traumatic separation of the epiphyses,* London, 1898, Smith, Elder.

72. Spiegel PG, Cooperman DR, Laros GS: Epiphyseal fractures of the distal ends of the tibia and fibula, *J Bone Joint Surg* 60A:1046, 1978.

73. Bishop PA: Fractures and epiphyseal separation fractures of the ankle, *AJR* 28:491, 1932.

74. Holland CT: Radiographical note on injuries to the distal epiphyses of radius and ulna, *Proceedings of the Royal Society of Medicine* 22:695, 1929.

75. Werenskiold B: A contribution to the roentgen diagnosis of epiphyseal separations, *Acta Radiol* 8:4199, 1927.

76. Weber BG, Sussenbach F: Malleolar fractures. In Weber BG, Brunner C, Freuler F, editors: *Treatment of fractures in children and adolescents,* p 350, New York, 1980, Springer.

77. Crenshaw AH: Injuries of the distal tibial epiphysis, *Clin Orthop* 41:98, 1965.

78. Dias LA, Tachdjian MO: Physeal injuries of the ankle in children, *Clin Orthop* 136:230, 1978.

79. Lauge-Hansen N: Fractures of the ankle: analytic historic survey as the basis of new experimental roentgenologic and clinical investigations, *Arch Surg* 56:259, 1948.

80. Dias LS: Fractures of the tibia and fibula. In Rockwood CA, Wilkins KE, King RE, editors, *Fractures in children,* vol 3, p 983, Philadelphia, 1984, Lippincott.

81. Ogden JA: *Skeletal injury in the child,* Philadelphia, 1982, Lea & Febiger.

82. MacNealy GA, Rogers LF, Hernandez R, Poznanski AK: Injuries of the distal tibial epiphysis: systematic radiographic evaluation, *AJR* 138:683, 1982.

83. Pott P: *Some few general remarks on fractures and dislocations,* London, 1768, Haives, Clark and Collins. Reprinted by *Medical Classics* 1:329, 1936.

84. Dupuytren G: Of fractures of the lower extremity of the fistula and luxations of the foot, *Medical Classics* 4:151, 1939 [reprint].

85. Von Volkmann R, *Beitrage zur chirurgie,* Leipzig, 1875, Breitkopf und Hartel.

86. Cotton FJ: A new type of ankle fracture, *JAMA* 64:318, 1915.

87. Heppenstall RB: Injuries of the ankle. In Heppenstall RB, editor: *Fracture treatment and healing,* p 803, Philadelphia, 1980, Saunders.

88. Maisonneuve JC: Recherches sur la fracture du perone, *Arch Gen Med* 7:165, 1840.

89. Pankovich AM: Maisonnueve fracture of the fibula, *J Bone Joint Surg* 58A:337, 1976.

90. Tillaux P: Recherche cliniques et experimentales sur les fractures malleolaires, rapport par Gosselin, *Bull Acad Med* (Paris) 21:817, 1872.

91. Chaput V: *Les fractures malleolaires due cou-de-pieds et les accidents du travail,* Paris, 1907, Masson et Cie.

92. Wagstaffe WW: An unusual form of fracture of the fibula, *St. Thomas Hosp Rep* 6:43, 1873.

93. Ruch HA, Downey MS, Malay DS: Ankle fractures. In McGlamry ED, editor: *Comprehensive textbook of foot surgery,* vol 2, p 936, Baltimore, 1987, Williams & Wilkins.

94. LeFort L: Note sur une variete indecrite de la fracture verticale de la malleole externe par arrachement. Cited in Lauge-Hansen N: Fractures of the ankle, *Arch Surg* 56:259, 1948.

95. Bauer M, Johnell O, Reldlund-Johnell I, Johnsson K: Ankle fractures, *Foot & Ankle* 8:231, 1987.

96. Woersdorfer O, Weber BG: Diaphyseal fractures of both bones of the lower leg with associated injury of the ankle mortise, *Arch Orthop Trauma Surg* 98:293, 1981.

97. Weber BG: Lengthening osteotomy of the fibula to correct a widened mortice of the ankle after fracture, *Int Orthop* 4:2891, 1981.

98. Ashurst APC, Bromer RS: Classification and mechanism of fractures of the leg bones involving the ankle, *Arch Surg* 4:51, 1922.

99. Kleiger B: Mechanisms of ankle injury, *Orthop Clin North Am* 5:127, 1974.

100. Arimoto HK, Forrester DM: Classification of ankle fractures: an algorithm, *AJR* 135:1057, 1980.

101. Henderson MS: Fractures of the ankle, *WMJ* 31:684, 1932.

102. Husfeldt E: Treatment of malleolar fractures, *Hospitalstid* 81:717, 1938.

103. Lauge-Hansen N: Fractures of the ankle. II. Combined experimental-surgical and experimental-roentgenologic investigations, *Arch Surg* 60:957, 1950.

104. Lauge-Hansen N: Fractures of the ankle. III. Genetic roentgenologic diagnosis of fractures of the ankle, *AJR* 71:456, 1954.

105. Lauge-Hansen N: Fractures of the ankle. IV. Clinical use of genetic roentgen diagnosis and genetic reduction, *Arch Surg* 64:488, 1952.

106. Lauge-Hansen N: Fractures of the ankle. V. Pronation-dorsiflexion fracture, *Arch Surg* 67:813, 1953.

107. Yde J: The Lauge-Hansen classification of malleolar fractures, *Acta Orthop Scand* 51:181, 1980.

108. Ala-Ketola L, Peranan J, Kovivisto E, Pupera M: Arthrography in the diagnosis of ligament injuries and classification of ankle injuries, *Radiology* 125:63, 1977.

109. Edwards GS, DeLee JC: Ankle diastasis without fracture, *Foot & Ankle* 4:305, 1984.

110. Ovadia DN, Beals RK: Fractures of the tibial plafond, *J Bone Joint Surg* 68A:543, 1986.

111. Coonrad RW: Fracture-dislocations of the ankle joint with impaction injury of the lateral weight-bearing surface of the tibia, *J Bone Joint Surg* 52A:1337, 1970.

112. Danis R: *Theorie et pratique de l'osteosynthese,* Paris, 1949, Desoer et Masson.

113. Weber BG: Die verletzungen des oberen sprunggelenkes. In *Aktuelle probleme in der chirurgie,* ed 2, Bern, Stuttgart, Vienna, 1972, Hans Huber.

114. Weber BG, Simpson LA: Corrective lengthening osteotomy of the fibula, *Clin Orthop* 199:61, 1985.

115. Muller ME, Allgower M, Schneider R, Willenegger H: *Manual of internal fixation,* New York, 1979, Springer.

116. Yablon IG, Heller FG, Shouse L: The key role of the lateral malleolus in displaced fractures of the ankle, *J Bone Joint Surg* 59A:1691, 1977.

117. Blanchard KS, Finlay DBL, Scott DJA et al: A radiological analysis of lateral ligament injuries of the ankle, *Clin Radiol* 37:247, 1986.

118. Gudas CJ: Current concepts in the management of ankle repair. In Marcus SA, editor: *American College of Foot Surgeons: Complications in foot surgery,* ed 2, p 357, Baltimore, 1984, Williams & Wilkins.

119. Weiss L, Docks G, Freedland JA: Lauge Hansen classification: a clockwork injury, *J Foot Surg* 22:192, 1983.

## Suggested Readings

Cotton FJ: Ankle fractures: a new classification and a new class, *N Engl J Med* 201:753, 1929.

Kelikian H, Kelikian AS: *Disorders of the ankle,* Philadelphia, 1985, Saunders.

Perlman M, Leveille D, DeLeonibus J, Hartman R, Klein J et al: Inversion lateral ankle trauma: differential diagnosis, review of the literature, and prospective study, *J Foot Surg* 26:95, 1987.

Perlman MD, Leveille D, Gale B: Traumatic classifications of the foot and ankle, *J Foot Surg* 28:551, 1989.

Von Laer L: Classification, diagnosis, and treatment of transitional fractures of the distal part of the tibia, *J Bone Joint Surg* 67A:687, 1985.

# CHAPTER 20

# Osteonecrosis and Osteochondrosis

RANDY E. COHEN • ROBERT A. CHRISTMAN

Osteonecrosis and osteochondrosis are two radiographically similar disorders associated with multiple etiologies. Overlap between these disorders often confuses the novice. Osteonecrosis, also referred to as ischemic necrosis of bone, can affect either epiphyseal or nonepiphyseal bone and demonstrates distinct pathologic features. Trauma is probably the most common etiology of osteonecrosis in the foot. Osteochondrosis, however, represents a group of disorders with similar radiographic features affecting epiphyses and apophyses only; they have been characterized by three "pathologies": osteonecrosis, trauma without underlying osteonecrosis, and variant ossification.[1]

## OSTEONECROSIS

Osteonecrosis, or bone death, is caused by bone ischemia. Several terms have been used as synonyms for *osteonecrosis*, including *ischemic necrosis, avascular necrosis, aseptic necrosis*, and *bone infarct*. Ischemic necrosis is the death of tissue from lack of blood.[2] This is caused either by interruption of the arterial supply or by occlusion of the venous drainage, resulting in stasis and oxygen deprivation.[3] Osteonecrosis is "the death of bone in mass, as distinguished from molecular death, or relatively small foci of necrosis in bone."[2] Bone death is followed by attempts at repair, which include revascularization, reossification, and the resorption of dead bone. All osteonecroses undergo this sequence of events.[4]

Dead bone has no vascular supply, so its density does not change radiographically. It is the healing process that causes the subsequent radiographic changes.[5] Initially, before the healing process has begun, the necrotic bone appears the same density as the viable surrounding bone. No appreciable changes have yet occurred radiographically. If hyperemia is present, the viable bone becomes osteopenic. The necrotic bone does not change density. However, the necrotic fragment appears more radiodense than the osteopenic bone surrounding it.

Healing varies radiographically depending on the anatomic site and vascular status of the area. In general, as revascularization and resorption occur around the area of necrosis, a radiolucent rim appears. Fibroblastic ingrowth within the necrotic bone may appear as irregular radiolucencies. This may give the radiographic appearance of fragmentation. New bone being laid down on necrotic trabeculae gives an absolute increased bone density and appears denser than normal bone. If the dead trabeculae are reabsorbed, the bone regains its normal density.[3-6]

Ischemic necrosis of bone occurs most commonly within the epiphyseal and the metaphyseal/diaphyseal marrow cavities of adult long tubular bones. The femoral and humeral heads are common epiphyseal sites, but the lesser-metatarsal heads are also affected.[7] Osteonecrosis also involves irregular bones such as the talus and calcaneus. They each vary in etiology, size of area affected, and age predilection.

Radiographically, diametaphyseal osteonecrosis (also referred to as bone infarct) differs significantly from epiphyseal osteonecrosis. Diametaphyseal infarcts show nothing radiographically for weeks or months. As necrotic bone is reabsorbed, an area of serpiginous calcification and ossification surrounds a lucent region (Figures 20-1 and 20-2). The entire area often calcifies[4] (Figure 20-3). Epiphyseal infarcts, in contrast, affect the weight-bearing capacity of the joint, with concomitant changes of the articulating cartilage and underlying subchondral bone. The radiographic appearance of epiphyseal osteonecrosis varies depending on its stage of repair. Initially radiographs are normal. Early findings include osteopenia mixed with sclerosis (Figure 20-4). A radiolucent fracture line that parallels the subchondral bone plate, referred to as the crescent line (Figure 20-5), occasionally follows. The weakened subchondral bone collapses, with subsequent deformity of the epiphysis (Figure 20-6).

452

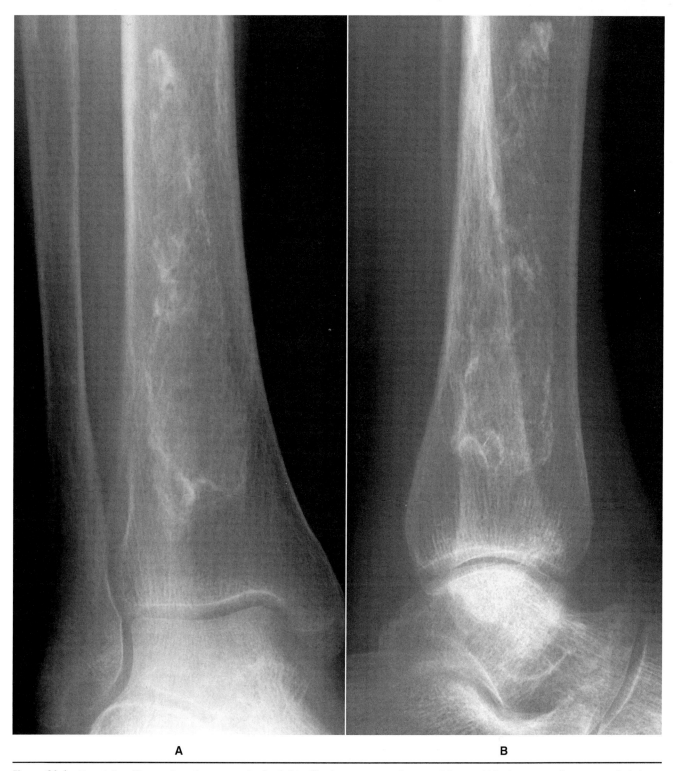

**A**                                                    **B**

Figure 20-1    Bone infarct/diametaphyseal osteonecrosis, distal tibia. Classic appearance, a large, serpiginous calcification surrounding an area of relative lucency. **A**, Mortise view. **B**, Lateral view.

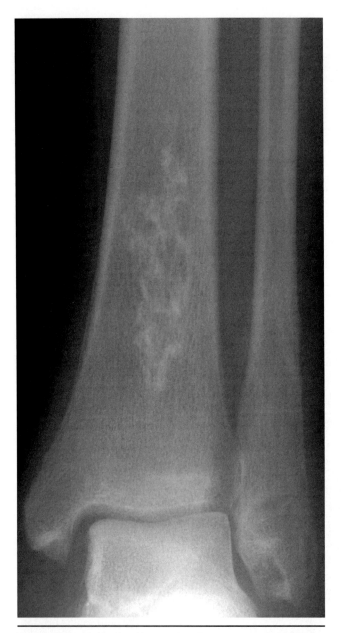

**Figure 20-2** Bone infarct/diametaphyseal osteonecrosis, distal tibia. Stippled calcification, somewhat serpiginous in outline.

Osteoarthritis develops secondarily (Figure 20-7). Osteonecrosis of irregular bone may be radiographically similar to the appearance of a bone infarct in diametaphyseal bone (Figures 20-8 and 20-9). However, post-traumatic osteonecrosis in certain bones, such as the talus and navicular, eventually demonstrate osteopenia following normal radiographs. In the traumatized talus, with patent vascularity, a linear radiolucency parallels the articular surface of the talar dome, referred to as Hawkins' sign (Figure 20-10). Healed post-traumatic osteonecrosis appears as a region of sclerosis (Figure 20-11).

Causes of osteonecrosis include trauma, alcoholism, steroid therapy, pancreatitis, Cushing disease, gout, systemic lupus erythematosus, caisson disease, Gaucher's disease, Fabry's disease, hemoglobinopathy, hyperlipidemia, and irradiation.[7,8]

Dysbaric osteonecrosis (caisson disease), which occurs in people who work with compressed air (high-pressure environments), was first described by Bornstein and Plate.[9] Bone infarction occurs during decompression, when at the lower atmospheric pressure nitrogen leaves solution and forms bubbles in its gaseous state. These nitrogen bubbles can occlude vessels and are thought to cause the characteristic bilateral osseous lesions.[3] Histopathologic changes suggest that a disturbance of blood supply caused by platelet aggregation, red cell sludging, and thrombosis associated with intravascular air bubble formation is related to the occurrences of osteonecrosis in divers.[10] Radiographic studies show large bilateral and symmetrical serpentine lesions. The lesion is initially radiolucent with a calcific or ossific rim and usually calcifies over time.[4] Juxta-articular lesions may progress to fragmentation and structural failure of the subchondral plate, resulting in symptomatology and osteoarthritis.[11]

The use of steroids and alcohol have been implicated in causing osteonecrosis. Most theories on the etiology involve alterations of lipid metabolism with either fat emboli causing vascular occlusion, or sludging and hemorrhage, or a systemic buildup of lipid in the marrow, compromising vascular space. The elevated cholesterol content in the necrotic tissues may contribute to cell death by altering membrane metabolism.[12] The radiographic findings are similar to those described for diametaphyseal osteonecrosis.

Gaucher's disease is a metabolic disorder in which cerebrosides are deposited in the cells of the reticuloendothelial system. The skeletal changes are caused by the infiltration of the marrow with cerebrosides, occluding the vessels and producing an osteonecrosis.[13] Radiographically, early changes consist of osteonecrosis of the femoral head, or osteoporosis of the distal femur progressively expanding the cortex distally to a contour resembling an Erlenmeyer flask.[13,14]

The hemoglobinopathies are subdivided into two groups. The first group, sickle cell anemia, results from an inherited structural alteration in one of the globin chains. The second group, the thalassemias, results from inherited defects in the rate of synthesis of one or more of the globin chains.[15]

In sickle cell disease the fundamental abnormality resides in the abnormal structure of the globin portion of the hemoglobin molecule. Sickle cell hemoglobin (hbA) is much less soluble than normal adult hemoglobin (hbS) in the deoxygenated state. In erythrocytes the insoluble hemoglobin molecules aggregate, which distorts the shape of the red cells, producing the characteristic sickle cell deformity.[16]

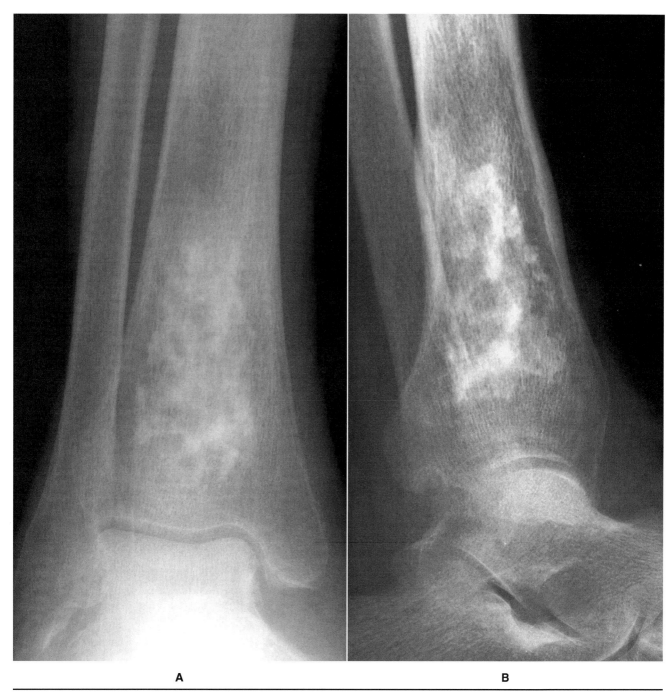

**A**                                                                                     **B**

Figure 20-3    Bone infarct/diametaphyseal osteonecrosis, distal tibia. Nearly solid calcification. **A,** AP view. **B,** Lateral view.

Sickle cell disease and the other hemoglobinopathies can cause either epiphyseal or metaphyseal and diaphyseal infarcts.[16] Sludging of sickled erythrocytes within the sinusoidal vascular bed results in occlusion.[4] The painful vaso-occlusive crisis is probably caused by infarction of bone marrow. Signs of acute long-bone infarction in children are common and can resemble those of acute bacterial osteomyelitis. Acute long-bone infarction is at least 50 times more common than bacterial osteomyelitis in sickle cell disease.[17] In older patients infarcts appear in long and flat bones. Roentgenograms do not show the infarcts for several weeks. Lesions in long bones often affect the femoral and humeral heads.[16]

The thalassemias are a group of anemias that are hereditary and manifest hypochromic microcytic anemia with a decreased synthesis of one or more of the constituents

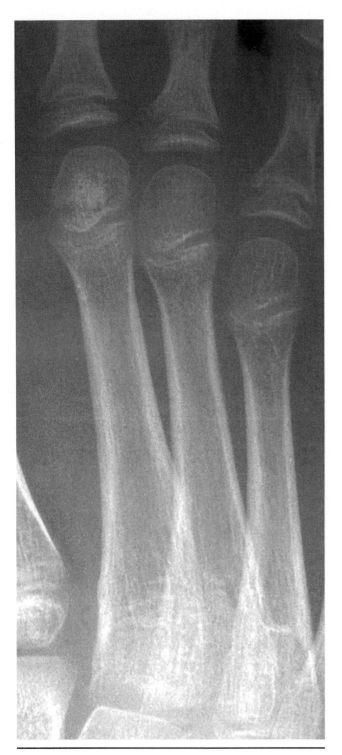

Figure 20-4    Epiphyseal osteonecrosis, second metatarsal. Centralized sclerosis mixed with ill-defined rarefaction.

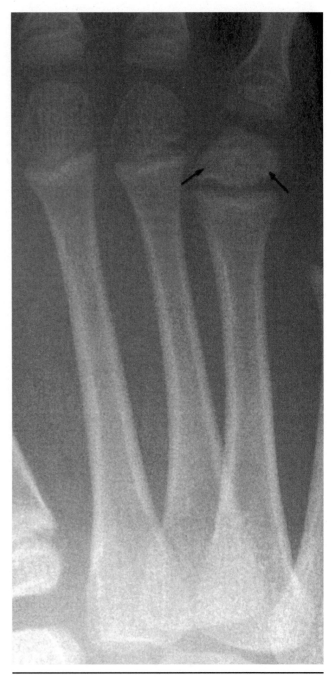

Figure 20-5    Epiphyseal osteonecrosis, fourth metatarsal. Collapse of subchondral bone; an ill-defined curvilinear radiolucency parallels the subchondral surface, the "crescent" sign (arrows).

of hemoglobin.[15] Cooley's anemia is the homozygous form of the disease inherited from both parents. Thalassemia minor is the heterozygous form, inherited from one parent.[18] Thalassemia minor varies in severity.[19] Usually these patients have only mild anemia and no significant skeletal changes. Adults may have vertebral osteoporosis and some diploic widening in the skull.[4,18] In Cooley's anemia, where children rarely survive past adolescence, the peripheral skeleton is affected. The small bones, including the metatarsals and phalanges, appear rectangular, with a

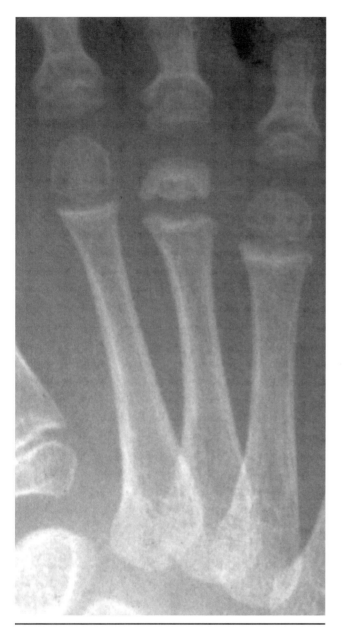

Figure 20-6    Epiphyseal osteonecrosis, third metatarsal

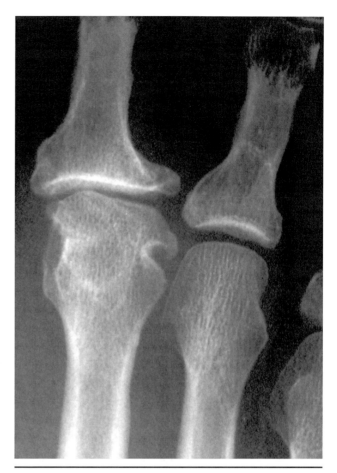

Figure 20-7    Old, healed epiphyseal osteonecrosis, second metatarsal, and secondary osteoarthritis. The second metatarsal head and proximal phalangeal base are flattened, along with osteophyte formation and uneven joint space narrowing.

loss of the normal concavity of the shaft and with cortical thinning.[17] Trabecular resorption occurs, the remaining trabeculae appearing coarsened[4] (Figure 20-12).

## ■ OSTEOCHONDROSIS

The osteochondroses are defined as idiopathic self-limited conditions characterized by disorderliness of osteochondral ossification, including both chondrogenesis and osteo-genesis, that comes on a formerly normal growth process.[20] Some of the so-called osteochondroses are in fact normal

variations, others are true osteonecroses, and some are growth disturbances with no evidence of necrosis.[5]

Historically, three separate descriptions of a similar abnormality affecting the hip joint were published in the early 1900s. Most classic descriptions of epiphyseal osteonecrosis focus on the hip. Legg-Calvé-Perthes disease affects the capital femoral epiphysis in young children; it is characterized by necrosis followed by a regenerative process that is variable and that depends on the patient's age, the adequacy of treatment, and the rapidity with which it is instituted.[21] This is a true osteonecrosis that occurs between infancy and age 16 with the greatest incidence at age 5. It occurs six times more frequently in boys than girls and is rarely seen in blacks.[4] Roentgenographic changes consist of initial joint space swelling with lateral displacement of the hip.[22] Fatigue fracture of the necrotic fragment often occurs early. The subchondral fracture shows up radiographically as a subchondral radiolucent line and is called the crescent or rim sign. This is visible only before collapse of the articular

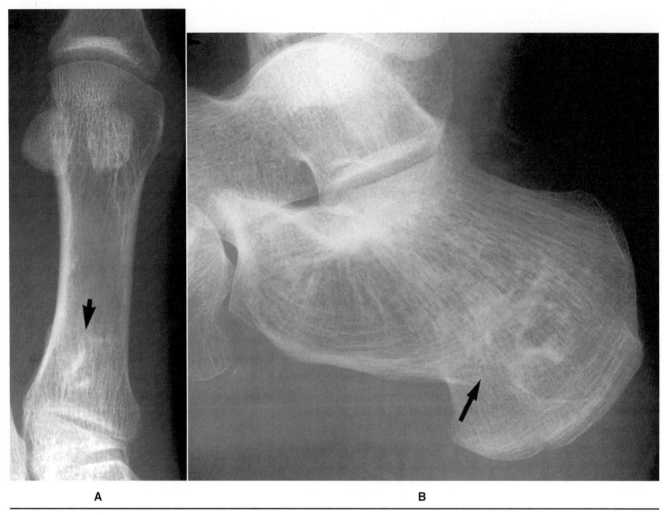

**Figure 20-8**  Osteonecrosis of diametaphyseal and irregular bones. **A**, First metatarsal. **B**, Calcaneus.

cartilage and attached necrotic cancellous bone.[23] The epiphysis undergoes density changes and flattening. Flattening of the head and neck of the femur often occurs, with resultant osteoarthritis.[5]

Freiberg's disease is a true osteonecrosis of the metatarsal head seen most commonly in the second metatarsal. It is much more prevalent in females than males and occurs most commonly between the ages of 10 and 15.[24] Freiberg's disease undergoes a radiographic sequence of events consistent with an osteonecrosis, resulting from a subchondral bone fatigue fracture.[25] Braddock showed, using cadavers, that in this age group the weakest area in the metatarsals was the epiphyseal area, which was the area most likely to fracture.[26] This fracture of the metatarsal is thought to occur secondary to repeated trauma.[27] Clinically, pain, swelling, and tenderness about the metatarsal head area are noted. Range of motion at the metatarsophalangeal joint is often decreased.[24] The radiographic features of Freiberg's disease have varying presentations depending on its stage of healing

(see Figures 20-4 through 20-7). An early radiographic finding often is flattening of the metatarsal head, with possible joint widening. A fracture in the subarticular necrotic bone may present as a crescent-shaped radiodensity.[23] Flattening and fragmentation of the head accompany apparent joint space widening (Figure 20-13). The shaft and neck of the metatarsal thicken cortically, with widening of the bone. The base of the proximal phalanx often widens and molds to the abnormally shaped metatarsal head.[4] The end result is secondary osteoarthritic changes from damage to the articular cartilage.[27] The classic radiographic picture of Freiberg's disease in the adult represents an old, healed osteonecrosis with secondary osteoarthritis (see Figure 20-7). Treatment during the acute stages consists of early immobilization to prevent the deformation of the articular cartilage and the subsequent arthritic changes.

True osteonecrosis of the navicular (Köhler's disease) is extremely uncommon. It occurs more frequently in males than females, typically between the ages of 3 and 7.

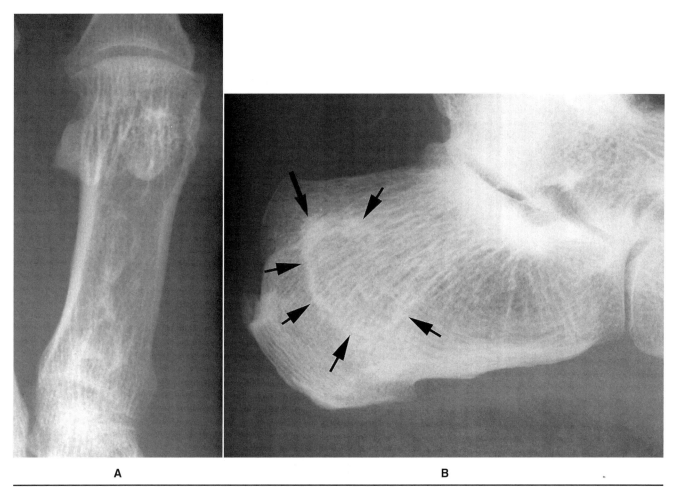

Figure 20-9    Alcoholic bone infarct. **A,** First metatarsal. **B,** Calcaneus.

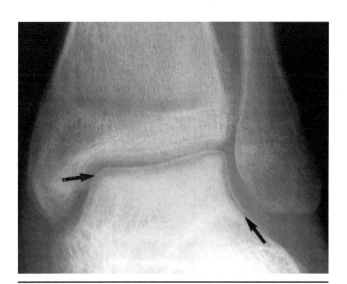

Figure 20-10    Hawkins' sign. Note the linear radiolucency that parallels the talar dome outline, just beneath the subchondral bone plate.

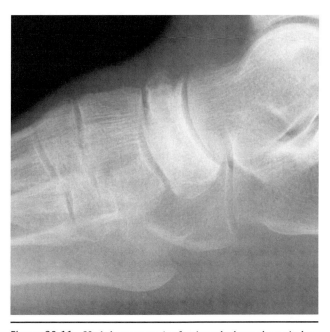

Figure 20-11    Healed osteonecrosis of an irregular bone, the navicular. It is sclerotic and deformed.

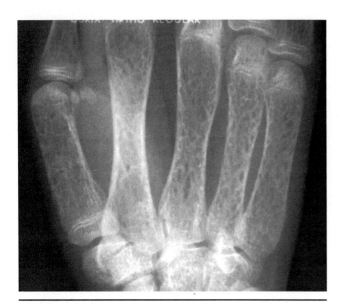

**Figure 20-12**  Thalassemia major.

Unilateral involvement is present 75% to 80% of the time.[7] According to Ozonoff, the diagnosis can only be made by showing that a normal navicular was present before the development of sclerosis and fragmentation or by showing that progressive bone resorption followed by progressive bone repair is on serial x-ray studies.[6] Much more common is an anatomic variation resulting from a delayed appearance of the ossification center of the navicular.[28] This often results in a navicular that appears radiographically as sclerotic, fragmented, and narrowed in its anteroposterior (AP) diameter with a hazy outer border (Figure 20-14). Ferguson found irregular ossification of the navicular in about one third of normal children.[28] McCauley used a bone scan to evaluate a possible Köhler's.[29] He found decreased uptake on the symptomatic navicular, which he argued supported a diagnosis of true osteonecrosis. Brower[5] suggests that the decreased uptake was probably caused by delayed ossification at the growth center. She goes on to argue that because a true osteonecrosis must involve a hypervascular state, to support the diagnosis the scan should be hot at some point. Weston demonstrated an increased focal uptake of scanning agent in a true Köhler's.[30] True osteonecrosis requires immobilization to prevent collapse of the navicular. The anatomic variation generally ossifies normally regardless of treatment.

Sever's disease, or osteochondrosis of the calcaneal apophysis, is not a true osteochondrosis. A normal calcaneal apophysis is sclerotic and often fragmented because of multiple ossification centers[27] (Figure 20-15). It has been shown that increased density of the calcaneal apophysis is normal and attributed to weight bearing and is absent in children without normal weight bearing.[31] Pain is not caused by the calcaneal apophysis, or so-called apophysitis.

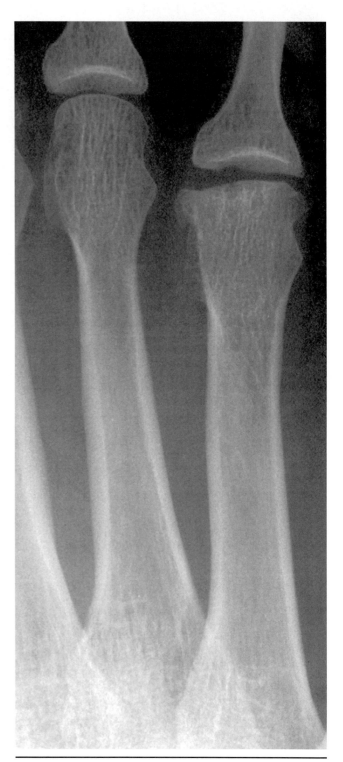

**Figure 20-13**  Healing osteonecrosis of the second-metatarsal head. Note the apparent widening of the joint space.

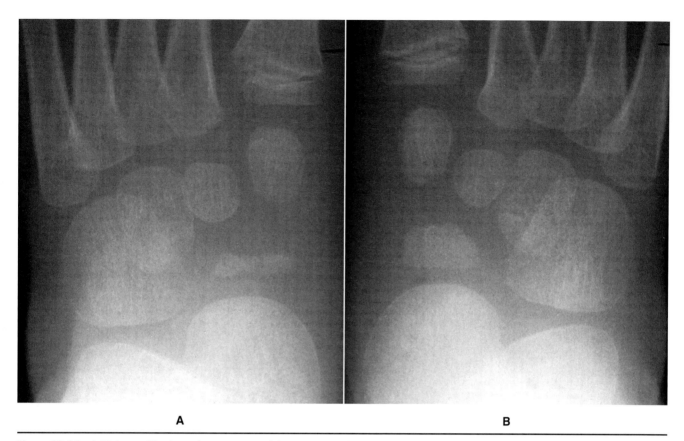

**A**                                                                                           **B**

Figure 20-14   **A,** Variant ossification and segmentation of the navicular ossification center mimicking Köhler's disease. **B,** Opposite foot, same patient.

Painful heels in children are usually related to plantar fasciitis, Achilles tendonitis, or a prominent posterosuperior calcaneus.[5,27,28]

Iselin's disease is traditionally thought of as an osteochondrosis of the base of the fifth metatarsal. It is actually an apophysitis of the base with no osteonecrosis noted. Although the apophysis may be fragmented, this is a normal finding, not pathology (Figure 20-16). Limiting physical activity and removing shoe pressure from the base of the fifth metatarsal usually alleviates symptoms.[32]

Buschke's disease (osteochondrosis of the tarsal cuneiforms) is not a true osteonecrosis. The reversible nature of the so-called irregular size, shape, and trabecular density of the cuneiforms regardless of treatment is a strong indication that this disorder is nothing more than a normal variation in endochondral ossification[33] (Figure 20-17).

Blount's disease is not a true osteonecrosis. It is a growth disturbance of the posteromedial part of the proximal tibial metaphysis and epiphysis. Bony necrosis is not evidenced. The growth of the epiphyseal cartilage is arrested, resulting in varus medial torsion of the tibia and a degree of flexion of the diaphysis on the upper tibial epiphysis.[34] Blount[35] described two types of the disease, infantile and adolescent. The infantile form occurs between ages 1 and 3 and is much

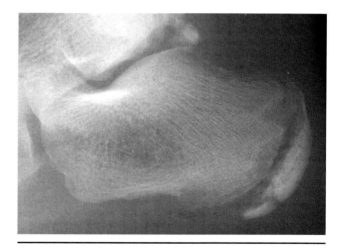

Figure 20-15   Variant ossification and segmentation of the calcaneal apophyseal ossification center once referred to as Sever's disease. Also note the jagged appearance of the adjacent metaphysis, a variant of normal development.

more common and much more severe. The adolescent form occurs between ages 6 and 13 and is rare in comparison.[36] Blount's is common in black children.[37] The radiographic study shows that the medial part of the epiphysis is poorly developed and shows a beak on the posteromedial aspect of

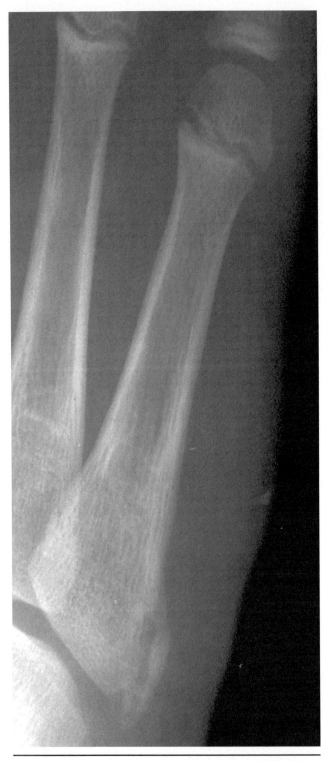

Figure 20-16 Variant ossification and segmentation of the fifth-metatarsal basal apophyseal ossification center mimicking Iselin's disease.

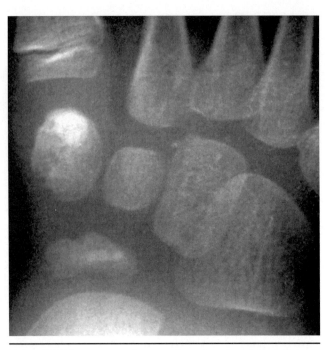

Figure 20-17 Variant ossification and segmentation of the medial cuneiform ossification center mimicking Buschke's disease.

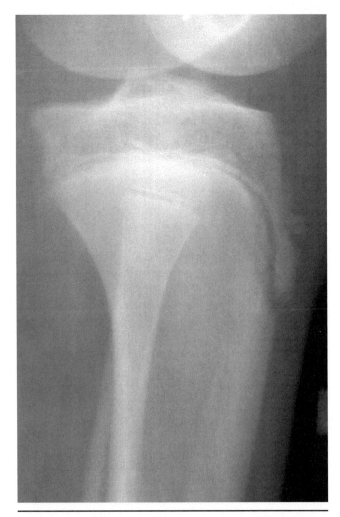

Figure 20-18 Variant ossification and segmentation of the tibial tubercle ossification center mimicking Osgood Schlatter's disease. This patient was asymptomatic at that location.

the metaphysis. These changes are progressive.[34] The sharply angular appearance of infantile Blount's differs from the gradual curve in physiologic bowed legs. The nature and severity of the osseous changes are highly variable.[7]

Osgood Schlatter's disease, or osteochondrosis of the tibial tubercle, does not show osteonecrosis. It is seen most commonly in boys between the ages of 11 and 15, when the ossification center of the proximal tibial tubercle appears.[4] Pain, swelling, and tenderness over the tibial tubercle are noted.[5] Pain is exacerbated by physical activity such as running, going up or down steps, or squatting. Osgood Schlatter's is caused by the pull of the patella tendon at its insertion.[24] This results in a traumatic avulsion of the quadriceps tendon or a tendonitis of the tendon with heterotopic new bone formation.[5,38,39]

The normal tibial tubercle is often fragmented and sclerotic (Figures 20-18 and 20-19). More than one ossification center is often evident. Osgood Schlatter's cannot be diagnosed from a radiograph. Although soft tissue swelling over the tibial tubercle is noted, Osgood Schlatter's remains a clinical diagnosis.

Renander[40] was the first to report aseptic necrosis of the first-metatarsal sesamoids, which he described as an osteochondropathy. This true osteonecrosis occurs most commonly in young adult women. The radiograph shows fragmentation, mottling, and irregularity of the sesamoid[41] (Figure 20-20). The sesamoid axial view is the best view for isolating the sesamoids (Figure 20-21). The three phase bone scan is useful in diagnosing true osteonecrosis. Treatment consists of balance padding to take the weight off the sesamoid. Casting is also useful to alleviate symptoms

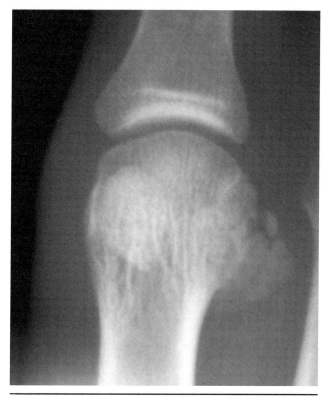

Figure 20-20    Osteonecrosis of the fibular sesamoid, dorsoplantar view. Note significant fragmentation with mixed rarefaction.

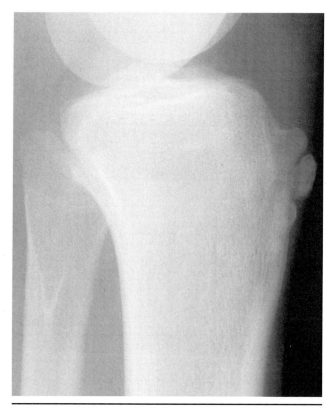

Figure 20-19    Prominent tibial tubercle with fragmentation associated with positive clinical symptomatology consistent with osteochondrosis of the tibial tubercle or Osgood Schlatter's disease.

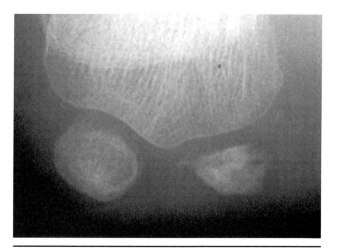

Figure 20-21    Osteonecrosis of the fibular sesamoid, sesamoid axial view. Note the fragmentation, deformity, and sclerosis.

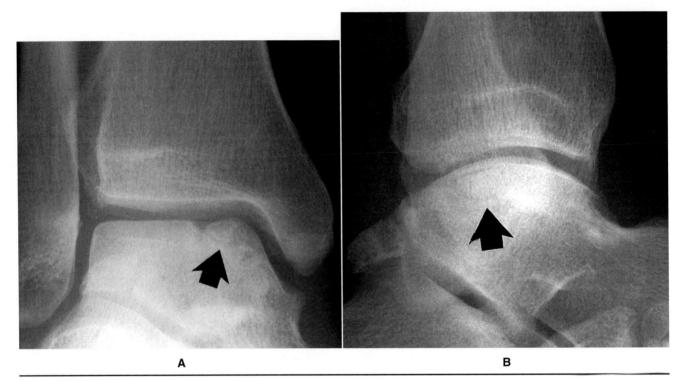

Figure 20-22    Osteochondritis dissecans, talar dome, superomedially. **A,** Mortise view. **B,** Lateral view.

and to speed healing. Sesamoidectomy has been proven effective for unresponsive cases.[41]

## ■ OSTEOCHONDRITIS DISSECANS

Osteochondritis dissecans appears to be a localized ischemic necrosis that occurs more frequently in young men and boys.[4] Tachdjian believes the etiology is multifactorial, including heredity, constitution predisposition, ischemia, and trauma. The necrosis of the subchondral bone is followed by destruction of the underlying cartilage.[24] Osteochondritis dissecans occurs most commonly in the knee at the lateral aspect of the medial femoral condyle.

The characteristic radiographic picture is a button of subchondral bone surrounded by a radiolucent line.[4,24] Tomography, bone scanning, arthrography, computed tomography (CT) scanning, and especially magnetic resonance imaging (MRI) have all been shown useful in identifying and staging osteochondral lesions.[42-44]

Osteochondritis of the talus is fairly common and occurs in either the upper medial or lateral aspect of the dome[45] (Figures 20-22 and 20-23). Although the lateral lesion is thought to be caused by trauma, experts debate the etiology of the medial lesion.[24] O'Farrell and Costello proposed that if the foot were plantarflexed during inversion, a medial lesion would result from compression of the medial talar dome by the tibia.[45] If the foot were dorsiflexed, a lateral

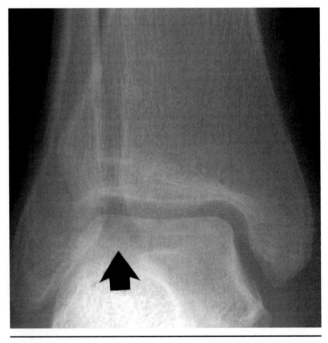

Figure 20-23    Osteochondritis dissecans, talar dome, superolaterally.

lesion would result from shearing forces by the fibula. Treatment is aimed at preventing the lesion from detaching.[24] If detachment occurs, surgery is often required, which consists of drilling the base of the defect and excising the fragment.[45]

## References

1. Resnick D: *Bone and joint imaging*, Philadelphia, 1989, Saunders.

2. *Stedman's medical dictionary*, ed 25, Baltimore, 1990, Williams & Wilkins.

3. Solomon, L: Mechanisms of idiopathic osteonecrosis, *Orthop Clin North Am* 16:655, 1985.

4. Edeiken J, Dalinka M, Karasick D: *Edeiken's Roentgen diagnosis of disease of bone*, ed 4, vol 1, Baltimore, 1990, William & Wilkins.

5. Brower AC: The osteochondroses, *Orthop Clin North Am* 14:99, 1983.

6. Ozonoff MB: *Pediatric orthopedic radiology*, Philadelphia, 1979, Saunders.

7. Resnick D, Niwayama G: *Diagnosis of bone and joint disorders*, Philadelphia, 1981, Saunders.

8. Boettcher WG et al: Nontraumatic necrosis of the femoral head, *J Bone Joint Surg* 52A:312, 1970.

9. Bornstein A, Plate E: Über chronische gelenkveränderungen, entstandendurch presslufterkrankung, *Fortschr Geb Roentgenstr Nuklearmed* 18:197, 1911.

10. Kawashima M et al: Pathological review of osteonecrosis in divers, *Clin Orthop* 130:107, 1978.

11. Heard JL, Schneider CS: Radiographic findings in commercial divers, *Clin Orthop* 130:179, 1978.

12. Boskey AL et al: Changes in the bone tissue lipids in persons with steroid and alcohol induced osteonecrosis, *Clin Orthop* 172:289, 1983.

13. Amstutz HC: The hip in Gaucher's disease, *Clin Orthop* 90:83, 1973.

14. Rourke JA, Weslin JD: Gaucher's disease, *AJR* 94:621, 1965.

15. Williams WJ et al: *Hematology*, New York, 1977, McGraw-Hill.

16. Piggs LW: Bone and joint lesions in sickle cell disease, *Clin Orthop* 52:119, 1967.

17. Kelley K, Buchanan GR: Acute infarction of long bones in children with sickle cell anemia, *J Pediatr* 101:170, 1982.

18. Juhl JW et al: *Essentials of radiologic imaging*, Philadelphia, 1987, Lippincott.

19. Meschan I: *Roentgen signs in diagnostic imaging*, vol 2, Philadelphia, 1985, Saunders.

20. Siffert RS: Classification of the osteochondroses, *Clin Orthop* 158:10, 1981.

21. Jacobs BW: Early recognition of osteochondrosis of capital epiphysis of femur, *JAMA* 172:527, 1960.

22. Caffey J: The early roentgenographic changes in essential coxa plana: their significance in pathogenesis, *AJR* 103:620, 1968.

23. Kenzora JE, Glimcher MJ: Pathogenesis of idiopathic osteonecrosis: the ubiquitous crescent sign, *Orthop Clin North Am* 16:681, 1985.

24. Tachdjian MO: *Pediatric orthopedics*, vol 2, Philadelphia, 1990, Saunders.

25. Gauthier G, Elbaz R: Freiberg's infraction: a subchondral bone fatigue fracture, *Clin Orthop* 142:93, 1979.

26. Braddock GTF: Experimental epiphyseal injury and Freiberg's disease, *J Bone Joint Surg* 41B:154, 1959.

27. Forrester DM, Kricun ME, Kerr R: *Imaging of the foot and ankle*, Rockville, Md, 1988, Aspen.

28. Ferguson AB, Gingrich RM: The normal and the abnormal calcaneal apophysis and tarsal navicular, *Clin Orthop* 10:87, 1957.

29. McCauley MB, Kahn PC: Osteochondritis of the tarsal navicular, *Radiology* 22:332, 1978.

30. Weston WJ: Köhler's disease of the tarsal scaphoid, *Aust Radiol* 22:332, 1978.

31. Shopfner CE, Coin CG: Effect of weight bearing on the appearance and development of the secondary calcaneal epiphysis, *Radiology* 86:201, 1966.

32. Schwartz B, Jay RM, Schoenhaus HB: Apophysitis of the fifth metatarsal base, *JAMA* 81:128, 1991.

33. Leeson MC, Weiner DS: Osteochondrosis of the tarsal cuneiforms, *Clin Orthop* 196:260, 1985.

34. Golding JSR, McNeil-Smith JDG: Observations on the etiology of tibia vara, *J Bone Joint Surg* 45B:320, 1963.

35. Blount WP: Tibia vara, *J Bone Joint Surg* 19:1, 1937.

36. Langenskiöld A: Tibia vara: osteochondrosis deformans tibiae, *Clin Orthop* 158:77, 1981.

37. Bathfield CA, Beighton PH: Blount disease, *Clin Orthop* 135:29, 1978.

38. Ogden JA, Southwick WD: Osgood Schlatter's disease and tibial tubercle development, *Clin Orthop* 116:180, 1976.

39. Bowers KD Jr: Patellar tendon avulsion as a complication of Osgood Schlatter's disease, *Am J Sports Med* 9:356, 1981.

40. Renander A: Two cases of typical osteochondropathy of the medial sesamoid bone of the first metatarsal, *Acta Radiol* 2:521, 1924.

41. Ogata K et al: Idiopathic osteonecrosis of the first metatarsal sesamoid, *Skeletal Radiol* 15:141, 1986.

42. Davies AM, Cassar-Pullicino VN: Demonstration of osteochondritis dissecans of the talus by coronal computed tomographic arthrography, *BJR* 62:1050, 1989.

43. Anderson IF et al: Osteochondral fractures of the dome of the talus, *J Bone Joint Surg* 71A:1143, 1989.

44. DeSmet AA et al: Value of MR imaging in stating osteochondral lesions of the talus (osteochondritis dissecans): results in 14 patients, *Am J Roentgenology* 154:555, 1990.

45. O'Farrel TA, Costello BG: Osteochondritis dissecans of the talus, *J Bone Joint Surg* 64B:494, 1982.

# CHAPTER 21

# Bone Infection

MARIE WILLIAMS

Bone infection requires appropriate clinical and radiographic diagnosis to prevent debilitating disease. Accurate clinical and radiographic evaluation of the patient with bone infection depends on age of patient, route of infection, type of organism involved, and the nature of the disease process. Early diagnosis of bone infection allows appropriate treatment and diminishes the risk of long-term sequelae and complications. This chapter discusses how infecting organisms cause bone and joint destruction. To thoroughly understand the etiology of bone infection, the clinician must first have a basic understanding of bone pathophysiology and how infecting organisms invade bone and joints. When the vascular supply to bone is disrupted, physiological changes take place within the Haversian and Volkmann systems affecting osteoblastic and osteoclastic function, which are responsible for normal bone function. Correlating clinical findings with radiographic findings can give the practitioner a greater comprehension of the disease process.

## DEFINITION OF TERMS

The terms used to describe bone infection must be understood before one can understand the disease process. The term *osteomyelitis* is used to describe infection of bone and bone marrow.[1] Osteomyelitis is classified as acute, subacute, and chronic. The infection is also described according to transmission route of the organisms. The term *infectious periostitis* is used for infection that invades the periosteum but does not affect the bone and bone marrow. With infectious periostitis the changes are subtle and may be identified from a periosteal reaction (Figure 21-1). As the infection penetrates to the cortex but does not invade medullary bone, the term *infectious osteitis* is used (Figure 21-2).[1] Once the infection involves both cortex and bone marrow, the more accurate term is *osteomyelitis* (Figure

21-3). Radiographically, it can be difficult to differentiate infectious osteitis and osteomyelitis, because a lag separates clinical presentation and radiographic signs.[1-3] Most researchers believe that 30 to 60% of bone demineralizes before radiographic evidence is noted.[1,3-6] Also, approximately 10-14 days of lag time separate clinical disease and radiographic changes caused by the infectious process. Bone scintigraphy is valuable in early diagnosis of osteomyelitis if no other underlying pathology is present (Figure 21-4).

Radiographically, the fascial planes of the plantar and dorsal midfoot and tarsus normally can be identified in the lateral view. As soft tissues become infiltrated with the infecting organism, the fascial planes disappear. This disappearance can be the initial radiographic sign of impending bone infection and should alert the practitioner to institute early proper treatment of the infection. Occasionally gas or air is seen in the affected area (Figures 21-5 and 21-6). Digital soft tissue infection is seen radiographically as an increased soft tissue density and volume (Figure 21-7). If inappropriately treated, soft tissue infection can lead to bone infection.[1-3,5,6]

Osteomyelitis has been classified as acute, subacute, and chronic in nature (Box 21-1). Acute osteomyelitis is clinically identified by an insidious onset of pain localized to bone, with soft tissue swelling and erythema of the involved area. A patient may develop fever, malaise, irritability, and marked increase in pain. During the initial stage of infection, it is difficult to ascertain the infectious process radiographically. Soft tissue swelling and obliteration of fascial planes may be the only radiographic signs.[7] Early on, subperiosteal new bone may appear; this may be the only radiographic change so far, because at least 10 to 14 days elapse before radiographically visible changes occur.[1,6,8] The term *rarefaction* is used to describe localized loss of bone density. It is one of the earliest findings of osteomyelitis (Figure 21-8).[1,2,4,6] The term *osteolysis* applies to a more destructive process or resorption of bone (Figure 21-9).

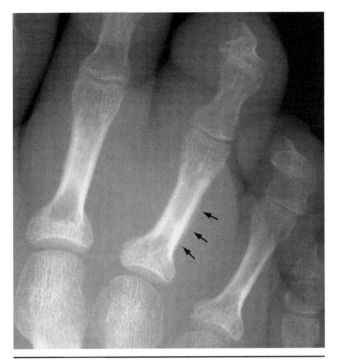

Figure 21-1    Infectious periostitis. A subtle, linear periosteal reaction *(arrows)* can be seen along the lateral aspect of the third-toe proximal phalanx. Note the associated soft tissue increase in density and volume affecting the third and fourth toes.

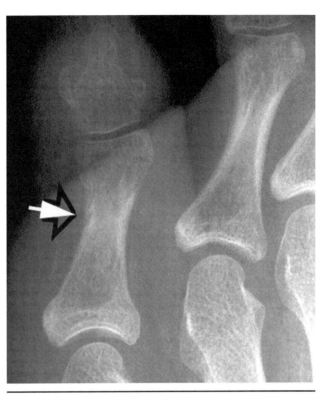

Figure 21-2    Infectious osteitis. Erosion *(arrow)* can be identified along the lateral aspect of the fifth-toe proximal phalanx distal diametaphysis. No rarefaction or other lysis is seen radiographically that would suggest medullary involvement.

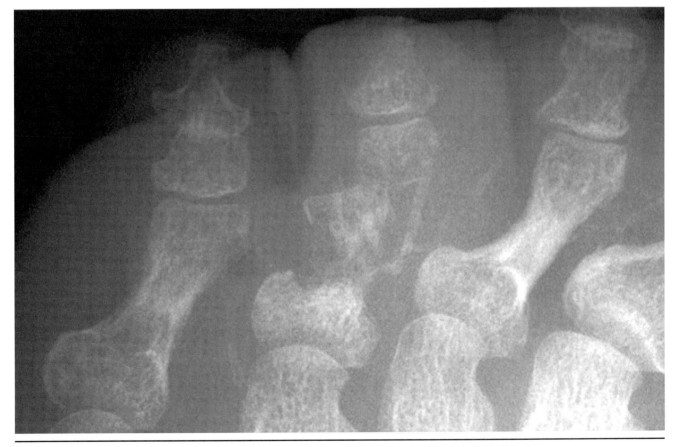

Figure 21-3    Osteomyelitis, fourth-toe proximal phalanx. Infection involves the entire bone, resulting in loss of its form.

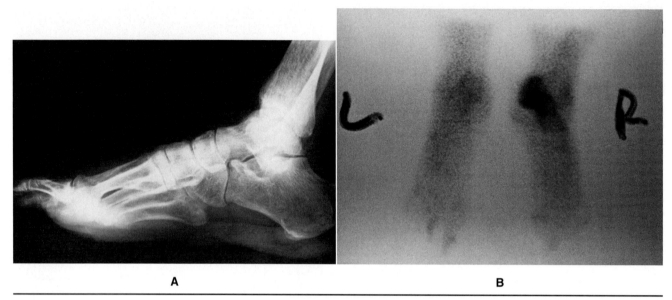

**A**                                                           **B**

Figure 21-4   Early calcaneal osteomyelitis. **A,** Soft tissue density has increased along the plantar aspect of the calcaneus and subtle rarefaction in the calcaneal body, but these findings alone are not specific for osteomyelitis. **B,** Bone scan. Focal increased uptake is seen in the heel. In the proper clinical setting this is very suggestive of osteomyelitis.

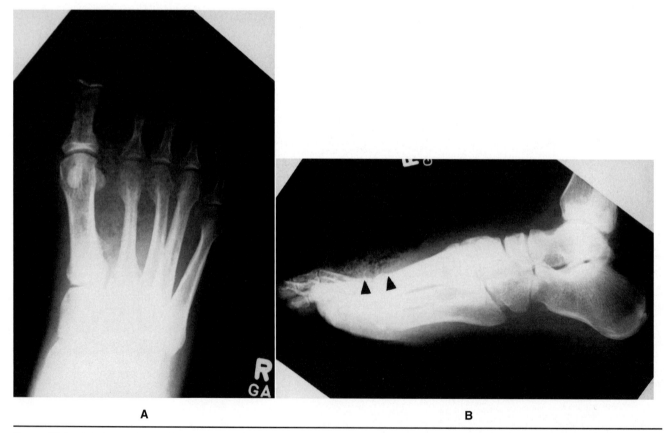

**A**                                                           **B**

Figure 21-5   Soft tissue infection: Gas gangrene. **A,** Dorsoplantar view. Air/gas shows in the soft tissues of the forefoot. **B,** The lateral view shows loss of fascial planes dorsally as well as air/gas (arrows) in the soft tissues.

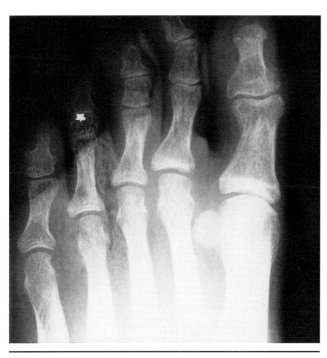

Figure 21-6    Soft tissue infection secondary to gas-forming bacteria. Note the multiple airlike densities in the fourth ray.

### BOX 21-1    Classification of Osteomyelitis

| CLINICAL SIGNS | RADIOGRAPHIC SIGNS |
| --- | --- |
| **ACUTE OSTEOMYELITIS** | |
| Insidious onset with pain, malaise, fever. Cellulitis. | No radiographic findings initially. Early findings may be periostitis, rarefaction, and soft tissue swelling. Obliteration of fascial planes. |
| **SUBACUTE OSTEOMYELITIS** | |
| Low-grade pain with no systemic signs. Occasional pain around the affected area. | Well-defined lytic lesion in bone with dense sclerotic rim usually 1 to 4 cm in diameter (Brodie's abscess). |
| **CHRONIC OSTEOMYELITIS** | |
| Pain localized to the affected area, with soft tissue swelling and localized cellulitis. Ulceration and draining. Sinus may be present. | Bone lysis and malformation with involucrum, cloaca, and sequestrum. |

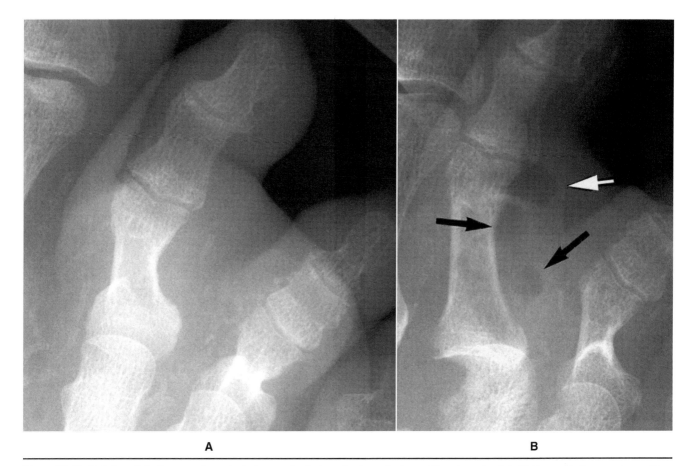

A                                                                B

Figure 21-7    Soft tissue infection, second toe. **A,** An increased soft tissue density and volume affects the entire digit. **B,** Four weeks later, gas is noted in the same digit *(arrows).*

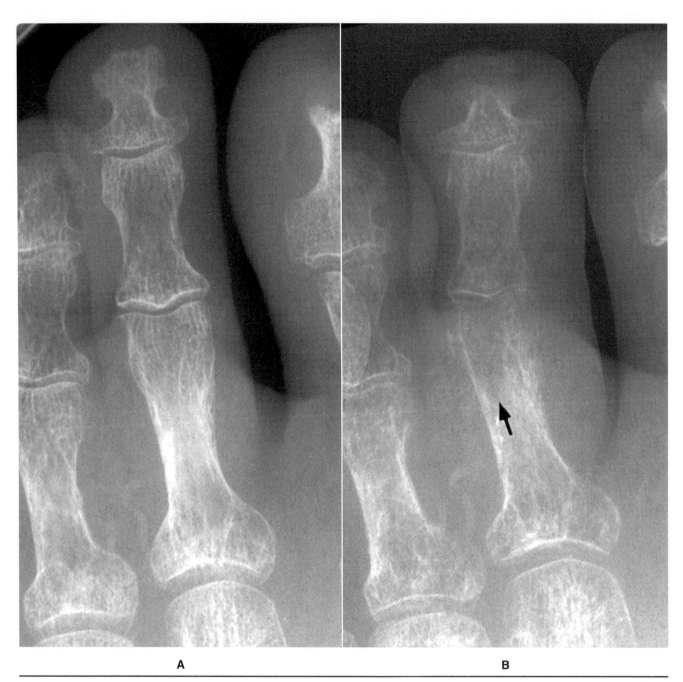

**Figure 21-8**  Early osteomyelitis. **A,** Normal second toe before infection. **B,** Significant rarefaction *(arrow)* is seen in the head of the proximal phalanx. Notice that the form of the phalanx is still intact.

The term *subacute osteomyelitis* is used to describe a well-defined lytic lesion in bone that is caused by an infectious organism of low virulence.[1,3] The walled-off abscess in bone known as Brodie's abscess was first described by Sir Benjamin Brodie in 1832.[9] A Brodie's abscess as seen on radiograph must be differentiated from a benign bone cyst. They differ radiographically in that an abscess appears as a lytic area of bone with a dense, sclerotic rim that fades

peripherally as the eburnated trabeculae gradually return to normal size (Figure 21-10).[4] The abscess may vary in size from 1 to 4 cm in diameter and is commonly found in metaphyseal bone.[2]

Chronic osteomyelitis develops when an acute infection is inappropriately treated or therapy has been inadequate. During the chronic process, viable new bone is laid down around dead bone, developing a periosteal envelope that can

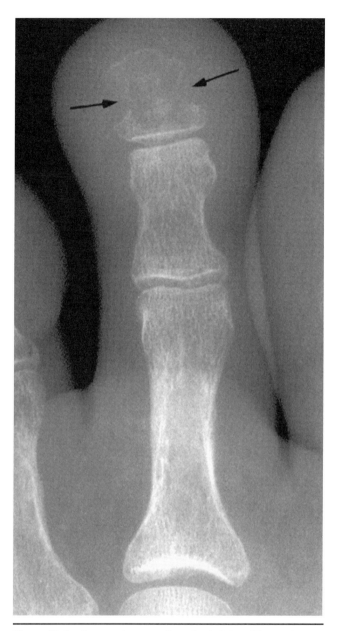

**Figure 21-9**   Osteomyelitis, second-toe distal phalanx. The rarefaction has progressed to osteolysis (loss of form); the medial and lateral cortices are not intact *(arrows)*, and the ungual tuberosity is now separate from the remainder of the phalanx. Bone fragments can be seen centrally.

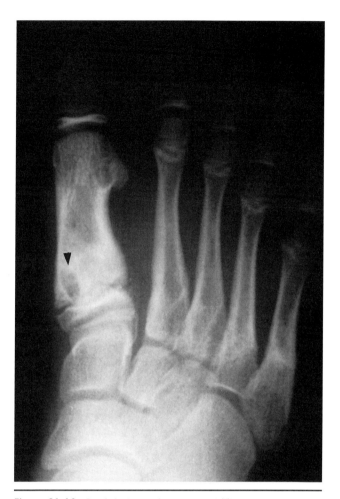

**Figure 21-10**   Brodie's abscess, first metatarsal. This is an 8-year-old boy 11 months after metatarsus adductus surgery with a painful first metatarsal. A geographic, lytic lesion lies at the medial aspect of the first-metatarsal proximal metaphysis *(arrowhead)*. This lesion represents a bone abscess. Note that the epiphysis is spared and the lesion has a sclerotic rim that fades peripherally away from the epiphyseal plate.

surround the entire shaft. This covering is called an involucrum (Figure 21-11).[1,3,6] The involucrum surrounds dead bone, which may be seen as an irregular or jagged area. Long-standing chronic osteomyelitis results in significant bone deformity (Figure 21-12). Dead bone that is detached from the cortex and appears sclerotic relative to the surrounding area is known as sequestrum. Sequestrum is one of the most important findings in the assessment of chronic osteomyelitis. The presence of dead, necrotic bone

represents active infection during the chronic stage of the disease (Figure 21-13).[1,3,6] The term *cloaca* refers to a defect in the cortex that allows pus and nonviable bone to be expelled from the bone. A fistula or sinus tract is an opening that allows the sequestrum or pus to move through the soft tissues.

The term *septic arthritis* is used to describe infection of a joint. Joint infection erodes cartilage and decreases joint mobility.[1,10] Radiographically, septic arthritis appears similar to rheumatoid arthritis or gouty arthritis. The initial juxta-articular osteoporosis leads to a more lytic process than does other arthritis. Septic arthritis causes erosion within and at the margins of the joint (Figure 21-14) and can later lead to bony ankylosis.

Sclerosing osteomyelitis of Garré is a chronic form of osteomyelitis caused by organisms of low virulence. The

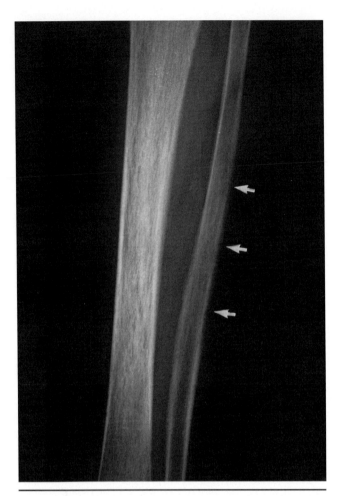

**Figure 21-11**    Involucrum, fibular mid-diaphysis. Periosteal new bone *(arrows)* is evident along the lateral shaft of the midfibula. When associated with chronic bone infection, this collar of new bone is known as an involucrum. Notice the normal cortex at both the distal and proximal ends of the fibula.

disease is nonsuppurative and usually affects a single bone. Radiographically the bone appears sclerotic and shows marked cortical thickening with very little evidence of a draining sinus or osteolysis. This entity must be differentiated from Ewing sarcoma, which is a more destructive lesion showing scalloping of the periosteum.[1,3,6,11]

### ■ CLASSIFICATION OF OSTEOMYELITIS

Many authors have classified bone infection according to the route of contamination.[1,2,6] Trueta has classified osteomyelitis into three types according to variations in blood supply to bone in different age groups, and that schema is discussed in more detail later. Different routes of contamination that cause osteomyelitis include hematogenous

osteomyelitis; osteomyelitis secondary to contiguous soft tissue; puncture wounds or implantation devices such as pins, wires, screws, or staples from surgery; and postoperative wound infections.[1]

The route of contamination is important radiographically because the findings may appear differently depending on route. Hematogenous osteomyelitis is infection in which the bone is infected from blood-borne organisms that are themselves seen in medullary and metaphyseal regions of bone. Metaphyseal bone is most often affected, because of impairment in the vascular anatomy.[12,13] Metaphyseal bone is very vascular and is affected because the sluggish, venous sinusoidal blood flow provides a good medium for bacterial growth and enhances localization of the organisms in the metaphysis and marrow. It is especially true in children, where nutrient arteries are relatively large, and the branches to the marrow, cortex, and metaphysis are small end arteries or capillaries that are relatively stagnant.[12] Intraosseous pressure rapidly increases with infection, leading to marked necrosis and demineralization. If the infection persists, exudate continues to expand and spread through the Volkmann and Haversian systems of bone. Blood flow is increasingly disrupted, leading to advanced necrosis, destruction, resorption, and possibly sclerosis. As the infection advances, it crosses the cortex, with ensuing periosteal proliferation. Subperiosteal abscess formation and subsequent irritation may lead to new bone formation or involucrum.[4,7,12] Superperiosteal proliferation may be noted as early as 5 to 7 days in children, whereas in adults it may appear in 10 to 14 days. Subperiosteal proliferation is usually a more common finding because the child's bone has a loosely attached periosteum. In addition, large areas of dead bone may be surrounded by granulation tissue and may be walled off from adjacent viable bone. This sclerotic fragment of bone is known as the sequestrum. It is important to fully understand the route of contamination clinically because radiographically the bony destruction presents itself somewhat differently depending on route, as noted earlier.

Osteomyelitis secondary to contiguous soft tissue or direct extension to bone gives a somewhat different appearance from that of hematogenous osteomyelitis. In the lower extremity and foot, hematogenous osteomyelitis is rather rare.[2] Changes consistent with contiguous soft tissue or direct extension osteomyelitis are more common. Osteomyelitis secondary to direct extension is caused by an organism invading bone from the outside source via a portal of entry.[4,6] Because of the invading organism from an outside source, the bone infection is seen initially as an infectious periostitis, which then leads to an infectious osteitis. Once the periosteum is invaded and the cortex is destroyed, a full-blown osteomyelitis occurs. Radiographic findings associated with contiguous soft tissue infection, puncture wounds, and surgery are soft tissue swelling,

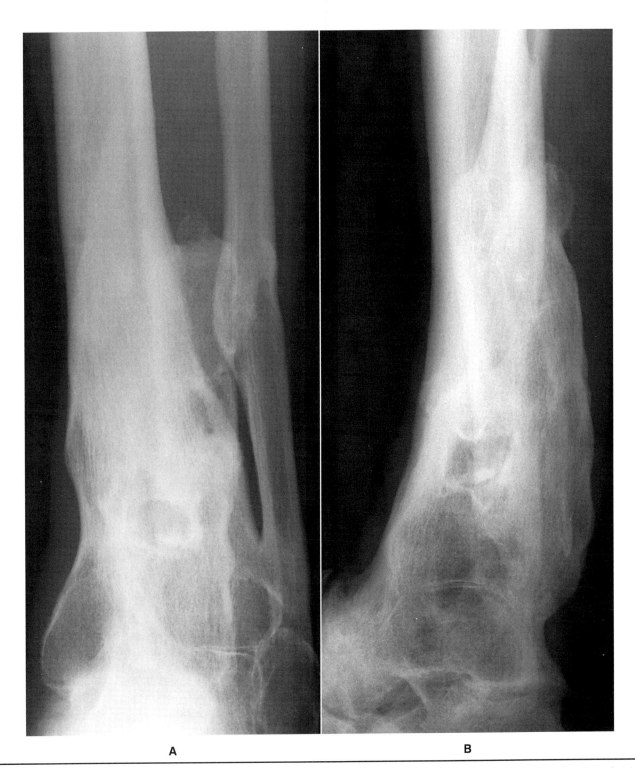

**A**    **B**

**Figure 21-12**  Chronic osteomyelitis, distal leg. **A,** Anteroposterior, and **B,** lateral views. After many years, the periosteal remodeling (involucrum) yields severe bone deformity.

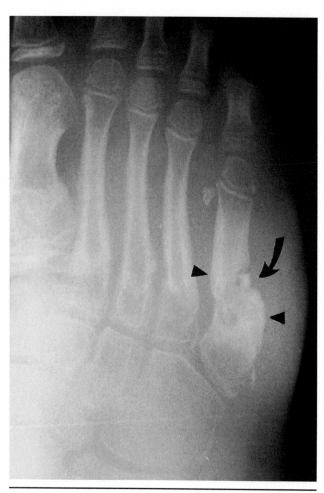

**Figure 21-13** Chronic, active osteomyelitis. Note the well-defined lytic lesion within the base of the fifth metatarsal. Also note the extensive periosteal new bone *(arrowheads)*, representing an involucrum. The involucrum surrounds or walls off the sequestrum within the cystlike lesion. A small piece of bone is exiting through a cloaca *(curved arrow)*.

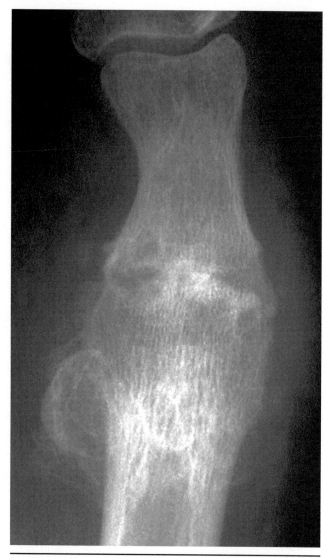

**Figure 21-14** Septic arthritis, first metatarsophalangeal joint, left foot. Significant joint space narrowing and erosions are seen along both sides of the first metatarsophalangeal joint.

obliteration of fascial planes, and eventual invasion of the bone and/or joint. Radiographic abnormalities from soft tissue infection differ from hematogenous osteomyelitis in that the initial phase of infection is seen as soft tissue swelling with obliteration of fascial planes. As the infection invades the periosteum, evidence appears of periostitis secondary to lifting of the periosteum from bone by pus. Once the cortex becomes involved, cortical erosions are noted. These represent subcortical abscess formation. As the infection invades the Haversian and Volkmann canals, cortical erosion and rarefaction occur. As the bone marrow becomes affected, pus can infiltrate the vascular supply to the medullary bone. The circulation to bone becomes more sluggish, and bone lysis occurs. Osteomyelitis from puncture wounds, including human and animal bites, are radiographically the same except that the soft tissue swelling is

more commonly related to inflammation secondary to trauma than from the infection itself.[1]

Osteomyelitis is difficult to differentiate in the postoperative patient because of the proliferation of normal healing bone associated with periosteal reaction and bone callous formation (Figure 21-15). Early diagnosis is very important, to prevent an acute osteomyelitis or periostitis from becoming a chronic problem. Other diagnostic modalities, such as bone scintigraphy, magnetic resonance imaging (MRI), or computed tomography (CT), may help differentiate periosteal reaction secondary to bone healing or a periostitis from infection. Increased osseous and/or cartilaginous destruction with radiolucency around an

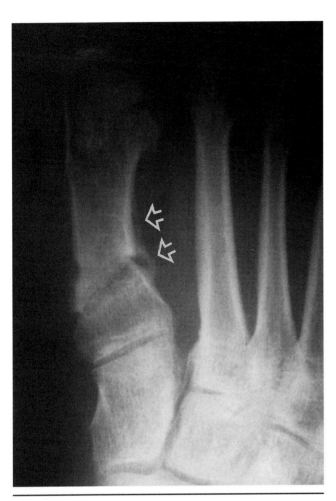

Figure 21-15   Normal postoperative periostitis. A periosteal reaction is seen along the lateral aspect *(open arrows)* of the first-metatarsal proximal metadiaphysis. The patient is 13 weeks after a base wedge osteotomy with screw fixation. The screw was removed because it loosened. The periosteal reaction could represent infection, although this example is a uninfected periostitis secondary to normal healing.

implant or prosthesis should alert the clinician to possible bone infection.[1]

Some authors have identified osteomyelitis according to vascular metaphyseal blood supply to the bone in different age groups.[5,12] Metaphyseal vascular anatomy is age dependent and subsequently affects a patient's susceptibility to osteomyelitis. Understanding the metaphyseal vascular anatomy is important when differentiating osteomyelitis in children, infants, and adults (Figure 21-16). As noted, Trueta[12] has described three distinct patterns of osteomyelitis based on metaphyseal blood supply in different age groups. An infantile pattern is described in children less than 1 year of age. Metaphyseal vessels penetrate the epiphyseal growth plate in the infant to supply the epiphysis. Subsequently, metaphyseal infection may cross the growth plate,

invading contiguous joint spaces, and results in sepsis. Neonatal osteomyelitis rapidly transgresses the growth plate, leading to joint infection, which can destroy the joint as well as bone.[5,12,14] Involvement of the epiphyseal plate may lead to a decrease in the length of the affected limb. When the epiphyseal plate is spared, hyperemia may lead to accelerated growth rate, with early maturation and closure of the plate.[6] A juvenile pattern has been described as affecting children from 1 year of age to the closure of the physis. No vascular penetration of the growth plate occurs during this period, and the plate may act as a "barrier" confining the infection to the metaphyseal region. The infection may spread laterally, however, perforating the cortex and eventually elevating the loosely adhered periosteum. In the juvenile pattern, periosteum is loosely attached to bone and may show an extensive periosteal reaction and lifting (Figure 21-17).

After growth plate closure the adult pattern is evident. Once the epiphyseal plate has closed, penetration into the epiphysis can occur and joint sepsis is more likely. Because in adults the periosteum adheres more firmly to the underlying bone, radiographic studies of adults may also show less subperiosteal elevation and advancement.

## ◼ DIABETIC OSTEOMYELITIS VERSUS OSTEOLYSIS

Another classification has also been proposed for osteomyelitis. This category includes hematogenous osteomyelitis, osteomyelitis secondary to contiguous soft tissue infection, and osteomyelitis in association with peripheral vascular disease.[14,15] Hematogenous osteomyelitis and osteomyelitis secondary to contiguous soft tissue infection have already been discussed. Osteomyelitis secondary to peripheral vascular disease is important because of the fact that conditions such as diabetes fall in this category. The most common age group affected with osteomyelitis caused by peripheral vascular disease is the group aged 50 to 70 years. Osteomyelitis with concurrent vascular disease and diabetes usually develops from a localized infection or ulceration of the skin. Radiography of a patient with severe peripheral vascular disease may show very little destructive change except for osteopenia caused by poor perfusion to bone in general. Osteomyelitis can be difficult to differentiate from diabetic osteolysis and Charcot joint disease[16,17] (Figure 21-18).

Diabetic osteomyelitis is often associated with an ulcer or skin infection. Radiographs show soft tissue swelling present with or without gas or air in the tissue, depending on the type of organism present. Gas-producing organisms such as Clostridium and Bacteroides can lead to soft tissue necrosis and ultimately to gas gangrene. Obliteration of fascial planes is a radiographic sign of soft tissue swelling associated with

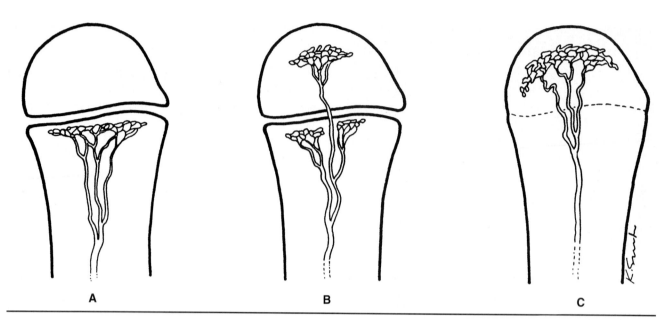

**Figure 21-16** Normal vascular patterns of a tubular bone in the child, infant, and the adult. **A**, In the child, the capillaries of the metaphysis turn sharply, without violating the open growth plate. **B**, In the infant, some metaphyseal vessels may penetrate the open growth plate, ramifying in the epiphysis. **C**, In the adult, with closure of the growth plate, a vascular connection between metaphysis and epiphysis can be recognized. (Courtesy Resnick D: *Diagnosis of bone and joint disorders*, Philadelphia, 1981, Saunders, p. 2048 [Figure 60-2].)

cellulitis. Osteolysis, periosteal new bone formation, cortical erosion, sequestrum, and involucrum can occur, as with exogenous osteomyelitis. Radiographic evaluation of osteomyelitis in the diabetic with underlying peripheral neuropathy and/or vascular disease can be confusing, because the radiographic features overlap (Figure 21-19). Furthermore, osteopmyelitis and neuropathic osteoarthropathy can easily coexist (Figure 21-20).

The radiographic picture of diabetic neuropathic osteoarthropathy has been widely described[16-19] and is discussed in Chapter 22. Nuclear medicine and MRI can play an important role in differentiating osteomyelitis from neuropathic (Charcot) joint disease and can be used if the question arises.

## ■ COMMON ORGANISMS CAUSING BONE INFECTION

Organisms most commonly causing acute hematogenous osteomyelitis usually stem from a single organism such as staphylococcus or streptococcus. In patients under 2 years old the most common organism from a hematogenous source causing osteomyelitis has been found to be *Haemophilus influenzae*. In young adults *Staphylococcus aureus* is considered the primary infecting organism, whereas in the elderly gram-negative rods are most commonly isolated.

*Pseudomonas aeruginosa* and methicillin-resistant staph are frequently found in the intravenous (IV) drug abuser.

Osteomyelitis secondary to contiguous soft tissue or by direct extension depends on the route of infection. For example, a puncture wound is most commonly affected by staph or pseudomonas, whereas an animal bite from a dog or a cat can cause an infection from *Pasteurella multocida*.

Diabetics tend to contract polymicrobial wound infections leading to osteomyelitis. Aerobes as well as anaerobes must be considered. The primary infecting organism is most commonly isolated by bone biopsy. A culture from the sinus tract or ulcer is usually affected with mixed flora and can be unreliable for proper diagnosis and treatment of the bone infection.[20]

Chronic osteomyelitis can be caused by many organisms, including bacteria, fungi, mycobacteria, and the spirochete *Treponema pallidum* (which causes syphilis). Osteomyelitis secondary to mycobacterial tuberculosis can be identified radiographically as well as clinically because of the chronicity of the disease. Clinically the patient has pain, stiffness, mild-to-moderate swelling, and erythema of the affected part. The soft tissues are affected by a granulomatous reaction leading to severe soft tissue destruction. The soft tissue destruction is characterized by mononuclear cell infiltrates, giant cell inflammatory infiltrates, fibroblast proliferation, mild edema, and small vessel congestion.[21,22]

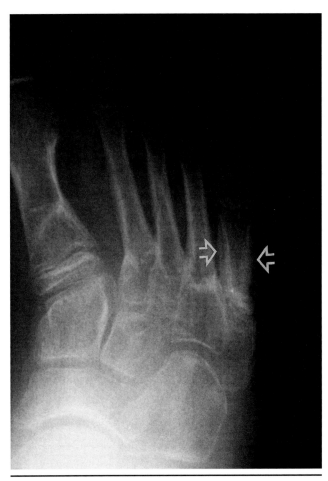

**Figure 21-17** Extensive periostitis in a child secondary to osteomyelitis. Patient is shown several weeks after base wedge osteotomies of the metatarsals. Note the extensive periosteal reaction along the medial and lateral shaft of the fifth metatarsal *(open arrows)*.

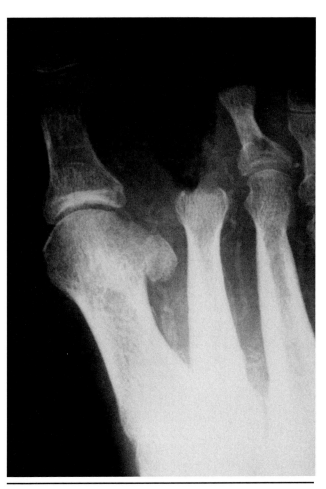

**Figure 21-18** Osteomyelitis versus neuropathic osteopathy, second-metatarsal head. This diabetic patient previously had amputation of the second toe because of severe vascular compromise. Erosion is now evident along the distal aspect of the metatarsal head. In most cases, diabetic osteopathy cannot be easily differentiated from osteomyelitis radiographically.

Radiographic findings of osteomyelitis secondary to mycobacterial tuberculosis include soft tissue changes early on followed by bone destruction. Bone destruction is usually evident, because of the chronic nature of the disease. Bone changes include subchondral osteoporosis followed by irregular areas of destruction with minimal marginal sclerosis. Periosteal reaction is characteristically minimal. Joint changes may occur, and spaces between joints may narrow. Damage to epiphyseal plates can cause growth abnormalities in children. Sequestrum is much less common with mycobacterial tuberculosis than in osteomyelitis from a bacterial origin.[23,24]

Fungal osteomyelitis may mimic bacterial or tuberculosis infection of bone both clinically and radiographically. Clinicians usually consider the possibility of a fungal infection of bone when a patient has not responded well to

antibiotic therapy for a bacterial infection or bacteria have been isolated from the bone culture.[22]

Syphilitic osteomyelitis can be either congenital or acquired with tertiary syphilis. In the fetus, the newborn, or young infant, bone destruction can develop. A syphilitic osteochondritis can occur, causing changes in endochondral ossification. This leads to broad, horizontal radiolucent bands on a radiograph. Metaphyseal abnormalities can appear, leading to epiphyseal separation. Diaphyseal osteomyelitis can appear in the untreated newborn or infant. Osteolytic lesions with bony eburnation and underlying periostitis are found in the diaphyseal bone. Periostitis can also be seen in congenital syphilis. It is diffuse, symmetric, and widespread.[1]

Acquired syphilis can cause bone destruction as well. The bone changes usually occur in the tertiary stage of the

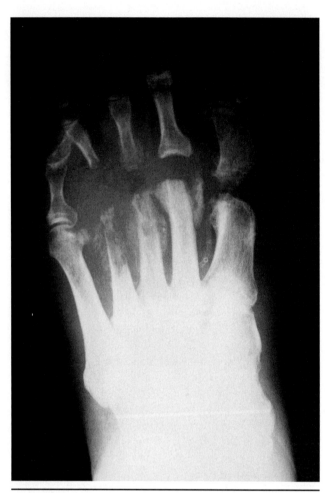

**Figure 21-19** A diabetic patient with severe peripheral vascular disease. In the proper clinical setting, soft tissue edema, rarefaction, osteolysis, erosion, and periosteal new bone production all suggest osteomyelitis.

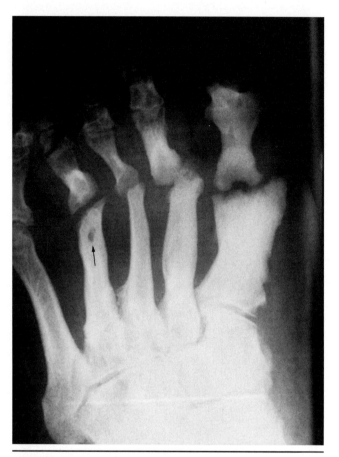

**Figure 21-20** Mixed long-standing osteomyelitis and neuropathic osteopathy in a diabetic patient. Exuberant remodeling is seen affecting the first four metatarsals and adjacent proximal phalanges. The geographic, lytic lesion surrounded by diffuse sclerosis in the fourth-metatarsal distal diaphysis is a bone (Brodie's) abscess *(arrow)*.

disease. Irregular cortical thickening may be present. The tibia and femur are the most commonly affected bones in the lower extremity. The irregular cortical thickening of the anterior tibia has been described as a "saber shin" appearance.[11] Periosteal reaction may be irregular or lacelike and show spicules radiating perpendicular to the shaft of the bone, mimicking osteogenic sarcoma.[1,11]

### ■ SPECIAL IMAGING MODALITIES

This section provides an overview of special imaging studies and their application to skeletal infection in the foot. Special imaging studies have been discussed in Chapters 16 and 17, and the reader is encouraged to refer to them for further information.

In cases showing a distinct bone and soft tissue infection or underlying neuropathic disease and/or postoperative

infection, radiographic evaluation can be difficult. Special imaging methods are extremely helpful in differentiating osteomyelitis from soft tissue infection, underlying neuropathic disease, or postoperative bone healing, which all may mimic osteomyelitis with soft tissue swelling, periosteal proliferation, erosion, or osteolysis. Radionucleotide techniques are now commonly used for the early detection of osteomyelitis. Also, CT and MRI are available to aid in the diagnosis of osteomyelitis. Radionucleotides that can be used for detecting osteomyelitis include technetium-99 ethylene diphosphonate (99mTc-MDP), gallium-67 citrate, and indium-111 (In-111).

Localization of Tc-99 is related to both osteoblastic activity and skeletal vascularity. A technetium bone scan can often be positive 24 hours after the onset of symptoms and 10 to 14 days before any radiographically visible changes have occurred.[25] A positive scan shows a well-defined, localized, increased uptake of Tc-99 in an area of inflammation or infection. Increased uptake of Tc-99 is referred to as a "hot spot." A hot spot shows an accumulation of radionucleotide in the affected region of bone. A positive bone scan does not prove that osteomyelitis is present, because Tc-99 uptake is relative to osteoblastic activity and therefore anything that causes increased osteoblastic activity produces a positive scan. Occasionally, 1 to 2 days after development of symptoms from infection a technetium scan may be normal or show an area of decreased uptake or a "cold spot" because the medullary microcirculation is compressed by intraosseous pus.[7] A cold spot shows up as a lack of radionucleotide accumulation in the affected bone area. The triphasic bone scan includes the angiogram, blood pool phase, and the actual bone scan. The angiogram is done within the first few minutes after injection and represents the radioisotope flowing through the vascular tree. The blood pool phase is performed approximately 2 to 4 hours after injection. The radioisotope is bound to portions of bone with increased osteoblastic activity at this time.[2] Triphasic bone scintigraphy cannot differentiate osteomyelitis from other causes of active bone remodeling such as recent fracture, neoplasm, loose prosthesis, septic arthritis, or diabetic osteoarthropathy.[26] For this reason, other nuclear scans have been used with technetium to help in making a diagnosis.

Gallium-67 scan is another modality that can be useful in detecting osteomyelitis. Gallium has several possible mechanisms of concentration in a lesion: granulocyte uptake, direct bacterial uptake, lactoferrin binding at the site of injection, or uptake of gallium in reactive bone.[25] Gallium was initially proposed as a bone-scanning agent, because it showed increased uptake in areas of increased bone turnover. Because gallium accumulated in leukocytes and bacteria uptake can occur in infected bone or with soft tissue infection, osteomyelitis cannot be differentiated by gallium scan alone. To improve the specificity of gallium imaging at the site of pre-existing skeletal disease, investigators have compared gallium scans with triphasic bone scans.[2,26] If a gallium scan is negative in light of a positive technetium scan, most likely no osteomyelitis is present. In cases of osteomyelitis, a gallium scan should show a local increase uptake that is equal to or greater than technetium uptake. A positive gallium scan in association with a negative technetium scan may suggest cellulitis. Gallium can be positive as early as 30 minutes after its injection in the presence of an active bone infection.[27] It is very useful in detecting soft tissue abscesses throughout the body. By showing a decreased uptake as infection improves, gallium can be used as a prognosticator in determining clinical response and termination of antibiosis in treatments of osteomyelitis. Gallium uptake was found to parallel the clinical course, with scans reverting to normal after successful antibiotic therapy.[27]

Indium-111 leukocyte imaging can be useful for detecting both acute and chronic osteomyelitis. However, it is much more reliable in acute osteomyelitis. To perform an indium scan, blood must be taken from the patient. Leukocytes that are separated from the whole blood are then labeled with In-111. The labeled leukocytes are then reinjected into the patient, and images are obtained at 2 to 4 hours and again at 24 hours after injection. The labeled cells aggregate at the site of infection because leukocytes respond in the act of healing. The main drawback to the use of In-111 is the more complex preparation, high cost, and relatively high radiation dose to the spleen.[25,28] Because leukocytes labeled with In-111 are not usually incorporated into areas of increased bone turnover, they are reported to be specific for infection in cases where osteomyelitis is superimposed on diseases that also cause increased bone turnover.[25,28] According to Seabold and associates,[26] combined technetium and indium scan imaging improves the specificity over indium alone. Indium-labeled WBC (white blood cell) scan is the best diagnostic technique to exclude the diagnosis of osteomyelitis. When differentiating a soft tissue infection from bone infection or postoperative infection, indium combined with technetium is more specific and permits a more reliable diagnosis. False positives have been reported, caused by early fractured callus, acute bone infarct, heterotrophic bone formation, inflammatory arthritis, and rare neoplasms. Also, indium localization has been reported in uninfected fractures for up to 3 months.[26]

Recently technetium has been used like indium-111 by labeling leukocytes to identify superficial and deep wound infection. Leukocytes have been labeled with Tc99m using hexamethylpropyleneamine oxine (HMPAO) or with exametazime. Tc99 HMPAO has been used, in a manner similar to that used with indium-111, to detect inflammatory change as well as an infectious process.[29,30] Tc-exametazime has also been used in detecting focal infection, abdominal abscesses, inflammatory bowel disease, osteomyelitis, sepsis, and pyrexia of unknown origin.[29] Tc99m-labeled leukocytes have some advantages over indium-111 in that Tc99 has a shorter half-life of six hours, compared with a 2.8-day half-life for indium. Technetium images are said to have better resolution, the process is less expensive, and the patient is exposed to less radiation.[30] Although Tc99m-labeled leukocytes appear to have many advantages, very little research has been done regarding this method for detecting osteomyelitis in the foot. Further research must be evaluated to justify this approach as an accurate diagnosis for osteomyelitis.

CT scans have a definite use in the diagnosis of osteomyelitis and can be used in conjunction with plain radiographs to evaluate patients both for acute and chronic osteomyelitis. CT scans show reliable detection or cortical destruction, periosteal proliferation, and soft tissue extension even when radiographs are normal.[31] It is a sensitive method to detect sequestrum. Sequestrum appears as isolated bony fragments completely separated from adjacent bone or as free fragments within the medullary cavity. The detection of a sequestrum is very important when planning surgical intervention. In chronic osteomyelitis the presence of sequestrum represents an active infection. CT scans are also useful to detect cortical defects leading to subcutaneous sinus tracts through which pus, granulation tissue, or sequestrum are excreted. Soft tissue defects in abscess formation can be seen on CT more readily than on plain radiographs.

Although CT scanning is a reliable indicator of osteomyelitis, in many institutions MRI has become a more standard test for osteomyelitis than are CT scans.[31] MRI represents the latest technological advance in the diagnosis of osteomyelitis. MRI gives more accurate, detailed information than do plain radiographs or CT.[25,28] It can detect signal alterations in soft tissue and determine the extent of disease in both bone and soft tissue. MRI is at least equal to if not better than CT scans in disclosing sinus tracts and associated soft tissue masses and in visualizing active foci of infection in osteomyelitis.

Radiographic follow-up of the treated patient is helpful. If antibiotic therapy is adequate in the acute phase of osteomyelitis, further destruction should be arrested. Clinical improvement usually precedes radiographic changes consistent with healing of the affected site. In a chronic case, after surgical debridement one can use radiographs to follow bone remodeling or to watch for signs of chronic osteomyelitis.

## References

1. Resnick D, Niwayama G: *Diagnosis of bone and joint disorders*, ed 2, Philadelphia, 1988, Saunders.
2. Christman R: The radiographic presentation of osteomyelitis in the foot, *Clin Podiatr Med Surg* 7(3):443-446, 1990.
3. Edeiken J: *Roentgen diagnosis of diseases of bone*, Baltimore, 1981, Williams & Wilkins.
4. Bravo AA, Bruskoff BL, Perner R: A review of osteomyelitis with case presentation, *J Am Podiatr Med Assoc* 75(2):83-89, 1985.
5. Bonakdapour A, Baines V: The radiology of osteomyelitis, *Orthop Clin North Am* 14(1):21-37, 1983.
6. Kehr LE, Zulli LP, McCarthy DJ.: Radiographic factors in osteomyelitis, *J Am Podiatr Assoc* 67(10):716-732, 1977.
7. Septimus EJ, Muscher DM: Osteomyelitis: recent clinical and laboratory aspects, *Orthop Clin North Am* 10(2):347-359, 1977.
8. Schneider R, Freidberger RH, Ghelman B et al: Radiologic evaluation of painful joint prosthesis, *Clin Orthop* 170:156-168, 1982.
9. Williams ML, Fleetor M: Radiographic evaluation of subacute osteomyelitis in children, *J Cur Podiatr Med* 39(6):81-13, 1990.
10. Chusid MS, Jacobs WM, Sty JR: Pseudomonas arthritis following puncture wounds of the foot, *J Pediatr* 94(3):429-431, 1979.
11. Greenfield GB: *Radiology of bone diseases*, ed 4, Philadelphia, 1986, Lippincott.
12. Trueta J: Three types of acute hematogenous osteomyelitis: a clinical and vascular study, *J Bone Joint Surg* 41(B):671-680, 1959.
13. Robbins SL, Cotran RS: *Pathologic basis of disease*, ed 2, pp 1477-1486, Philadelphia, 1979, Saunders.
14. Waldvogel FA, Vassey H: Osteomyelitis: the past decade, *N Engl J Med* 303(8):360-370, 1980.
15. Waldvogel FA, Medoff G, Swartz NM: Osteomyelitis: a review of clinical features, therapeutic considerations and unusual aspects, *N Engl J Med* 282:198, 1970.
16. Frykberg RG: Osteoarthropathy, *Clin Podiatr Med Surg* 4(2):351-359, 1987.
17. Kaschok TJ, Laine W: Radiology of the diabetic foot, *Clin Podiatr Med Surg* 5(4):849-857, 1988.
18. Kozak GO, Hoar Jr CS, Rowbothan JL et al: *Management of diabetic foot problems, Joslin Clinic & New England Deaconess Hospital*, Philadelphia, 1984, Saunders.
19. Levin ME, O'Neal LW: *The diabetic foot*, ed 4, St. Louis, 19884, Mosby.
20. Joseph WS: *Handbook of lower extremity infections*, New York, 1990, Churchill-Livingstone.
21. Schlossberg D: *Orthopedic infection: chronic infective arthritis*, pp 76-92, New York, 1988, Springer.
22. Waldvogel FA, Medoff G, Swartz MN: Osteomyelitis: clinical features, therapeutic considerations, and unusual aspects, pp 78-82, Springfield, Ill, 1971, Charles C Thomas.
23. Somerville FW, Wilkinson MC: *Girdlestone's tuberculosis of bone and joint*, ed 3, pp 152-159, New York, 1965, Oxford University Press.
24. Nielsen F, Helmeg O, de Caraulho A: Case Report 533, *Skeletal Radiol* 18:153-155, 1989.
25. Schauwecker DS, Park HM, Mock BH et al: Evaluation of complicating osteomyelitis with Tc-99m MDP, In-111 granulocytes, and Ga-67 citrate, *J Nucl Med* 25:849-853, 1984.
26. Seabold JE, Nepola JV, Conrad GR et al: Detection of osteomyelitis at fracture nonunion sites: comparison of two scintigraphic methods, *AJR* 152:1021-1027.
27. Visser HJ, Jacobs AM, Oloff L et al: The use of differential scintigraphy in the clinical diagnosis of osseous and soft tissue changes affecting the diabetic foot, *JFS* 23(11):74-85, 1984.

28. Schauwecker DS, Braunstein EM, Wheat JL: Diagnostic Imaging of osteomyelitis, *Infect Dis Clin North Am* 4(3):441-463, 1990.

29. Sampson CB, Solanki C, Barber RW: 99Tcm-exametazime-labeled leukocytes: effect of volume and concentration of exametazime or labeling efficiency: multi-dose radiolabeling, *Nucl Med Commun* 12:719-723, 1991.

30. Reynolds JH, Graham D, Smith FW: Imaging inflammation with 99Tcm HMPAO labeled leukocytes, *Clin Radiol* 42:195-198, 1990.

31. Wang A, Weinstein D, Greenfield L et al: MRI and diabetic foot infections, *Magn Reson Imaging* 8:805-809, 1990.

## Suggested Readings

Al-Sheikh W, Sfakianakis GN, Mnaymneh W et al: Subacute and chronic bone infections: diagnosis using In-111, Ga-67, and Tc-99m MDP bone scintigraphy, and radiography, *Radiology* 155:501-506, 1985.

Bamberger DM, Davis GP, Gerding DN: Osteomyelitis in the feet of diabetic patients, *Am J Med* 83:653-660, 1987.

Beltran J, McGhee RB, Shaffer PB et al: Experimental infections of the musculoskeletal systems: scintigraphy, *Radiology* 167:167-172, 1988.

Beltran J, Noto AM, McGhee RB et al: Infections of the musculoskeletal system: high field strength MR imaging, *Radiology* 164:449-454, 1987.

Buze BH, Hawkins RA, Marcus CS: Technetium-99m white blood cell imaging: false negative result in salmonella osteomyelitis associated with sickle cell disease, *Clin Nucl Med* 14:104-106, 1989.

Chandnani VP, Beltran J, Morris C et al: Acute experimental osteomyelitis and abscess: detection with MR imaging vs CT, *Radiology* 174:233-236, 1990.

Donohue TW, Kanat IO: Radionuclides: their use in osteomyelitis, *J Am Podiatr Med Assoc* 77(6):284-289.

Ewing R, Fainstein V, Musher D et al: Articular and skeletal infections caused by *Pasteurella multocida, South Med J* 73(10):1349-1352, 1980.

Gelfand MJ, Silberstein EB: Radionuclide imaging use in the diagnosis of osteomyelitis in children, *JAMA* 237:245-247, 1977.

Ingerman J, Abrutyn E: Osteomyelitis: a conceptual approach, *J Am Podiatr Med Assoc* 7(69):487-492, 1986.

Jacobs AM, Oloff LM: Osteomyelitis. In McGlamry ED (editor): *Comprehensive textbook of foot surgery*, vol 2, Baltimore, 1987, Williams and Wilkins.

Jacobson HG: Musculoskeletal applications of magnetic resonance imaging, *JAMA* 262(17):2420-2426, 1989.

Kinberg P: Osteomyelitis of an epiphyseal region, *JFS* 22(3):251-256, 1983.

Laitinen R, Tahtinen J, Lantto T, Vorne M: Tc99m labeled leukocytes in imaging of patients with suspected acute abdominal inflammation, *Clin Nucl Med* 15:597-602, 1990.

Lisbona R, Rosenthall L: Observations on the sequential use of 99MTC-phosphate complex and 67Ga imaging in osteomyelitis, cellulitis and septic arthritis, *Radiology* 123:123-129, 1977.

Mader JT, Calhoun JH: Long bone osteomyelitis: an overview, *JAMA* 79(10):476-481, 1989.

Mansor IA: Typhoid osteomyelitis of the calcaneus due to direct inoculation, *J Bone Joint Surg* 49A(4):732-734, 1967.

Miller ER, Semian DW: Gram negative osteomyelitis following puncture wounds of the foot, *J Bone Joint Surg* 57A(4):535-537, 1975.

Quinn SF, Murray W, Clark RZ et al: MR imaging of chronic osteomyelitis, *J Comput Assist Tomogr* 12(1):113-117, 1988.

Stone RA, Lehlman RA, Zeichner AM: Acute hematogenous osteomyelitis: a case report, *J Am Podiatr Assoc* 72(1):31-34, 1982.

Varzos P, Galinski A, Gelling WJ et al: Osteomyelitis associated with monofilament wire fixation, *JFS* 22(3):212-217, 1983.

Vorne M, Salo S, Anttolainen I et al: Septic *Haemophilus influenzae*. Polyarthritis demonstrated best with Tx-99m HMPAO labeled leukocytes, *Clin Nucl Med* 15:883-886, 1990.

Vorne M, Lanatto IS, Paakkinen S: Technetium 99m HMPAO labeled leukocytes in detection of inflammatory lesion: comparison with gallium-67 citrate, *J Nucl Med* 30:1332-1336, 1989.

Wheat J: Diagnostic strategies in osteomyelitis, *Am J Med* 78:218-224, 1985.

Wing VW, Jeffrey RB, Federle MP et al: Chronic osteomyelitis examined by CT, *Radiology* 171-174, 1985.

Yuh WT, Corson JD, Baraniewski HM et al: Osteomyelitis of the foot in diabetic patients: evaluation with plain film, 99m Tc-MDP bone scintigraphy, and MR imaging, *Am J Roentgen* 152:795-800, 1989.

Zeiger LS, Fox IM: Use of indium-111 labeled white blood cells in the diagnosis of diabetic foot infections, *JFS* 29(1):46-51, 1990.

22

# Joint Disease

## ROBERT A. CHRISTMAN

Several arthritides (types of arthritis) have a predilection for the foot (Box 22-1). Without question, osteoarthritis is the most common, primarily because of the mechanical wear and tear that weight-bearing activities place on cartilage. However, it is not unusual for the inflammatory rheumatic diseases (rheumatoid arthritis, psoriatic arthritis, ankylosing spondylitis, and Reiter's syndrome) to first appear or be diagnosed in the feet. Furthermore, gouty arthritis and diabetic neuropathic osteoarthropathy target have a predilection for the foot.

The archetypal radiographic presentations of joint disorders that have been described in the literature are not necessarily what the clinician encounters in everyday practice. The classic picture is typically the patient who was diagnosed with the joint disease many years or even decades ago. In contrast, the patient with acute symptomatology may initially come for help at the onset of disease or soon thereafter. In such a case, the radiographic findings are frequently subtle and nonspecific, the clinical findings are vague, and the diagnosis is often elusive. Furthermore, atypical cases are common. The challenge therefore is to identify the subtle, early radiographic findings, because the classic features of a particular joint disorder do not manifest until many years later. To maximize the detection of early arthritis, you "must know how to look, where to look, and what to look for."[1]

Then, along with the clinical and other laboratory findings, you must list and consider the probable differential diagnoses.

## ■ SYSTEMATIC APPROACH TO DIFFERENTIATING JOINT DISORDERS

A detailed, systematic approach for evaluating pedal joints entails three considerations[2] (Box 22-2). For obvious reasons, the symptomatic joint or joints are assessed first. The asymptomatic joints of both extremities should also be evaluated, for two reasons: Most joint disorders target both

---

**BOX 22-1  Joint Disorders Affecting the Foot**

Osteoarthritis
Rheumatoid arthritis
Psoriatic arthritis
Reiter's syndrome
Ankylosing spondylitis
Gouty arthritis
Neuropathic osteoarthropathy
Septic arthritis

---

**BOX 22-2  A Systematic Approach to Evaluating Joint Disease**

Roentgen features at or adjacent to involved joints
  Primary findings
    Osseous erosion
    New bone formation
    Joint space alteration
  Secondary findings
    Soft tissue edema
    Calcification
    Geographic rarefaction
    Alignment abnormalities
Roentgen features at sites distant from involved joints
  Erosion
  Enthesopathy
  Soft tissue mass
Patterns of joint disease according to distribution of roentgen findings
  Joints involved
    Targeted joints
      Bilateral versus unilateral
      Symmetry versus asymmetry
  Extra-articular sites involved

---

**BOX 22-3    Causes of Joint Disease**

Monoarticular
  Trauma
  Infection
  Crystal deposition
    Gout
    CPPD
  Rheumatoid monoarthritis
  Pigmented villonodular synovitis
Polyarticular
  Osteoarthritis
  Rheumatoid arthritis
  Seronegative arthritis
  Chronic tophaceous gout
  Neuropathic osteoarthropathy
  Pigmented villonodular synovitis (midfoot)
  Multiple reticulohistiocytosis

---

**BOX 22-4    Categories of Joint Disease (based on underlying pathology)**

Degenerative
  Osteoarthritis
Inflammatory
  Rheumatoid arthritis
  Seronegative arthritis
    Psoriatic arthritis
    Reiter's disease
    Ankylosing spondylitis
  Septic arthritis
Metabolic
  Gouty arthritis

---

**BOX 22-5    Categories of Joint Disease (based on radiographic features)**

Hypertrophic joint disease
  Osteoarthritis
  Detritus arthritis
    Post-traumatic arthritis
    Tarsus and midfoot neuropathic osteoarthropathy
Atrophic joint disease
  Rheumatoid arthritis
  Seronegative arthritis
    Psoriatic arthritis
    Ankylosing spondylitis
    Reiter's disease
  Septic arthritis
  Forefoot neuropathic osteoarthropathy
Associated with adjacent soft tissue mass and preservation of joint space
  Gouty arthritis
    Multiple reticulohistiocytosis
    Pigmented villonodular synovitis

---

extremities, and joints may be affected that are clinically asymptomatic. (Joint disease is one of the few conditions that warrants performing a bilateral radiographic study.) The examination doesn't stop here, however. Sites distant from involved joints, osseous and soft tissue are also considered. Abnormal findings at the calcaneal entheses and heel pain, for example, can be associated with joint disease. Finally, the distribution of radiographic findings must be assessed for specific patterns.[3] Many articular disorders demonstrate characteristic patterns of joint involvement that help distinguish one disease from another.

Articular disorders affecting the foot may involve one or multiple joints. Monoarticular joint disease is generally attributed to either trauma, infection, or acute gouty arthritis (Box 22-3). Less common causes of pedal monoarticular disease include rheumatoid monoarthritis and pigmented villonodular synovitis. Examples of polyarticular joint disorders affecting the foot include osteoarthritis, rheumatoid arthritis, seronegative arthritis (psoriatic arthritis, ankylosing spondylitis, and Reiter's syndrome), neuropathic osteoarthropathy, and chronic tophaceous gout.

Differentiation of joint disorders can be simplified by applying a general classification system to the presenting features. One categorization of arthritis has been based on underlying pathologic processes: degenerative, inflammatory, and metabolic[4] (Box 22-4). This classification, unfortunately, does not include neuropathic osteoarthropathy. In 1904, Goldthwaite used radiographic criteria to distinguish between osteoarthritis and rheumatoid arthritis.[5] These criteria can be expanded to include the remaining forms of pedal arthritis.

Joint disorders affecting the foot can be divided into two radiographic categories, based on the *predominant* radiographic feature: hypertrophic and atrophic (Box 22-5).

Hypertrophic joint disease features bone overgrowth and enlargement. The characteristic findings are subchondral sclerosis and osteophyte formation at the margin of a joint. Detritus arthritis, a subcategory of hypertrophic arthritis, includes those disorders that exhibit fragmentation in addition to exaggerated hypertrophic features. The loss of bone substance, primarily through erosion, and joint space narrowing, with or without periarticular osteoporosis, characterize the atrophic joint disorders. A subdivision of this group is commonly associated with an adjacent soft tissue mass clinically and the preservation of joint space. Forrester and Brown have used the term "lumpy-bumpy" joint disease to characterize this latter group.[4]

Neuropathic osteoarthropathy is divided into two subtypes: forefoot, and the combined midfoot and tarsus. Its radiographic features vary depending on location: Forefoot sites exhibit findings characteristic of atrophic joint disease;

the midfoot and tarsal sites display features of detritus (hypertrophic) arthritis.

Each of the roentgen features associated with joint disease is discussed individually in the following sections. Remember the radiographic categories of joint disorders; you can recognize associations between certain roentgen findings and arthritis categories, improving your diagnostic acumen.

## Roentgen Features at Involved Joints: Primary Findings

**Osseous erosion.**    Bone erosion is a primary feature of all joint disorders except hypertrophic joint disease. Generally speaking, erosion associated with active atrophic joint disease appears small, ill defined, and irregular (Figure 22-1). This characterization contrasts with the larger, well-defined C-shaped erosion classically seen in the disorders associated with an adjacent soft tissue mass (Figure 22-2). Erosion associated with gouty arthritis, however, is indistinguishable early in the disease process, but preservation of joint space and target involvement of the first metatarsophalangeal joint differentiate gouty arthritis from the other inflammatory rheumatic disease in the proper clinical setting. The presence of an erosion excludes osteoarthritis as a primary diagnosis; however, both a trauma-induced

subchondral bone defect and a subchondral bone cyst can mimic the appearance of an erosion (Figure 22-3).

Erosion is an early finding in the course of an inflammatory joint disease. The erosions are intra-articular and typically begin along the medial or lateral margins of the joint. Between where the cartilage ends and the joint capsule inserts is a bony surface covered only by periosteum or perichondrium.[3] This surface is in contact with the synovium and its fluid and is known as the "bare" area. The inflamed synovium, known as pannus, invades the bone; on a radiograph, the outer margin of subchondral bone quickly disappears. Initially this disappearance may be as subtle as a "dot-dash" appearance or "skipping" along the thin white line that comprises the subchondral bone plate (Figure 22-4). Eventually the localized loss of marginal bone (decreased density) progresses so far that the form of the affected bone appears abnormal. These findings may be recognized days or weeks after the onset of symptoms and contribute to the erosion's ill-defined and irregular appearance.

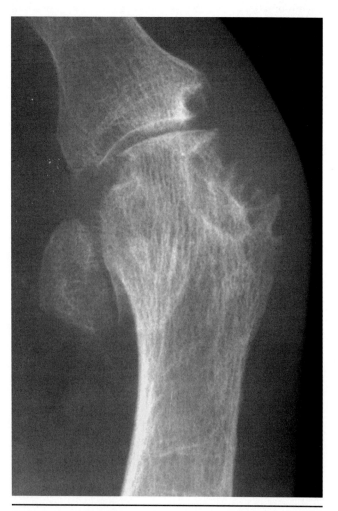

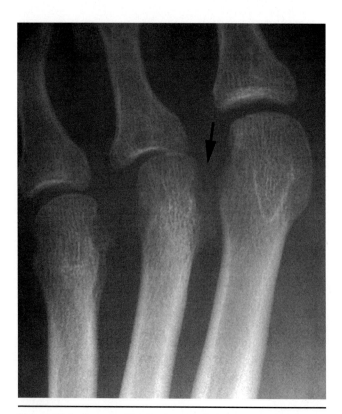

Figure 22-1    Irregular, ill-defined erosion (ankylosing spondylitis).

Figure 22-2    Well-defined, C-shaped erosion (gouty arthritis).

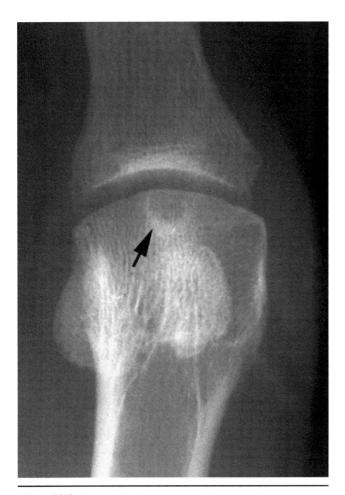

Figure 22-3   Subchondral bone cyst mimicking an erosion.

The well-defined erosion, in contrast, appears radiographically several months or years after the initial onset of symptoms. It frequently results from chronic pressure atrophy secondary to direct apposition of a soft tissue mass with concomitant infiltration and replacement of bone (see Figure 22-2). It may or may not be intra-articular in location. Or it may result months or years after an acute, ill-defined erosion remodels.

Erosions that involve both margins of any metatarsophalangeal or interphalangeal joint can result in a condition known as arthritis mutilans. Arthritis mutilans, also called *resorptive arthropathy*, is characterized by concentric bone resorption and primary joint destruction.[4] Bone resorption may even expand to include the nearby metadiaphyseal cortex. This has figuratively been described by several terms, most commonly the "pencil-in-cup" deformity. Other terms used to describe arthritis mutilans are listed in Box 22-6. This presentation has characteristically been associated with psoriatic arthritis (Figure 22-5). However, forefoot neuro-

---

**BOX 22-6** Arthritis Mutilans

Figurative terms
 Pencil-in-cup deformity
 Mortar and pestle
 Sucked candy stick
 Whittling
Differential diagnosis
 Psoriatic arthritis
 Forefoot neuropathic osteoarthropathy
 Rheumatoid arthritis (fifth metatarsophalangeal joint)

---

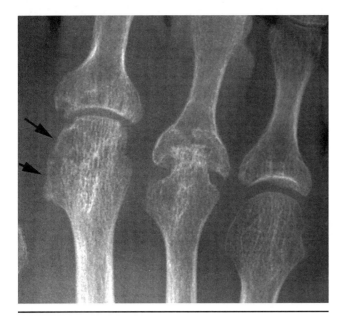

Figure 22-4   Early rheumatoid arthritis: Dot-dash or skip pattern.

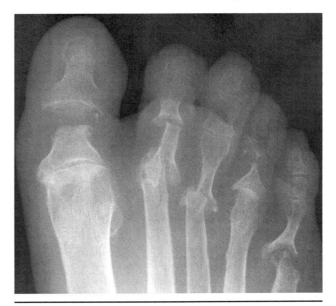

Figure 22-5   Arthritis mutilans: Psoriatic arthritis.

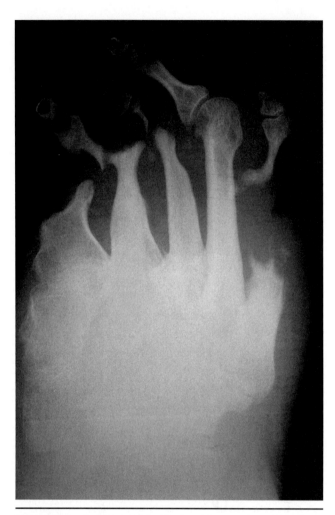

Figure 22-6    Arthritis mutilans: Neuropathic osteoarthropathy.

pathic osteoarthropathy and rheumatoid arthritis at the fifth metatarsophalangeal joint (Figures 22-6 and 22-7) present similar pictures.

**New bone formation.** The predominant feature of hypertrophic joint disease is bone production. Osteophytosis and subchondral sclerosis are characteristic radiographic findings. Bone production, however, can show other forms, including periostitis, whiskering, and cortical and trabecular thickening. This latter group of examples is not seen with hypertrophic joint disease but is frequently associated with seronegative arthritis. New bone production is rarely seen at joints affected by rheumatoid arthritis. An overhanging margin of new bone is frequently associated with the C-shaped erosions encountered with gouty arthritis. Box 22-7 lists the varying forms of bone production and associated joint disorders.

An osteophyte is a spur at the margin of a joint (Figure 22-8). It is a classic feature of osteoarthritis. Numerous figurative terms have been applied to this lesion, including

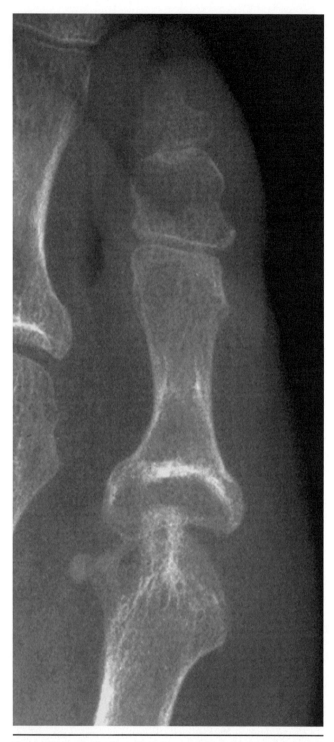

Figure 22-7    Arthritis mutilans: Rheumatoid arthritis (fifth-metatarsophalangeal joint).

*dorsal flag* (along the first-metatarsal head), *lipping* (if at both sides of the joint), and *beaking*.

Subchondral sclerosis is also referred to as eburnation (see Figure 22-8). It is, rarely, seen in the absence of joint space narrowing. Subchondral sclerosis represents bone

---

| BOX 22-7 | Forms of Bone Production and Associated Joint Disorders |
|---|---|

Osteophyte
   Osteoarthritis
Subchondral sclerosis
   Osteoarthritis
   Neuropathic osteoarthropathy (midfoot and tarsus)
Periostitis
   Seronegative arthritis
      Psoriatic
      Reiter's
   Septic arthritis
   Forefoot neuropathic osteoarthropathy
Overhanging margin (Martel's sign)
   Gouty arthritis
Whiskering
   Psoriatic arthritis
Ivory phalanx
   Psoriatic arthritis

production and is not a primary feature of the atrophic and soft tissue erosive joint disorders.

The presence of periostitis near the metaphysis of a symptomatic metatarsophalangeal or interphalangeal joint is highly suggestive of seronegative arthritis (Figure 22-9). Unfortunately the periostitis is short-lived: Within a few weeks it quickly remodels and become continuous with the bony margin. Periostitis may also be seen with septic arthritis and forefoot neuropathic osteoarthropathy. The latter disease is difficult to differentiate from infection.

A variation of periostitis seen particularly with psoriatic arthritis is referred to as "whiskering," because it resembles the stubble of new beard growth.[6] Its spiculated appearance radiates away from the bone margin, and it is characteristically seen at the hallux and, less frequently, the lesser-digit distal interphalangeal joints (Figure 22-10). Ill-defined sclerosis accompanies this finding. Whiskering appears to

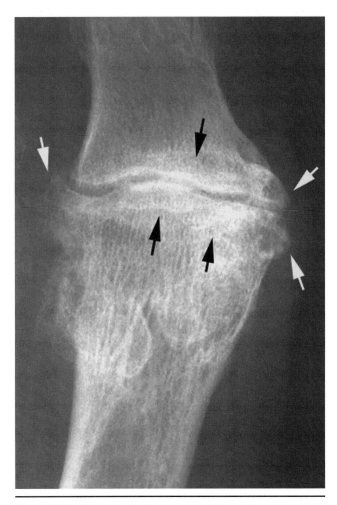

Figure 22-8   Osteoarthritis, first metatarsophalangeal joint. Osteophytes *(white arrows)* and subchondral sclerosis *(black arrows)*.

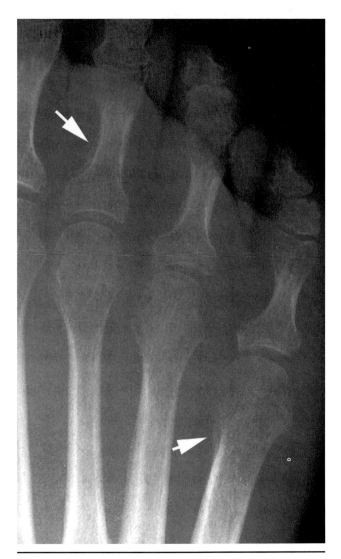

Figure 22-9   Psoriatic arthritis: Periostitis.

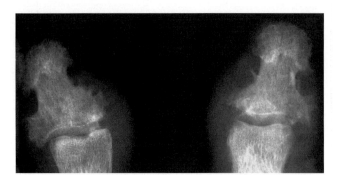

Figure 22-10    Psoriatic arthritis: Whiskering at hallux.

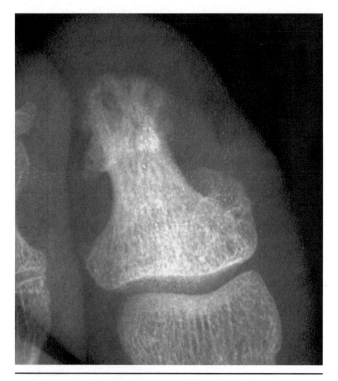

Figure 22-11    Psoriatic arthritis: Ivory phalanx.

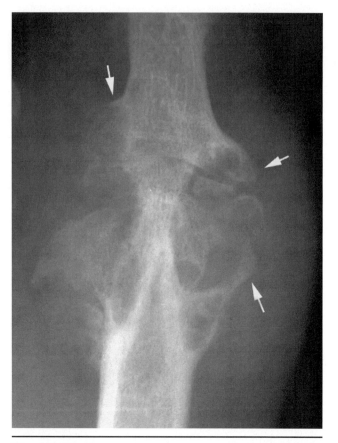

Figure 22-12    Gouty arthritis: Martel's sign.

From Kaye JJ: *Radiology* 177(3):601, 1990.

---

| BOX 22-8 | Grouping of Joint Disease Based on Joint Space Alteration |
| --- | --- |

| JOINT SPACE | ARTHRITIS |
| --- | --- |
| Nonuniform narrowing | Degenerative arthritis |
| Uniform narrowing | Inflammatory arthritis |
| Normal or near normal joint space | Miscellaneous arthritis |

---

represent concomitant new bone formation and erosion at the capsular and ligamentous entheses.

Occasionally the distal phalanx of an affected digit becomes quite dense or sclerotic relative to normal bone density. This is seen especially in the hallux (Figure 22-11). Known as the "ivory" phalanx, it is another presentation associated, in the proper clinical setting, with psoriatic arthritis.[7]

The well-defined erosions of gouty arthritis occasionally have an overhanging margin of new bone (Figure 22-12). This finding, described by Martel,[8] represents new bone production at the margin of an erosion. The body seems to be responding to the presence of the tophus and attempting to encapsulate it or wall it off. The overhanging margin of bone is not an uncommon finding. Its presence strongly suggests gouty arthritis. Another finding sometimes associated with the erosions of gouty arthritis is surrounding sclerosis.

**Joint space alteration.**    Normal, widened, or narrowed joint spaces may be seen with articular disorders. Kaye has correlated the types of joint space alteration with three groups of arthritides[9] (Box 22-8). This box, along with the remaining radiographic and clinical information, offers valuable information that can lead to diagnosis of the arthritis in question.

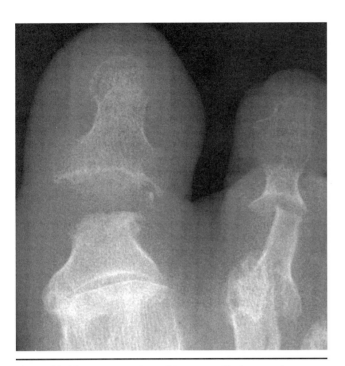

Figure 22-13   Psoriatic arthritis: Joint space widening secondary to erosion.

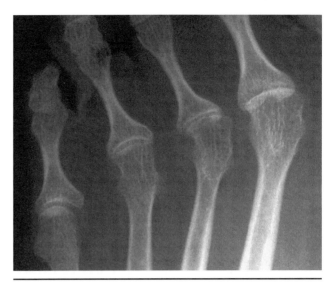

Figure 22-14   Rheumatoid arthritis: Even joint space narrowing.

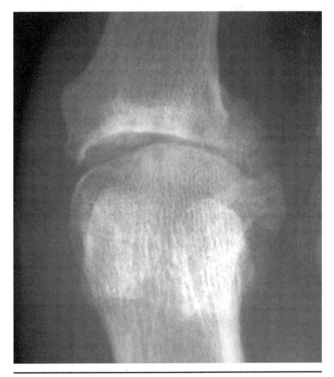

Figure 22-15   Osteoarthritis: Uneven joint space narrowing.

Excess fluid accumulates in a joint that is acutely inflamed. To accommodate this fluid, the capsule becomes stretched and the opposing bones are distracted. Radiographically this may appear as widening of the joint space. Unfortunately, joint space widening secondary to acute synovitis is a very subtle finding. Furthermore, the finding is short-lived; its radiographic presence is a hit-or-miss incident.

Extensive erosion of subchondral bone also gives the appearance of joint space widening (Figure 22-13). Erosion and subsequent fibrous tissue deposition between bones contribute to the widening seen in psoriatic arthritis.[2]

The joint space seen radiographically corresponds to the cartilage lining each bony surface. Erosion or lysis of the articular cartilage eventually appears as joint space narrowing, as the two opposing surfaces retract on one another. This is an early radiographic finding with inflammatory joint disorders such as rheumatoid or septic arthritis. Joint space narrowing may be either even or uneven. The narrowing seen with inflammatory arthritis usually is even or uniform across the joint (Figure 22-14). This is because inflammatory pannus is found throughout the joint and affects all cartilage. In contrast, osteoarthritis secondary to wear and tear or trauma usually only involves a segment of the cartilage or subchondral bone, not the entire surface. As a result, narrowing of the joint space has an uneven or nonuniform presentation radiographically (Figure 22-15). The unaffected joint segment has normal spacing.

The presence of a normal joint space associated with periarticular erosion is characteristic of joint disorders associated with soft tissue masses (Figure 22-16). Chronic tophaceous gout, for example, is not primarily an inflammatory disorder. Although intense inflammation is clinically seen with acute attacks of gout, these symptoms

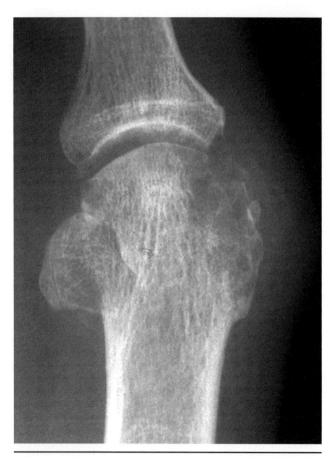

Figure 22-16   Gout: Sparing of joint space despite erosive disease.

last only a short period of time. Several years may lapse before radiographic evidence of joint disease is evident. Furthermore, many of the erosions associated with gouty arthritis are periarticular, outside the capsule. Therefore cartilage may not be directly involved until much later in the course of disease. As a result, the presence of normal joint space in light of obvious erosion is a characteristic finding. This is in strict contrast to inflammatory joint disease. The aggressive nature of this latter group of disorders and associated intense synovitis quite rapidly cause bone and cartilage destruction.

Bony or fibrous ankylosis may occur between two joint surfaces as an end stage of some joint diseases. This is especially true of the inflammatory joint disorders. Bony ankylosis is more commonly associated with seronegative arthritis and septic arthritis. The interphalangeal joints are targeted in psoriatic arthritis. Midfoot ankylosis may be seen in the rheumatoid foot (Figure 22-17). Ankylosis is seldom seen with gouty arthritis and is not associated with pedal osteoarthritis. However, the superimposition of osteophytes and joint space narrowing may simulate bony ankylosis.

## Roentgen Features at Involved Joints: Secondary Findings

**Soft tissue edema and masses.**    Soft tissue edema may be generalized throughout the foot, regional, or localized to a joint or other site. It is viewed radiographically as an increased soft tissue density and/or volume relative to normal expectation. Generalized soft tissue edema can be related to abnormal systemic conditions (cardiac disease, acromegaly), diffuse inflammatory states (cellulitis), or peripheral vascular disease (venous insufficiency, lymphedema).[4] It is not, however, a primary finding in joint disorders. Many patients with pedal joint disease have concomitant generalized soft tissue edema that is secondary to the conditions just noted.

Regional soft tissue edema is confined to a smaller segment of the body. An entire digit, for example, may be edematous from acute inflammatory conditions including infection, seronegative arthritis (the so-called sausage toe), and gout. The edema associated with an acute gouty attack at the first metatarsophalangeal joint may extend to the midfoot. This clinical presentation may certainly mimic an infectious process. Post-traumatic states also can show regional soft tissue edema. Neuropathic osteoarthropathy of the midfoot and tarsus shows either regional or diffuse edema.

Localized soft tissue edema may be related to synovial inflammation or to a mass. The edema associated with synovitis surrounds the joint and is quite well defined radiographically. Increased soft tissue density and volume secondary to synovitis is known as joint effusion. This condition, although nonspecific, is highly associated with inflammatory joint disease. However, synovitis secondary to trauma, either acute or chronic and repetitive, appears radiographically identical to that caused by inflammatory rheumatic disease (rheumatoid and seronegative arthritis). In acute attacks of gout, the edema is pronounced. It often mimics the diffuse edema associated with infection.

Periarticular soft tissue masses are associated with a few joint disorders. The most common example is the gouty tophus. Tophi are well-defined masses that are found adjacent to joints or at extra-articular sites (Figure 22-18). They occasionally exhibit calcification (see following discussion). Lesions are distributed asymmetrically in the foot.

Tophi may be seen several years after the initial onset of symptoms. They are a characteristic feature of chronic tophaceous gout and may or may not be associated with erosions; the latter develop adjacent to tophi. It has been reported that the clinical presence of tophi are strongly associated with the characteristic radiographic features of gouty arthritis.[10]

Another soft tissue erosive joint disorder is multiple reticulohistiocytosis. These masses radiographically appear similar to those seen in gout. However, masses associated

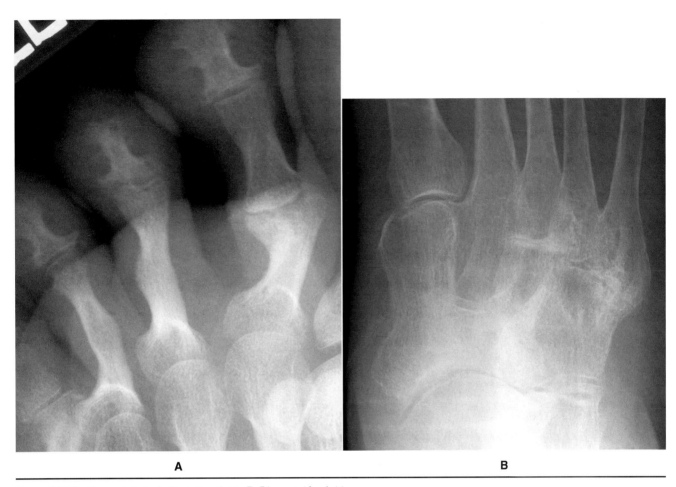

Figure 22-17    Bony ankylosis. **A,** Psoriatic arthritis. **B,** Rheumatoid arthritis.

with multiple reticulohistiocytosis are widespread, symmetric, and noncalcifying.

Soft tissue masses are occasionally seen with rheumatoid arthritis. Rheumatoid nodules are seldom found in the foot but, when present, may radiographically appear indistinguishable from a gouty tophus except that the former rarely calcifies.[11]

Soft tissue tumors and tumorlike lesions may manifest in periarticular locations and cause articular erosions. Although not common, an example of one such lesion occurring in the foot is pigmented villonodular synovitis. As a rule, it is monoarticular. However, a rare, polyarticular manifestation can appear in the midfoot (Figure 22-19). This is probably related to the unique synovial compartmentalization in this anatomic region. Well-defined erosions develop adjacent to soft tissue masses.

**Calcification.**    Numerous disorders are associated with soft tissue calcification in the foot. Widespread soft tissue calcification in otherwise normal tissues is associated with disorders that demonstrate elevated calcium or phosphate

levels in the serum. Hyperparathyroidism, for example, may cause diffuse periarticular, capsular, and vessel calcification. The majority of soft tissue calcifications seen in the foot, however, are probably dystrophic or idiopathic. Dystrophic calcifications occur in soft tissues that are damaged or altered but have no underlying disturbance in calcium or phosphorus metabolism.[12,13]

Soft tissue calcifications, when associated with joint disease, may be diagnostic for a group of disorders known as the crystal deposition diseases. They are monosodium urate crystal deposition disease (gouty arthritis), calcium pyrophosphate dihydrate (CPPD) deposition disease, and hydroxyapatite crystal deposition disease (HADD). Calcifications can be found in the periarticular tissues, joint capsule, or cartilage.

The crystals associated with gouty arthritis may be deposited in the joint capsule, synovium, cartilage, subchondral bone, or periarticular tissues.[14] A collection of monosodium urate crystals in the soft tissues is known as a tophus. In the foot, radiographic visualization of calcified crystals is best appreciated in the periarticular soft tissues.

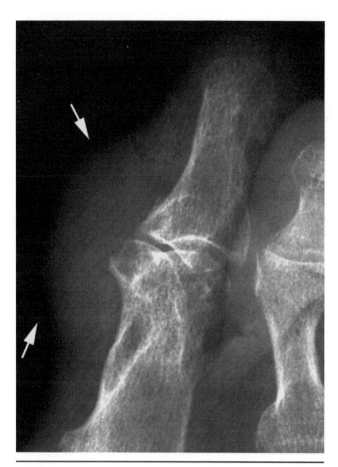

Figure 22-18   Gout: Tophus at hallux interphalangeal joint.

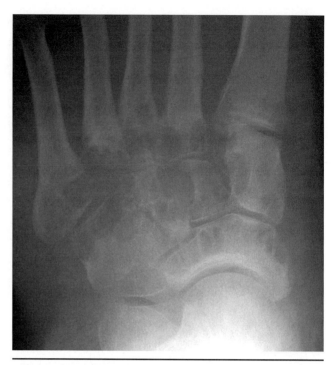

Figure 22-19   Pigmented villonodular synovitis, tarsus.

Tophus calcification is occasionally seen with tophaceous gout. Although not a pathognomonic finding, calcification of a periarticular soft tissue mass, especially if situated adjacent to an erosion, is highly suggestive of gouty arthritis in the proper clinical setting. Small, punctate calcifications can be identified in the soft tissue mass (Figure 22-20).

Calcium pyrophosphate dihydrate (CPPD) deposition disease is associated with several patterns of joint involvement.[15] In general, radiographic features include soft tissue calcification, joint space narrowing, subchondral sclerosis, and fragmentation. The latter findings are known as pyrophosphate arthropathy when associated with CPPD deposition. Calcifications can occur in articular and periarticular soft tissues. However, cartilage calcification, or chondrocalcinosis, has received the most attention. The primary crystal associated with chondrocalcinosis appears to be CPPD.

Little has been reported in the literature regarding pedal CPPD involvement. Perhaps this is because microscopic examination for crystals is not performed routinely for the workup of acutely symptomatic joints. However, the literature refers to metatarsophalangeal, tarsal, and ankle joint involvement.[16] Chondrocalcinosis is not readily recognized at the tarsal joints, because other bones are superimposed. Magnification radiography using high-detail industrial x-ray film may be necessary to see the subtle metatarsophalangeal joint calcifications.[17]

Calcification of periarticular structures, including tendons and bursae, is also seen with hydroxyapatite crystal deposition disease (HADD).[18] The clinical course may mimic the single-joint symptomatology seen with gout and pseudogout.[19] The radiographic presentation of HADD, also referred to as calcifying tendonitis, consists of round or oval calcifications within the course of a tendon.[20] Linear or punctate calcific densities may be seen along the margins of affected joints. Another presentation can be a rather large, amorphous calcification adjacent to a joint.

Calcifications and ossifications may be seen in the joint itself and are referred to as loose bodies. Loose osseous bodies ("joint mice") vary considerably in size and architecture. They are not uncommon in osteoarthritic joints (Figure 22-21). Trauma can cause osteophytes or subchondral bone with overlying cartilage to break off. These fragments of bone and/or cartilage can float or become wedged within the joint or synovium. Because many of these loose bodies contain cartilage, faint calcifications may be identified. They tend to enlarge over time. Large osseous bodies or fragments and concomitant severe hypertrophic joint disease in tarsal joints are suggestive of either post-traumatic arthritis or neuropathic osteoarthropathy (Figure 22-22).

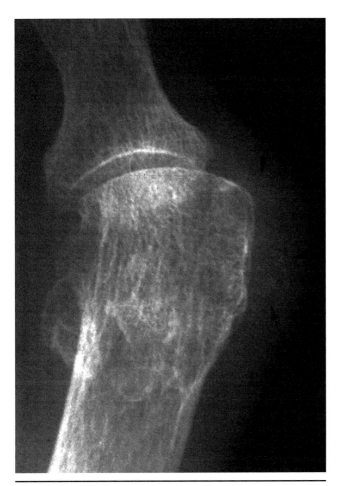

Figure 22-20    Gout: Calcified tophus.

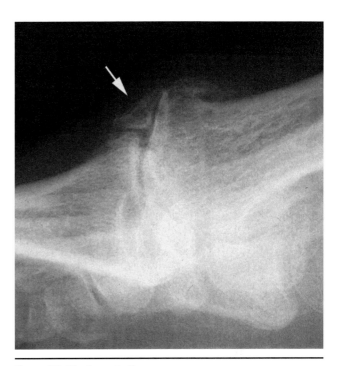

Figure 22-21    Loose bodies.

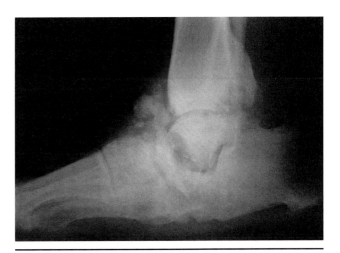

Figure 22-22    Detritus arthritis: Tarsal neuropathic osteoarthropathy.

**Geographic rarefaction.**    Subchondral bone cysts occasionally accompany arthritis. They appear as geographic, lytic lesions and may mimic erosions viewed en face. This is especially true along the medial aspect of the first-metatarsal head. The typical subchondral cyst with sclerotic margin is commonly associated with degenerative joint disease[21] (see Figures 22-3 and 22-15). Its pathogenesis is controversial; the two probable mechanisms are bone contusion[22] and synovial intrusion.[23] Subchondral cystic lesions have also been associated with rheumatoid arthritis (Figure 22-23). They have been referred to as pseudocysts. Their radiographic appearance is identical to the degenerative cyst but lacks a sclerotic margin.[17] The mechanism of formation is thought to be pannus invading the subchondral bone.[24]

Monosodium urate crystals, typically deposited in the soft tissues in patients with gout, may also be deposited in bone.[25] This deposition has been associated with chronic tophaceous gout. Multiple focal, geographic areas of bone loss (rarefaction) are seen at these sites (see Figure 22-16). I have observed in a retrospective study of a large group of

patients that localized rarefaction at the first metatarsophalangeal joint with the absence of erosion is frequently an early radiographic finding in gouty arthritis. The rarefaction is localized in the medial and superior aspects of the first-metatarsal head (Figure 22-24). Although this finding is nonspecific, in the proper clinical setting it suggests gouty arthritis.

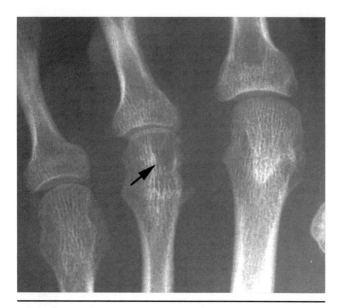

Figure 22-23    Rheumatoid arthritis: Pseudocyst.

**Alignment abnormalities.**    Positional deformities may be encountered with joint disorders. Abnormalities range from nonspecific misalignment of two bones to subluxation and dislocation.

A finding commonly associated with rheumatoid arthritis is fibular deviation of the digits, especially the hallux (Figure 22-25, *A*). This finding generally does not involve the fifth digit, however. The constraints of shoe gear probably prevent lateral deviation of this toe. Erosion may or may not accompany misalignment. Digital deviation in a fibular direction is not found in all instances of rheumatoid arthritis. Tibial deviation may also be encountered (Figure 22-25, *B*). It is important to note that hallux abductovalgus and lesser-toe deformities are nonspecific; these abnormalities are frequently seen in the absence of rheumatoid arthritis.

Subluxation and dislocation are frequently encountered in the rheumatoid forefoot. These changes especially affect the lesser metatarsophalangeal joints. The digits dislocate superiorly; superimposition of the proximal phalanx base on the metatarsal head may appear as ankylosis in the dorsoplantar view (Figure 22-26). Metatarsophalangeal joint dislocation is best appreciated with the lateral view, although it is difficult to visualize the joint structures because the adjacent osseous structures are superimposed.

Midfoot joint subluxation and dislocation are a characteristic feature of tarsal neuropathic osteoarthropathy. This change is especially noteworthy at the tarsometatarsal joints, although it can also occur at the intertarsal joints (Figure 22-27). The forefoot dislocates superolaterally relative to the rearfoot. Posterosuperior calcaneal displacement is noted when the talocalcaneal joint is involved.

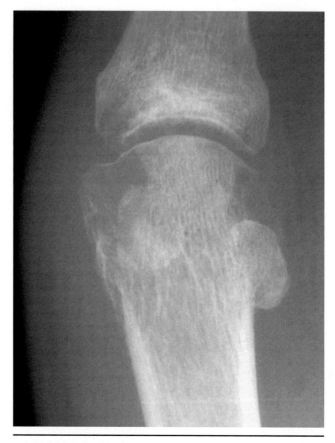

Figure 22-24    Early gout: Rarefaction first-metatarsal head.

Misalignment between two articular surfaces can result in cartilage damage and subsequent osteoarthritis. Examples include hallux abductovalgus and other medial column misalignments associated with pes planus and pes cavus.

Pes planovalgus is a frequent deformity in the rheumatoid arthritis midfoot. It is also seen with neuropathic osteoarthropathy. Alignment abnormalities are not commonly observed with seronegative and gouty arthritis.

## Roentgen Features at Sites Distant from Involved Joints

**Erosion.**    With rheumatoid and seronegative arthritis, erosions may also be found at sites distant from involved joints. The calcaneus is a common location. The site most frequently affected is the bursal projection (posterosuperior aspect). The retrocalcaneal bursa lays over this portion of bone. The bursa is lined by synovium, and the bursal projection is covered with cartilage.[26] The bursitis accompanying rheumatoid arthritis and the seronegative arthritides frequently causes rarefaction and erosion of the adjacent calcaneus (Figure 22-28). The erosion may be bounded by sclerosis in some instances. Retrocalcaneal

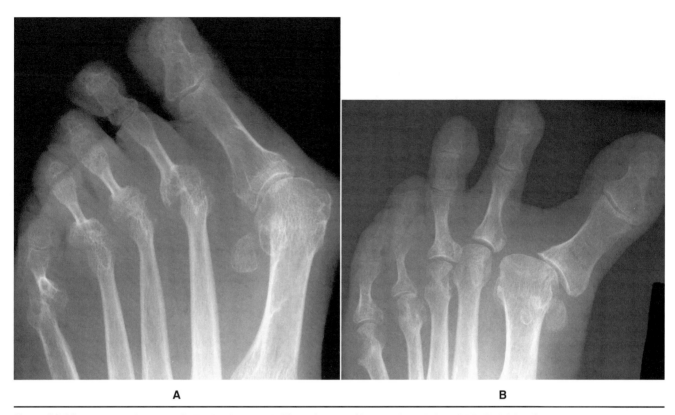

**Figure 22-25**    Rheumatoid arthritis. **A,** Fibular deviation. **B,** Tibial deviation. (Courtesy Irwin Juda, D.P.M., Philadelphia)

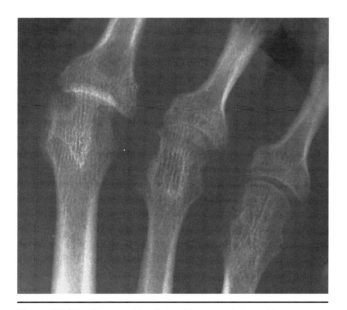

**Figure 22-26**    Rheumatoid arthritis: Metatarsophalangeal joint dislocation simulating ankylosis.

bursitis caused by local trauma or irritation should not in turn cause underlying bone pathology in the absence of infection or systemic inflammatory rheumatic disease. Erosion along the inferior surface of the medial tuberosity

can also be encountered. Rarely, calcaneal erosions are seen associated with gout.

Psoriatic arthritis can erode the hallux ungual tuberosity. This may be an isolated finding. The outline of the tuberosity appears irregular and sometimes spiculated (Figure 22-29). This finding alone is not pathognomonic for psoriatic arthritis: One variation of normal appears similar.

**Enthesopathy.**    Enthesopathy represents an alteration at any ligamentous or tendonous attachment to bone (that is, enthesis). It may present as spur formation, erosion, or a combination thereof. Enthesopathy has been associated with many joint disorders[27] (Box 22-9). Common sites of enthesopathy in the foot are the inferior calcaneal tuberosities and the posterior calcaneus. The fifth-metatarsal tuberosity is infrequently affected.

Inferior calcaneal spur formation associated with degenerative joint disease and rheumatoid arthritis is generally well defined. Degenerative spurs commonly are pointed and sometimes hook shaped. However, early spur development, regardless of etiology, may be ill defined. Calcaneal spur formation related to seronegative arthritis tends to be large and irregular. Ill-defined erosion and adjacent sclerosis frequently accompany these spurs (Figure 22-30). Inferior calcaneal spurs may be seen with gout. They are smaller and ill defined.

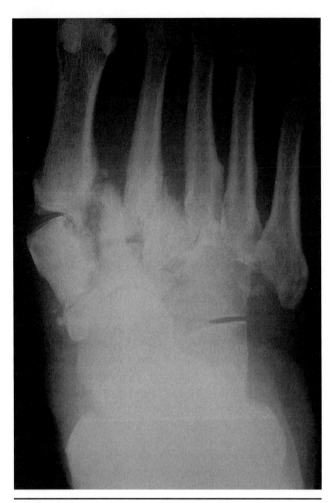

Figure 22-27    Neuropathic osteoarthropathy: Midfoot subluxation and dislocation.

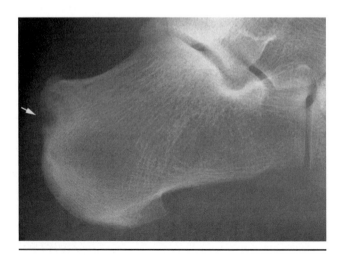

Figure 22-28    Rheumatoid arthritis: Enthesopathy.

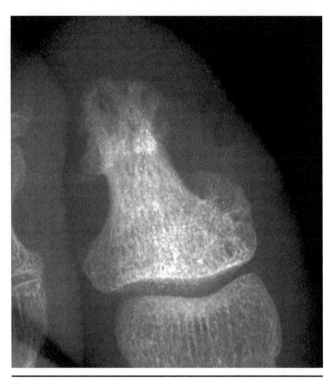

Figure 22-29    Psoriatic arthritis: Ungual tuberosity erosion.

---

**BOX 22-9    Differential Diagnosis of Enthesopathy in the Foot**

Trauma
Degenerative disease
   Osteoarthritis
   Diffuse idiopathic skeletal hyperostosis
Inflammatory joint disease
   Rheumatoid arthritis
   Seronegative arthritis
Crystal deposition disease
   CPPD (probable)
   HADD (probable)
   Gout (possible)
Endocrine disorders
   Diabetes mellitus

---

**Soft tissue mass.**    Gouty tophi may be found anywhere in the foot, not just intra- or periarticular. Rheumatoid nodules are rarely encountered in radiographs of the foot but could appear similarly at extra-articular sites.

## Patterns of Joint Disease and Distribution of Roentgen Findings

**Joints involved.**    Each of the joint disorders consistently target specific sites in the foot. Furthermore, joints may be

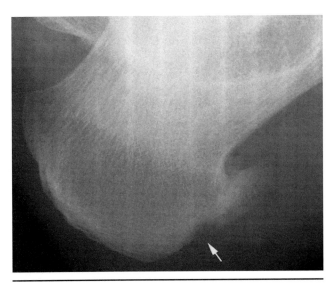

**Figure 22-30**    Rheumatoid arthritis: Enthesopathy—spur and erosion *(arrow)*.

involved that are clinically asymptomatic. Radiographs of both feet (dorsoplantar and lateral views, at a minimum) are needed to assess the pattern of joint disease and distribution of roentgen findings. Box 22-10 lists the primary joints targeted by the more common pedal disorders. The patterns of joint involvement and distribution of roentgen findings are discussed in more detail with the following characteristic descriptions of each joint disorder.

**Extra-articular sites involved.**    The calcaneus is not an uncommon site of involvement associated with joint disease. Both spur and erosion may be encountered at inferior and retrocalcaneal locations. For this reason, lateral views should always be included with dorsoplantar views of the feet when evaluating for joint disease. It is unusual to see erosions of the calcaneus unless they are associated with inflammatory rheumatic disease or infection. Occasionally an erosion may be encountered with gouty arthritis at an enthesis, adjacent to a tophus.

## ■ CHARACTERISTIC (AND UNCHARACTERISTIC) PRESENTATIONS

Table 22-1 summarizes and differentiates the characteristic radiographic features of joint disorders seen in the foot.

### Osteoarthritis

Osteoarthritis is by far the most frequently encountered pedal joint disorder. It is not just a disease of the elderly population; in the foot and ankle, regardless of age, it is

| BOX 22-10 | Target Joints |
|---|---|
| Osteoarthritis | First MPJ |
| Rheumatoid arthritis | All MPJs |
| Psoriatic arthritis | Lesser MPJs, hallux IPJ, DIPJs |
| Gout | First MPJ |
| Neuropathic osteoarthropathy | Tarsometatarsal and intertarsal joints |

*MPJ,* Metatarsophalangeal joint; *IPJ,* interphalangeal joint; *DIPJ,* distal interphalangeal joint.

more likely secondary to abnormal wear and tear to a particular joint (biomechanical abnormality, for example) or is post-traumatic.

The term *osteoarthritis* is misleading, because the disease is not primarily inflammatory in nature. It has also been referred to as *degenerative joint disease (DJD), degenerative arthritis,* and *osteoarthrosis.* The general term *degenerative joint disease* pertains to synovial and nonsynovial locations.[28] Osteoarthritis is degenerative joint disease at a synovial articulation. The disorder is one of chronic cartilage and subchondral bone deterioration; if inflammation is present, it is mild in severity and not a primary pathologic feature. Because the term *osteoarthritis* is widely accepted, I will use it in this discussion.

Another misnomer is use of the term *destructive* to denote a late-stage osteoarthritic joint. I distinguish the terms *destructive* and *degenerative* as follows: *Degenerative* implies a slow or chronic "wear and tear" process, whereas *destructive* reflects an aggressive, acute, and lytic process. Because the latter term may have different connotations, its use should be avoided.

Osteoarthritis targets joints along the medial column of the foot (Box 22-11). Its distribution is typically asymmetric, but it is not uncommon to see the same joint or joints affected in both feet; in the latter case the findings may not be symmetric in severity. It is unusual to see osteoarthritis at the remaining pedal joints unless related to previous trauma.

Osteoarthritis has been classified by its etiology as follows[29]: (1) abnormal concentration of force on normal articulation (for example, direct trauma, accumulation of repetitive microtrauma, misalignment) and (2) normal concentration of force on abnormal articulation (an underlying cartilage or subchondral bone abnormality, such as osteonecrosis).

Radiographic evidence of osteoarthritis typically takes years to develop. The characteristic features (Figure 22-31) include (collectively or individually):

1. *Osteophytosis.* An osteophyte is a bony outgrowth (spur) at the margin or margins of the affected joint. It frequently is an isolated finding but can present in

**TABLE 22-1**    "Classic" Presentation of Each Joint Disorder in the Foot

| | Target Joint(s) | Bone Production | Erosion | Joint Space | Soft Tissue Swelling | Soft Tissue Calcification/ Ossification | Positional Deformity | Bilateral Symmetry |
|---|---|---|---|---|---|---|---|---|
| Osteoarthritis | First MPJ | Osteophyte; subchodral sclerosis | None (subchondral bone cyst may mimic erosion) | Nonuniform narrowing | None | Loose osseous body ("joint mouse") | Associated with hallux abductovalgus | No (if post-traumatic) |
| Rheumatoid arthritis | Lesser MPJs and hallux IPJ | None | Medial aspects | Uniform narrowing | Not significant | None | Deviation of toes laterally; sublux/ luxation | Yes |
| Psoriatic arthritis | Lesser MPJs and IPJs; varies | Occasionally periostitis; whiskering and ivory phalanx | Medial/ lateral/ central | Widening (relative) | Diffuse; sausage toe | None | Nothing specific | No |
| Gouty arthritis | First MPJ | Overhanging edge (Martel's sign) | Medial (more common) and/or lateral margins | Normal | Lumpy-bumpy | Small, punctate calcifications | No | No |
| Neuropathic arthropathy (tarsus) | Tarsal-metatarsal joints | Diffuse Sclerosis | Subchondral resorption | Narrowing or relative widening | Diffuse | Fragmentation of bone | Subluxation/ dislocation | No |

**BOX 22-11**    **Target Joints: Osteoarthritis**

Hallux interphalangeal
First metatarsophalangeal
First and second metatarsocuneiform
Naviculocuneiform
Talonavicular

combination with any or all of the following four findings, especially in more severe cases.

2. *Joint space narrowing.* The joint space narrowing typically is uneven (or nonuniform). Narrowing occurs at the focus of the applied abnormal force or at the site of cartilage or subchondral bone abnormality; however, uniform narrowing may be seen if the entire cartilaginous surface is affected.

3. *Subchondral sclerosis (also called eburnation).* This finding is represented by periarticular increased bone density. Subchondral sclerosis is frequently found adjacent to the site of joint space narrowing. In more severe cases, its appearance is diffuse.

4. *Subchondral cyst formation.* A subchondral (or "degenerative") cyst is a geographic, radiolucent lesion frequently associated with the osteoarthritic joint. It characteristically has a thin, sclerotic margin. The location of this lesion at the margin of a bone may be mistaken for an erosion; however, erosion is not a characteristic feature of osteoarthritis and its presence suggests an underlying inflammatory condition.

5. *Loose osseous body (or "joint mouse").* The loose body appears as a bone fragment or ossicle within the joint or along its margins. It more than likely is related to a traumatic event, which the patient may not ever recall; it could be an osteochondral bone fragment that initiates osteoarthritis (a subchondral defect may be identified) or can represent a fractured osteophyte in an already existing osteoarthritic joint.

**Interphalangeal joints.** Unlike the hands, osteoarthritis seldom affects the interphalangeal joints of the lesser toes. Joint space narrowing and osteophyte formation are the usual findings; however, joint space narrowing is difficult to ascertain in most cases, because of digital contracture. Furthermore, the tubercles along the margins of the phalangeal bases may appear as osteophytes, because of the adductovarus position of the toe.

Hallucal interphalangeal osteoarthritis is frequently post-traumatic in nature and affects the medial aspect of this joint; radiographic findings generally are limited to irregular joint space narrowing. Loose osseous bodies and small subchondral cysts are occasionally associated with osteoarthritis at this site.

**First-metatarsophalangeal joint.**  The first metatarso-phalangeal joint is by far the most commonly affected pedal joint and may demonstrate few or all of the classic roentgenographic features of osteoarthritis (see Figure 22-31).

Mild osteoarthritis typically features an osteophyte, small or large, but with only minimal uneven joint space narrowing. Osteophytes, typically found at the margins of the first-metatarsal head, may also present along the adjacent proximal phalangeal base. Osteophytes may be seen in several locations: superiorly in the lateral view, laterally in the dorsoplantar view, dorsomedially in the medial oblique view, or dorsolaterally in the lateral oblique view. A larger superior osteophyte may be associated with medial enlargement of the metatarsal head. Joint space narrowing is best appreciated in the dorsoplantar view. Loose osseous bodies are more commonly associated with severe osteo-arthritis but also can be seen in mild disease. They typically present superiorly and are therefore best visualized in the lateral view. An osteochondral defect is infrequently seen centrally in the first-metatarsal head.

Mild to moderate osteoarthritis demonstrates progressive joint space narrowing and osteophytosis in varying degrees. Loose osseous bodies are also more frequent. Mild sub-chondral sclerosis may become evident. A well-defined, increased density is normally present along the hallux proximal phalanx base centrally and may be mistaken for eburnation. The eburnation associated with osteoarthritis is typically ill defined and diffuse in appearance. Osteo-chondral defects and/or subchondral cyst formation are infrequent but may appear exaggerated relative to the other radiographic findings.

Significant joint space narrowing, osteophytosis, and eburnation are seen with moderate to severe osteoarthritis. Subchondral cyst formation, at either side of the joint or within the hypertrophied medial eminence, is also frequent.

Gross joint deformity is seen in severe osteoarthritis. The first-metatarsal head and proximal phalanx base are hyper-trophied both medially and laterally. Subchondral sclerosis is diffuse, and subchondral lucent lesions and loose osseous bodies are predominant.

Metatarsosesamoid osteoarthritis is not uncommon and is best visualized in the sesamoid axial view. Irregular joint space narrowing and small osteophytes may be seen. Similar findings may be seen in the lateral view but are unlikely, because numerous osseous structures are superimposed.

**Lesser metatarsophalangeal joints.**  Lesser meta-tarsophalangeal joint osteoarthritis is generally not seen

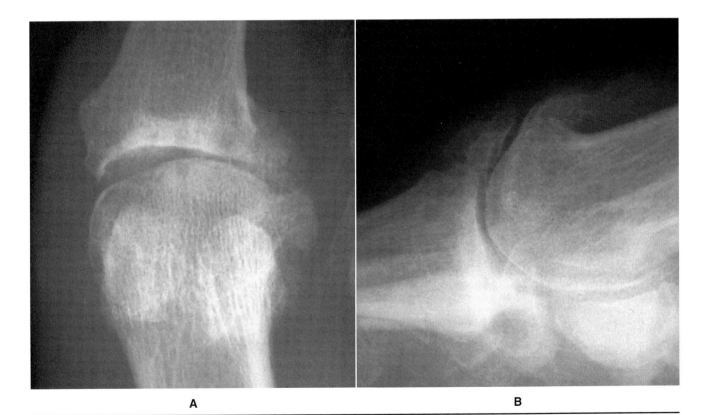

|          A          |          B          |

Figure 22-31   Osteoarthritis, first metatarsophalangeal joint. **A**, Dorsoplantar view. **B**, Lateral view.

unless the patient has had epiphyseal osteonecrosis (Freiberg's disease) or a history of injury to the joint. Gross deformity of the metatarsal head and proximal phalangeal base are predominant findings.

### Metatarsocuneiform joints.

Osteophytosis, subchondral sclerosis, and joint space narrowing can be visualized in both the dorsoplantar and lateral views. Osteoarthritis of the first metatarsocuneiform joint is frequently associated with osteoarthritis of the second metatarsocuneiform joint; however, the converse is not.

Osteoarthritis of the second metatarsocuneiform joint is best identified in the lateral view. The primary finding is superior bone hypertrophy (osteophytosis); lack of visualization of a joint space and subchondral sclerosis may also be apparent. Joint disease is not easily visualized in the dorsoplantar or medial oblique views unless the arthritis is severe.

Osteoarthritis of the third metatarsocuneiform joint is not frequently encountered. When present, joint space irregularity and eburnation are best noted in the medial oblique and lateral views.

### Naviculocuneiform joints.

Osteoarthritis of the medial naviculocuneiform joint primarily consists of joint space irregularity and subchondral sclerosis, with or without mild osteophytosis. These findings are best seen in the dorsoplantar view, although joint space narrowing can also be seen along the inferior aspect of this joint in the lateral view.

Intermediate naviculocuneiform osteoarthritis is best visualized in the lateral view and is characterized by dorsal osteophytosis, joint margin irregularity, and eburnation. Similar findings may be seen in the medial oblique view; the dorsoplantar view seldom is useful for assessment at this location. Intermediate naviculocuneiform osteoarthritis is frequently associated with osteoarthritis of the second metatarsocuneiform and medial naviculocuneiform joint.

### Talonavicular joint.

Talonavicular joint osteoarthritis is best appreciated in the lateral view. Radiographic findings vary from large osteophyte formation superiorly with normal joint space to significant joint narrowing with subchondral sclerosis. It is not uncommon to see an osteochondral defect along the navicular's posterior articular surface associated with osteoarthritis at the talonavicular joint.

### Calcaneocuboid joint.

Osteoarthritis is seldom seen at the calcaneocuboid joint. The typical finding, when present, includes an enlarged, hooklike exostosis laterally, originating from the calcaneus, seen primarily in the dorsoplantar view; the joint space is relatively spared, and the lateral view appears normal. When more pronounced, eburnation and joint space narrowing can also be seen in both the dorsoplantar, medial oblique, and lateral views.

### Talocalcaneal joint.

The middle and posterior talocalcaneal joints are not easily visualized with plain films, and osteoarthritis is not common. However, posterior talocalcaneal osteoarthritis may be recognized in the medial oblique and lateral ankle views by joint space narrowing and osteophyte production, and less frequently with calcaneal axial views at varying degrees of tubehead angulation.

### Ankle joint.

Ankle osteoarthritis is nearly always associated with a previous history of fracture or significant ankle trauma. In contrast, the painful ankle in a geriatric patient with no prior history of trauma seldom demonstrates radiographic evidence of osteoarthritis, or mild at best. Post-traumatic ankle arthritis demonstrates varied radiographic features, depending on the type of injury and its extent. Findings may include osteophytosis (best seen in the lateral view), uneven joint space narrowing, subchondral sclerosis, and subchondral lucency (related either to the fracture site itself, an osteochondral defect, or degenerative cyst formation).

## Rheumatoid Arthritis

Rheumatoid arthritis targets synovial tissue, especially of the feet and hands. The acute synovitis and associated pannus results in lysis of intra-articular structures, including cartilage and subchondral bone. Capsular and ligamentous laxity also occurs. Clinically the onset is insidious, and its course demonstrates periods of remission and exacerbation. The majority of these patients are seropositive for rheumatoid factor.

The appearance of early rheumatoid arthritis differs from its well-established form. The latter classically involves all metatarsophalangeal joints bilaterally and occasionally the hallux interphalangeal joints. In contrast, early rheumatoid arthritis of the foot is often monoarticular or polyarticular but asymmetric. The fifth metatarsophalangeal joint is frequently the first joint affected. Findings at the first metatarsophalangeal joint are generally subtle or unremarkable. Although rheumatoid arthritis may involve the tarsal, especially the subtalar, joints, early recognition is difficult with plain films. Computed tomography may be necessary for further evaluation of these joints. Unlike the situation with hands, it is rare to see involvement of the lesser-toe proximal interphalangeal joints.

The radiographic features of rheumatoid arthritis include the following:

1. *Erosion.* Erosions typically are seen along the medial side of affected forefoot joints; lateral involvement is infrequent except at the fifth metatarsophalangeal joint, which is common. Erosion may also be seen along the posterosuperior aspect of the calcaneus in the lateral

view adjacent to the retrocalcaneal bursal recess. It is not unusual to see erosion along the inferior aspect of the calcaneal medial tuberosity, with or without adjacent spur formation.

2. *Joint space narrowing.* This early feature of an affected joint often is evenly distributed (or uniform) across the joint. However, mild subluxation can occur simultaneously, giving the appearance of uneven narrowing.

3. *Osteopenia.* This term refers to generalized radiolucency of bones. Objective features that can be recognized include thinning of cortexes, intracortical tunneling, and prominence of primary trabeculations standing out in relief. Osteopenia is a characteristic finding of rheumatoid arthritis in association with erosion and joint space narrowing; but osteopenia found alone is a nonspecific finding.

4. *Digital misalignment and joint subluxation/dislocation.* All toes (except the fifth) generally deviate in a fibular direction relative to the metatarsals; however, do not be surprised to see deviation in a tibial direction. As the disease progresses, the proximal phalangeal bases may only partially appose their respective metatarsal heads (subluxation) and can further result in dislocation (0% apposition).

5. *Cyst (or pseudocyst).* Geographic, subchondral radiolucent lesions occasionally are seen centrally at affected joints.

6. *Ankylosis.* In the later stages of rheumatoid arthritis, the joint space may disappear entirely and the two bones appear united as one. Ankylosis appears more frequently in the tarsus but can also affect the first ray.

**Classic forefoot rheumatoid arthritis.**    The classic radiographic picture of pedal rheumatoid arthritis is bilateral and symmetric (Figure 22-32): medial erosions at the first through fourth metatarsophalangeal and the hallux interphalangeal joints, and medial and lateral erosion at the fifth metatarsophalangeal joint; fibular deviation of the toes (with the exception of the fifth toe) at the metatarsophalangeal joints; uniform joint space narrowing at affected joints, but subluxation and/or dislocation prevents this from being visualized in many cases; and osteopenia.

**Metatarsophalangeal joints.**    Initial findings in early rheumatoid arthritis may present as monoarticular or oligoarticular and unilateral. Erosion is frequently identified early in the disease at the fifth metatarsophalangeal joint. Or, only two or three metatarsophalangeal joints may be affected. Asymmetric, bilateral joint involvement is also seen. Figures show many different early presentations.

The erosions of rheumatoid arthritis tend to target the medial margins of the metatarsophalangeal joints. Tenosynovitis, ligamentous laxity, and resultant fibular

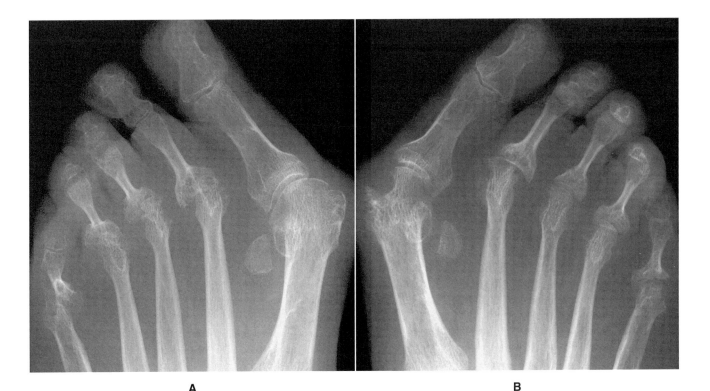

|                                  A                                  |                                  B                                  |

Figure 22-32    Rheumatoid arthritis. **A,** Left foot. **B,** Right foot.

deviation of digits associated with this disease leave the medial margins of the joints unprotected from the destructive pannus; it is believed that this accounts for the medial erosions.[28] However, one of the earliest sites for erosion in the rheumatoid foot is the lateral aspect of the fifth-metatarsal head. The fifth digit usually does not deviate laterally, because of the constraints within the shoe. This may allow equal distribution of the pannus along both margins. Marginal erosions eventually progress to involve the entire subchondral surface.

Bursitis is a characteristic clinical feature of rheumatoid arthritis. It is interesting to note that several small bursae are found adjacent to all metatarsal heads: Subcutaneous bursae are found along the dorsomedial and dorsolateral aspects of the first- and fifth-metatarsal heads, respectively; subfascial synovial bursae are located between the medial collateral ligaments of the lesser-metatarsal heads and the interosseous tendons; another bursa is found between the abductor tendon and the fifth-metatarsal head.[30] Coexisting bursitis may contribute to the specific marginal erosions.

**Hallux interphalangeal joint.** Erosions, when found at the hallux interphalangeal joint, are typically along the medial aspect. It is not an isolated finding and usually appears in association with metatarsophalangeal joint involvement.

**Tarsometatarsal and intertarsal joints.** Occasionally the tarsometatarsal and intertarsal joints are afflicted, frequently without associated forefoot involvement. Typical radiographic features are even joint space narrowing and, occasionally, large geographic lucent lesions or pseudocysts. Eventually ankylosis results (see Figure 22-17, *B*). Subchondral sclerosis and osteophytosis may be a secondary finding (that is, secondary osteoarthritis). To recognize involvement of the talocalcaneal joints, cross-sectional imaging studies may be necessary.

**Ankle joint.** Radiographic findings are often nonspecific at the ankle joint. Increased soft tissue density and volume at the ankle (joint effusion) may be the only feature. Eventually even joint space narrowing and irregular subchondral surfaces are recognized. Secondary osteoarthritis, including subchondral sclerosis and osteophytes, frequently accompany these findings.

**Calcaneal bursal projection.** Retrocalcaneal bursitis is often associated with rheumatoid arthritis. Radiographically, erosion may be seen along the posterosuperior aspect of the calcaneus adjacent to this bursa (see Figure 22-28). As time progresses, sclerosis is seen at the margins of the erosion.

## Psoriatic arthritis

Psoriatic arthritis affects all forefoot joints, that is, metatarsophalangeal and interphalangeal. Pathologically, synovial involvement is similar to rheumatoid arthritis but is not as intense. The presence of psoriatic arthritis is frequently associated with psoriatic skin and/or nail involvement.[31] Most of these patients are seronegative for rheumatoid factor but show strong association with the HLA-B27 antigen.[32] Psoriatic arthritis has several different clinical features that may overlap[33] (Box 22-12); features selective for the foot are discussed in more detail next.

Characteristic radiographic features vary but include the following:

1. *Bone proliferation.* Several forms of new bone production may be seen with psoriatic arthritis, including whiskering, "ivory phalanx," and periostitis. Whiskering and the ivory phalanx typically affect the hallux distal phalanx; whiskering appears as small spicules of bone arising perpendicular from the phalanx shaft, and ivory phalanx appears as overall increased density of the phalanx. Periosteal new bone production is seen adjacent to affected metatarsophalangeal joints.

2. *Erosion.* Loss of the marginal subchondral bone plate may appear no different from that seen in rheumatoid arthritis. In contrast to rheumatoid arthritis, however, erosions frequently affect the medial and lateral margins of the metatarsophalangeal and hallux interphalangeal joints. Erosion can also occur centrally within the joint and can be quite destructive visually, leading to joint space widening of interphalangeal joints or arthritis mutilans of metatarsophalangeal joints (see item 5).

3. *Joint space widening.* Central joint erosion especially affects the interphalangeal joints and results in a relative widening of the joint space. Aggressive erosion along the medial and lateral aspects of a metatarsal head also results in apparent joint space widening (see discussion of arthritis mutilans, item 5).

---

| **BOX 22-12** | **Clinical Presentations of Psoriatic Arthritis** |
|---|---|

1. Polyarticular DIPJ involvement ("classic" psoriatic arthritis)
2. Osteolysis (arthritis mutilans) (associated with sacroiliitis)
3. Symmetric MPJ involvement (similar to rheumatoid arthritis)
4. Asymmetric MPJ and IPJ involvement with associated swelling ("sausage toe"); the most common presentation
5. Spondylitis

*DIPJ*, Distal interphalangeal joint; *MPJ*, metatarsophalangeal joint; *IPJ*, interphalangeal joint.

4. *Joint space narrowing.* Narrowing of joint spaces is more frequently seen early in the disease at the metatarsophalangeal joints.

5. *Arthritis mutilans.* Excessive bone erosion along both the medial and lateral margins of a metatarsophalangeal joint can result in an appearance that has frequently been described by the following figurative terminology: *pencil-in-cup deformity, mortar-in-pestle, sucked candy,* and *whittling.* Severe osteolysis mutilates the joint, thus the term *arthritis mutilans.*

**Lesser-toe distal interphalangeal joints.** Psoriatic arthritis may target the lesser-digit distal interphalangeal joints (Figure 22-33). It can affect one or multiple joints. Findings include erosion at the margins of the joint, progressing to osteolysis of the entire articular surface(s). Adjacent sclerosis may accompany the erosion.

**Hallux distal phalanx and interphalangeal joint.** The hallux distal phalanx and interphalangeal joint are common sites of involvement. Erosions, frequently accompanied with new bone production, present along the medial and lateral aspects of the joint (Figure 22-34). This helps to differentiate psoriatic from rheumatoid arthritis; the latter generally affects only the medial aspect of this joint.[34] Furthermore, rheumatoid arthritis rarely has new bone production associated with hallux interphalangeal joint erosions. New bone production (whiskering and the ivory phalanx) frequently accompanies hallucal psoriatic arthritis (see Figure 22-10). Ungual tuberosity erosion may be an isolated radiographic finding (Figure 22-35).

**Ray involvement.** Another presentation of psoriatic arthritis targets the joints of an entire ray. The metatarsophalangeal and proximal and distal interphalangeal joints are affected (Figure 22-36). This is commonly associated with the clinical presentation of a "sausage" toe. Periostitis may also be seen near affected joints.

**Metatarsophalangeal joints.** Psoriatic arthritis frequently involves multiple metatarsophalangeal joints. One extremity alone may be affected. If bilateral, the distribution usually is asymmetric; for example, the second and third metatarsophalangeal joints may be affected in the right foot and only the fourth metatarsophalangeal joint in the left foot. Erosions may be medial only, but typically affect both sides of the joint. This can give the appearance of arthritis mutilans. Severe osteolysis is rare (see Figure 22-5). Metatarsophalangeal joint findings are frequently associated with adjacent periostitis and digital involvement (see Figure 22-9).

The radiographic features of ankylosing spondylitis and Reiter's disease mimic psoriatic arthritis in the foot.

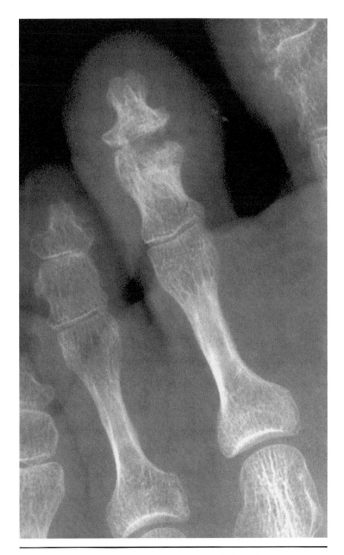

Figure 22-33    Psoriatic arthritis: Distal interphalangeal joints.

Ankylosing spondylitis, although seldom affecting the foot, has a predilection for multiple metatarsophalangeal and interphalangeal joints, symmetric or asymmetric. Reiter's disease, although it can involve any forefoot joint, affects fewer joints than do psoriatic arthritis and ankylosing spondylitis. Periostitis near affected joints and hallux interphalangeal joint involvement are not uncommon.

**Calcaneus.** Calcaneal pathology—that is, enthesopathy—frequently is associated with the seronegative arthropathies. In the proper clinical setting, erosion along the inferior calcaneus is a particularly suggestive finding (see Figure 22-30).

## Gouty Arthritis

The clinical presentation of acute gout is quite dramatic. Findings include severe swelling, redness, and pain at the

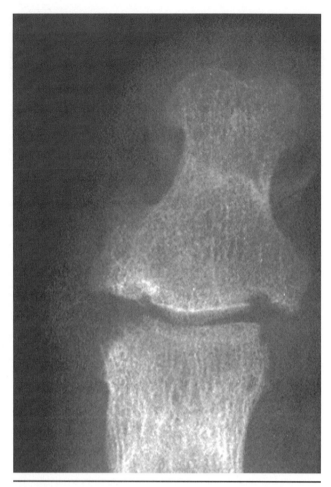

Figure 22-34    Psoriatic arthritis: Medial and lateral margin erosions.

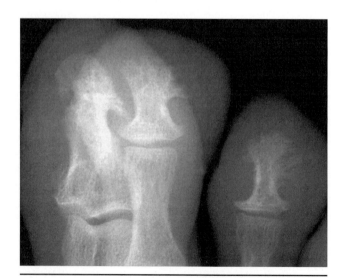

Figure 22-35    Psoriatic arthritis: Ungual tuberosity erosion.

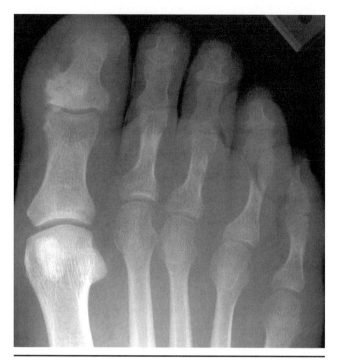

Figure 22-36    Psoriatic arthritis: Ray involvement.

affected joint. Patients with gout may exhibit elevated levels of uric acid in the blood (hyperuricemia). Monosodium urate crystals can be deposited in joints, bone, and soft tissue near or distant to a joint. The irritation and inflammation secondary to synovial urate deposition results in the classic clinical picture just described.

Gouty arthritis targets the first metatarsophalangeal joint; however, this disorder may present at any foot articulation. Joint involvement is asymmetrically distributed. Characteristic radiographic findings are not seen for several years after the initial onset of symptoms.

Characteristic radiographic features of gouty arthritis include the following:

1. *Erosion.* Initial erosions are ill defined but eventually become well defined and **C**-shaped over an extended period of time. They tend to target the medial aspect of the first metatarsophalangeal and hallux interphalangeal joints. Gouty erosions are found adjacent to tophi, which are sodium urate deposits.
2. *Overhanging margin of new bone.* This feature (described by Martel[35]) is seen at the periphery of the erosion and appears to represent new bone production forming around the soft tissue tophus. This finding is very characteristic of gouty arthritis.
3. *Normal joint space.* In contrast to the inflammatory joint diseases (rheumatoid, psoriatic, and septic arthritis), the

joint space is relatively spared. Joint space narrowing does not occur until much later in the disease. Furthermore, secondary osteoarthritis commonly occurs with subsequent joint space narrowing.

4. *Soft tissue calcification.* Small, speckled, increased densities may be recognized in the soft tissue tophus. This finding is uncommon.

**First metatarsophalangeal joint.**    The earliest finding associated with acute gout is an increased soft tissue density and volume medial to the first-metatarsal head. A rarefaction of the first-metatarsal head's medial aspect may or may not be associated. Soft tissue calcification is infrequently encountered.

Pre-erosions are commonly seen along the dorsomedial aspect of the first-metatarsal head in the medial oblique view. Bloch and associates described the appearance as a "lace pattern."[36] Medial head erosions are not always clearly isolated in the dorsoplantar view; they may appear as geographic lucent lesions, that is, cysts (see Figure 22-24). The sesamoid axial view may prove valuable in recognizing the erosion in these cases.

Erosions associated with gouty arthritis are classically described as being C-shaped (see Figure 22-2). This certainly is the case in chronic disease. An overhanging margin of bone (Martel's sign) accentuates this presentation (see Figure 22-12). However, developing erosions frequently are ill defined (see Figure 22-16). Notice in Figure 22-2 that despite the significant presence of erosions, the joint space is relatively spared. Joint space narrowing is frequently a result of secondary osteoarthritis or long-standing intra-articular involvement.

The sesamoids inferior to the first-metatarsal head can also be affected.

**Interphalangeal joints.**    Medial marginal erosion, similar to that seen at the first metatarsophalangeal joint, affects the hallux interphalangeal joint. Well-defined soft tissue density and volume presents adjacent to this finding. However, large geographic defects frequently involve the lesser-toe interphalangeal joints (Figure 22-37) and occasionally the hallux.

**Lesser metatarsophalangeal joints.**    Lesser metatarsophalangeal joint involvement is rare, but, when present, it often is selective for the fifth metatarsophalangeal joint. Findings may mimic rheumatoid arthritis or cause large geographic defects in the metatarsal head.

**Tarsometatarsal and intertarsal joints.**    Tarsal bone involvement is atypical but demonstrates profound findings when it occurs. Large geographic defects are seen, frequently affecting multiple bones.

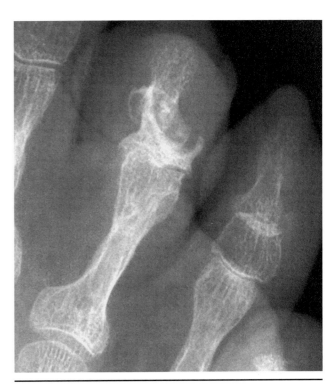

**Figure 22-37**    Gouty arthritis: Distal interphalangeal joint.

## Neuropathic Osteoarthropathy

Neuropathic osteoarthropathy (also called Charcot joint) is most commonly associated with diabetes mellitus in the foot, although it can also be seen in patients with a history of alcoholism or leprosy. Its etiology is not well understood, but appears related in part to either neurogenic disease, hypervascularity, or both.

Cofield and associates listed three target areas in the foot for neuropathic osteoarthropathy associated with diabetes mellitus: the metatarsophalangeal joints, the tarsometatarsal joints, and the combined talonavicular, naviculocuneiform, and intercuneiform joints.[37] However, any foot joint can be affected. The most common presentation is at the tarsometatarsal joints. The talonavicular and naviculocuneiform joints predominate in the tarsal region. Forefoot neuropathic osteoarthropathy is not as prevalent as in the midfoot and tarsus. Bone resorption predominates in the forefoot; this is in gross contrast to the hypertrophic arthritis seen in the neuropathic tarsus and midfoot.

The primary radiographic features of forefoot neuropathic osteoarthropathy include the following:

1. *Fracture and fragmentation.* Acute involvement, especially at a metatarsophalangeal joint, mimics osteonecrosis. Focal osteolysis and fragmentation are the primary findings (Figure 22-38). The metatarsal

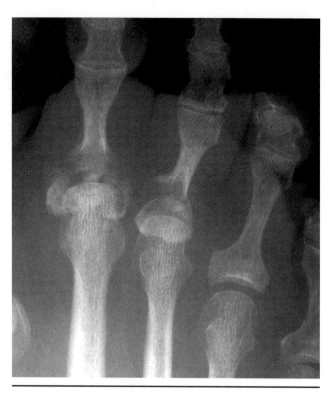

Figure 22-38  Forefoot neuropathic osteoarthropathy: Acute, early involvement.

head may collapse and be accompanied by underlying sclerosis.

2. *Periostitis.* Periosteal new bone production accompanies acute manifestations (see Figure 22-6, fifth metatarsal).

3. *Arthritis mutilans.* Osteolysis is typically more pronounced than that seen in psoriatic arthritis. A large portion of bone, affecting phalanges and metatarsals alike, seemingly disappears, individually or en masse (see Figure 22-6).

The primary radiographic features of neuropathic osteoarthropathy at the intertarsal and tarsometatarsal joints (Figure 22-39) include the following:

1. *Diffuse sclerosis.* Increased density is seen at all affected joints and bones.

2. *Subchondral resorption (early).* Not easily visualized because of the diffuse sclerosis, resorption at articular margins is particularly important when differentiating between early neuropathic osteoarthropathy and osteoarthritis.

3. *Subluxation and dislocation.* Loss of apposition eventually occurs at affected joints and progresses to gross dislocation.

4. *Fragmentation.* Bone fragments are seen, typically associated with the subluxation and dislocation. The fragments may be quite large.

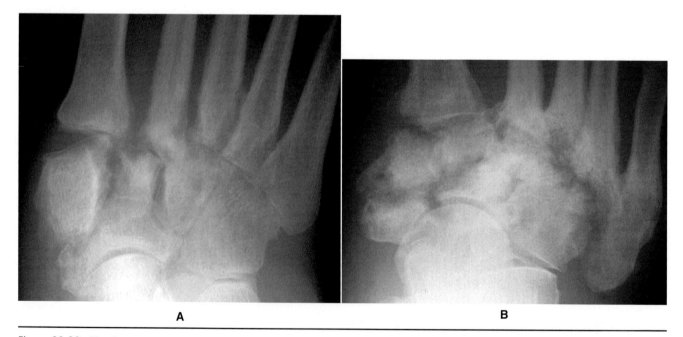

**A**          **B**

Figure 22-39  Tarsal neuropathic osteoarthropathy. **A,** Early manifestations include subchondral resorption (second and third metatarsocuneiform joints), mild sclerosis (intermediate cuneiform and second metatarsal base), and subluxation (first and second metatarsocuneiform joints). **B,** In a different patient, additional findings include diffuse sclerosis and fragmentation of the navicular and cuneiform bones.

## References

1. Rubin DA: The radiology of early arthritis, *Semin Roentgenol* 31(3):185, 1996.

2. Christman RA: A systematic approach for radiographically evaluating joint disease in the foot, *J Am Podiatr Med Assoc* 81(4):174, 1991.

3. Resnick D: The target area approach to articular disorders: a synopsis. In Resnick D, Niwayama G: *Diagnosis of bone and joint disorders*, ed 2, p 1913, Philadelphia, 1988, Saunders.

4. Forrester DM, Brown JC: The radiographic assessment of arthritis: the plain film, *Clin Rheum Dis* 9(2):291, 1983.

5. Goldthwaite JE: The differential diagnosis and treatment of the so-called rheumatoid disease, *Boston Med Surg J* 151:529, 1904. (Cited by Benedek TG, Rodnan GP: A brief history of the rheumatic diseases, *Bull Rheum Dis* 32(6):59, 1982.)

6. Edeiken J, Dalinka M, Karadick D: *Edeiken's roentgen diagnosis of diseases of bone*, ed 4, p 693, Baltimore, 1990, Williams & Wilkins.

7. Resnick D, Broderick TW: Bony proliferation of terminal toe phalanges in psoriasis. The "ivory" phalanx, *Can Assoc Radiol J* 28:187, 1977.

8. Martel W: The overhanging margin of bone: a roentgenologic manifestation of gout, *Radiology* 91:755, 1968.

9. Kaye JJ: Arthritis: roles of radiography and other imaging techniques in evaluation, *Radiology* 177(3):601, 1990.

10. Barthelemy CR, Nakayama DA, Carrera GF et al: Gouty arthritis: a prospective radiographic evaluation of sixty patients, *Skeletal Radiol* 11:1, 1984.

11. Keil H: Rheumatic subcutaneous nodules and simulating lesions, *Medicine* 17:261, 1938.

12. Edeiken J, Dalinka M, Karadick D: *Edeiken's roentgen diagnosis of diseases of bone*, ed 4, p 1369, Baltimore, 1990, Williams & Wilkins.

13. Greenfield GB: *Radiology of bone diseases*, ed 4, p 688, Philadelphia, 1986, Lippincott.

14. Jaffe HL: *Metabolic, degenerative, and inflammatory diseases of bones and joints*, Philadelphia, 1972, Lea & Febiger.

15. McCarty DJ: Diagnostic mimicry in arthritis: patterns of joint involvement associated with calcium pyrophosphate dihydrate crystal deposits, *Bull Rheum Dis* 25:804, 1974-1975.

16. Resnick D, Niwayama G, Goergen TG, Utsinger PD, Shapiro RF, Haselwood DH, Wiesner KB: Clinical, radiographic, and pathologic abnormalities in calcium pyrophosphate dihydrate deposition disease (CPPD): pseudogout, *Radiology* 122:1, 1977.

17. Resnick D, Niwayama G: *Diagnosis of bone and joint disorders*, ed 2, p 1696, Saunders, Philadelphia, 1988.

18. Gruneberg R: Calcifying tendinitis in the forefoot, *BJR* 36:378, 1963.

19. Bonavita JA, Dalinka MK, Schumacher HR: Hydroxyapatite deposition disease, *Radiology* 134:621-625, 1980.

20. Yochum TR, Rowe LJ: *Essentials of skeletal radiology*, Baltimore, 1987, Williams & Wilkins.

21. Bullough PG, Bansal M: The differential diagnosis of geodes, *Radiol Clin North Am* 26(6):1165, 1988.

22. Ondrouch AS: Cyst formation in osteoarthritis, *J Bone Joint Surg* 45(B):755, 1963.

23. Resnick D, Niwayama G, Coutts RD: Subchondral cysts (geodes) in arthritic disorders: pathologic and radiographic appearance of the hip joint, *AJR* 128:799, 1977.

24. Magyar E, Talerman A, Feher M, Wouters HW: The pathogenesis of the subchondral pseudocysts in rheumatoid arthritis, *Clin Orthop* 100:341, 1974.

25. Resnick D, Broderick TW: Intraosseous calcifications in tophaceous gout, *AJR* 137:1157-1161, 1981.

26. Resnick D, Feingold ML, Curd J, Niwayama G, Goergen TG: Calcaneal abnormalities in articular disorders: rheumatoid arthritis, ankylosing spondylitis, psoriatic arthritis and Reiter syndrome, *Radiology* 125:355, 1977.

27. Resnick D, Niwayama G: Entheses and enthesopathy: anatomical, pathological, and radiological correlation, *Radiology* 146:1, 1983.

28. Resnick D: *Bone and joint imaging*, Philadelphia, 1989, Saunders.

29. Mitchell NS, Cruess RL: Classification of degenerative arthritis, *CMAJ* 117:763, 1977.

30. Sarrafian SK: *Anatomy of the foot and ankle*, pp 256-259, Philadelphia, 1983, Lippincott.

31. Bartolomei FJ: Pedal radiographic manifestations of the seronegative spondyloarthritides. II. Psoriatic arthritis, *J Am Podiatr Med Assoc* 76(5):266, 1986.

32. Kettering JM, Towers JD, Rubin DA: The seronegative spondyloarthropathies, *Semin Roentgenol* 31(3):220, 1996.

33. Moll JMH, Wright V: Psoriatic arthritis, *Semin Arthritis Rheum* 3:55, 1973.

34. Resnick D: The interphalangeal joint of the great toe in rheumatoid arthritis, *Can Assoc Radiol J* 26:255, 1975.

35. Martel W: The overhanging margin of bone: a roentgenologic manifestation of gout, *Radiology* 91:755, 1968.

36. Bloch C, Hermann G, Yu TF: A radiologic reevaluation of gout: a study of 2,000 patients, *AJR* 134:781-787, 1980.

37. Cofield RH, Morrison MJ, Beabout JW: Diabetic neuroarthropathy in the foot: patient characteristics and patterns of radiographic change, *Foot & Ankle* 4(1):15, 1983.

# CHAPTER 23

# Bone Tumors and Tumorlike Lesions

JEFFREY E. SHOOK • LAWRENCE S. OSHER • ROBERT A. CHRISTMAN

## ■ SYSTEMATIC EVALUATION OF SOLITARY BONE LESIONS

Solitary bone lesions are occasionally encountered in the foot and distal leg. Fortunately, most of these lesions are benign. Examples include the solitary bone cyst, enchondroma, and bone island. Some lesions have characteristic radiographic features. However, many appear similar to one another or only demonstrate subtle differences; it may be impossible to distinguish between them by plain film radiography alone.

An efficient, reliable approach is needed to assess these lesions. The radiographic features must first be recognized. These features can be used not only as diagnostic clues but also for determining the growth rate or aggressiveness of the lesion. A list of potential differential diagnoses can then be formulated based on these radiographic findings.

Ten diagnostic clues are used for assessing a solitary bone lesion (Table 23-1). Eight of these clues are radiographic

<table>
<tr><td colspan="2">TABLE 23-1 Diagnostic Indicators for Evaluating the Solitary Bone Lesion</td></tr>
</table>

**Radiographic Clues**
*1. Destructive pattern
*2. Size and shape
*3. Cortical involvement
*4. Periosteal reaction
 5. Anatomic position (transverse and longitudinal planes)
 6. Skeletal location
 7. Trabeculation
 8. Matrix production

**Nonradiologic Clues**
1. Clinical course
2. Age of patient

*Features useful for determining a lesion's growth rate or aggressiveness.

features. Of these eight, four are valuable for determining the aggressiveness or growth rate of the lesion. Two nonradiologic diagnostic clues complete the initial assessment: the patient's age and clinical course. These ten criteria (eight radiographic and two clinical) should be considered when evaluating any solitary bone lesion. After these data are collected, differential diagnoses are determined.

### Destructive Pattern

Three types of destructive (that is, lytic) patterns have been described in the literature pertaining to solitary bone lesions: geographic, moth-eaten, and permeative[1] (Figure 23-1). A geographic lytic lesion has a recognizable form (Figure 23-2). These recognizable lesions are often referred to as "cystic." However, the term *cystic* should not be used, because it implies that the lesion is not solid; a greater percentage of cases are solid.[9] The lesion's outline may be well defined or ill defined; well-defined geographic lesions have less aggressive—that is, slower growth activity—than ill-defined lesions. Examples of geographic lesions include bone island, enchondroma, giant cell tumor, and fibrocortical defect. If, over sequential studies, the margin becomes increasingly less defined, increased biologic activity should be suspected.[2]

A well-defined geographic bone lesion that is bounded by a sclerotic margin has very slow growth activity (Figure 23-3). The sclerotic margin represents the surrounding normal bone's attempt to wall off the lesion. Normal bone cannot be deposited quickly enough around an aggressive moth-eaten or permeative lesion to be visible radiographically. Sclerotic margins, therefore, are only seen around lesions with geographic destructive patterns and are almost always benign.[3]

Moth-eaten and permeative destructive patterns do not have a definite form or shape (Figure 23-4). Multiple, small, lytic lesions appear to spread across the affected area of

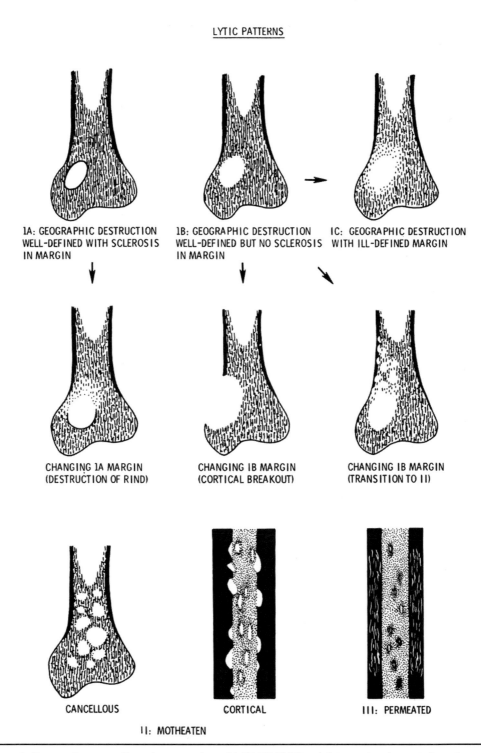

**Figure 23-1**   Schematic diagram of patterns of bone destruction (types IA, IB, IC, II, III) and their margins. Arrows indicate the most frequent transitions or combinations of these margins. Transitions imply increased activity and a greater probability of malignancy. (Courtesy Madewell JE, Ragsdale BD, Sweet DE: *Radiol Clin North Am* 19[4]:722, 1981, figure 6)

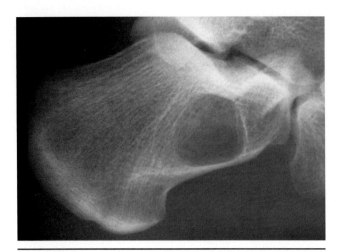

**Figure 23-2**   Calcaneal bone cyst demonstrating geographic type IB destruction.

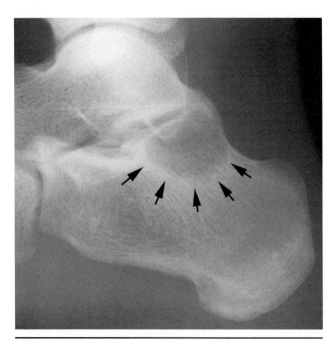

**Figure 23-3**   Calcaneal lesion demonstrating a geographic type IA destructive pattern; arrows indicate the sclerotic margin.

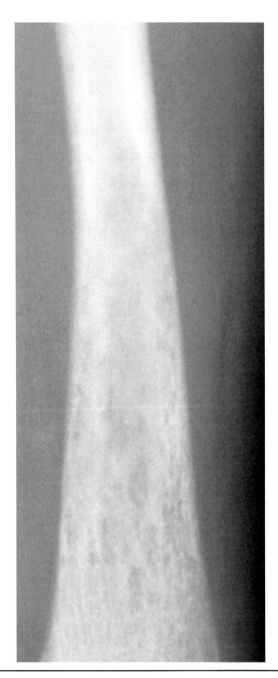

**Figure 23-4**   Permeated (type III) destruction involves the entire distal tibial diametaphysis, characteristic of fast growth rate.

bone. A moth-eaten pattern appears as multiple, small holes in cancellous or medullary bone; the permeative pattern typically presents as multiple, small streaks running through cortical bone. Lesions with either of these destructive patterns highly suggest aggressive activity. Examples include Ewing's sarcoma, osteosarcoma, and untreated osteomyelitis. Acute osteopenia can also demonstrate a permeative or moth-eaten appearance, except it involves multiple bones (Figure 23-5).

## Size and Shape

Generally speaking, aggressive lesions tend to be larger in size than slowly growing lesions. Regarding shape, a slowly growing lesion appears elongated in the diaphysis of a tubular bone (Figure 23-6); its length is at least 1½ times its width. This lesion is contained by the cortex, which acts as a wall; the lesion extends along the path of least resistance, that is, the medullary cavity.

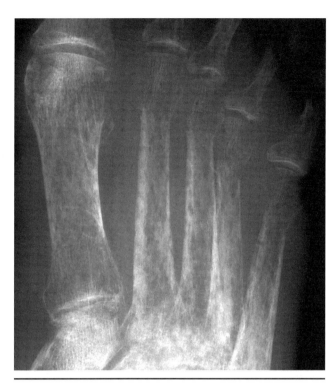

Figure 23-5    An excellent example of cortical, moth-eaten (type II) destruction in a patient with acute osteoporosis.

## Cortical Involvement

A solitary bone lesion's growth rate also can be estimated by the pattern of resorption along the adjacent cortex. Slow growth may only cause scalloping of the endosteal surface (Figure 23-7). With increasing growth rate, the cortex may be nearly fully resorbed yet still intact adjacent to the lesion. As endosteal resorption occurs, subperiosteal apposition may accompany it, giving the cortex an "expanded" appearance (Figure 23-8). A more aggressive lesion penetrates or breaks through the cortex and invades the soft tissues.

## Periosteal Reaction

Periosteal reactions can have many different presentations (Figure 23-9). They generally do not accompany lesions demonstrating slow growth. When a periosteal reaction is present, a degree of aggressiveness does exist. The growth rate can be further estimated by the type of periosteal reaction present (Box 23-1). For example, lesion that are accompanied by a continuous periosteal reaction are less aggressive than those demonstrating interrupted periosteal reactions. The most aggressive lesions typically are associated with complex periosteal reactions.[4]

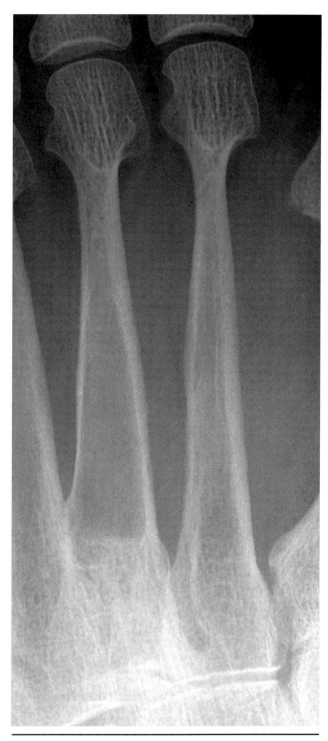

Figure 23-6    A geographic type IB destructive lesion of the third metatarsal; note the elongated shape of this slow-growing lesion involving nearly two thirds of the diaphysis.

## Anatomic Position

The anatomic position of the lesion in a tubular bone can provide valuable diagnostic information. Many tumors occur

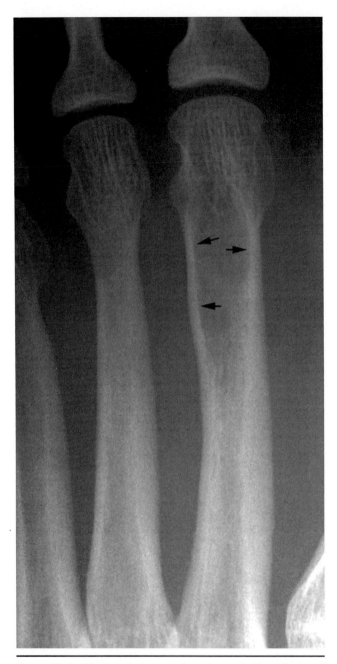

**Figure 23-7**  This lesion's slow growth rate has resulted in scalloping of the endosteal surface of the cortex *(arrows)*.

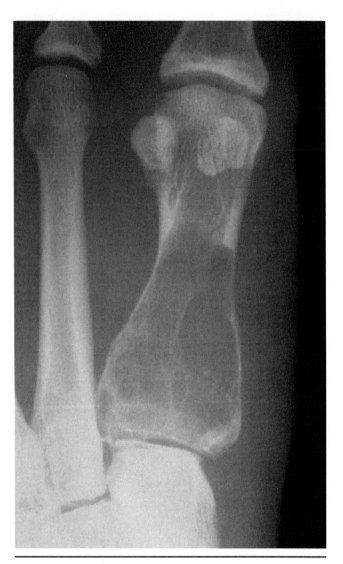

**Figure 23-8**  Chronic endosteal resorption caused by a slow-growing lesion and subsequent periosteal apposition results in the appearance of an "expanded" cortex.

only in specific anatomic sites. Position can be assessed in two planes of the film, horizontal and vertical (Figure 23-10). In the horizontal plane, the center of the lesion can have a position that is central (solitary bone cyst, enchondroma), eccentric (fibrous cortical defect), cortical (osteoid osteoma), or parosteal (osteoma). A lesion's vertical position can either be epiphyseal (chondroblastoma), metaphyseal (giant cell tumor, enchondroma), diametaphyseal (chondromyxoid fibroma), or diaphyseal (fibrous dysplasia, Ewing's sarcoma).

## Skeletal Location

Some solitary bone lesions have a predilection for certain bones. For example, enchondroma is frequently found in the phalanges of the hand and sometimes the foot. Osteoid osteoma is not uncommonly found in the talar neck. Intraosseous lipoma and the solitary bone cyst are frequently seen in the calcaneal body.

## Trabeculation

Trabeculation, when present, is found with only a few lesions (Table 23-2). Also, the type of trabeculation may further narrow the choice of diagnoses. Fine, delicate trabeculation is associated with giant cell tumor; horizontally oriented fine,

# PERIOSTEAL REACTIONS

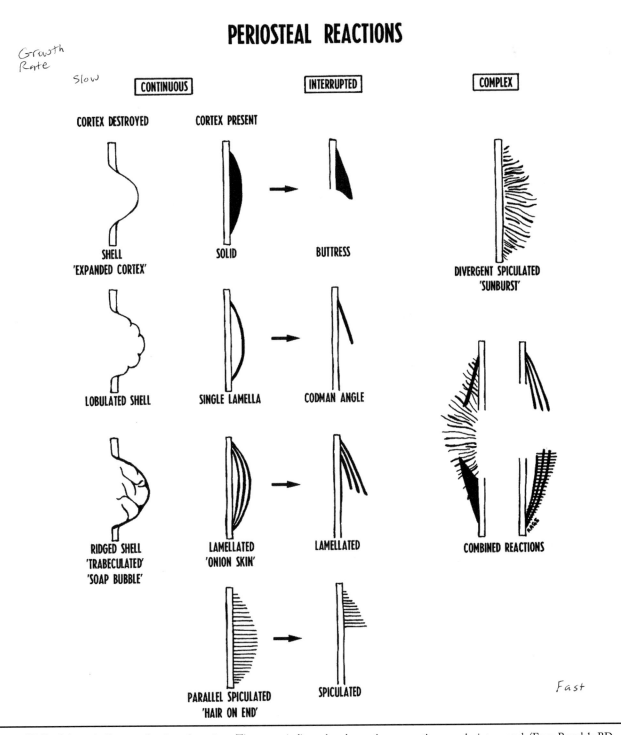

**Figure 23-9** Schematic diagram of periosteal reactions. The arrows indicate that the continuous reactions may be interrupted. (From Ragsdale BD, Madewell JE, Sweet DE: *Radiol Clin North Am* 19[4]:751, 1981, figure 2).

delicate trabeculae are a feature of aneurysmal bone cyst; coarse, thick trabeculations are seen with chondromyxoid fibroma; fibrous cortical defect has lobulated trabeculations that appear as "soap bubbles" (Figure 23-11); and radiating trabeculations are seen with hemangioma.[5]

## Matrix Production

Most tumors do not produce a radiographically visible matrix. However, when present, matrix mineralization can narrow the list of differential diagnoses for any particular lesion to a specific category of primary bone tumors.[6]

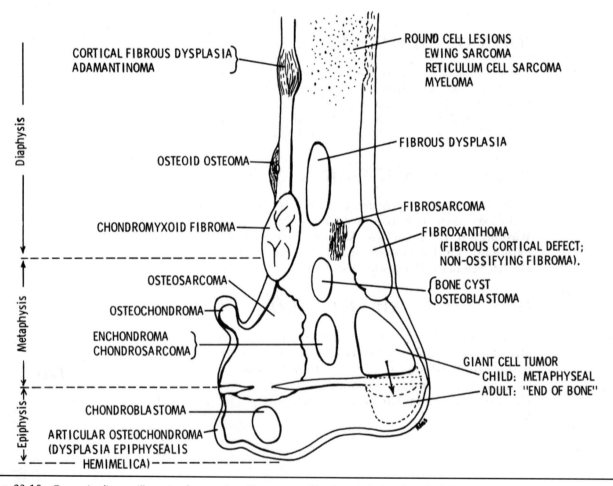

Figure 23-10   Composite diagram illustrating frequent sites of bone tumors. The diagram depicts the end of a long bone that has been divided into the epiphysis, metaphysis, and diaphysis. The typical sites of common primary bone tumors are labeled. Bone tumors tend to predominate in those ends of long bones that undergo the greatest growth and remodeling; hence, they have the greatest number of cells and amount of cell activity (shoulder and knee regions). When small tumors, presumably detected early, are analyzed, preferential sites of tumor origin become apparent within each bone (as shown in this illustration), suggesting a relationship between the type of tumor and the anatomic site affected. In general, a tumor of a given cell type arises in the field where the homologous normal cells are most active. These regional variations suggest that the composition of the tumor is affected or may be determined by the metabolic field in which it arises. (From Madewell JE, Ragsdale BD, Sweet DE: *Radiol Clin North Am* 19[4]:716, 1981, figure 1).

**TABLE 23-2**  **Tumors Demonstrating Trabeculation**

Giant cell tumor
Aneurysmal bone cyst
Chondromyxoid fibroma
Hemangioma
Fibrous cortical defect

Mineralized matrix either has a solid, homogeneous appearance or a speckled, stippled appearance (Figure 23-12). Solid matrix production is typically seen with osteoblastic tumors, including osteoid osteoma, osteoblastoma, and osteosarcoma. Stippled or speckled matrix production is a feature of the chondroblastic tumor group. Examples include enchondroma (Figure 23-13), osteochondroma, chondroblastoma, and chondrosarcoma. Occasionally,

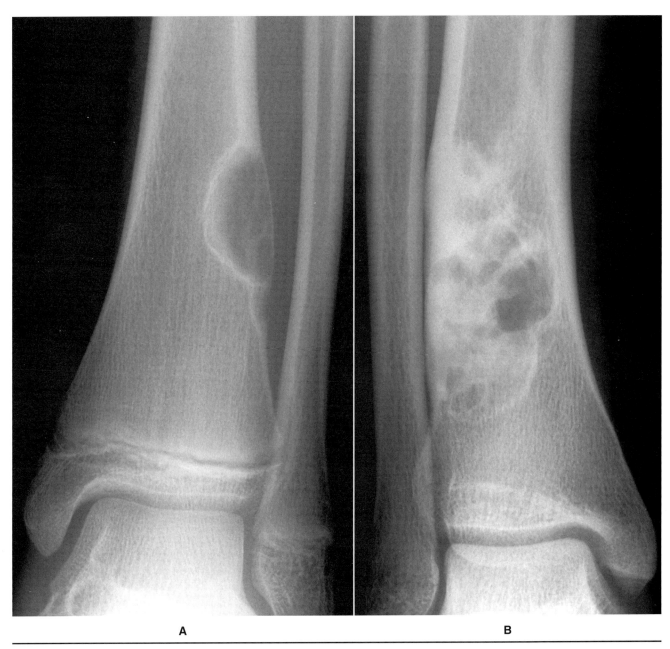

**A**                                                                                **B**

Figure 23-11   Examples of fibrocortical defects (nonossifying fibromas) at varying stages of development. **A,** The trabeculations appear fine and delicate in early stages. **B,** In an older patient, the lesion remodels, and the "soap bubble" appearance is more obvious.

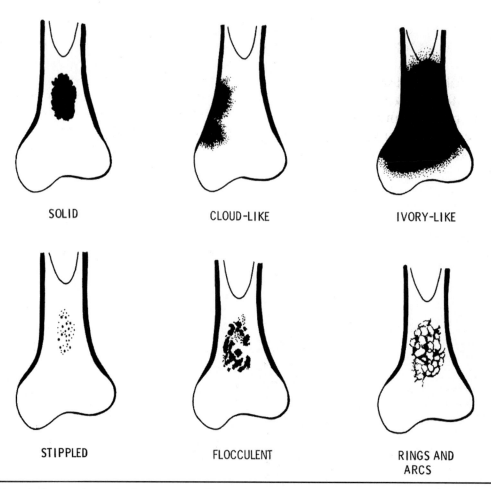

**SOLID**          **CLOUD-LIKE**          **IVORY-LIKE**

**STIPPLED**          **FLOCCULENT**          **RINGS AND ARCS**

**Figure 23-12**  Schematic diagram of mineralized matrix patterns. Tumor osteoid appears as increased density with a solid (sharp-edged) or cloudy to ivory-like (ill-defined edge) pattern. Tumor cartilage creates stippled, flocculent, and solid density patterns. Rings and arcs represent bony rims around tumor cartilage lobules. Dystrophic mineralization and ischemic osteoid tend to mimic the stippled, flocculent, or patchy solid density pattern. (From Sweet DE, Madewell JE, Ragsdale BD: *Radiol Clin North Am* 19[4]:788, 1981, figure 1.)

chondroblastic lesions may have matrix mineralization that appears as "rings and arcs." Fibroblastic lesions, especially fibrous dysplasia, occasionally demonstrate an intermediate type of mineralization frequently referred to as a "ground glass" appearance.

## Clinical Course

Some tumors have a characteristic clinical presentation that can aid in differentiation from other lesions. For example, osteoid osteoma has been reported as presenting with night pain that is relieved by aspirin. However, the clinical course generally is nonspecific and not helpful in differentiating between tumors.

## Age of Patient

Most bone tumors characteristically present in specific age ranges, especially those that are malignant[7] (Table 23-3). For example, Ewing's tumor, simple bone cyst, and chondro-blastoma are found in the first two decades of life. In contrast, multiple myeloma, fibrosarcoma, and metastasis present in the fifth to seventh decade.

## ■ OVERVIEW OF PEDAL INVOLVEMENT

Bone tumor and tumorlike conditions rarely occur in the foot, and most reports range from approximately 2% to 3.5%. Experience suggests that the phalanges are the most frequently involved bones (osteochondromas). However, if one excludes osteochondromas, then metatarsal bones and the calcaneus are the next most frequent sites, followed by the talus. Neoplasms of the midfoot bones are the least frequent sites. The frequency of pedal enchondromas in the small tubular bones is probably overestimated, because these lesions are far more commonly encountered in the hands. Of the primary malignant bone tumors, chondrosarcomas are

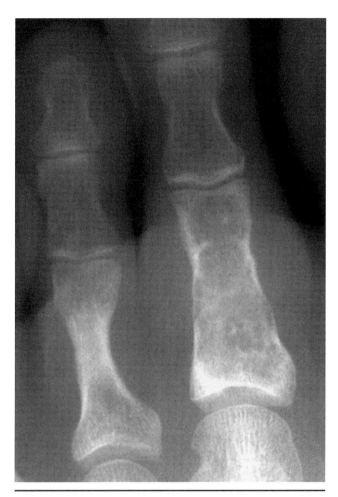

**Figure 23-13**  Enchondroma, second toe proximal phalanx, demonstrating a rings-and-arcs mineralized matrix pattern. (Courtesy Gary F. Bjarnason, Roanoke Rapids, North Carolina.)

| TABLE 23-3 | Age Ranges: Outline of Bone Tumor Age Distribution |
| --- | --- |
| Tumor | Peak Age Range (years) |
| **Benign Tumors** | |
| Osteoma | 15 to 45 |
| Osteoid osteoma | 10 to 23 |
| Benign osteoblastoma | 10 to 30 |
| Osteochondroma | 10 to 30 |
| Central chondroma | 10 to 40 |
| Chondroblastoma | 10 to 20 |
| Chondromyxoid fibroma | 10 to 30 |
| Eosinophilic granuloma | 5 to 10 |
| Nonosteogenic fibroma | 10 to 20 |
| Desmoplastic fibroma | 10 to 30 |
| Intraosseous lipoma | 30 to 50 |
| Neurilemoma | 10 to 30 |
| Hemangioma | 40 to 50 |
| Giant cell tumor | 25 to 40 |
| Simple bone cyst | 5 to 20 |
| Aneurysmal bone cyst | 10 to 30 |
| Enchondroma | 30s |
| **Primary Malignant Tumors** | |
| Osteogenic sarcoma | 10 to 20 |
| Parosteal osteosarcoma | 20 to 40 |
| Chondrosarcoma | 30 to 60 |
| Fibrosarcoma | 30 to 40 |
| Malignant giant cell tumor | 30 to 50 |
| Adamantinoma | 10 to 30 |
| Hemangioendothelioma | 30 to 40 |
| Ewing sarcoma | 10 to 20 |
| Reticulum cell sarcoma | 30 to 60 |
| Myeloma | 50 to 80 |
| Chordoma | 30 to 60 |
| **Other Tumors** | |
| Leukemia | |
| Acute | 2 to 6 |
| Chronic | 40 to 70 |
| Metastatic neuroblastoma | Under 4 |
| Metastatic carcinoma | 40 to 80 |

Modified after Dahlin DC, Unni KK: *Bone tumors: general aspects and data on 8542 cases*, ed 4, Springfield, Ill, 1986, Charles C Thomas.

among the most frequent in adults. One could argue that secondary osseous involvement associated with synovial sarcoma is a more frequent pedal event.

Metastases distal to the knee are not common. When acrometastatic lesions to the foot occur, they are most frequently secondary to lung carcinomas or aggressive visceral tumors. Associated hypertrophic pulmonary osteoarthropathy not uncommonly extends to the ankles and may present with ankle pain and swelling. Tumors with metastatic extension to the vertebral bodies may also travel distal to the knee (hypothetically via Batson's vertebral plexus). In long bones, metastatic lesions may be lytic, blastic, or more frequently mixed lytic-blastic with a propensity to demonstrate moth-eaten destruction. In addition, periosteal reactions not uncommonly comprise part of the overall picture. In contradistinction, acrometastases are more likely to manifest gross lysis without periostitis. When acrosclerotic lesions occur, the differential diagnosis should

include SLE (systemic lupus erythematosus), seronegative arthritis, and intraosseous sarcoidosis.

Matrix evaluation and an appreciation of cardinal radiographic characteristics with respect to patterns of internal bony lysis, periosteal reactions, and cortical erosions are used in approaching bone tumors. Beyond this, probabilities in diagnosis frequency rest on epidemiologic data such as patient age and specific tumor location.

Clinical examinations generally yield nonspecific findings of pain of variable character (often begins insidiously with an intermittent character. Progression to a severe, constant pain can occur with the more aggressive neoplasms.

Other findings may include the following:

> Swelling and/or palpable mass
> Variable signs of inflammation and local venous dilation
> Effusion into the adjacent joint
> Pathologic fracture
> Occasional constitutional symptoms

## ■ MALIGNANT BONE TUMORS

The "big three" mesenchymal malignancies (osteosarcoma, chondrosarcoma, Ewing sarcoma) are rarely encountered in the foot.

### Osteogenic Sarcoma (OS)

Osteogenic sarcoma (OS) is a malignant bone tumor characterized by profound osteoid elaboration by sarcomatous cells. Osteogenic sarcomas occur approximately three times as frequently as Ewing tumors. Pathologically, the osteoid may be admixed with cartilage and/or fibrous tissue of varying amounts, which can have radiologic consequences. Histologic grading is associated with the following classification:

> *Intraosseous*
> Conventional (osteoblastic, fibroblastic, chondroblastic)
> Telangectasia
> Small cell
> Low grade
> Cortical
> *Surface*
> Periosteal
> High-grade periosteal
> Juxtacortical (parosteal)
> *Extraosseous*
> Secondary
> Multicentric

**Epidemiology.** Because pedal involvement is exceedingly rare (occurring in about 1% of all osteogenic sarcomas), most of the data pertain to conventional osteogenic sarcomas. If one looks at OS in the whole body, it is considered to be the second most common primary bone sarcoma, with multiple myeloma the most frequent. Males are twice as likely than females to develop OS. Age data show peak incidence in adolescence, with a median of about 17 years for tubular bones and 25 for flat bones. A second, older age peak exists for secondary osteosarcomas and is associated with Paget's disease, irradiated bone, or degeneration of a pre-existing osteochondroma.

**Metastases.** Most commonly osteosarcomatous metastases occur to the lungs, but occasionally they occur to the viscera or other parts of the skeletal system. Rarely metastasis occurs via lymphatics, with regional lymph node involvement.

Approximately 65% occur about the knee, with the distal femur approximately twice as frequent as the proximal tibia. The origin is usually metaphyseal, occasionally diaphyseal (10% to 20%), and rarely epiphyseal (<1%). Despite these preferences of sites of origin, extension of OS into either the diaphysis or epiphysis is not uncommon (15% to 30%). Although epiphyseal extension occurs more commonly after physeal closure, *it is a mistake* to think that penetration of the physis by OS is rare.

**Location.** The majority of pedal OS (about 70%) is located within the tarsal bones, with the os calcis the most frequent site. Metatarsal and phalangeal locations do occur, and in some instances have been confused with osteomyelitis in children. Probably because of a combination of the large size of lesion at time of discovery and small bone size, pedal osteosarcomas are generally reported as occurring in either diaphysis or metaphyses.

**Radiography.** Osteosarcomas may present with bony lesions that are either densely sclerotic (25%), osteolytic (25%), or (most frequently) mixed lytic-sclerotic (50%). Signs of an ossific matrix are therefore present in around 75% or cases. Inasmuch as the bony cortex is freely penetrated/permeated, periosteal reactions are typically present. In contradistinction, articular cartilage presents a significant barrier to penetration, and the joint is usually violated only in advanced cases. However, direct penetration through a physis is not uncommon.

1. Ossific matrix patterns result in densely sclerotic or mixed lytic-sclerotic changes to bone in most pedal cases. Although this reflects the amount of neoplastic osteoid elaboration, the more homogenous the radiographic density or advanced the state, the greater the difficulty in distinguishing new bone formation from a reactive sclerotic response of normal bone. Despite being generally associated with chronic inflammatory bony processes, reports of Ewing sarcoma in tarsal bones suggest that reactive medullary sclerosis is typical, and therefore radiographic distinction from OS can be problematic in the absence of soft tissue ossification.

2. Aggressive periosteal reaction patterns, classically complex spiculated "sunburst" type, characterize OS. "Hair on end" periosteal spiculation is also seen, as well as multilaminated reactions. The Codman angle (interrupted single lamella) periosteal reaction is typical at sites of extraosseous extension.

3. Internal destruction—evidence of moth-eaten or, less commonly, permeative destruction may be apparent, but this is often obscured once as matrix ossification progresses. Geographic IC margination is occasionally observed.
4. Cortical erosion is not uncommon.
5. Soft tissue invasion is typical. The soft tissues may be quite ossified.

## Chondrosarcoma

Chondrosarcoma is a malignant tumor (somewhat slow-growing) that elaborates pure hyaline cartilage. Two general types based on location are recognized, central and peripheral. Unfortunately, primary and secondary forms of the lesion have also been described, and therefore considerable confusion exists as to what this means. The following definitions are helpful:

*Central:* Within the medullary canal
*Peripheral:* Arising in and around the cortical surfaces
*Primary:* Arising as malignant lesion, occasionally in children
*Secondary:* Malignant degeneration of a pre-existing benign lesion, often cartilaginous (for example, osteocartilaginous exostosis, hereditary multiple exostoses enchondromas, or in Pagetic bone)

**Clinical data.**    The male:female ratio is 1.5:1; chondrosarcomas are the third most common of the primary malignant tumors (about 10% or all primary bone tumors, they occur about half as often as osteosarcoma). Research finds a decided tendency for older age involvement (50% of central chondrosarcomas over the age of 40), the peak age range is 30 to 60 years. Chondrosarcomas are rarely found in children. Hand and foot involvement is quite rare (about 3%). Nonetheless, it is still probably the most common malignant bone tumor of the hand or foot in the middle-aged patient. Hand involvement is predictably greater than foot (degeneration of enchondroma). Dull pain and gradual swelling are the most common presenting symptoms of chondrosarcoma, without antecedent trauma. Tumor growth is usually slow (unless high grade) with late bloodstream metastasis. Pathologic fractures are uncommon and are usually seen in the higher-grade tumors.

**Location.**    Chondrosarcomas of the foot have been found in toes, metatarsals, and tarsal bones. Overall, the calcaneus appears to be most frequently involved, followed by the talus. Most chondrosarcomas are the central type in tubular bones, and typically involve the metaphysis and meta-diaphyseal areas (mesenchymal cell lesions). Epiphyseal/apophyseal involvement is rare.

**Radiography.**    Unless an origin from a pre-existing lesion such as a sessile osteochondroma can be established or a calcific matrix pattern exists, the picture is somewhat general, albeit suggestive of malignancy. The following features may be seen:

1. Lytic lesion of bone with poorly defined margins, and often thinned overlying cortex with expansion
2. Evidence of calcified matrix, that is, punctate/stippled, "fluffy," flocculant, or curvilinear patterns ("ring and arc" formations) in about 65% of lesions. In some cases, calcification can be so dense so as to be confused with a more homogenous ossific matrix of osteosarcoma or reactive sclerosis of Ewing tumor (especially os calcis).
3. Endosteal erosive changes, scalloping.
4. Soft tissue mass occasionally present with or without calcification.
5. Pathologic fracture uncommon.

## Ewing Sarcoma

Ewing sarcoma is a malignant neoplasm thought to be derived from primitive marrow elements, vascular endothelium, or possibly neural tissue. Along with myeloma and non-Hodgkin's lymphoma (reticulum cell sarcoma), Ewing sarcoma is classified as a non–matrix-producing, round-cell tumor. Despite its ranking as sixth most common malignant bone tumor, pedal Ewing sarcoma is quite rare, with about 0.5% arising in the foot.

**Location.**    Almost any bone in the body can be involved, but a decided tendency for long bones, greatest in lower-extremity bones. In the foot, most cases appear split between the calcaneus and metatarsals. Nonetheless, cases in the toes and other tarsal bones have been reported. In the os calcis, which is the most frequent pedal attack site for Ewing sarcoma, the lesion frequently has its epicenter at the junction of the posterior body and greater tuberosity (where vestigial red marrow may occur in some adults).

**Clinical data.**    Pain, often becoming severe and recalcitrant, is usual. With extension of the neoplasm into the soft tissues, swelling becomes apparent. Ewing sarcoma is predominantly a young person's tumor, with a predilection for Caucasians. The peak age incidence is 15 years old, with a range between 5 and 30 years old. Under age 5 years old, metastatic neuroblastoma should be suspected. In a patient over age 30, one should suspect reticulum cell sarcoma. The tumor shows a 3:2 male:female ratio.

**Radiography**

1. Radiography shows diaphyseal to metadiaphyseal involvement. Permeative bone destruction is visible, as

is type III growth rate assessment most apparent with cortical bony involvement.

2. In about 10%, a patchy type (generally nonhomogeneous) of reactive bony sclerosis is noted, with or without mottled destruction. This appearance is most characteristic of flat bones and seems quite frequent when tarsal bones (especially the os calcis) are involved. In the calcaneus (as well as other tarsal bones), lytic changes may not be very obvious. Instead, a mixed lytic-sclerotic appearance or complete reactive sclerosis is typical. In this respect, the tumor shows some radiographic similarities with chronic osteomyelitis.

3. Periosteal reactions are present in up to 50% of patients, especially in tubular and long bones. Classically, they appear as multilamellar "onion skin," "lace like," or spiculated "hair on end" types. Nevertheless, it is important to note that, as with osteomyelitis, periosteal reactions are generally blunted when tarsal (cancellous) bones are involved.

4. Soft tissue mass in up to 90% of cases

5. Pathologic fracture is not uncommon and may be the presenting complaint. The differential of Ewing tumor consists of osteomyelitis, eosinophilic granuloma of bone, and osteogenic sarcoma.

## ■ BENIGN BONE TUMORS

The following benign bone tumors are those more commonly encountered in the foot and ankle.

## Nonossifying Fibroma (Nonosteogenic Fibroma, or NOF) and Fibrous Cortical Defects (FCD)

Nonossifying fibroma (nonosteogenic fibroma, or NOF) and fibrous cortical defects (FCD) are two benign fibrous lesions of bone that are (1) histologically identical, (2) identical in that the lesional tissue does not produce bone (unlike ossifying fibromas and fibrous dysplasia), and (3) most likely represent developmental defects rather than true neoplasms, possibly in continuum with one another. The primary differences between the two concern their intraosseus location, clinical and epidemiologic data, and radiographic features.

**Clinical data.** FCDs are generally asymptomatic and discovered as incidental findings. NOFs are also generally asymptomatic but may become painful with increasing size and certainly show pain with pathologic fracture. Both kinds of tumors may regress spontaneously.

**Epidemiology.** FCDs are very common and may occur in 30% of the normal population. NOFs are much less common; both lesions have been reported as having a slight male preponderance.

**Age Incidence**

*NOF:* Generally NOF tumors arise in the first two decades, with a 13-year-old average age (range 4 to 40 years old).

*FCD:* Generally discovered between ages 4 and 8, FCD is rare after age 14.

**Location.** Lower extremities are the most common, especially the knees and bones of the distal legs, and are often appreciated with ankle films. They are, however, very rare lesions within the foot, ranging from about 0.5% to 3.0% of primary bone tumors of the foot.

## Radiography

**FCD** (Figure 23-14).

1. The round to oval radiolucent intracortical lesions typically erode the outer cortical surface.

2. Sharply marginated with a sclerotic lining or "rind."

3. Metaphyseal location of long bones, with distal tibia and fibula quite common. Calcaneal involvement has been noted posterosuperiorly, growing away from the apophyseal region. The inner rind of the lesion may cause convexity of the internal cortex with impingement of the medullary canal.

4. Size ranges from 1.0 to 4.0 cm (1.0 to 2.0 is typical), long axis parallel to bony shaft.

5. Regressed/healed lesions may present as nontender, nonprogressive areas of focal cortical thickening.

**NOF** (Figure 23-15).

1. NOF tumors are round to oval geographic (Type IA) lesions.

2. Eccentric intramedullary location, typically metaphyseal. Just like unicameral bone cysts, the lesion may grow into the diaphysis. The epiphysis is usually not involved.

3. Multiloculated, "bubbly," "bundle of grapes" appearance is classic.

4. May attain large size and cause generally mild cortical "shell" expansion and thinning.

5. Medullary margins of the lesions are sclerotic, with sharp outer definition.

6. Pathologic fracture possible, especially when size is greater than or equal to 50% of the diameter of the involved bone.

7. Inner cortical concave "scalloping" favors diagnosis of NOF. Inner cortical "convex" or "bubbling" remodeling favors diagnosis of FCD.

8. Healed lesions chronologically display progressive medullary sclerosis of lytic zone(s). Residual lesions

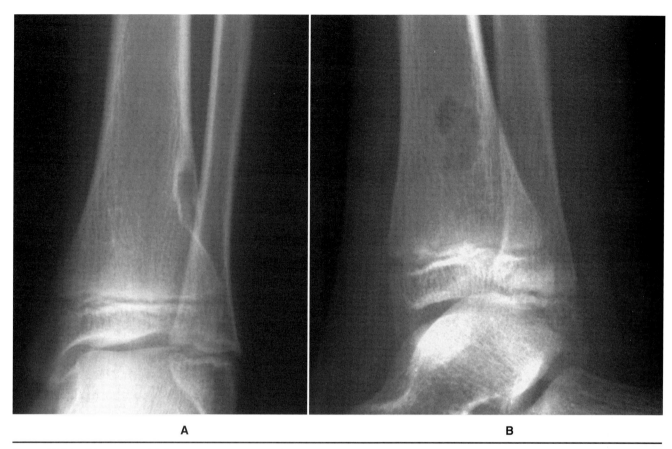

**A**                                                                                          **B**

Figure 23-14   Fibrous cortical defect in 9-year-old male. **A,** Anteroposterior study of ankle reveals eccentric, oval metaphyseal lesion eroding the lateral cortical surface of the distal tibia. A well-delineated sclerotic reactive margin is obvious. **B,** Lateral ankle study of same lesion reveals polylobular outline.

therefore appear as focal osteosclerotic lesion of the metadiaphysis, often with scalloped outlines.

9. Periosteal new bone formation generally lacking.

### Solitary Osteochondroma (Osteocartilaginous Exostosis)

Solitary osteochondroma (osteocartilaginous exostosis) is a benign, slow-growing juxtacortical, cartilaginous-capped neoplasm with a trunklike osseous attachment to the underlying bone. Known to arise in virtually any bone preformed in cartilage, osteochondromas are generally considered the most common benign cartilaginous tumor of the skeletal system. Cartilaginous cap varies in thickness from 1 to 6 mm.

Two different types are encountered:

1. *Pedunculated:* Mushroom-shaped exostosis on a narrowed osseous stalk joining the cap to underlying bone
2. *Sessile:* Flared or broad-based attachment, appearing rounded, lobulated, or "plateaulike" in shape, and with a higher incidence of malignant degeneration

**Location.** Predominantly lower extremity, especially knee/distal femur. The tibia is involved in about 20% of cases. When the femur is involved, the lesion must be differentiated from parosteal osteosarcoma (veil-like, pasted-on appearance) and fibrous dysplasia (intramedullary, "ground glass" appearance). However, fibrous dysplasia and parosteal OS are rare pedal encounters. Distal tibial/ankle locations are more frequent locations for parosteal myositis ossificans. In the foot, lesions typically are found on small tubular bones and/or bones with epiphyses or apophyses; however, any pedal bone (preformed in cartilage) can theoretically give rise to an osteochondroma. Typical sites include the dorsomedial aspect of the hallucal distal phalanx, the distal metatarsals, calcaneus, dorsal talus, and distal tibia. Osteochondromas typically originate in the metaphysis and then can continue to grow along with longitudinal growth into the diaphysis. Lesions stop growing coincident with the cessation of longitudinal bone growth.

**Clinical data.** The male:female incidence is 2:1. About 75% of patients present in the first two decades of life.

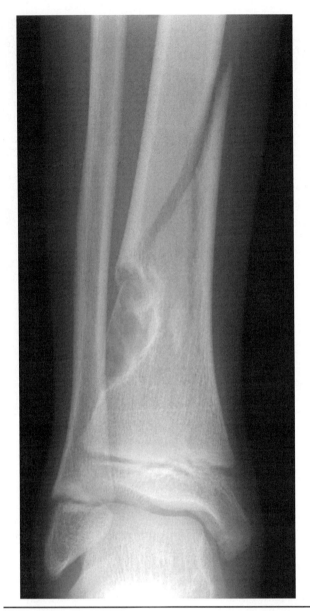

**Figure 23-15**  Evolution of fibrous cortical defect to an eccentric nonossifying fibroma has resulted in pathologic fracture. A spiral oblique fracture of the tibial midshaft can be seen emanating from the superior aspect of the lesion. The risks of pathologic fracture are increased with lesions that approximate 50% of the bony diameter.

Generally ranges from asymptomatic to slow-growing "bump" or "growth." Pedal osteochondromas may be discovered in the workup relating to chronic paronychia or in suspected nerve compression. A bursa occasionally develops over the cap portion of the lesion. Rarely, first-metatarsal osteochondromas may present as an enlarging hallux valgus deformity. Although this may seem paradoxical inasmuch as there is no growth plate in the area, it must be remembered that double metatarsal epiphyses are a relatively common finding in the pediatric population.

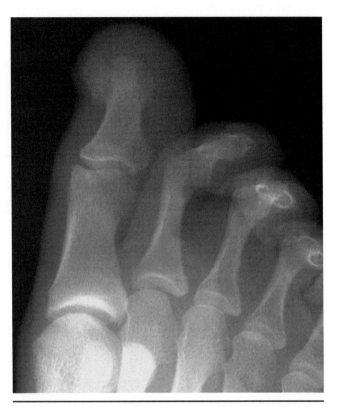

**Figure 23-16**  Pedunculated osteochondroma. Medial oblique view of a 23-year-old male patient presenting with chronic paronychia. An anvil-shaped lesion is noted, with only mildly constricted pedicle. Although many of these lesions are not true osteochondromas, this case suggests the probability of medullary confluence, which was eventually confirmed with CT scans.

## Radiography

1. Radiography shows a protruding, mushroom-shaped exostosis with either a constricted pedicle (Figure 23-16) or a sessile base attaching to the underlying bony cortex (Figure 23-17). Key point: *The cortex of the lesion generally flares into the cortex of the underlying bone (and vice versa).* Absence of this flaring increases the possibility of post-traumatic "look-alike" exostotic juxtacortical/parosteal lesions: a continuum of lesions from florid reactive periostitis to Nora's lesion to acquired osteochondroma (turret exostosis) to subungual (Dupuytren's) exostosis (Figure 23-18). Generally these lesions lack medullary (spongiosal) confluence and flaring of the cortex.

2. Predominantly metaphyseal, although occasionally the diaphyseal cortex flares into the osteochondroma.[8]

3. Multiple views demonstrate medullary/spongiosa confluence with the host bone.

4. Tumor tends to point away from the nearest joint, toward the midshaft.

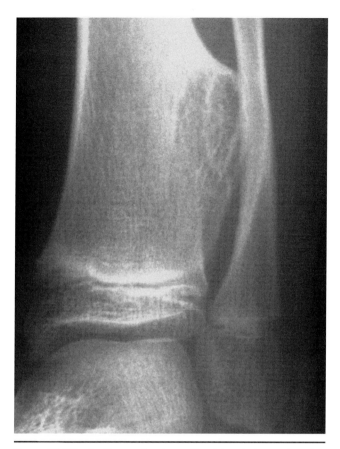

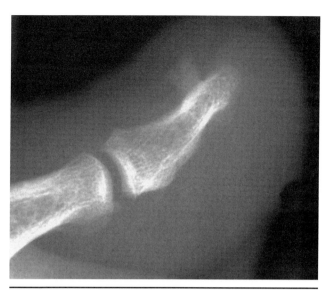

Figure 23-18    Dupuytren's exostosis: Lateral study of hallux demonstrates small, distal dorsal subungual exostotic lesion without medullary confluence or any evidence of corticolesional flaring. The odds are against this being a true osteochondroma. Note that this does not exactly match the typical appearance of exostoses of the distal phalanx associated with hallux limitus, presumably the result of chronic soft tissue compression (with or without shoe-box trauma). These lesions emanate from the most distal-dorsal aspect of terminal tuft and are almost never constricted.

Figure 23-17    Sessile osteochondroma: Broad-based, plateau-shaped lesion involving the distal lateral tibial metaphysis-metadiaphysis of a 7-year-old female. The cortex is flared, and medullary confluence is obvious. A mild angular deformity of the distal tibia is noticeable. Consistent pressure of this slow-growing lesion has resulted in "saucerized" remodeling of the adjacent cortex of the distal-medial fibula along with lateral bowing of the fibular diaphysis. *Note:* The edges of a broad-based exostotic lesion viewed in line with its axis may impart the erroneous appearance of a geographic type IA margin to a pseudolytic lesion. Multiple views should always be obtained.

5. Dystrophic calcification beneath the cartilaginous cap is not uncommon.
6. Growth ceases with closure of the epiphysis.
7. Resorptive or erosive changes, rapid enlargement, and occasionally cap calcification may reflect malignant degeneration to chondrosarcoma.

## Bizarre Osteochondromatous Proliferation (Nora's Lesion)

Bizarre osteochondromatous proliferation (Nora's lesion) is an exostotic lesion generally derived from the parosteal tissues with a high frequency for the small bones of the hands and feet. The lesion consists of cartilage, bone, and fibrous tissue and often has a cartilaginous cap. This lesion probably represents one spectrum of post-traumatic cortical lesions (florid reactive periostitis, turret exostoses, subungual exostoses/Dupuytren's exostosis) derived from subperiosteal hematoma and/or inflammatory changes in and/or around the periosteum. Pathologically, nuclear atypia are common in the cartilaginous components, simulating malignancy.

**Clinical data.**    The incidence ratio is 1:1 male:female; most cases are discovered in an age range from the mid 20s through the fourth decade (slightly older than osteochondroma). Patients predictably complain of a painful dactylitis, generally without a history of trauma or underlying arthropathy. Virtually all cases involve the small bones of the hands and feet.

### Radiography

Bizarre osteochondromatous proliferation mimics osteochondroma but with several significant differences:

1. Well-defined ossified mass arising from the cortical surface
2. May appear pedunculated, attached by a pedicle
3. No flaring of the underlying bony cortex
4. Absence of medullary confluence
5. Periosteal reaction typical

## Simple Bone Cyst (Unicameral or Solitary Bone Cyst)

Simple bone cyst (unicameral or solitary bone cyst) is a non-neoplastic, fluid-filled intramedullary cavity lined by a thin fibrovascular connective tissue membrane and/or osteoid. If fractured, cyst cavities may contain straw-colored serous, serosanguineous, or frank blood.

**Epidemiology.**    Simple bone cysts appear to arise in growing bone and are relatively common in childhood and early adolescence, with a peak incidence in the first two decades. The male:female ratio is 2:1 to 3:1.

**Clinical data.**    The lesions are mostly asymptomatic unless pathologic fracture occurs. Limitation of joint motion has been reported, as well as pain and swelling in tubular bones.

**Location.**    Metaphyseal and, less commonly, diaphyseal regions of the proximal humerus and the femur are affected. Simple bone cysts are the most common tumor and tumorlike lesions of the os calcis and characteristically occupy the neutral triangle area. Occasionally tarsal bones and tubular bones, especially metatarsals, are affected. In long bones, simple cysts typically abut against the metaphyseal side of the physis and demonstrate centripetal growth into the diaphysis.

### Radiography

1.  Solitary, centrally located oval geographic lesion of the metaphysis, metadiaphysis, or diaphysis of a long bone, classically with type IA (see Figure 23-1) growth rate characteristics (that is, sharply delineated margins and a thin, well-delineated sclerotic halo).
2.  Unilocular, although occasionally multilocular, without endosteal scalloping.
3.  May be moderately expansile in tubular and long bones, but never penetrate the cortex—no soft tissue extension.
4.  Central Types IA to IB (see Figure 23-1) marginated lesion of the neutral triangle of the calcaneus with relatively straight anterior and rounded posterior edges (Figure 23-19).
5.  Pathologic fracture with large lesions, where periosteal reactions may be seen. Ossific fragments are known to gravitate to the bottom of the cyst in long bones ("fallen fragment" sign) and this is considered pathognomonic.
6.  Pathologic fracture is unusual in os calcis.

**Differential diagnosis.**    Differential diagnoses include pseudocystic neutral triangle and aneurysmal bone cyst. In older patients, differential diagnoses may be intraosseous lipoma and, rarely, aggressive vascular lesions such as hemangioendothelioma and hemangiopericytoma.

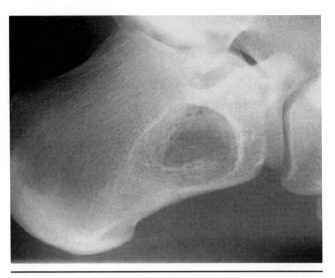

**Figure 23-19**    Lateral study of suspected unicameral bone cyst: Lateral view demonstrates somewhat triangular geographic IA lesion occupying the neutral triangle area of the os calcis. No calcification is apparent. This is the typical location for a unicameral bone cyst in the foot. Differentials include intraosseous lipoma (seen in older patients) and vascular lesions (especially ABC). In fact, this was a 61-year-old female patient, an age that favored what proved the correct diagnosis: intraosseous lipoma.

## Aneurysmal Bone Cyst (ABC)

Probably a reactive process (to trauma or another underlying bone lesion) and not a true neoplasm, aneurysmal bone cysts (ABCs) are rapidly expansile bone lesions consisting of multiple blood-filled cystic cavities with walls made of fibrous tissues and various amounts of osteoid, chondroid, and multinucleated giant cells. These tumors are often (30% to 50%) seen in association with giant cell tumors (GCTs), nonossifying fibromas, chondromyxoid fibromas (CMFs), and other benign bone neoplasms.

**Epidemiology.**    Aneurysmal bone cysts are benign but often locally aggressive. About 80% occur within the age range of 5 to 20 years old. Females are slightly more frequently affected than males.

**Clinical data.**    Rapid onset of pain and swelling. Limitation of joint motion is not uncommon, and dactylitis is typical. Pathologic fracture is possible.

**Location.**    Primary lesions can involve almost any solitary site, with the most frequent involvement of the vertebrae and the metaphyses of long bones, especially around the knee. There may also be an increased tendency to involve the distal fibula, and up to 15% may involve the small tubular bones of the hands and feet. In our experience, the proximal phalanges and distal fibula have been the most frequent pedal sites. Secondary lesions occur in the locale of the host lesion.

**Radiography.**   Classic findings include the following:

1. Oval, metaphyseal "blowout" lesion (Figure 23-20) with "soap bubble" trabeculation in its stable phase; it is important to realize that four radiographic phases have been identified[9]:
   a. *Incipient:* Small, eccentric geographic Type IB lesion with no expansion
   b. *Growth:* Rapid destruction with cortical lysis, no perceivable cortex
   c. *Stable:* Classic—grossly expanded, trabeculated lesion with a thin surrounding cortical shell that overlaps normal diaphyseal cortex ("finger in balloon" sign)
   d. *Healing:* Progressive ossification of lesion

*Note:* Geographic margination admixed with moth-eaten or permeative destruction can be seen in growth phase (type II growth rate), thereby simulating malignant degeneration.

2. "Finger in balloon" sign: Cortex protrudes into lytic zone.
3. Codman's angles (see Figure 23-9) appear during rapid growth phases. Generally, however, an underlying aggressive periosteal pattern *cannot* be identified.

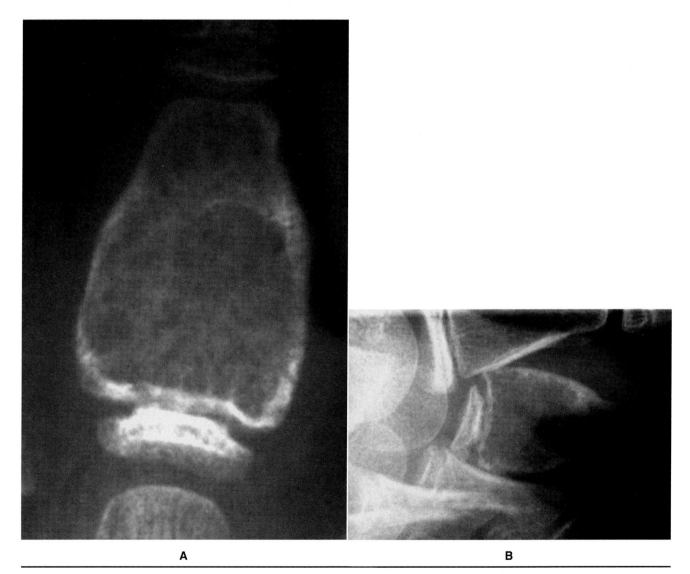

**A**                                              **B**

Figure 23-20   **A,** AP and, **B,** lateral views of an aneurysmal bone cyst (ABC). A non–matrix-forming, expansile geographic lesion involving the proximal metaphysis and the entire diaphysis of a second proximal phalanx in an 8-year-old female patient. Expansion (cortical replacement) is concentric and has produced the appearance of a finely pseudoseptate "shell." In the absence of adequate imaging, the septa can appear smudgy or resemble ground glass. The appearance of an open epiphysis and a nonepiphyseal location argue against giant cell tumor and in favor of an ABC.

4. Septation often not uniformly packed (unlike GCT) and somewhat coarser than giant cell tumors.
5. No propensity to spread to the subarticular cortex or cross physis.
6. Cortical breakthrough with soft tissue invasion possible.

## Giant Cell Tumor of Bone (GCT, Osteoclastoma)

An uncommon tumor of marrow connective tissue origin, giant cell tumor of bone (GCT, osteoclastoma) may be more common in the foot than once thought. Histopathologically, GCTs are characterized by multinucleated giant cells against a background of mononuclear spindle-shaped stromal cells. The ratio of stroma to giant cells has been associated with the relative aggressiveness.

**Epidemiology.** GCTs are benign but often locally aggressive. In our experience, this is one of the more common pedal tumors in the adult foot. Of all GCTs, 75% occur in the 15- to 40-year-old age range (the mean is in the 30s), and they almost always occur in a skeletally mature individual. Males and females show about equal incidence.

**Clinical data.** The chief presenting symptom is a dull ache, possibly associated with a palpable, tender mass. In the toes, dactylitis is typical. Adjacent joints are commonly symptomatic. Pathologic fracture is probably not as frequent as reported in some studies (inasmuch as the lesion typically demonstrates cortical breakthrough) and is a complication in 10% to 35% of cases.

**Location.** GCT primarily arises around the knee in up to 50% of patients, followed by the distal radius. In the feet, the phalanges and metatarsal bones (predictably, the first-metatarsal base and lesser-metatarsal heads) appear the most frequent, followed by the talus and posterior calcaneus. Some studies report midfoot bones (for example, the navicular). In tubular bones, GCTs are characteristically eccentric lesions of the metaphysis (epicenter) with subsequent centrifugal epiphyseal extension.

**Radiography.** Classic findings include the following:

1. Tumors show geographic lysis, are morphologically round, and lack marginal sclerotic reactivity (IB prototype of "punched-out" lesion). In small tubular bones, GCTs often present as a rapidly expansile radiolucent lesion. Although textbook lesions are classically eccentric, metaphyseal with spread to the subarticular cortex, in the foot a central (on axis) location is typical in the digits, metatarsals, and talar body and may indeed may involve the entire width of the bone.

2. Paucity of periosteal reaction; that is, continuous periosteal new bone formation with the underlying cortex grossly intact. Technically, all cortical expansion can be thought of as replacement of the original cortex (which has been destroyed/resorbed) by a newly formed, albeit thinned periosteal shell—and cortical expansion with GCTs is common.
3. Expansile and (pseudo-)trabeculated, especially in phalanges and metatarsals. This expansion can occur rapidly in 6 to 9 months, simulating other "blowout" lesions such as aneurysmal bone cysts and desmoplastic fibromas. or involving the entire width of the bone (Figure 23-21).
4. Marked propensity for spread to the subarticular cortex; however, spread across the joint or through an open physis is unusual (Figure 23-22).
5. Cortical breakthrough with soft tissue invasion possible.
6. Absent matrix.

**Standard differentials.** Differential diagnoses include aneurysmal bone cyst (younger age), enchondroma (same age range, lobulated IA metaphyseal lesion generally lacking septation). Other epiphyseal lesions include arthropathic geodes (for example, intraosseous ganglion, intraosseous gouty tophus), chondroblastoma, occasionally CMF, infection, rarely benign fibrous histiocytoma, and clear-cell chondrosarcoma.

## Enchondroma

As the name suggests, enchondromas are benign, hyaline cartilage tumors of intramedullary origin. Long considered one of the more common pedal tumors, their incidence is probably not as high as some early studies indicated.

**Epidemiology.** Although clearly enchondroma is the most common tumor of the phalanges, the frequency is much higher in the hands (6:1 hand:foot ratio) and much higher in the proximal phalanges. The typical age range is similar to that of GCT (ages 10 to 35), with a peak in the mid 30s, although enchondroma can occur in skeletally immature individuals. Male:female incidence is the same.

**Clinical data.** Although frequently asymptomatic, the patient may complain of nonspecific pain, and swelling. Pain is often associated with pathologic fracture. Although enchondromas are benign, sarcomatous malignant transformation may occur and should be suspected when local pain occurs in the absence of pathologic fracture. Malignant transformation is much more common in more proximal lesions or in multiple enchondromatosis.

**Location.** Enchondroma is almost exclusively a tumor of the appendicular skeleton; about 50% primarily arise in the

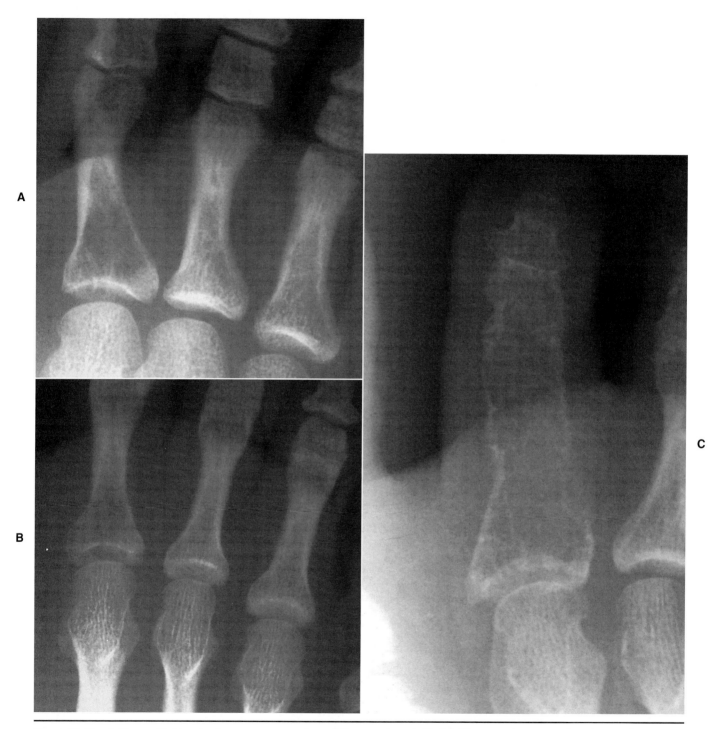

Figure 23-21    A 31-year-old visits a local urgent care center after stubbing second toe. **A,** Medial oblique view demonstrates hyperlucency of second proximal phalangeal base, extending from the subarticular cortex. The lesion is poorly delineated, suggestive of geographic IC-type margins, and virtually invisible on DP study **(B).** Differential diagnoses include intraosseous hemorrhage and GCT. Nevertheless, these radiographs are read as normal. **C,** Same patient 9 months later. Virtually the entire cortex of the proximal phalanx has been replaced by a pseudoseptated periosteal shell. Trabeculation is uniform. No hint of lobulation or endosteal scalloping is apparent. Final pathologic diagnosis after amputation was aggressive giant cell tumor.

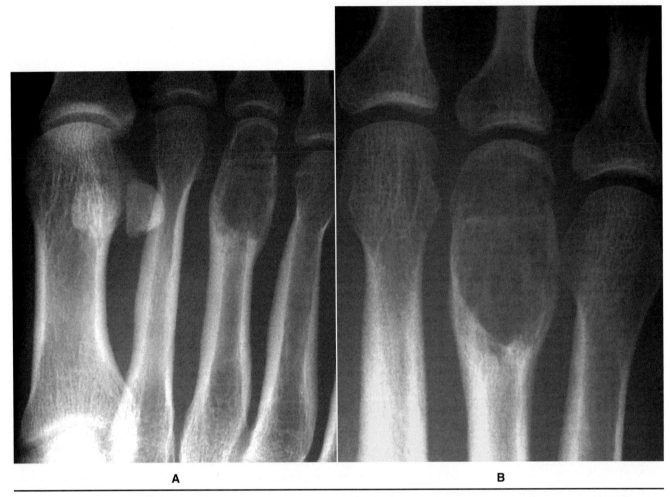

**A**                                             **B**

**Figure 23-22** A 24-year-old patient presented with symptomatic lesion. **A,** Medial oblique view. **B,** DP view. An expansile, geographic type IB lesion with metaphyseal epicenter is noted in the distal third-metatarsal bone. The lesion extends to the subarticular cortex but is without transarticular spread. Sparse epiphyseal septation is noted. Close-up evaluation demonstrates the presence of several smaller holes, suggesting possible motheaten destruction (type II destructive pattern) and therefore degeneration of a benign process. The transverse linear sclerotic zone of the proximal epiphyseal area suggests fracture. Final diagnosis was aggressive giant cell tumor.

small bones of hands, and about 20% around the knee. The distal is involved in up to 50% of patients, followed in frequency by the distal radius. The majority of lesions have their epicenter in the metaphysis, centrally located in long bones and eccentric in tubular bones.

**Radiography.** Classic findings include the following (Figure 23-23):

1. Central intramedullary oval geographic lesion with sharp margination and a thin rim of reactive sclerosis. Less commonly, enchondromas may manifest with unreactive IB margins and/or eccentric locations. Enchondromas are typically located in the metaphysis, metadiaphysis, or—less frequently—diaphysis of a tubular bone. Epiphyseal involvement is distinctly uncommon (Figure 23-24).

2. Frequent endosteal *"scalloping"*—lobulated resorption of the inner cortex.
3. Matrix calcification—flocculent, punctate, occasionally annular internal densities.
4. Pathologic fracture in small tubular bones.

**Imaging nuances.** CT scan is best for analyzing matrix densities and cortical integrity, whereas MR scanning is best for evaluating nonmineralized matrix and marrow involvement.

**Ollier's disease.** In Ollier's disease, multiple enchondromas arise, especially involving the hands and feet, which can result in marked expansile deformities and shortened bones. This is a nonheritable, dyschondroplasia and generally presents at an earlier age than do solitary enchondromas.

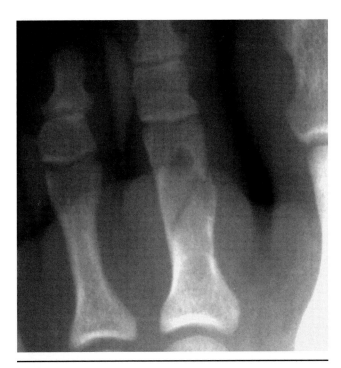

Figure 23-23  Pathologic fracture through an enchondroma in a 25-year-old male patient. Obvious dactylitis of second digit along with the oval-shaped, lobulated lesion demonstrates geographic Type IA destruction of the proximal phalanx. The lesion extends from proximal to distal metaphysis, and is centrally located. Despite this on-axis location, the distal medial diaphysis demonstrates eccentric lobulated shell expansion. No matrix calcification is apparent. Benign cartilaginous lesions such as chondromyxoid fibroma should also be considered.

**Radiography.**    Lesions often display a somewhat more aggressive appearance than solitary enchondroma, often with overt cortical lysis and thickened "strands" emanating from craterlike defects. Typically one extremity is much more affected than the other. Chondrosarcomatous degeneration appears in up to 30% of patients with Ollier's disease. The presence of extensive soft tissue masses should suggest Maffucci's syndrome.

**Maffucci's syndrome.**    Multiple enchondromas and soft tissue hemangiomas characterize Maffucci's syndrome. Radiographically this syndrome may demonstrate multiple phleboliths.

## Chondromyxoid Fibroma (CMF)

Chondromyxoid fibroma (CMF) is a benign tumor characterized by lobules of myxoid and/or chondroid tissue separated by fibrous septa.

**Clinical data.**    The clinical findings are not specific to the disease. Mild pain of long duration is not uncommon. Soft-tissue mass develops on occasion.

**Epidemiology.**    CMF shows a 2:1 male:female incidence ratio, and is most frequent in first two decades.

**Location.**    CMF involves the lower extremities, especially knees, with the proximal tibia most frequent. Talus and plantar mid-calcaneus are most frequent pedal locations, followed by the small tubular bones.

### Radiography

1.  Markedly eccentric, oval geographic lesion of the metaphysis or metadiaphysis in a long bone. As with enchondromata, contours are often lobulated. In tubular bones, a more central location with round shape is likely. Appears on inferior surface of the calcaneus.
2.  Intralesional calcifications rare.
3.  Buttress periosteal reaction ("periosteal collarette"[81]), especially with eccentric oval lesions. Otherwise, there is no tendency toward periosteal new bone formation. When detected, medullary involvement and lack of matrix calcification favors CMF as opposed to juxtacortical chondroma.
4.  Dramatic expansion with or without eccentric cortical resorption.

## Juxtacortical (Periosteal) Chondroma

Juxtacortical (periosteal) chondroma is an uncommon, benign neoplasm composed of mature cartilage. Juxtacortical chondromas are largely cortical lesions in that they typically erode the outer surface of the cortex but generally do not significantly extend into the medullary cavity.

**Clinical data.**    Clinical findings are not specific to the disease. Dactylitis is a symptom when the tumor is located around toes. Mild pain of long duration (1 to 5 years) is not uncommon. Soft tissue mass is found on occasion.

**Epidemiology.**    Juxtacortical chondromas have 2:1 male:female ratio, and are most frequent in the first three decades.

**Location.**    These tumors affect the appendicular skeleton, phalanges, and metatarsal bones in the foot. Femur and humerus are the most frequent sites overall.

### Radiography

1.  Well-delineated, craterlike cortical erosion, simulating an eccentric IA-type oval geographic lesion with epicenter in either the metaphysis or metadiaphysis (Figure 23-25). Contours are smooth.
2.  Intralesional calcifications are common in about 50%, which typically present as a calcified soft tissue mass.

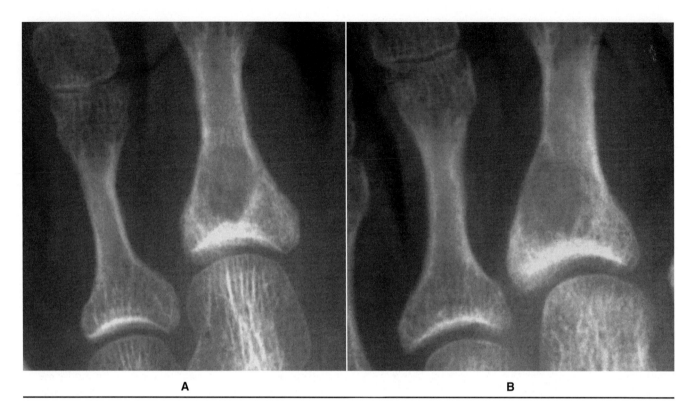

**Figure 23-24** **A,** AP and, **B,** medial oblique views of biopsy-proven enchondroma: Smooth, round geographic B lytic lesion base of second proximal phalanx occupying a somewhat eccentric location in a 33-year-old male patient. No septa are obvious. The lesion has its epicenter in the proximal metaphysis, and the lateral cortex demonstrates mild expansion. The proximal abutment on the subarticular cortex suggests that giant cell tumor (GCT) should be strongly considered. Strangely, even though GCTs are generally eccentric in origin, small tubular bone lesions may have a central predilection. In contradistinction, cartilaginous lesions of the small tubular bones may be more prone to display eccentric (off-axis) expansion at some aspect. (Courtesy Daniel Callahan, D.P.M., Vandalia, Ohio.)

3. Buttress periosteal reaction ("periosteal collarette"). When detected, medullary involvement and lack of matrix calcification favors chondromyxoid fibroma (CMF) as opposed to juxtacortical chondroma.
4. Endosteal cortical surface convexity. This helps distinguish the juxtacortical chondroma from the CMF.

## Chondroblastoma

Chondroblastoma is an uncommon primary bone tumor with a predilection for epiphyseal involvement in younger patients. Unlike enchondromas, chondroblastomas consist of a proliferation of immature cartilage cells.

**Epidemiology.** Ranging from 4% to 7% of all primary bone tumors that involve the foot, about 10% (mean) of all chondroblastomas involve the foot. Incidence follows a 1.4:1 male:female ratio.

**Location.** Chondroblastoma is generally found around the knee (distal femur and proximal tibia). Given the

predilection for this tumor to involve epiphyses with cartilage matrix formation, one might hypothesize that tarsal bones (preformed in cartilage and largely surrounded by joints) would be most frequently involved. This is, in fact, the case. The calcaneus followed by the talus are most frequently involved, followed by the metatarsal bones. Within the calcaneus, chondroblastomas tend to occur peripherally in either juxta-apophyseal or juxta-articular subtalar joint or calcaneocuboid joint locations. In contradistinction, talar lesions tend to arise in the mid-body at the time of discovery (basically abutting ankle and subtalar joints). The cuboid, navicular, cuneiform, or phalanges are uncommonly reported pedal locations.

**Clinical data.** Pain is a consistent initial finding, typically associated with progressive joint symptomatology. The pain may be present for months or even years, and association with joint effusion is not uncommon.

**Radiography.** Sharply demarcated oval or round, centrally located lytic epiphyseal or apophyseal defect

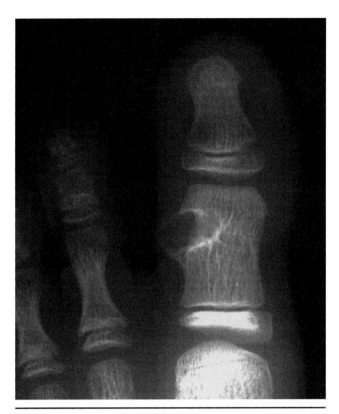

**Figure 23-25**   Biopsy-proven juxtacortical chondroma, 9-year-old female. Shallow cortical erosive change centered over the distal lateral diametaphysis of the proximal hallucal phalanx. A sclerotic reactive margin is noted, with characteristic "buttress" interrupted periosteal reaction (periosteal "collarette" formation). Despite the frequent appearance of matrix calcification in these lesions, none is observed. In theory, when an eccentric lesion appears to be intramedullary (in this age-group and metaphyseal) and manifests with buttress reactions, chondromyxoid fibroma is most likely. However, anecdotally these lesions are much more likely to be located centrally when discovered in small tubular bones.

surrounded by a rim of sclerotic bone (geographic Type IA margination). Occasional IB lesions are encountered. Fine trabeculation is rarely present, as are punctate/stippled calcifications (about 7% of all pedal lesions). In our experience, talar lesions can be mildly expansile. Lesser-tarsal and metatarsal chondroblastomas may demonstrate significant expansion (especially true of metatarsal bones, occasionally simulating osteoblastomas). As with most benign tumors involving the short tubular bones of the hands and feet, even though chondroblastomas may originate in an epiphyseal location by the time of discovery they frequently involve most of the bone.

## Osteoid Osteoma

Osteoid osteoma is an osteoblastic lesion consisting of a small central area of active new bone formation known as the nidus. The nidus is composed of richly vascular con-

nective tissue, interlacing trabeculae of osteoid and calcified bone surrounded by osteoblasts, along with small, unmyelinated nerve fibers. Pedal osteoid osteomas are notorious for causing chronic pain without obvious radiographic findings when greater or lesser tarsal bones are involved, whereupon the index of suspicion is frequently confirmed with ancillary CT (or MR) scan findings.

**Epidemiology.**   Osteoid osteomas comprise about 11% of all benign bone tumors and about 3% of all osseous neoplasia. Reports of foot and ankle involvement generally range between 3% and 15% (7.5% average). Therefore, although pedal involvement is decidedly not common, it probably should not be considered rare.

**Age and sex.**   Statistically most frequent in the first 2½ decades, 75% of osteoid osteomas occur in an ages ranging between 5 and 25 years, with a 2:1 male:female ratio.

**Location.**   Osteoid osteoma is generally found in the femur (mostly proximal) and diaphysis of the tibia. The talus (especially neck) is clearly the most commonly involved pedal bone (also true of osteoblastoma), followed by the os calcis. Otherwise, the hallux has been involved in a number of case reports, as well as the metatarsals and tarsals. The frequency of subtalar joint involvement parallels that of the talocrural joint.

**Clinical data.**   Patients typically complain of a dull, aching pain, localized to the region of involvement, that is generally worse at night. Occasionally the onset of symptoms can be correlated with antecedent trauma. Regional swelling is common, especially when the toes are involved (dactylitis). Classically the pain is relieved by aspirin/salicylates (probably related to local prostaglandin vasodilatory activity). It is important to note that this relief does not always occur. Periarticular locations may present as a monoarticular arthritis with pain, swelling, and limited range of motion, (occasionally simulating tarsal coalition). When the lesion is in one of the phalanges, dactylitis is typical. Marked hypertrophy of the nail plate has been reported in cases that involve the distal phalanx (differential includes osteochondroma, intraosseous glomus, inclusion cyst, and enchondroma).

Inasmuch as pedal lesions can present with few radiographic findings, diagnosing foot and ankle osteoid osteomas can be quite difficult. Numerous case reports show that patients were limping with chronic pain for 6 months to 2 years before the diagnosis was made. Talar lesions typically present with either ankle or subtalar joint pain.

**Radiography.**   The appearance of osteoid osteomas are best described as "pleomorphic," based on their location.

Specifically, the extent of perilesional reactive new bone formation and/or periostitis varies with the origin of the nidus. Three different types are generally appreciated:

1. Cortical
2. Medullary
3. Subperiosteal

Although cortical osteoid osteomas are "textbook" lesions, recent literature employing MR and CT scans has demonstrated that a number of cortical lesions are actually subperiosteal in nature.[10] Indeed, medullary and subperiosteal/para-articular osteoid osteomas are far more common in the foot. They aptly belong in the classification of "targetoid" lesions. (A targetoid lesion is a central area of radiolucency surrounded by a zone of uniform bone sclerosis).

1. *Cortical:* Intracortical lucency that evokes marked new bone formation resulting in cortical thickening and/or sclerosis. The inner cortex typically expands and may encroach on the medullary canal. Despite representing the classic osteoid osteoma, the cortical type is least often encountered in the foot. When present, most cortical osteoid osteomas occur within the metatarsals and only rarely in the phalanges. Within the small tubular bones of the forefoot, the entire bone may appear enlarged or expanded secondary to periosteal new bone formation.
   a. Small, round intracortical nidus generally between 0.5 and 1.5 cm (should not exceed 1.5 cm, otherwise consider osteoblastoma). The nidus may be variably calcified and is often surrounded by a 1- to 2-mm radiolucent, fibrovascular zone.
   b. Cortical thickening or new bone formation can commonly obscure the nidus.
   c. Overlying solid periosteal reaction is common (60%).
   d. MRI and CT or conventional tomography can help image nidus.
2. *Medullary (cancellous):* Most common type encountered in the foot, most frequently in the tarsal bones. The talus is the most common site, followed by the calcaneus. The radiographic appearance is more typical of a so-called annular sequestrum with a central opaque nidus, a perinidal vascular lucent ring that is ultimately limited by a thin rim of reactive sclerosis (Figure 23-26).
   a. Small "bull's-eye" or "target" lesion of bone. Medullary osteoid osteomas do not evoke new bone formation to the degree that cortical lesions do. Variable amounts of peripheral sclerosis may be present, with well-defined inner border. Occasionally a thick sclerotic capsule with poorly defined outer margins (geographic "Type D" lesion) is encountered, mimicking chronic bone abscess.
   b. Central nidus may be lucent or opaque (more commonly opaque at the time of discovery (Figure 23-27).

c. Thin, perinidal lucent zone frequently surrounded by a faint zone of reactive sclerosis that is blunted in comparison to the cortical type.
   d. Minimal to absent periosteal new bone formation.
   e. Typically requires ancillary imaging for diagnosis.
3. *Subperiosteal/para-articular/intra-articular:* As noted, it is now apparent that the subperiosteal, para-articular, and intra-articular osteoid osteomas are fairly common in the foot, as elsewhere in the body. Our experience has been that subperiosteal osteoid osteomas present as symptomatic, shallow surface erosions with a faint sclerotic halo (hence "targetlike") when intracapsular. In contradistinction, when located outside of the joint (especially when they are larger than 3 cm), they can evoke variable amounts of periosteal new bone. This bone may be exuberant and solid when the bone is diaphyseal. In contradistinction, tarsal bony involvement is more likely to have mild periostitis or even a symptomatic "spur." This can be especially misleading when the dorsal talar neck is involved. In fact, osteophyte-like spurring and joint space narrowing have occasionally been associated with articular osteoid osteomas, thereby simulating degenerative arthritis. In other instances, a small, irregular erosion near the chondro-osseous junction and capsular attachments exists, mimicking septic arthritis.

Given that most of the superior, anterior, and inferior aspects of the talus (most common pedal site) are either articular or juxta-articular, the erosive variety is predictably more frequent. Osteoid osteomas of the os calcis generally are medullary or erosive subperiosteal (occasionally retrocalcaneal areas). This pattern seems to be true for the os calcis, even though much of the bone is nonarticular.
   a. *Subperiosteal articular:* May occur within joint, at marginal bare area or at capsular attachments
      (1) Talar lesions often barely visible or not visible on plain film studies.
      (2) Bulk of lesions sits on top of cortex.
      (3) Small traction spur may be present at anterior ankle.
      (4) Limited new bone formation, absent sclerosis (probably caused by the lack of intracapsular periosteum).
      (5) Occasionally presents as a small, irregular erosion of the chondro-osseous junction and/or capsular attachments.
      (6) Fine-cut CT or MR scanning are the best imaging modalities; bone scanning generally helps localize occult lesions.
   b. *Subperiosteal nonarticular*
      (1) Eccentric lesion that sits on top of cortex, although many times this is most obvious with CT scanning.
      (2) Periostitis, sometimes exuberant, that is generally less compact or dense.

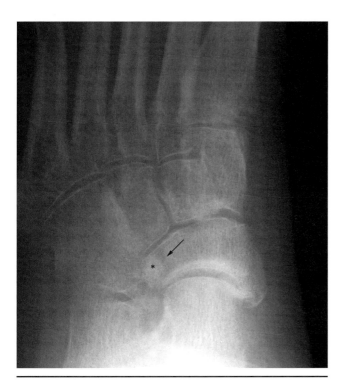

**Figure 23-26** Plain film medial oblique view, osteoid osteoma lateral navicular. Small "target" lesion consisting of osteosclerotic nidus *(asterisk)* and subtle perinidal lucent ring *(arrow)*. This is a rather typical appearance of intra-articular and medullary osteoid osteomas in that they lack the dramatic reactive bone formation/medullary sclerosis of diaphyseal lesions.

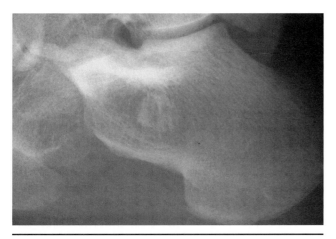

**Figure 23-27** Medullary osteoid osteoma, midbody calcaneus. Lateral study demonstrates focal osteosclerotic lesion neutral triangle of os calcis. Mild "targetoid" appearance noted. Dramatic medullary sclerosis is lacking. Periostitis, however, would best be evaluated with an axial study of the calcaneus. Standard differential diagnoses include enostosis; ossified osteoblastoma; osteoma; old, healed fibrous lesion of bone; dystrophic calcinosis within an intraosseous lipoma; nutrient foramen; and annular sequestrum in bone abscess. The smooth outline (as well as location) argues against medullary infarct and osteoblastic metastasis (rare below knee).

(3) Can mimic healing stress fracture, osteomyelitis, eosinophilic granuloma, and even Ewing's tumor and osteosarcomas.

**Imaging strategies.**    Bone scintigraphy can localize the lesion by demonstrating focal uptake on delayed image bone scans. In contradistinction, enostoses do not take up the tracer. Only a few cases of negative bone scans associated with osteoid osteomas have been reported. Fine-cut (3.0 mm) CT scans are generally considered the best modality for evaluating pedal osteoid osteomas (despite limited ability to acquire direct sagittal-plane images of the foot).

**Differential diagnosis.**    Brodie's abscess, osteoblastoma, enostosis, intraosseous ganglion, and erosive monoarticular arthritis are the differential diagnoses.

## Enostosis (Solitary "Bone Island")

Enostosis, or solitary "bone island," is a discrete, intramedullary sclerotic zone comprised of compact bone, surrounded by normal spongiosa. Bone islands are completely benign. Although commonly discovered in adults, experience suggests that the lesions may arise during periods of bony growth and probably represent a developmental variation or defect and not neoplasia. Some suggest that these are normal variants.

**Clinical data.**    Bone islands are asymptomatic, indolent, and therefore incidental radiologic discoveries.

**Epidemiology.**    With the exception of the skull, bone islands can be found in any bone of the body with a predilection for the femur, pelvis, and ribs. Although the literature is somewhat confusing, experience suggests that enostoses are frequently discovered in the foot and around the ankle. In the foot, although virtually any bone may be involved, the posterior calcaneus, lesser-metatarsal heads, talar neck, and distal tibia are most frequent. Males may predominate slightly.

### Radiography

1.  Most commonly discovered incidentally as a small round or oval intramedullary osteosclerotic lesion found almost exclusively in cancellous bone. When located in epiphyseal regions of long bones, enostoses are typically round, whereas outside of the epiphyseal area they tend to be oval. This argues strongly that enostoses arise in growing bone, thereby at an earlier age.
2.  Smooth, small, well-defined, round to oval osteosclerotic lesion in cancellous bone.
3.  Margins appear well defined at a distance, and the lesion appears uniformly dense and not "targetoid."

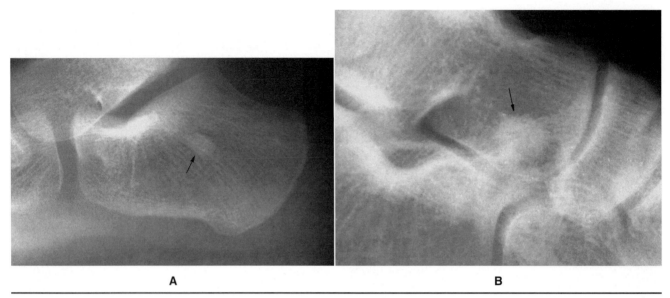

**Figure 23-28  A,** Typical enostosis is located in the greater thalamic compressive patterns of the calcaneus and is concordantly oval. **B,** Enostosis located in the inferior talar neck, with obvious "brush" border.

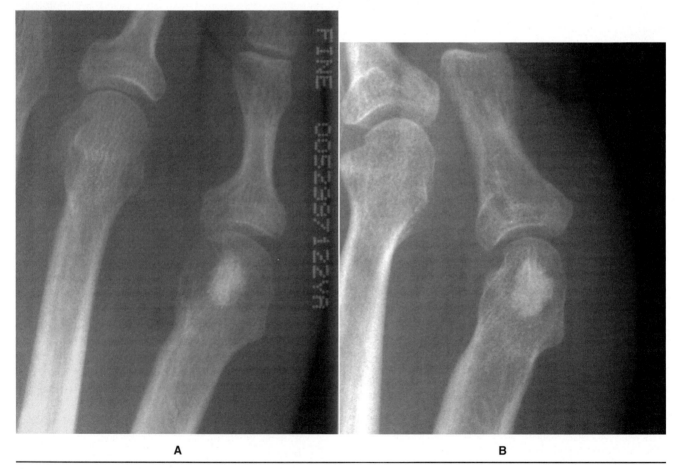

**Figure 23-29  A,** DP and, **B,** medial oblique views of a round enostosis located in the head of the fifth metatarsal demonstrates minimal displacement between these two studies (lesion must be central, near axis), thereby ruling out possible ossicle or lesser sesamoid bone. Note presence of brush border on medial oblique view **(B).**

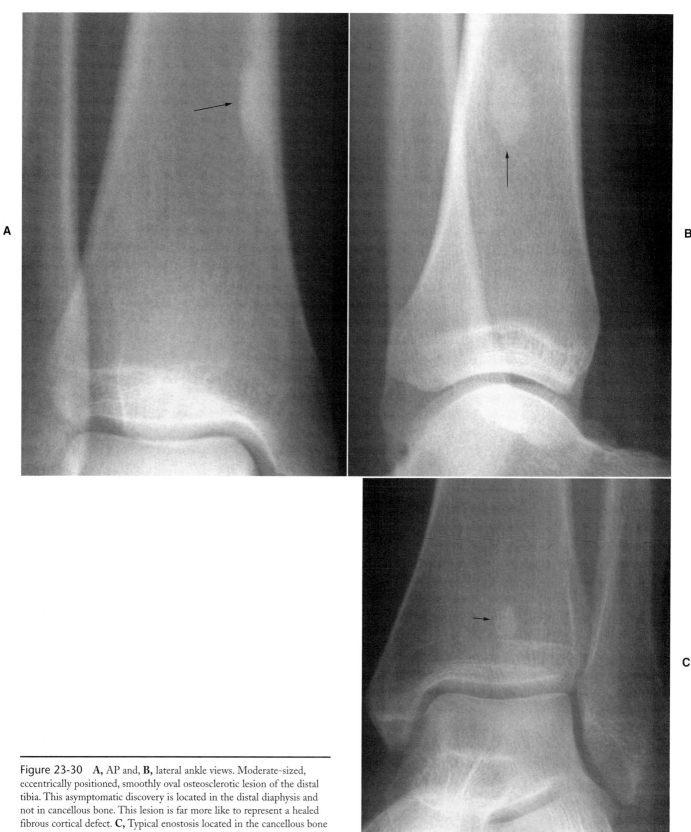

Figure 23-30  **A,** AP and, **B,** lateral ankle views. Moderate-sized, eccentrically positioned, smoothly oval osteosclerotic lesion of the distal tibia. This asymptomatic discovery is located in the distal diaphysis and not in cancellous bone. This lesion is far more like to represent a healed fibrous cortical defect. **C,** Typical enostosis located in the cancellous bone of the epiphyseal region of the distal tibia. Not subject to longitudinal bony growth, this lesion is round and not oval.

However, magnification commonly reveals the presence of a characteristic "thorny" or "brush" border.

4. No periosteal reactions, absence of any destruction within or around lesion.

5. Frequently found in tarsal bones (Figure 23-28) or within the ends of tubular bones (especially the fourth- or fifth-metatarsal heads (Figure 23-29).

6. The axis of oval lesions typically parallels compressive trabecular patterns.

7. Diameter is usually 1.0 centimeter or less (average range from 2 mm to 2 cm), but may be larger ("giant lesions range from 2.0 to 4.5 cm). Larger lesions may resemble the "cumulus cloud" appearance of osteosarcoma.

8. Absence of cortical expansion, periosteal reactions, lucent rimming or bony destruction.

9. Virtually never produce positive bone scan once stable or mature (no longer increasing in size).[11]

On occasion enostoses are known to increase or decrease in size, and in either of these cases bone scans have been positive. The possibility of a malignant process (with positive bone scan) necessitates serial radiographic evaluation. True bone islands generally should not grow more than 25% in 6 months or more than 50% in one year.[8] Suspicious changes should be reviewed at repeat intervals of 1, 3, 6, and 12 months. *Growth exceeding one of these two parameters merits a bone biopsy.*

**Differential diagnosis.** Focal sclerotic lesions, including osteoid osteoma, solitary bone abscess, osteoma, osteoblastoma, healed fibrous lesion of bone (Figure 23-30), focal bony infarct (Figure 23-31) or necrosis, sesamoid/ossicle (bony overlap); osteoblastic metastasis. Focal or patchy sclerotic calcaneal lesions without sharp delineation or uniform shape—consider Ewing sarcoma.

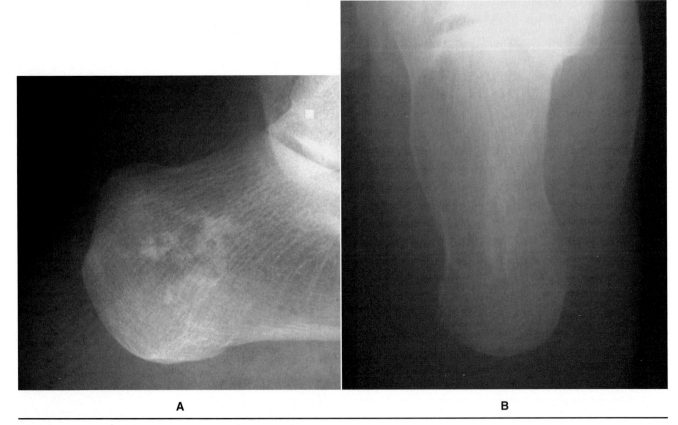

**A**                                                **B**

**Figure 23-31** **A,** Lateral view. Focal sclerotic lesion of the posterior calcaneal tuberosity with flocculent morphologic appearance. The lesion was not symptomatic. Obviously not a bone island, most likely differential diagnoses include enchondroma and medullary infarction. **B,** Calcaneal axial view of same lesion demonstrates narrow, somewhat serpiginous outline of lesion, without overt lysis. This strongly favors the diagnosis of medullary infarct. Past medical history for this patient revealed a long history of steroid use. Other common differentials include chronic alcoholism, collagen vascular disease, and sickle cell anemia.

## References

1. Madewell JE, Ragsdale BD, Sweet DE: Radiologic and pathologic analysis of solitary bone lesions. I. Internal margins, *Radiol Clin North Am* 19(4):715, 1981.

2. Moser RP, Madewell JE: An approach to primary bone tumors. *Radiol Clin North Am* 25(6):1049, 1987.

3. DeSantos LA: The radiology of bone tumors, *CA* 30(2):66, 1980.

4. Ragsdale BD, Madewell JE, Sweet DE: Radiologic and pathologic analysis of solitary bone lesions. II. Periosteal reactions, *Radiol Clin North Am* 19(4):749, 1981

5. Resnick D, Niwayama G: *Diagnosis of bone and joint disorders*, ed 2, Philadelphia, 1988, Saunders.

6. Sweet DE, Madewell JE, Ragsdale BD: Radiologic and pathologic analysis of solitary bone lesions. III. Matrix patterns, *Radiol Clin North Am* 19(4):785, 1981.

7. Edeiken J: *Roentgen diagnosis of diseases of bone*, ed 3, Baltimore, 1981, Williams & Wilkins.

8. Mirra JM, editor, in collaboration with Picci P, Gold RH: *Bone tumors: clinical, radiologic and pathologic correlations*, ed 2, vols 1-2, Philadelphia, 1989, Lea & Febiger.

9. Fechner RE, Mills SE: *Tumors of the bones and joints*, Washington, DC, Armed Forces Institute of Pathology; Bethesda, Md, under the auspices of Universities Associated for Research and Education in Pathology Inc., 1993.

10. Kayser F, Resnick D, Haghighi P, Pereira ER, Greenway G, Schweitzer M, Kindynis P: Evidence of the subperiosteal origin of osteoid osteomas in tubular bones: analysis by CT and MR imaging, *AJR* 170(3):609-614, 1998.

11. Go RT, El-Khoury GY, Wehbe MA: Radionuclide bone image in growing and stable bone island, *Skeletal Radiol* 5:15-18, 1980.

### Additional References

Bernstein AL, Jacobs AM, Oloff LM, Gilula L: Cyst and cystlike lesions of the foot, *JFS* 24:3, 1985.

Brien EW, Mirra JM, Luck JV Jr: Benign and malignant cartilage tumors of bone and joint: their anatomic and theoretical basis with an emphasis on radiology, pathology and clinical biology. II. Juxtacortical cartilage tumors, *Skeletal Radiol* 28:1-20, 1999.

Burgener FA, Kormano M: *Differential diagnosis in conventional radiology*, ed 2, New York, 1991, Thieme Medical.

Coley BL, Higinbotham NL: Tumors primary in bones of hand and feet, *Surgery* 5:112, 1939.

Dahlin DC: *Bone tumors*, ed 4, Springfield, Ill, 1986, Charles C Thomas.

Dahlin DC, Unni KK: *Bone tumors: general aspects and data on 8542 cases*, ed 4, Springfield, Ill, 1986, Charles C Thomas.

Dorfman HD, Czerniak B: *Bone tumors*, St. Louis, 1998, Mosby.

Edeiken J, Dalinka M, Karasick D: *Edeiken's roentgen diagnosis of diseases of bone*, ed 4, Baltimore, 1990, Williams & Wilkins.

Feldman F: The radiographic approach to solitary lesions of bone, *Postgraduate Radiology* 2:3, 1982.

Ghelman B: Radiology of bone tumors, *Orthop Clin North Am*, 20:287, 1989.

Greenfield GB: *Radiology of bone diseases*, ed 5, New York, 1990, Lippincott.

Greenspan A, Klein MJ: Radiology and pathology of bone tumors. In Lewis MM, editor: *Musculoskeletal oncology: a multidisciplinary approach*, Philadelphia, 1992, Saunders.

Greenspan A, Remagen W: *Differential diagnosis of tumors and tumor-like lesions of bones and joints*, Philadelphia, 1998, Lippincott-Raven.

Huvos AG: *Bone tumors: diagnosis, treatment, and prognosis*, ed 2, Philadelphia, 1991, Saunders.

Kransdorf MJ, Jelinek JS, Moser RP Jr: Imaging of bone and soft tissue tumors, *Radiol Clin North Am* 31(2): 359, 1993.

Kricun ME: Radiographic evaluation of solitary bone lesions, *Orthop Clin North Am* 14:39-64, 1983.

Kricun M[E]: *Imaging of bone tumors*, Philadelphia, 1993, Saunders.

Madewell JE, Ragsdale BD, Sweet DE: Radiologic and pathologic analysis of solitary bone lesions. I. Internal margins, *Radiol Clin North Am* 19(4):715, 1981.

Marcove RD, Arlen M: *Atlas of bone pathology: with clinical and radiographic correlations*, Philadelphia, 1992, Lippincott.

McLeod, RA: Bone and soft tissue neoplasms. In Berquist TH, editor: *Radiology of the foot and ankle*, New York, 1989, Raven Press

Moser RP, Madewell JE: An approach to primary bone tumors, *Radiol Clin North Am* 25(6):1049-1093, 1987.

Murari TM, Callaghan JJ, Berrey BH, Sweet DE: Primary benign and malignant neoplasms of the foot, *Foot & Ankle* 10:68, 1989.

Neff JR: Tumors of the foot. In Evarts CM, editor: *Surgery of the musculoskeletal system*, ed 2, vol 5, New York, 1990, Churchill-Livingstone.

Nelson SW: Some fundamentals in the radiologic differential diagnosis of solitary bone lesions, *Semin Roentgenol* 1:244-66, 1966.

Pettersson H, Springfield DS, Enneking WF: *Radiologic management of musculoskeletal tumors*, New York, 1987, Springer.

Ragsdale BD, Madewell JE, Sweet DE: Radiologic and pathologic analysis of solitary bone lesions. II. Periosteal reactions, *Radiol Clin North Am* 19(4):749-783, 1981.

Resnick D, Kyriakos M, Greenway GD: Tumors and tumorlike lesions of bone: imaging and pathology of specific lesions. In Resnick D, Niwayama G, editors: *Diagnosis of bone and joint disorders*, ed 2, vol 6, Philadelphia, 1988, Saunders.

Schajowicz F: *Tumors and tumorlike lesions of bone and joints*, New York, 1981, Springer.

Spjut HJ, Dorfman HD, Fechner RE, Ackerman LV: Tumors of bone and cartilage. In Spjut HJ, Dorfman HD, Fechner RE, Ackerman LV: *Atlas of tumor pathology*, series 2, fascicle 5, Washington, DC, 1970, Armed Forces Institute of Pathology.

Stewart JR, Dahlin DC, Pugh DG: The pathology and radiology of solitary benign bone tumors, *Semin Roentgenol* 1:268, 1966.

Sweet DE, Madewell JE, Ragsdale BD: Radiologic and pathologic analysis of solitary bone lesions. III. Matrix patterns, *Radiol Clin North Am* 19(4):785, 1981.

Turcotte RE, Wold LE, Sim FH: Primary cystic and neoplastic diseases of bone. In Coe FL, Favus MJ, editors: *Disorders of bone and mineral metabolism*, New York, 1992, Raven Press.

Wilner D: *Radiology of bone tumors and allied disorders*, Philadelphia, 1982, Saunders.

Wu KK: Bone tumors and tumor-like malformations of the lower extremity. In DeValentine SJ, editor: *Foot and ankle disorders in children*, New York, 1992, Churchill-Livingstone.

Yeager KK, Mitchell M, Sartoris DJ: Diagnostic imaging approach to bone tumors of the foot, *JFS* 30:197-208, 1991.

Yeager KK, Mitchell M, Sartoris DJ, Resnick D: Diagnostic imaging of bone tumors in the foot, *Clin Podiatr Med Surg* 5:859, 1988.

Zulli LP, Cohen R: Tumors of the foot. In Weissman SD, editor: *Radiology of the foot*, ed 2, Baltimore, 1989, Williams & Wilkins.

## Suggested Readings

### Metastatic Bone Lesions

Abrams HL, Spiro R, Goldstein N: Metastases in carcinoma: analysis of 1000 autopsied cases, *Cancer* 3:74, 1950.

Batson OV: The function of the vertebral veins and their role in the spread of metastases, *Ann Surg* 112:138, 1940.

Gall RJ, Sim FH, Pritchard DJ: Metastatic tumors to the bones of the foot, *Cancer* 37:492, 1976.

Hattrup SJ, Amadio PC, Sim FH, Lombardi RM: Metastatic tumors of the foot and ankle, *Foot & Ankle* 8:243, 1988.

Healey JH, Turnbull AD, Miedema B, Lane JM: Acrometastases. A study of twenty-nine patients with osseous involvement of the hands and feet, *J Bone Joint Surg* 68A:743, 1986.

Kumar PP, Kovi J: Metastases to bones of the hands and feet, *J Natl Med Assoc* 70:836, 1978.

Leeson MC, Kamely JT, Carter JR: Metastatic skeletal disease distal to the elbow and knee, *Clin Orthop* 206:94, 1986.

Mulvey RB: Peripheral bone metastases, *AJR* 91:155-160, 1964.

Neff JR: Metastatic disease to bone. In Lewis MM, editor: *Musculoskeletal oncology: a multidisciplinary approach*, Philadelphia, 1992, Saunders.

Springfield DS: Mechanisms of metastasis, *Clin Orthop* 169:15, 1982.

Sundberg SB, Carlson WO, Jonnson KA: Metastatic lesions of the foot and ankle, *Foot & Ankle* 3(3):167, 1982.

Thrall JH, Burton IE: Skeletal metastases, *Radiol Clin North Am* 25(6):1155, 1987.

Vaezy A, Budson DC: Phalangeal metastases from bronchogenic carcinoma, *JAMA* 239:226, 1978.

Wilner D: *Radiology of bone tumors and allied disorders*, vol 4, chap 53, Philadelphia, 1982, Saunders.

Wu KK, Guise ER: Metastatic tumors of the foot, *South Med J* 71:807, 1978.

Zindrick MR, Young MP, Daley RJ, Light TR: Metastatic tumors of the foot: case report and literature review, *Clin Orthop* 170:219, 1982.

### Osteoid Osteoma

Aisen AM, Glazer GM: Diagnosis of osteoid osteoma using computed tomography, *J Comput Tomogr* 8:175, 1984.

Alkalay I, Grunberg B, Daniel M: Osteoid osteoma in an ossicle of the big toe, *JFS* 26:246, 1987.

Apple DF, Loughlin EC: Osteoid osteoma of the ankle in an athlete, *Am J Sports Med* 9:254, 1981.

Bordelon RL, Cracco A, Book MK: Osteoid osteoma producing premature fusion of the epiphysis of the distal phalanx of the big toe, *J Bone Joint Surg* 57A:120, 1975.

Bullough PG: *Atlas of orthopedic pathology with clinical and radiologic correlations*, ed 2, sec 14.15-14.17, New York, 1992, Gower Medical.

Byers PD: Solitary benign osteoblastic lesions of bone: osteoid osteoma and benign osteoblastoma, *Cancer* 22:43, 1968.

Capanna R, Van Horn JR, Ayala A, Picci P, Bettelli G: Osteoid osteoma and osteoblastoma of the talus: A report of 40 cases, *Skeletal Radiol* 15:360, 1986.

Cohen MD, Harrington TM, Ginsburg WW: Osteoid osteoma: 95 cases and a review of the literature, *Semin Arthritis Rheum* 12:265, 1983.

de Souza Dias L, Frost HM: Osteoid osteoma: osteoblastoma, *Cancer* 33:1075, 1974.

Edeiken J, DePalma AF, Hodes PJ: Osteoid osteoma (roentgenologic emphasis), *Clin Orthop* 49:201, 1966.

Fehring TK, Green NE: Negative radionuclide scan in osteoid osteoma, *Clin Orthop* 185:245, 1984.

Freiberger RH, Loitman BS, Helpern M, Thompson TC: Osteoid osteoma: a report on 80 cases, *AJR* 82:194, 1959.

Gagnon JH, Roy A, Dumas JM: Osteoid osteoma in cancellous bone, *Can Assoc Radiol J* 30:60, 1979.

Gitelis S, Schajowicz F: Osteoid osteoma and osteoblastoma, *Orthop Clin North Am* 20(3):313, 1989.

Golding JSR: The natural history osteoid osteoma: with a report of twenty cases, *J Bone Joint Surg* 36B:218, 1954.

Goranson K, Johnson RP: Osteoid osteoma of os calcis: diagnosis is made by computerized tomography, *Orthopaedic Review* 15:81, 1986.

Gould N: Articular osteoid osteoma of the talus: a case report, *Foot & Ankle* 1:284, 1981.

Hamilos DT, Cervetti RG: Osteoid osteoma of the hallux, *JFS* 26:397, 1987.

Healey JH, Ghelman B: Osteoid osteoma and osteoblastoma: current concepts and recent advances, *Clin Orthop* 264:76, 1986.

Helms CA, Hattner RS, Vogler JB: Osteoid osteoma: radionuclide diagnosis, *Radiology* 151:779, 1984.

Herrlin K, Ekelund L, Lovdahl R, Persson B: Computed tomography in suspected osteoid osteoma of tubular bones, *Skeletal Radiol* 9:92, 1982.

Huvos AG: Bone tumors: *Diagnosis, treatment, and prognosis*, ed 2, Philadelphia, 1991, Saunders.

Jackson RP, Reckling FW, Mantz FA: Osteoid osteoma and osteoblastoma similar histologic lesions with different natural histories, *Clin Orthop* 128:305, 1977.

Jaffe HL: "Osteoid osteoma": a benign osteoblastic tumor composed of osteoid and atypical bone, *Arch Surg* 31:709, 1935.

Jaffe HL: Osteoid osteoma of bone, *Radiology* 45:319, 1945.

Jaffe HL, Lichtenstein L: Osteoid osteoma: further experience with this benign tumor of bone, *J Bone Joint Surg* 22A:645; 1940.

Kahn MD, Tiano FJ, Lillie RC: Osteoid osteoma of the great toe, *JFS* 22:325, 1983.

Kallio E: Osteoid osteoma of the metacarpal and metatarsal bones, *Acta Orthop Scand* 33:246, 1963.

Kendrick JI, Evarts CM: Osteoid osteoma: a critical analysis of forty tumors, *Clin Orthop* 54:51, 1967.

Kenzora JE, Abrams RC: Problems encountered in the diagnosis and treatment of osteoid osteoma of the talus, *Foot & Ankle* 2(3):172, 1981.

Lawrie TR, Aterman K, Path FC, Sinclair AM: Painless osteoid osteoma, *J Bone Joint Surg* 52A:1357, 1970.

Le Saout J, Kerboul B, Courtois B, Jaffres R, Chicault P: Osteoid osteoma of the toes: report on two cases, *J Chir (Paris)* 121:483, 1984.

Mahboubi S: CT appearance of nidus in osteoid osteoma versus sequestration in osteomyelitis, *J Comput Assist Tomogr* 10:457, 1986.

Makely J: Prostaglandins: a mechanism for pain mediation in osteoid osteoma, *Orthop Trans* 6:72, 1982.

Meissner PJ, Mauro G: Osteoid osteoma: a literature review and case report, *JFS* 20:25, 1981.

Patterson BT, Peters VJ: Osteoid osteoma of the fourth metatarsal, *J Am Podiatr Assoc* 71:328, 1981.

Schajowicz F, Lemos C: Osteoid osteoma and osteoblastoma: closely related entities of osteoblastic derivation, *Acta Orthop Scand* 41:272, 1970.

Schulman L, Dorfman HD: Nerve fibers in osteoid osteoma, *J Bone Joint Surg* 52A:1351, 1970.

Sevitt S, Horn JS: A painless and calcified osteoid osteoma of the little finger, *J Pathol* 67:571, 1954.

Shader AF, Schwartzerneld SA: Osteoid osteoma: report of a case, *JFS* 28:438, 1989.

Shereff MJ, Cullivan WT, Johnson KA: Osteoid osteoma of the foot, *J Bone Joint Surg* 65A:638, 1983.

Sherman MS: Osteoid osteoma: review of the literature and report of thirty cases, *J Bone Joint Surg* 29:918; 1947.

Sherman MS, McFarland G: Mechanism of pain in osteoid osteomas, *South Med J* 58:163, 1965.

Shilero J: Osteoid osteoma: two unusual case reports, *JFS* 28:20, 1989.

Short LA, Mattana GW, Benton VG: Osteoid osteoma in the medial malleolus, *JFS* 27:264, 1988.

Sim FH, Dahlin DC, Beabout JW: Osteoid osteoma: diagnostic problems, *J Bone Joint Surg* 57A:154, 1975.

Spinosa FA, Freundlich WA, Roy PP: Osteoid osteoma of the hallux, *JFS* 24:370, 1985.

Stapor DJ, Jacobs RL: Osteoid osteoma of the talus: a case study, *Bull Hosp Joint Dis* 47:273, 1987.

Swee RG, McLeod RA, Beabout JW: Osteoid osteoma: detection, diagnosis and localization, *Radiology* 130:117, 1979.

Wu K: Osteoid osteoma of the foot, *JFS* 30:190, 1991.

*Osteosarcoma*

Amini M, Colacecchi C: An unusual case of primary osteosarcoma of the talus, *Clin Orthop* 150:217, 1980.

Dahlin DC, Coventry MB: Osteogenic sarcoma: a study of 600 cases, *J Bone Joint Surg* 49A:101, 1967.

de Santos LA, Edeiken BS: Subtle early osteosarcoma, *Skeletal Radiol* 13:44, 1985.

Edeiken-Monroe B, Edeiken J, Jacobson HG: Osteosarcoma, *Semin Roentgenol* 24(3):153, 1989.

Harrelson JM: Tumors of the foot. In Jahss MH, editor: *Disorders of the foot and ankle: medical and surgical management*, ed 2, pp 1654-1677, Philadelphia, 1991, Saunders.

Hudson TM, Scheibler M, Hawkins IF, Enneking WF, Spanier SS: Radiologic imaging of osteosarcoma: role in planning surgical treatment, *Skeletal Radiol* 10:137, 1983.

Lane JM, Hurson B, Boland P, Glasser DB: Osteogenic sarcoma, *Clin Orthop* 204:93, 1986.

Lindbom A, Soderberg G, Spjut HJ: Osteosarcoma: review of 96 cases, *Acta Radiol* 56:1, 1961.

McKenna RJ, Schwinn CP, Soong KY, Higinbotham NL: Sarcomata of the osteogenic series (osteosarcoma, fibrosarcoma, chondrosarcoma, parosteal osteogenic sarcoma and sarcomata arising in abnormal bone): an analysis of 552 cases, *J Bone Joint Surg* 48A:1, 1966.

McLeod RA: Bone and soft tissue neoplasms. In Berquist TF, editor: *Radiology of the foot and ankle*, pp 247-276, New York, Raven Press, 1989.

Mirra JM, Kameda N, Rosen G, Eckhardt J: Primary osteosarcoma of toe phalanx: first documented case: review of osteosarcoma of short tubular bones, *Am J Surg Pathol* 12(4):300, 1988.

Ohno T, Abe M, Tateishi A et al: Osteogenic sarcoma: a study of 130 cases, *J Bone Joint Surg* 57A:397, 1975.

Sneppen O, Dissing I, Heerfordt J, Schiodt T: Osteosarcoma of the metatarsal bones: review of the literature and report of a case, *Acta Orthop Scand* 49:220, 1978.

Spjut HJ, Dorfman HD, Fechner RE, Ackerman LV: Tumors of bone and cartilage. In Spjut HJ, Dorfman HD, Fechner RE, Ackerman LV: *Atlas of tumor pathology*, series 2, fascicle 5, pp 141-162, Washington, DC, 1971, Armed Forces Institute of Pathology.

Uribe-Botero G, Russell WO, Sutow WW, Martin RG: Primary osteosarcoma of bone: a clinico-pathologic investigation of 243 cases, with necropsy studies in 54, *Am J Clin Pathol* 67:427, 1977.

Weinfeld MS, Dudley HR Jr: Osteogenic sarcoma: a follow-up study of 94 cases observed at the Massachusetts General Hospital from 1920-1960, *J Bone Joint Surg* 44A:269, 1962.

Wu KK: Tumor review: osteogenic sarcoma of the foot, *JFS* 26:269-271, 1987.

Wu K: Osteogenic sarcoma of the tarsal navicular bone, *JFS* 28:363, 1989.

### Cartilaginous Tumors

Giudici MA, Moser RP, Kransdorf MJ: Cartilaginous bone tumors, *Radiol Clin North Am* 31(2):238-240, 1993.

Sweet DE, Madewell JE, Ragsdale BD: Radiologic and pathologic analysis of solitary bone lesions. III. Matrix patterns, *Radiol Clin North Am* 19:802, 1981.

### Chondroma

Apfelberg DB, Druker D, Maser MR, Lash H: Subungual osteochondroma: differential diagnosis and treatment, *Arch Dermatol* 115:472-473, 1979.

Boriani S, Bacchini P, Bertoni F, Campanacci M: Periosteal chondroma: a review of twenty cases, *J Bone Joint Surg* 65A(2):205-212, 1983.

Coley BL, Santoro AJ: Benign central cartilaginous tumors of bone, *Surgery* 22:411-423, 1947.

deSantos LA, Spjut HJ: Periosteal chondroma: a radiographic spectrum, *Skeletal Radiol* 6:15, 1981.

Dohler R, Heinemann G, Busanny-Caspari W, Farrar MD: Chondrosarcoma of the first metatarsal: primary or secondary to endochondroma, *Acta Orthop Trauma Surg* 95:221-225, 1979.

Galinski AW, Vlahos M: Digital chondroma, *JFS* 28:524-526, 1989.

Gilmer WS, Kilgore W, Smith H: Central cartilage tumors of bone, *Clin Orthop* 26:81-102, 1963.

Giudici MA, Moser RP, Kransdorf MJ: Cartilaginous bone tumors, *Radiol Clin North Am* 31(2):240, 1993.

Greenspan A: Tumors of cartilage origin, *Orthop Clin North Am* 20:347-366, 1989.

Jaffe H[L]: Juxtacortical chondroma, *Bull Hosp Joint Dis* 17:20, 1956.

Jaffe HL, Lichtenstein L: Solitary benign enchondroma of bone, *Arch Surg* 46:480-493, 1943.

Jewusiak EM, Spence KF, Sell KW: Solitary benign enchondroma of the long bones of the hand, *J Bone Joint Surg* 53A:1587-1590, 1971.

Landry MM, Sarma DP: In-situ chondrosarcoma of the foot arising in a solitary enchondroma, *JFS* 29:324-326, 1990.

Levy WM, Aergeter EE, Kirkpatrick JA: The nature of cartilaginous tumors, *Radiol Clin North Am* 2:327-336, 1964.

McFarland Jr GB, Morden ML: Benign cartilaginous lesions, *Orthop Clin North Am* 8:737-749, 1977.

Milgram JW: The origins of osteochondromas and enchondromas: a histopathologic study, *Clin Orthop* 174:264-284, 1983.

Mirra JM, editor, in collaboration with Picci P, Gold RH: *Bone tumors: clinical, radiologic, and pathologic correlations*, vol 1, pp 450-519, Philadelphia, 1989, Lea & Febiger.

Mirra JM, Gold R, Downs J, Eckardt JJ: A new histologic approach to the differentiation of enchondroma and chondrosarcoma of the bones: a clinicopathologic analysis of 51 cases, *Clin Orthop* 102:214-237, 1985.

Murari TM, Callaghan JJ, Berrey BH, Sweet DE: Primary benign and malignant neoplasms of the foot, *Foot & Ankle* 10:68-80, 1989.

Noble J, Lamb DW: Enchondromata of bones of the hand: a review of 40 cases, *Hand* 6:275-284, 1974.

Perlman MD, Gold ML, Schor AD: Enchondroma: a case report and literature review, *JFS* 27:556-560, 1988.

Weissman SD: *Radiology of the foot*, pp 278-319, Baltimore, 1983, Williams & Wilkins.

Yaeger KK, Mitchell M, Sartoris DJ: Diagnostic imaging approach to bone tumors of the foot, *JFS* 30:197-208, 1991.

Yaeger KK, Mitchell M, Sartoris DJ, Resnick D: Diagnostic imaging of bone tumors in the foot, *Clin Podiatr Med Surg* 5:859-876, 1988.

### Osteochondroma

Apfelberg DB, Druker D, Maser MR, Lash H: Subungual

osteochondroma: differential diagnosis and treatment, *Arch Dermatol* 115:472-473, 1979.

Boardman KP: Talotibial impingement exostoses causing osteochondromatosis of the ankle, *Injury* 11:43-44, 1979.

Cavolo DJ, D'Amelio JP, Hirsch AL, Patel R: Juvenile subungual osteochondroma: case presentation, *J Am Podiatr Assoc* 71:81-83, 1981.

Chioros PG, Frankel SL, Sidlow CJ: Unusual osteochondroma of the foot and ankle, *JFS* 26:407-411, 1987.

Dorfman HD, Czerniak B: Bone tumors: in *reference to Nora's lesions, Dupuytren's exostosis, turret exostosis, and florid reactive periostitis*, St. Louis, 1998, Mosby.

Forster RA, Weinberg: Osteochondroma of the ankle: case history, *J Am Podiatr Assoc* 64:419-420, 1974.

Fox IM, Frank NG, Lasker A, Spatt JF: Solitary osteochondroma of a metatarsal: a case report, *J Am Podiatr Assoc* 72:162-164, 1982.

Greenberg D, Lenet MD, Sherman M: A large osteochondroma of the third toe, *J Am Podiatr Assoc* 73:208-211, 1983.

Greenspan A: Tumors of cartilage origin, *Orthop Clin North Am* 20:347-366, 1989.

Hudson TM, Springfield DS, Spanier SS, Enneking WF, Hamlin DJ: Benign exostoses and exostotic chondrosarcomas: evaluation of cartilage thickness by CT, *Radiology* 152:595-599, 1984,

Jones WT, Jones RO: Solitary osteochondroma of the ankle in a four-year-old, *JFS* 21:191-193, 1982.

Kapoor R, Saha MM: Large phalangeal exostosis in multiple cartilaginous exostoses (diaphyseal aclasia): a case report, *Aust Radiol* 31:212-213, 1987.

Kenney PJ, Gilula LA, Murphy WA: The use of computed tomography to distinguish osteochondroma and chondrosarcoma, *Radiology* 139:129-137, 1981.

Kent EJ, Weiner RH: Benign solitary osteochondroma: a case report, *JFS* 13:147-148, 1974.

Kricun M[E]: *Imaging of bone tumors*, pp 116-120, 204-205, 240, Philadelphia, 1993, Saunders.

Lange RH, Rao BK: Correlative radiographic, scintigraphic, and histological evaluation of exostoses, *J Bone Joint Surg* 66A:1454-1459, 1984.

McFarland Jr GB, Morden ML: Benign cartilaginous lesions, *Orthop Clin North Am* 8:737-749, 1977.

Milgram JW: The origins of osteochondromas and enchondromas: a histopathologic study, *Clin Orthop* 174:264-284, 1983.

Murari TM, Callaghan JJ, Berrey BH, Sweet DE: Primary benign and malignant neoplasms of the foot, *Foot & Ankle* 10:68-80, 1989.

Nora FE, Dahlin DC, Beabout JW: Bizarre parosteal osteochondromatous proliferations of the hands and feet, *Am J Surg Pathol* 7:245-250, 1983.

Perry GM: Multiple osteochondroma: a case report, *JFS* 13:105-107, 1974.

Rosen JS: Solitary osteochondroma of the metatarsal, *J Am Podiatr Assoc* 73:261-262, 1983.

Schajowicz F: *Tumors and tumorlike lesions of bones and joints*, pp 121-133, New York, 1981, Springer.

Warren MG, Reid JM: Osteochondroma of the first metatarsal bone: a case report, *J Am Podiatr Assoc* 72:469-470, 1982.

Wolf DS: Osteochondroma of the foot, *J Am Podiatr Assoc* 60:208-210, 1970.

Young CR, Solomon MG: Osteocartilaginous exostosis, *JFS* 19:95-97, 1980.

*Chondroblastoma*

Barbera C, Pinotti N, Klein MJ, Lewis MM: An unusual case of cystic chondroblastoma of the calcaneus: a case report, *Bull Hosp Joint Dis* 48:88, 1988.

Bloem JL, Mulder JD: Chondroblastoma: a clinical and radiological study of 104 cases, *Skeletal Radiol* 14:1-9, 1985.

Braunstein E, Martel W, Weatherbee L: Periosteal bone apposition in chondroblastoma, *Skeletal Radiol* 4:34-36, 1979.

Brower AC, Moser RP, Kransdorf MJ: The frequency and diagnostic significance of periostitis in chondroblastoma, *AJR* 154:309-314, 1990.

Coley BL, Santoro AJ: Benign central cartilaginous tumors of bone, *Surgery* 22:411-423, 1947.

Dahlin DC, Ivins JC: Benign chondroblastoma: a study of 125 cases, *Cancer* 30:401-413, 1972.

Edel G, Nakanishi J, Brinker KH, Roessner A, Blasius S, Vestring T, Muller-Miny H, Erlemann R, Wuisman P: Chondroblastoma of bone: a clinical, radiological, light and immunohistochemical study, *Virchows Archiv A Pathol Anat* 421:355-366, 1992.

Hatcher CH, Campbell JC: Benign chondroblastoma of bone: its histologic variations and a report of late sarcoma in the site of one, *Bull Hosp Joint Dis* 12:411-420, 1951.

Hudson TM, Hawkins IF: Radiologic evaluation of chondroblastoma, *Radiology* 39:1-10, 1981.

Huvos AG, Marcove RC, Erlandson RA, Mike V: Chondroblastoma of bone: a clinicopathologic and electron microscopic study, *Cancer* 29:760-771, 1972.

Huvos AG, Marcove RC: Chondroblastoma of bone: a critical review, *Clin Orthop* 95:300-311, 1973.

Jaffe HL, Lichtenstein L: Benign chondroblastoma of bone: reinterpretation of so-called calcifying or chondromatous giant cell tumor, *Am J Pathol* 18:969-991, 1942.

Kahmann R, Gold RH, Eckardt JJ, Mirra JM: Case report 337, *Skeletal Radiol* 14:301-304, 1985.

Kahn LB, Wood FM, Ackerman LV: Malignant chondroblastoma: report of two cases and review of the literature, *Arch Pathol* 88:371-376, 1969.

Kricun M[E]: *Imaging of bone tumors*, pp 51-54, 225-226, Philadelphia, 1993, Saunders.

Kricun ME, Kricun R, Haskin ME: Chondroblastoma of the

calcaneus: radiographic features with emphasis on location, *AJR* 128:613-616, 1977.

Kumar R, Matasar H, Stansberry S, Shirkhoda A, David R, Madewell, Swischuck LE: The calcaneus: normal and abnormal, *Radiographics* 11:415-440, 1991.

Kyriakos M, Land VJ, Penning HL, Parker SG: Metastatic chondroblastoma: report of a fatal case with a review of the literature on atypical, aggressive, and malignant chondroblastoma, *Cancer* 55:1770-1789, 1985.

McFarland Jr GB, Morden ML: Benign cartilaginous lesions, *Orthop Clin North Am* 8: 737-749, 1977.

McLeod RA, Beabout JW: The roentgenographic features of chondroblastoma, *AJR* 118:464-471, 1973.

Murari TM, Callaghan JJ, Berrey BH Jr, Sweet DE: Primary benign and malignant neoplasms of the foot, *Foot & Ankle* 10:68-80, 1989.

Nolan DJ, Middlemiss H: Chondroblastoma of bone, *Clin Radiol* 26:343-350, 1975.

Ohno T, Kadoya H, Park P, Yamanashi M, Wakayama K, Ihtsubo K, Tateishi A, Kijima M: Case report 382, *Skeletal Radiol* 15:478-483, 1986.

Schajowicz F: *Tumors and tumorlike lesions of bones and joints*, pp 135-148, New York, 1981, Springer.

Schajowicz F, Gallardo H: Epiphyseal chondroblastoma of bone: a clinico-pathologic study of sixty-nine cases, *J Bone Joint Surg* 52B:205-226, 1970.

Sherman RS, Uzel AR: Benign chondroblastoma of bone: its roentgen diagnosis, *AJR* 76:1132-1140, 1956.

Spjut HJ, Dorfman HD, Fechner RE, Ackerman LV: Tumors of bone and cartilage. In Spjut HJ, Dorfman HD, Fechner RE, Ackerman LV: *Atlas of tumor pathology*, series 2, fascicle 5, pp 33-50, Washington, DC, 1970, Armed Forces Institute of Pathology.

Sundaram TKS: Benign chondroblastoma, *J Bone Joint Surg* 48B:92-104, 1966.

*Chondromyxoid Fibroma*

Beggs IG, Stoker DJ: Chondromyxoid fibroma of bone, *Clin Radiol* 33:671-679, 1982.

Crisafulli JA, Adams D, Sakhuja R: Chondromyxoid fibroma of a metatarsal, *JFS* 29:164-168, 1990.

Dahlin DC, Wells AH, Henderson ED: Chondromyxoid fibroma of bone, *J Bone Joint Surg* 35A:831, 1953.

Feldman F, Hecht HL, Johnston AD: Chondromyxoid fibroma of bone, *Radiology* 94:249-260, 1970.

Gherlinzoni F, Rock M, Picci P: Chondromyxoid fibroma: the experience at the Instituto Ortopedico Rizzoli, *J Bone Joint Surg* 65A:198-204, 1983.

Jaffe HL, Lichtenstein L: Chondromyxoid fibroma of bone: distinctive benign tumor likely to be mistaken, especially for chondrosarcoma, *Arch Pathol* 45:541, 1948.

Kreicbergs A, Lonnquist PA, Willems J: Chondromyxoid fibroma: a review of the literature and a report on our own

experience, *APMIS* 93(A):189-197, 1985.

McFarland Jr GB, Morden ML: Benign cartilaginous lesions, *Orthop Clin North Am* 8:737-749, 1977.

Murari TM, Callaghan JJ, Berrey BH, Sweet DE: Primary benign and malignant neoplasms of the foot, *Foot & Ankle* 10:68-80, 1989.

Murphy NB, Price CHG: The radiological aspects of chondromyxoid fibroma of bone, *Clin Radiol* 22:261-269, 1971.

Perdiue RL, Mason WH, Schroeder KE, McGee TP: Chondromyxoid fibroma of the fourth metatarsal: case study and presentation, *J Am Podiatr Assoc* 69:385-388, 1979.

Rahimi A et al: Chondromyxoid fibroma: a clinico-pathologic study of 76 cases, *Cancer* 30:726-1095, 1972.

Ralph LL: Chondromyxoid fibroma of bone, *J Bone Joint Surg* 44B:7-24, 1962.

Schajowicz F, Gallardo H: Chondromyxoid fibroma (fibromyxoid chondroma) of bone: a clinico-pathologic study of thirty-two cases, *J Bone Joint Surg* 53B:198-216, 1971.

Sehayik S, Rosman MA: Malignant degeneration of a chondromyxoid fibroma in a child, *Can J Surg* 18:354, 1975.

Spjut HJ, Dorfman HD, Fechner RE, Ackerman LV: Tumors of bone and cartilage. In Spjut HJ, Dorfman HD, Fechner RE, Ackerman LV: *Atlas of tumor pathology*, series 2, fascicle 5, pp 50-59, Washington, DC, 1970, Armed Forces Institute of Pathology.

Strasberg Z, Tuttle RJ, Lamon CB: Quiz case, *J Can Assoc Radiol* 27:210-211, 1976.

Turcotte B, Pugh DG, Dahlin DC: The roentgenologic aspects of chondromyxoid fibroma of bone, *AJR* 87:1085-1095, 1962.

vanHorn JR, Lemmens JAM: Chondromyxoid fibroma of the foot: a report of a missed diagnosis, *Acta Orthop Scand* 57:375-377, 1986.

*Chondrosarcoma*

Dahlin DC, Beabout JW: Dedifferentiation of low-grade chondrosarcomas, *Cancer* 28:461-466, 1971.

Dahlin DC, Salvador AH: Chondrosarcomas of bones of the hands and feet: a study of 30 cases, *Cancer* 34:755-760, 1974.

Dohler R, Heinemann G, Busanny-Caspari W, Farrar MD: Chondrosarcoma of the first metatarsal-primary or secondary to endochondroma, *Acta Orthop Trauma Surg* 95:221-225, 1979.

Gilmer WS, Kilgore W, Smith H: Central cartilage tumors of bone, *Clin Orthop* 26:81-102, 1963.

Gitelis S, Bertoni F, Picci P, Campanacci M: Chondrosarcoma of bone: the experience at the Instituto Ortopedico Rizzili, *J Bone Joint Surg* 63A:1248-1257, 1981.

Greenspan A: Tumors of cartilage origin, *Orthop Clin North Am* 20:347-366, 1989.

Healey JH, Lane JM: Chondrosarcoma, *Clin Orthop* 204:119-129, 1986.

Henderson ED, Dahlin DC: Chondrosarcoma of bone: a study of two hundred and eighty-eight cases, *J Bone Joint Surg* 45A:1450-1458, 1963.

Hudson TM, Springfield DS, Spanier SS, Enneking WF, Hamlin DJ: Benign exostoses and exostotic chondrosarcomas: evaluation of cartilage thickness by CT, *Radiology* 152:595-599, 1984.

Kenney PJ, Gilula LA, Murphy WA: The use of computed tomography to distinguish osteochondroma and chondrosarcoma, *Radiology* 139:129-137, 1981.

Kricun M[E]: *Imaging of bone tumors*, pp 60-65, 196, 228, Philadelphia, 1993, Saunders.

Landry MM, Sarma DP: In-situ chondrosarcoma of the foot arising in a solitary enchondroma, *JFS* 29:324-326, 1990.

Levy WM, Aergeter EE, Kirkpatrick JA: The nature of cartilaginous tumors, *Radiol Clin North Am* 2:327-336, 1964.

Miki T, Yamamuro T, Oka M, Urushidani H, Itokazu M: Chondrosarcoma developed in the distal phalangeal bone of the third toe: a case report, *Clin Orthop* 136:241-243, 1978.

Mirra JM, Gold R, Downs J, Eckardt JJ: A new histologic approach to the differentiation of enchondroma and chondrosarcoma of the bones: a clinicopathologic analysis of 51 cases, *Clin Orthop* 102:214-237, 1985.

Murari TM, Callaghan JJ, Berrey BH, Sweet DE: Primary benign and malignant neoplasms of the foot, *Foot & Ankle* 10:68-80, 1989.

Nakajima H, Ushigome S, Fukuda J: Case report 482, *Skeletal Radiol* 17:289-292, 1988.

Norman A, Sissons HA: Radiographic hallmarks of peripheral chondrosarcoma, *Radiology* 151:589-596, 1984.

Pritchard DJ, Lunke RJ, Taylor WF, Dahlin DC, Medley BE: Chondrosarcoma: a clinicopathologic and statistical analysis, *Cancer* 45:149-157, 1980.

Reiter FB, Ackerman LV, Staple TW: Central chondrosarcoma of the appendicular skeleton, *Radiology* 105:525-530, 1972.

Sanerkin NG, Gallagher P: A review of the behaviour of chondrosarcoma of bone, *J Bone Joint Surg* 61B:395-400, 1979.

Terry DJ, Olson J: Solitary osteochondroma masquerading as a possible malignant lesion, *JFS* 21:305-315, 1982.

Wiss DA: Chondrosarcoma of the first metatarsal, *J Surg Oncol* 23:110-112, 1983.

Yaeger KK, Mitchell M, Sartoris DJ, Resnick D: Diagnostic imaging of bone tumors in the foot, *Clin Podiatr Med Surg* 5:859-876, 1988.

### Fibrocystic Tumors

#### Nonossifying Fibroma

Brenner RJ, Haltner RS, Lilien DL: Scintigraphic features of nonosteogenic fibroma, *Radiology* 131:727-730, 1979.

Greenfield GB: *Radiology of bone diseases*, pp 687-689, Philadelphia, 1990, Lippincott.

Greenspan A, Klein MJ: Radiology and pathology of bone tumors. In Lewis MM, editor: *Musculoskeletal oncology: a multidisciplinary approach*, pp 43-45, Philadelphia, 1992, Saunders.

Jaffe HL, Lichtenstein L: Non-osteogenic fibroma of bone, *Am J Pathol* 18:205, 1942.

Keats TE, Joyce JM: Metaphyseal cortical irregularities in children: a new perspective on a multi-focal growth variant, *Skeletal Radiol* 12:112-118, 1984.

Kricun M[E]: *Imaging of bone tumors*, pp 110-114, 203, 239, Philadelphia, 1993, Saunders.

Mirra JM: Fibrohistiocystic tumors of intramedullary origin. In Mirra JM, editor, in collaboration with Picci P, Gold RH: *Bone tumors: clinical, radiologic and pathologic correlations*, ed 2, pp 692-735, Philadelphia, 1989, Lea & Febiger.

Resnick D: Tumors and tumor-like lesions of bone: radiographic principles. In Resnick D, editor: *Bone and joint imaging*, pp 1144-1145, Philadelphia, 1989, Saunders.

Schajowicz F: *Tumors and tumorlike lesions of bones and joints*, pp 449-463, New York, 1981, Springer.

Skrede O: Non-osteogenic fibroma of bone, *Acta Orthop Scand* 41:369-380, 1970.

Spjut HJ, Dorfman HD, Fechner RE, Ackerman LV: *Tumors of bone and cartilage*, pp 254-259, Washington, DC, 1971, Armed Forces Institute of Pathology.

#### Bone Cyst

Baker DM: Benign unicameral bone cyst, *Clin Orthop* 71:140-151, 1970.

Campanacci M, Capanna R, Picci P: Unicameral and aneurysmal bone cysts, *Clin Orthop* 204:25-36, 1986.

Capanna R, Van Horn J, Ruggieri P, Biagini R: Epiphyseal involvement in unicameral bone cysts, *Skeletal Radiol* 15:428-436, 1986.

Chigira M, Maehara S, Arita S, Udagawa E: The aetiology and treatment of simple bone cysts, *J Bone Joint Surg* 65B:633-637, 1983.

Cohen J: Etiology of simple bone cyst, *J Bone Joint Surg* 52A:1493-1497, 1970.

Dahlin DC, Besse BE, Pugh DG, Ghormley RK: Aneurysmal bone cysts, *Radiology* 64:56-65, 1955.

Ewald FC: Bone cyst in a phalanx of a two-and-a-half-year-old child, *J Bone Joint Surg* 54A:399-401, 1972.

Huvos AG: *Bone tumors: diagnosis, treatment, and prognosis*, ed 2, pp 713-714, Philadelphia, 1991, Saunders.

Kricun M[E]: *Imaging of bone tumors*, pp 65-67, 228-229, Philadelphia, 1993, Saunders.

Kumar R, Matasar K, Stansberry S, Shirkhoda A, David R, Madewell JE, Swischuck LE: The calcaneus: normal and abnormal, *Radiographics* 11:415-440, 1991.

McGlynn FJ, Mickelson MR, El-Khoury GY: The fallen fragment sign in unicameral bone cyst, *Clin Orthop* 156:157-159, 1981.

Mirra JM: Cysts and cystlike lesions of bone. In Mirra JM, editor, in collaboration with Picci P, Gold RH: *Bone tumors: clinical, radiologic and pathologic correlations*, vol 2, pp 1233-1334, Philadelphia, 1989, Lea & Febiger.

Murari TM, Callaghan JJ, Berrey BH, Sweet DE: Primary benign and malignant osseous neoplasms of the foot, *Foot & Ankle* 10:68-80, 1989.

Norman A, Schiffman M: Simple bone cysts: factors of age dependency, *Radiology* 124:779-782, 1977.

Reynolds J: The fallen fragment sign in the diagnosis of unicameral bone cyst, *J Radiol* 92:949-953, 1962.

Schajowicz F: *Tumors and tumorlike lesions of bones and joints*, pp 417-424, New York, 1981, Springer.

Schajowicz F, Aiello CL, Slullitel I: Cystic and pseudocystic lesions of the terminal phalanx with special reference to epidermoid cysts, *Clin Orthop* 68:84, 1970.

Smith RW, Smith CF: Solitary unicameral bone cyst of the calcaneus: a review of twenty cases, *J Bone Joint Surg* 56A:49-56, 1974.

Spjut HJ, Dorfman HD, Fechner RE, Ackerman LV: Tumors of bone and cartilage. In Spjut HJ, Dorfman HD, Fechner RE, Ackerman LV: *Atlas of tumor pathology*, series 2, fascicle 5, pp 347-353, Washington, DC, 1971, Armed Forces Institute of Pathology.

Tillman BP, Dahlin DC, Lipscomb PR, Stewart JR: Aneurysmal bone cyst: an analysis of ninety-five cases, *Mayo Clin Proc* 43:478-495, 1968.

Yaeger KK, Mitchell M, Sartoris DJ: Diagnostic imaging approach to bone tumors of the foot, *JFS* 30:197-208, 1991.

Yaeger KK, Mitchell M, Sartoris DJ, Resnick D: Diagnostic imaging of bone tumors in the foot, *Clin Podiatr Med Surg* 5:859-876, 1988.

## Tumors of Marrow Origin

### Intraosseous Lipoma

Appenzeller J, Weitzner S: Intraosseous lipoma of os calcis: case report and review of literature of intraosseous lipoma of extremities, *Clin Orthop* 101:171-175, 1974.

Berlin SJ, Mirkin GS, Tubridy SP: Tumors of the heel, *Clin Podiatr Med Surg* 7:307-321, 1990.

Dickson AB, Ayres WW, Mason MW, Miller WR: Lipoma of bone of intra-osseous origin, *J Bone Joint Surg* 33A:257-259, 1951.

Dohler R, Harms D: Intraossare lipome, *Z Orthop Ihre Grenzgeb* 119:38-141, 1981.

Greenfield GB: *Radiology of bone diseases*, ed 5, p 712, New York, 1990, Lippincott.

Guntenberg B, Kindbolm LG: Intraosseous lipoma: a report of

two cases, *Acta Orthop Scand* 49:95-97, 1978.

Hall FM, Cohen RB, Grumbach K: Case report 377, *Skeletal Radiol* 15:401-403, 1986.

Hart JAL: Intraosseous lipoma, *J Bone Joint Surg* 55B:624-632, 1973.

Huvos AG: *Bone tumors: diagnosis, treatment, and prognosis*, ed 2, pp 762-766, Philadelphia, 1991, Saunders.

Leeson MC, Kay D, Smith BS: Intraosseous lipoma, *Clin Orthop* 181:186-190, 1983.

Milgram JW: Intraosseous lipomas: a clinicopathologic study of 66 cases, *Clin Orthop* 231:277-302, 1988.

Milgram JW: Intraosseous lipomas: radiologic and pathologic manifestations, *Radiology* 167:155-160, 1988.

Mirra JM, editor, in collaboration with Picci P, Gold RH: *Bone tumors: clinical, radiologic and pathologic correlations*, vol 1, pp 182-190, Philadelphia, 1989, Lea & Febiger.

Mueller MC, Robbins JC: Intramedullary lipoma of bone, report of a case, *J Bone Joint Surg* 42A:517, 1960.

Poussa M, Holmstrom T: Intraosseous lipoma of the calcaneus: report of a case and a short review of the literature, *Acta Orthop Scand* 47:570-574, 1976.

Resnick D, Kyriakos M, Greenway GD: Tumors and tumorlike lesions of bone: imaging and pathology of specific lesions. In Resnick D, editor: *Bone and joint imaging*, pp 3812-3814, Philadelphia, 1995, Saunders.

Schajowicz F: *Tumors and tumorlike lesions of bone and joints*, p 25, New York, 1981, Springer.

Smith WE, Feinberg R: Intraosseous lipoma, *Cancer* 10:1151, 1957.

Spjut HJ, Dorfman HD, Fechner RE, Ackerman LV: Tumors of bone and cartilage. In Spjut HJ, Dorfman HD, Fechner RE, Ackerman LV: *Atlas of tumor pathology*, series 2, fascicle 5, pp 197-198, Washington, DC, 1971, Armed Forces Institute of Pathology.

### Ewing Sarcoma

Bhansali SK, Desai PB: Ewing's sarcoma: observations on 107 cases, *J Bone Joint Surg* 45A:541-553, 1963.

Dahlin DC, Coventry MB, Scanlon PW: Ewing's sarcoma: a critical analysis of 165 cases, *J Bone Joint Surg* 43A:185-192, 1961.

Dahlin DC, Unni KK: *Bone tumors: general aspects and data on 8542 cases*, ed 4, pp 322-336, Springfield, Ill, 1986, Charles C Thomas.

Ewing J: Diffuse endothelioma of bone, *Proc Pathol Soc* 21:17-24, 1921.

Falk S, Alpert M: The clinical and roentgen aspects of Ewing's sarcoma, *Am J Med Sc* 250(5):492-508, 1965.

Garber CZ: Reactive bone formation in Ewing's sarcoma, *Cancer* 4:839-845, 1951.

Huvos AG: *Bone tumors: diagnosis, treatment, and prognosis*, ed 2, pp 523-552, Philadelphia, 1991, Saunders.

Kim TH, Zaatari G, Atkinson GO, McLaren JR, Ragab AH:

Ewing's sarcoma of a lower extremity in an infant: a therapeutic dilemma, *Cancer* 58:187-189, 1986.

Kricun M[E]: *Imaging of bone tumors*, pp 72-75, 197-198, 230-231, Philadelphia, 1993, Saunders.

Kumar R, Matasar K, Stansberry S, Shirkhoda A, David R, Madewell JE, Swischuck LE: The calcaneus: normal and abnormal, *Radiographics* 11:415-440, 1991.

Lichtenstein L, Jaffe HL: Ewing's sarcoma of bone, *Am J Pathol* 23:43-77, 1947.

Marcove RC, Charosky CB: Phalangeal sarcoma simulating infections of the digits: review of the literature and report of four cases, *Clin Orthop* 83:224-231, 1972.

Mirra JM, Picci P: Ewing's sarcoma. In Mirra JM, editor, in collaboration with Picci P, Gold RH: *Bone tumors: clinical, radiologic and pathologic correlations*, vol 2, pp 1087-1117, Philadelphia, 1989, Lea & Febiger.

Murari TM, Callaghan JJ, Berrey BH, Sweet DE: Primary benign and malignant osseous neoplasms of the foot, *Foot & Ankle* 10:68-80, 1989.

Ridings GR: Ewing's tumor, *Radiol Clin North Am* 2:315-325, 1964.

Schajowicz F: *Tumors and tumorlike lesions of bones and joints*, New York, 1981, Springer.

Sherman RS, Soong KY: Ewing's sarcoma: its roentgen classification and diagnosis, *Radiology* 66:529-538, 1956.

Shirley SK, Gilula LA, Siegal GP, Foulkes MA, Kissane JM, Askin FB: Roentgenographic-pathologic correlation of diffuse sclerosis in Ewing sarcoma of bone, *Skeletal Radiol* 12:69-78, 1984.

Swenson PW: The roentgenologic aspects of Ewing's tumor of bone marrow, *AJR* 50:343-353, 1943.

Taber DS, Libshitz HI, Cohen MA: Treated Ewing sarcoma: radiographic appearance in response, recurrence, and new primaries, *AJR* 140:753-758, 1983.

Vohra VG: Roentgen manifestations in Ewing's sarcoma: a study of 156 cases, *Cancer* 20:727-733, 1967.

Wang CC, Schulz MD: Ewing's sarcoma: a study of fifty cases treated at the Massachusetts General Hospital, 1930-1952 inclusive, *N Engl J Med* 248(14):571-576, 1953.

Wilkins RM, Pritchard DJ, Burgert EO, Unni KK: Ewing's sarcoma of bone: experience with 140 patients, *Cancer* 58:2551-2555, 1986.

Yaeger KK, Mitchell M, Sartoris DJ, Resnick D: Diagnostic imaging of bone tumors in the foot, *Clin Podiatr Med Surg* 5:859-876, 1988.

### Miscellaneous Tumors

#### Aneurysmal Bone Cyst

Beltran, Simon DC, Levy M, Herman L, Weis L, Mueller CF: Aneurysmal bone cysts: MR imaging at 1.5 T, *Radiology* 158:689-690, 1986.

Biesecker JL, Marcove RC, Huvos AG, Mike V: Aneurysmal bone cysts: a clinicopathologic study of 66 cases, *Cancer* 26:615-625, 1970.

Bonakdarpour A, Levy WM, Aegerter E: Primary and secondary aneurysmal bone cyst: a radiological study of 75 cases, *Radiology* 126:75-83, 1978.

Buirski G, Watt I: The radiological features of "solid" aneurysmal bone cysts, *BJR* 57:1057-1065, 1984.

Buraczewski J, Dabska M: Pathogenesis of aneurysmal bone cyst: relationship between the aneurysmal bone cyst and fibrous dysplasia of bone, *Cancer* 28:597-604, 1971.

Campanacci M, Capanna R, Picci P: Unicameral and aneurysmal bone cysts, *Clin Orthop* 204:30, 1986.

Carlson DH, Wilkinson RH, Bhakkaviziam A: Aneurysmal bone cysts in children, *AJR* 116:644-650, 1972.

Dahlin DC, Besse BE, Pugh DG, Ghormley RK: Aneurysmal bone cysts, *Radiology* 64:56-65, 1955.

Dahlin DC, McLeod RA: Aneurysmal bone cyst and other nonneoplastic conditions, *Skeletal Radiol* 8:243-250, 1982.

Dyer R, Stelling CB, Fechner RE: Epiphyseal extension of an aneurysmal bone cyst, *AJR* 137:172-173, 1981.

Hertzanu Y, Mendelsohn DB, Gottschalk F: Aneurysmal bone cyst of the calcaneus, *Radiology* 151:51-52, 1984.

Hudson TM: Fluid levels in aneurysmal bone cysts: a CT feature, *AJR* 141:1001-1004, 1984.

Huvos AG: *Bone tumors: diagnosis, treatment, and prognosis*, ed 2, pp 727-743, Philadelphia, 1991, Saunders.

Jaffe HL: Aneurysmal bone cyst, *Bull Hosp Joint Dis* 11:3, 1950.

Kricun M[E]: *Imaging of bone tumors*, pp 110-114, 203, 239, Philadelphia, 1993, Saunders.

Kumar R, Matasar K, Stansberry S, Shirkhoda A, David R, Madewell JE, Swischuck LE: The calcaneus: normal and abnormal, *Radiographics* 11:415-440, 1991.

Levine BS, Dorfman HD, Matles AL: Evolution of a post-fracture cyst of the fibula, *J Bone Joint Surg* 51A:1631-1637, 1969.

Lichtenstein L: Aneurysmal bone cyst: a pathological entity commonly mistaken for giant-cell tumor and occasionally for hemangioma and osteogenic sarcoma, *Cancer* 3:279-289, 1950.

Lichtenstein L: Aneurysmal bone cyst: observation of fifty cases, *J Bone Joint Surg* 39A:873-882, 1957.

Marcinko DE: Pediatric aneurysmal bone cyst of the ankle, *JFS* 29:429-431, 1990.

Mirra JM: Cysts and cyst-like lesions of bone. In Mirra JM, editor, in collaboration with Picci P, Gold RH: *Bone tumors: clinical, radiologic and pathologic correlations*, vol 2, pp 1267-1311, Philadelphia, 1989, Lea & Febiger.

Resnick D, Niwayama G: *Diagnosis of bone and joint disorders*, ed 2, pp 3617-3888, Philadelphia, 1988, Saunders.

Schajowicz F: *Tumors and tumorlike lesions of bones and joints*, pp 424-439, New York, 1981, Springer.

Sherman RS, Soong KY: Aneurysmal bone cyst: its roentgen diagnosis, *Radiology* 68:54-63, 1957.

Simon WH, Mayer DO, Schmidt RG, Brooks ML, Mitchell EI, Schwamm HA: Magnetic resonance imaging of calcaneal aneurysmal bone cyst, *JFS* 29: 448-451, 1990.

Slowick FA, Campbell CJ, Kettelkamp DB: Aneurysmal bone cyst: an analysis of thirteen cases, *J Bone Joint Surg* 50A:1142-1151, 1968.

Spjut HJ, Dorfman HD, Fechner RE, Ackerman LV: *Tumors of bone and cartilage*, pp 357-366, Washington, DC, 1971, Armed Forces Institute of Pathology.

Tillman BP, Dahlin DC, Lipscomb PR, Stewart JR: Aneurysmal bone cyst: an analysis of ninety-five cases, *Mayo Clin Proc* 43:478-495, 1968.

Yaeger KK, Mitchell M, Sartoris DJ: Diagnostic imaging approach to bone tumors of the foot, *JFS* 30:197-208, 1991. Yaeger KK, Mitchell M, Sartoris DJ, Resnick D: Diagnostic imaging of bone tumors in the foot, *Radiol Foot Ankle* 5:859-876, 1988.

*Giant Cell Tumor*

Campanacci M, Baldini N, Boriani S, Sudanese A: Giant-cell tumor of bone, *J Bone Joint Surg* 69A:106-114, 1987.

Carrasco CH, Murray JA: Giant cell tumors, *Orthop Clin North Am* 20:395-405, 1989.

Coley BL, Higinbotham NL: Giant-cell tumor of bone, *J Bone Joint Surg* 20A:870-884, 1938.

Dahlin DC: Giant cell tumor of bone: highlights of 407 cases, *AJR* 144:955-960, 1985.

Dhillon MS, Singh B, Gill SS, Walker R, Nagi ON: Management of giant cell tumor of the tarsal bones: a report of nine case and a review of the literature, *Foot & Ankle*, 14:265-272, 1993.

Eckhardt JJ, Grogan TJ: Giant cell tumor of bone, *Clin Orthop* 204:45-58, 1986.

Goldenberg RR, Campbell CJ, Bonfiglio M: Giant-cell tumor of bone, *J Bone Joint Surg* 52:619-664, 1970.

Hudson TM: Giant cell tumor. In Hudson TM, editor: *Radiologic-pathologic correlation of musculoskeletal lesions*, pp 209-213, Baltimore, 1988, Williams & Wilkins.

Hutter RVP, Foote FW, Frazell EL, Francis KC: Giant cell tumors complicaitng Paget's disease of bone, *Cancer* 16:1044-1056, 1963.

Jaffe HL: *Tumors and tumorous conditions of the bones and joints*, pp 18-43, Philadelphia, 1958, Lea & Febiger.

Jaffe HL, Lichtenstein L, Portis RB: Giant cell tumor of bone: its pathologic appearance, grading, supposed variants and treatment, *Arch Pathol* 30:993, 1940.

Johnson KA, Riley LH: Giant cell tumor of the bone: an evaluation of 24 cases treated at the Johns Hopkins Hospital between 1925 and 1955, *Clin Orthop* 62:188-191, 1969.

Kaufman SM, Isaac PC: Multiple giant cell tumors, *South Med J* 70:105, 1977.

Larsson SE, Lorentzon R, Boquist L: Giant-cell tumor of bone: a demographic, clinical, and histopathological study of all cases recorded in the Swedish Cancer Registry for the years 1958 through 1968, *J Bone Joint Surg* 57A:167-173, 1975.

Levine E, DeSmet AA, Neff JR: Role of radiologic imaging in management planning of giant cell tumor of bone, *Skeletal Radiol* 12:79-89, 1984.

Lichtenstein L: Aneurysmal bone cyst: a pathological entity commonly mistaken for giant-cell tumor and occasionally for hemangioma and osteogenic sarcoma, *Cancer* 279, 1950.

Manaster BJ, Doyle AJ: Giant cell tumors of bone, *Radiol Clin North Am* 31:299-323, 1993.

Marcove RC, Arlen M: Cyst formation and benign and malignant bone tumors. In Marcove RC, Arlen M, editors: *Atlas of bone pathology: with clinical and radiographic correlations*, pp 338-356, Philadelphia, 1992, Lippincott.

McDonald DJ, Sim FH, McLeod RA, Dahlin DC: Giant-cell tumor of bone, *J Bone Joint Surg* 68A:235-242, 1986.

McGrath PJ: Giant-cell tumor of bone: an analysis of fifty-two cases, *J Bone Joint Surg* 54B:216-229, 1972.

McInerney DR, Middlemiss JH: Giant-cell tumor of bone, *Skeletal Radiol* 2:195-204, 1978.

McLeod RA: Bone and soft tissue neoplasms. In Berquist TF, editor: *Radiology of the foot and ankle*, pp 247-276, New York, 1989, Raven Press.

Mechlin MB, Kricun ME, Stead J, Schwamm HA: Giant cell tumor of tarsal bones: report of 3 cases and review of the literature, *Skeletal Radiol* 11:266-270, 1984.

Mirra JM: Giant cell tumors. In Mirra JM, editor, in collaboration with Picci P, Gold RH: *Bone tumors: clinical, radiologic and pathologic correlations*, vol 2, pp 941-1020, Philadelphia, 1989, Lea & Febiger.

Murari TM, Callaghan JJ, Berrey BH, Sweet DE: Primary benign and malignant neoplasms of the foot, *Foot & Ankle* 10:68, 1989.

Peimer CA, Schiller AL, Mankin HJ, Smith RJ: Multicentric giant-cell tumor of bone, *J Bone Joint Surg* 62A:652, 1980.

Rietveld LA, Mulder JD, Brutel R: Giant cell tumor: metaphyseal or epiphyseal origin? *Diagnostic Imaging* 50: 289-293,1981.

Sherman M, Fabricus R: Giant-cell tumor in the metaphysis in a child: report of an unusual case, *J Bone Joint Surg* 43A:1225-1229, 1961.

Spjut HJ, Dorfman HD, Fechner RE, Ackerman LV: Tumors of bone and cartilage. In Spjut HJ, Dorfman HD, Fechner RE, Ackerman LV: *Atlas of tumor pathology*, series 2, fascicle 5, pp 293-314, Washington, DC, Armed Forces Institute of Pathology, 1971.

Sung HW, Kuo DP, Shu WP, Chai YB, Liu CC, Li SM: Giant-cell tumor of bone: analysis of two hundred and eight cases in Chinese patients, *J Bone Joint Surg* 64A(5):755, 1982.

Wu KK, Ross P, Mitchell DC, Sprague HH: Evolution of a case of multicentric giant cell tumor over a 23-year period, *Clin Orthop* 213 279-288, 1986.

*Enostoses*

Ferguson AB: Calcified medullary defects in bone, *J Bone Joint Surg* 29:598, 1947.

Go RT, El-Khoury GY, Wehbe MA: Radionuclide bone image in growing and stable bone island, *Skeletal Radiol* 5:15-18, 1980.

Greenspan A, Steiner G, Knutzon R: Bone island (enostosis): clinical significance and radiologic and pathologic correlations, *Skeletal Radiol* 20:85-90, 1991.

Mirra JM, editor, in collaboration with Picci P, Gold RH: *Bone tumors: clinical, radiologic and pathologic correlations*, ed 2, pp 182-190, Philadelphia, 1989, Lea & Febiger.

Onitsuka H: Roentgenologic aspects of bone islands, *Radiology* 123:607, 1977.

Smith J: Giant bone islands, *Radiology* 107:35-36, 1973.

# CHAPTER 24

# Miscellaneous Disorders

ROBERT A. CHRISTMAN

Many systemic disorders demonstrate associated radiographic findings in the lower extremity. Although these conditions typically are not clinically diagnosed by their foot or ankle manifestations, the practitioner should be familiar with these radiologic presentations so they are not misdiagnosed as other conditions. The metabolic diseases, in particular osteoporosis, include several endocrine and nutritional disorders (hyperparathyroidism, acromegaly, scurvy, and rickets, for example). Paget's disease may be localized in the lower extremity. Skeletal dysplasias present characteristic presentations that may be recognized as incidental findings; examples include osteopetrosis, osteopoikilosis, osteochondromatosis, and osteogenesis imperfecta. Finally, soft tissue manifestations of systemic disorders are frequently encountered in the foot and leg.

Decreased bone density, or increased radiolucency of bone,[1,2] is a prominent radiographic feature of numerous metabolic disorders. Misconceptions abound regarding the use of terms relating to this finding[3]; therefore, the following definitions are strictly adhered to in this chapter. The term *osteopenia* is used to refer to the nonspecific radiographic finding of decreased bone density. The terms *decalcification, undermineralization,* and *demineralization* are not used, because they refer more specifically to the underlying physiology and pathology of bone.[4] Moreover, the term *osteoporosis* is reserved for the clinical entity.

Generalized, diffuse osteopenia is a highly subjective radiographic finding; one must be careful with this "finding" because radiographic technique and/or processing can profoundly influence the visual appearance (that is, the darkness or lucency) of bones. For example, a dark film can result from high-kVp technique, high-mAs technique, increased time in developer, or raised developer temperature.

Instead, observe specific, more objective features involving the cortices and/or cancellous bone of the second, third, and fourth metatarsals in the dorsoplantar (DP) foot view. Patterns associated with cortical bone thinning in generalized (chronic, long-standing) osteopenia include endosteal resorption, intracortical tunneling, and/or subperiosteal resorption[1] (Figure 24-1). A cancellous bone pattern associated with generalized osteopenia is prominent primary trabeculations, which may stand out in relief because secondary trabeculae are resorbed and subsequent bone is laid down on the remaining primary trabeculae (Figure 24-2). Cortical and cancellous bone resorption is best identified using the DP foot view and concentrating on the second, third, and fourth metatarsals. The medial oblique view should not be used; striations that mimic intracortical tunneling normally are seen at the diametaphyseal region. Caution should be exercised so that these findings are not used to diagnose osteoporosis or other metabolic disease. Chronic osteopenia is commonly associated with systemic disorders, which are primarily diagnosed by other, more characteristic, radiologic features.

In contrast, the primary radiographic feature of acute osteopenia is spotty (mottled, moth-eaten) loss of bone density, particularly in periarticular regions. Acute osteopenia is associated with causes of regional osteoporosis (discussed next), such as immobilization or disuse.

## ◼ OSTEOPOROSIS

Osteoporosis is a metabolic disease that accompanies many other disease processes, including most of the endocrine and nutritional disorders discussed later in this chapter. It is

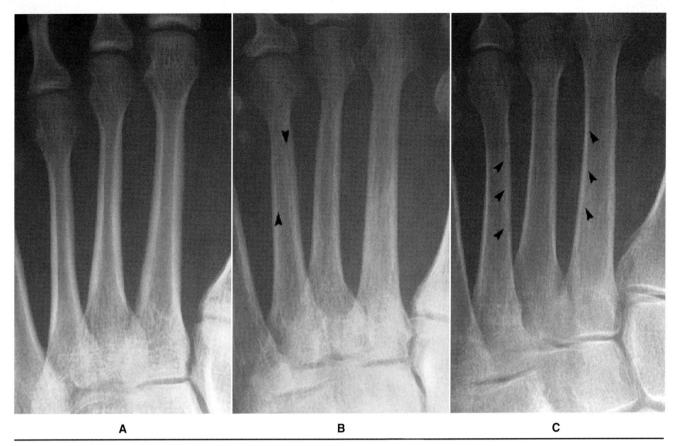

**Figure 24-1** Chronic osteopenia, cortical bone. **A,** Normally, the endosteal and subperiosteal surfaces of the cortex are well defined and continuous and the remainder of the cortex is radiopaque and homogeneous in density. **B,** In chronic cortical osteopenia, the endosteal surfaces are ill defined, and lucent striations (intracortical tunneling) may be seen running through the cortex, parallel to the shaft. **C,** Endosteal resorption, resulting in cortical thinning.

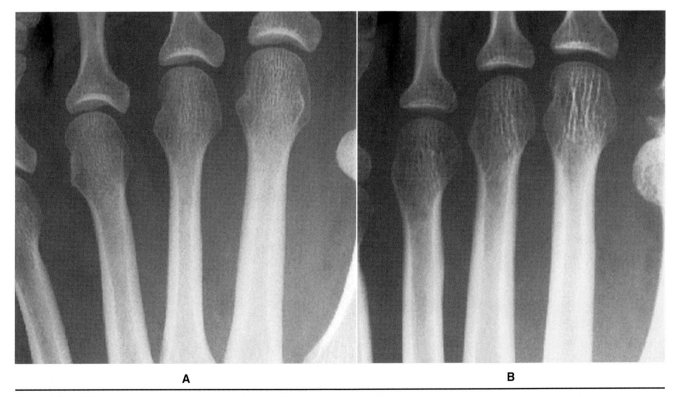

**Figure 24-2** Chronic osteopenia, cancellous bone. **A,** Cancellous bone is made of primary and secondary trabeculae. The primary trabeculae—also known as stress trabeculae—are found along lines of stress. Secondary trabeculae are found perpendicular or oblique to the primary or stress trabeculae. Secondary trabeculae give spongiosa a fine, homogeneous appearance. **B,** With chronic osteopenia, secondary trabeculae are resorbed, leaving the primary trabeculae to stand out in relief. As bone is laid down on the remaining primary trabeculae, they become coarse in appearance.

characterized by progressive loss of bone mass and may result in pathologic fracture. Osteoporosis is not easily diagnosed with plain films, because 30% to 50% of bone calcium must be lost before osteopenia is visually apparent. Quantitative methods are necessary to detect early osteoporosis; studies include single-energy x-ray absorptiometry (wrist and heel), radiographic absorptiometry (hand), single-photon absorptiometry (wrist), quantitative computed tomography (spine), and dual-photon absorptiometry (spine, hip, body). It has been suggested that the appearance of calcaneal trabecular patterns provide an index for assessing osteoporosis[5]; however, controversy exists as to whether or not these trabecular patterns correlate with actual bone density.[6] Osteoporosis has been classified according to its etiology: generalized, regional, and localized.[1]

*Generalized osteoporosis* affects the entire skeleton and is associated with aging (senile osteoporosis), postmenopause, medications (steroids), endocrine states (hyperparathyroidism, diabetes mellitus), deficiency states (scurvy, malnutrition), anemia, and alcoholism, to name a few. The radiographic features are more commonly visualized in the axial skeleton. Typical radiographic findings in the lower extremity (Figure 24-3) include one or any combination of the following:

Prominent primary trabeculations
Thinning of the cortices
Intracortical striations (tunneling)

Normal radiographic anatomy may be misinterpreted as osteopenia. For example, the trabeculations in the first-metatarsal head and neck are normally prominent and appear coarsened.

*Regional osteoporosis* affects one extremity. It is associated with disuse (immobilization) and reflex sympathetic dystrophy syndrome (RSD). Typical radiographic findings (Figure 24-4) include one or any combination of the following:

Spotty (moth-eaten, mottled, patchy) osteopenia in cancellous bone, especially periarticular regions
Ill-defined transverse bands of decreased density at subchondral or metaphyseal locations
Subperiosteal bone resorption (in severe cases, especially RSD)
Long-standing disuse (paralysis is often associated with coarse, prominent primary trabeculations and cortical thinning)

*Localized osteoporosis* affects one bone. Examples of pathology demonstrating localized osteoporosis include osteomyelitis, arthritis, and neoplasm. The medial aspect of the fifth-metatarsal head is normally radiolucent and should not be mistaken as pathology.

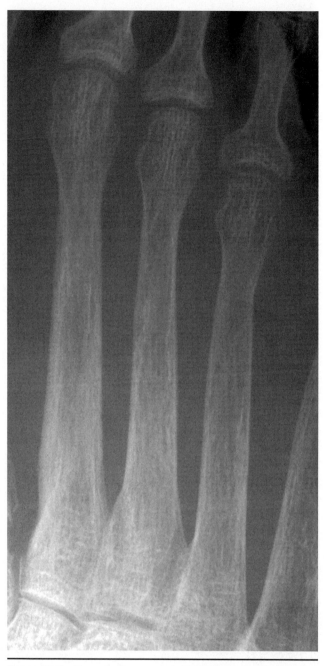

**Figure 24-3**  Generalized osteoporosis. This elderly, postmenopausal patient demonstrates the characteristic features of chronic osteopenia, including endosteal resorption, intracortical tunneling, and prominent, coarsened primary trabeculae.

## ■ OSTEOMALACIA AND RICKETS

Osteomalacia and rickets are characterized histologically as disorders with excessive amounts of uncalcified osteoid.[7] Etiologies include vitamin D deficiency and hypophosphatemia. When present in the adult skeleton, *osteomalacia* is the name given to this condition; in the

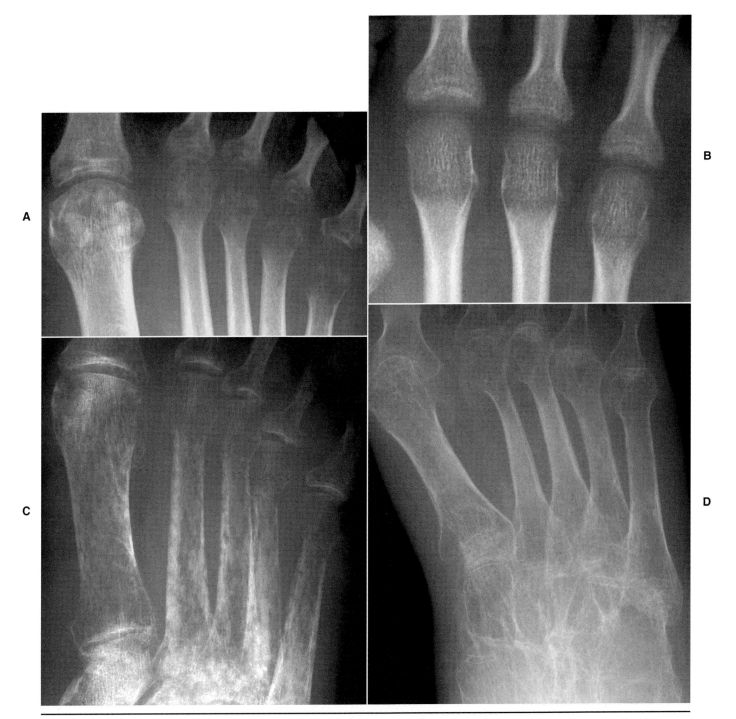

Figure 24-4    Regional osteoporosis. **A,** Periarticular, spotty (acute) osteopenia of cancellous bone at metatarsophalangeal joints. **B,** Metaphyseal ill-defined transverse bands of decreased density, all metatarsals (acute osteopenia). **C,** Severe acute osteopenia, with spotty, permeative decreased density of cancellous and cortical bone, and subperiosteal resorption. **D,** Severe osteopenia secondary to polio. Findings parallel those seen in chronic osteopenia (generalized osteoporosis).

growing skeleton of infancy and childhood, it is called rickets.

The radiographic features of osteomalacia are nonspecific, consisting primarily of osteopenia. Bowing deformity of long tubular bones may occur. Transversely oriented, incomplete radiolucencies, known as pseudofractures or Looser's zones, may be seen in tubular bones.[1]

The radiographic features of rickets consist of both nonspecific and characteristic findings (Figure 24-5). Nonspecific findings include general retardation of body growth, osteopenia, and bowing deformity of long tubular bones. Characteristic changes occur at the growth plate

region of tubular bones and include widening of the physis, decreased density at the zone of provisional calcification, irregularity of the physeal margin of the zone of provisional calcification (which has been described as "fraying" and a "paint-brush appearance"), and widening and cupping of the metaphysis.[1]

## HYPERPARATHYROIDISM

The general term *hyperparathyroidism* refers to increased levels of parathyroid hormone.[1] The characteristic feature of

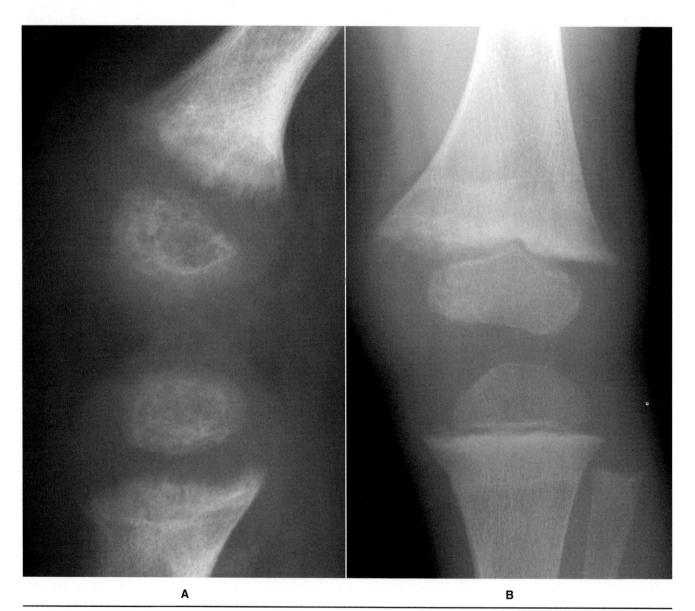

|            A            |            B            |

Figure 24-5  Rickets. **A,** Knee, lateral view. Characteristic features include an ill-defined, lucent and frayed zone of provisional calcification, with widening of the physis. **B,** Knee, anteroposterior (AP) view. Following treatment, the zone of provisional calcification has become more defined, although still irregular and ill-defined medially.

*Continued*

hyperparathyroidism is subperiosteal bone resorption (Figure 24-6). Other sites of bone resorption include peri-articular, intracortical, endosteal, subchondral, and at entheses.

Soft tissue calcification and geographic, lucent lesions known as Brown tumors may also be seen.

## ■ RENAL OSTEODYSTROPHY

Patients with chronic renal failure demonstrate bony abnormalities known as renal osteodystrophy.[1] The radiographic findings manifested may parallel those of hyperparathyroidism, osteoporosis, and osteomalacia (or rickets if in

the child). Calcification of soft tissue and vessels is a frequent finding (Figure 24-7).

## ■ ACROMEGALY

Excess pituitary somatotrophic growth hormone results in abnormal growth of bone, cartilage, and fibrous tissue.[7] In the adult, this is known as acromegaly; gigantism results in the child with open growth plates. Radiographically (Figure 24-8), the patient with acromegaly has an increase in skin volume; the heel pad thickness is greater than 25 mm in the male and 23 mm in the female (when local causes are

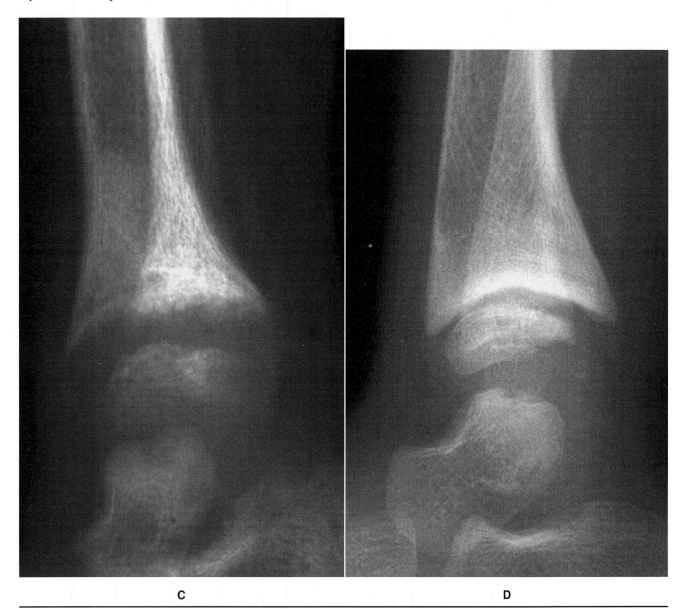

**C**                    **D**

Figure 24-5, cont'd    Rickets. **C,** Ankle, lateral view. Same date as *A;* similar findings demonstrated, with additional metaphyseal cupping. **D,** Ankle, lateral view. Metaphyseal cupping very prominent following treatment; also note defect along surface of talar dome.

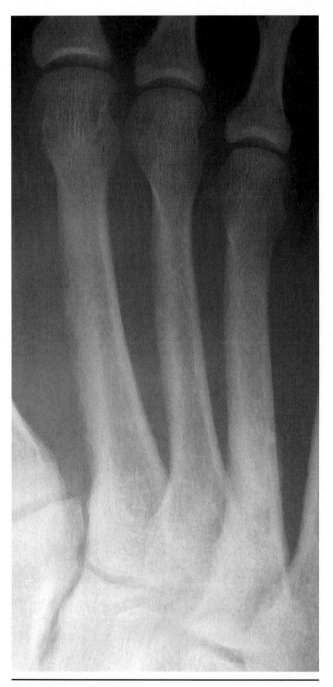

**Figure 24-6** Hyperparathyroidism. Subperiosteal bone resorption along the medial aspects of the metatarsal shafts.

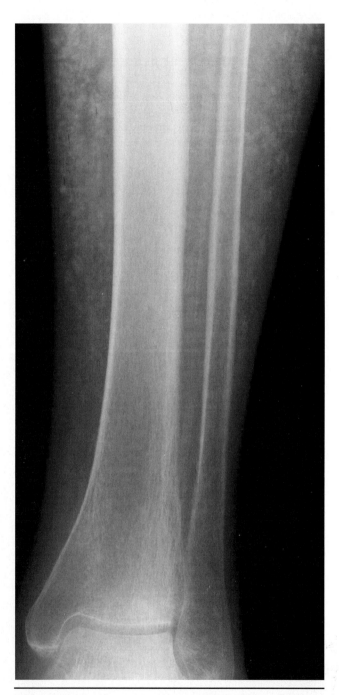

**Figure 24-7** Renal osteodystrophy. Soft tissue calcification throughout the leg.

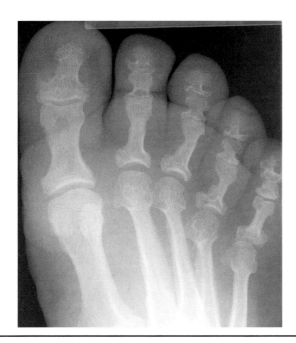

Figure 24-8    Acromegaly. Characteristic features include enlargement of bones (especially metatarsal heads and shafts and phalangeal bases) and soft tissue thickening (increased soft tissue density and volume).

excluded). The joint spaces are widened by cartilage thickening. Bones become prominent; the metatarsal heads and distal phalanx ungual tuberosities are enlarged, metatarsal shafts are thickened, and spurs are found at entheses. Interestingly, however, the proximal phalangeal shafts appear narrow in girth.

## ▬ HYPOVITAMINOSIS C (SCURVY)

Scurvy is caused by insufficient dietary intake of vitamin C.[8] The characteristic radiographic features (Figure 24-9) occur in the developing child. In the metaphyseal region they include a transverse line of increased density, a transverse line of decreased density adjacent to this line of increased density (the scurvy line), and a small, beaklike outgrowth of bone along the margins of the metaphysis. Extensive periostitis may be seen along the entire length of the bone. The epiphysis appears as an outer shell of increased density surrounding a central lucency (Wimberger's sign).[1]

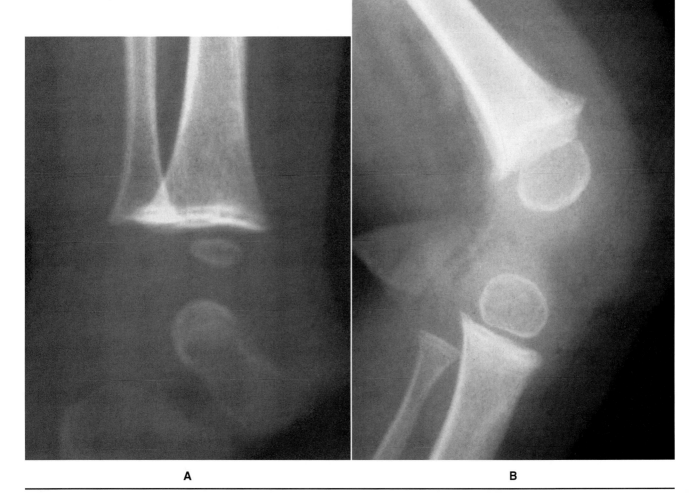

A                                                        B

Figure 24-9    Scurvy. **A,** Ankle. Note the transverse line of increased density along the metaphysis. **B,** Knee (different patient). In addition to the sclerotic line across the metaphysis, beaks are visible at the metaphyseal margins, and Wimberger's sign is evident.

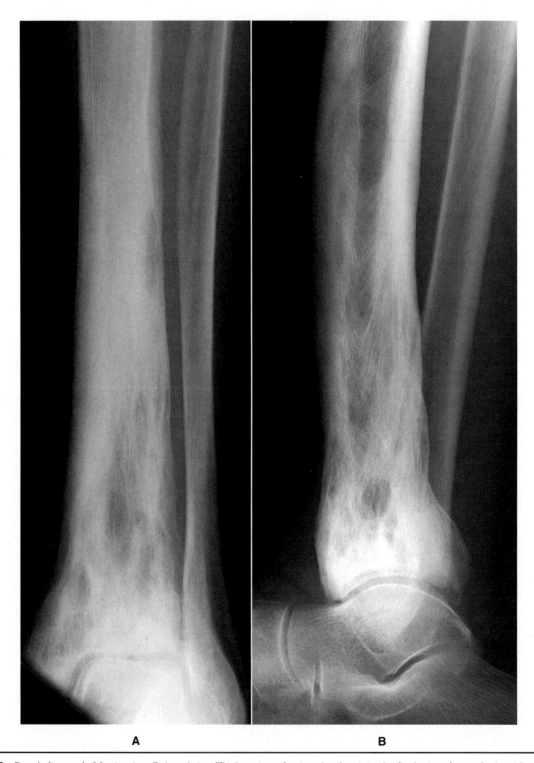

A

B

Figure 24-10    Paget's disease. **A,** Mortise view; **B,** lateral view. The bone is predominantly sclerotic in the diaphysis and metaphysis, with mixed well-defined lucent areas intermixed. Probably the third stage. (Accompanying text on following page.)

## ■ PAGET'S DISEASE (OSTEITIS DEFORMANS)

Paget's disease (Figure 24-10) is characterized by excessive and abnormal remodeling of bone.[1] Its etiology is unknown, and occurs more frequently in people who are 40 years and older. Paget's disease is typically asymptomatic in the foot, which may explain the infrequent reports at this location in the literature.[9] Four radiographic stages have been recognized. The first stage is described as osteolytic. It starts in the subchondral area, spreading to the metaphysis and eventually the diaphysis resulting in what has been described as a "blade of grass" appearance. The second stage demonstrates both osteolysis and osteosclerosis. The diaphysis appears lucent, whereas the epiphyseal and metaphyseal regions are sclerotic. Bone in the third stage is predominantly sclerotic. Findings include cortical thickening, bone enlargement, and coarsened trabeculae. The fourth phase is malignant degeneration, reported in 1% to 10% of patients.[8] Other complications associated with Paget's disease are fracture, osteomyelitis, and joint disease.[1]

## ■ HEREDITARY MULTIPLE EXOSTOSES (OSTEOCHONDROMATOSIS)

Hereditary multiple exostoses is a skeletal dysplasia resulting from a disturbance of chondroid production resulting in heterotopic proliferation of epiphyseal chondroblasts.[10] The individual lesions appear identical to the bone tumor osteochondroma, that is, multiple cartilage-capped exostoses adjacent to the diaphyseal side of the physis (Figure 24-11). This condition is autosomal dominant and appears in the first two decades of life as painless bumps near the ends of long bones. Its distribution is frequently symmetric, and it can cause bone deformity and shortening. Approximately 5 percent of these lesions transform into chondrosarcoma.[7]

## ■ OSTEOGENESIS IMPERFECTA

An inherited skeletal dysplasia that is the result of abnormal metaphyseal and periosteal ossification caused by deficient osteoid production is osteogenesis imperfecta.[10] Abnormal

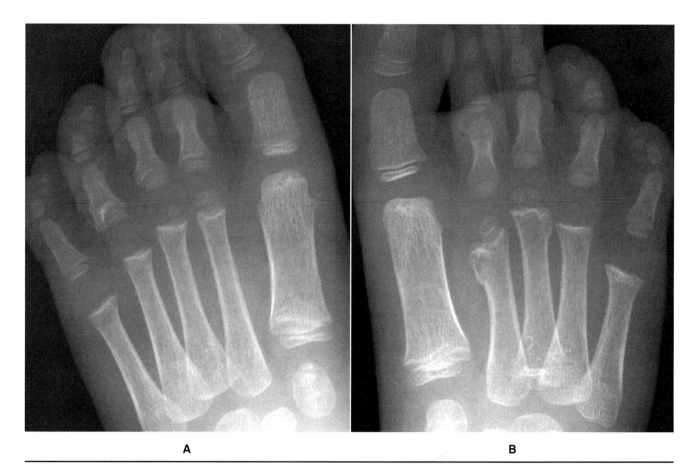

**A**                                                    **B**

Figure 24-11   Hereditary multiple exostoses. **A,** DP view, left foot. Small exostoses are becoming visible along the medial and lateral aspects of the first-metatarsal distal metadiaphysis and along the lateral aspects of the third- and fourth-toe proximal phalangeal bases. **B,** Same patient, DP view, right foot. Significant involvement of the second and third metatarsals, with shortening of the second.

*Continued*

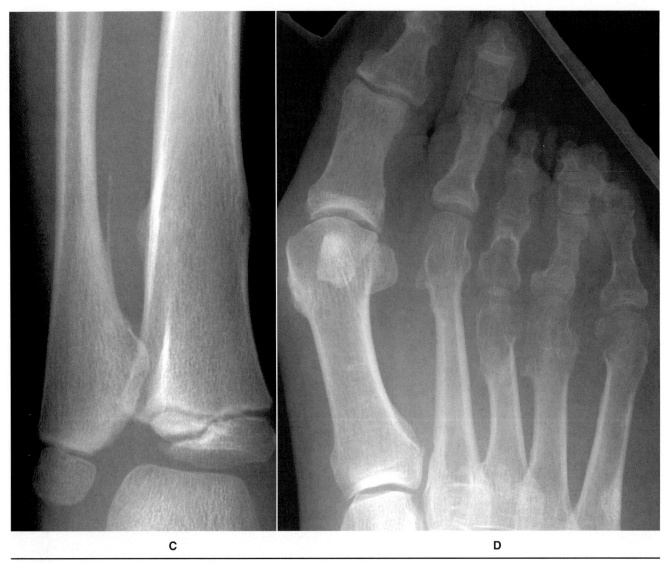

C                                                D

Figure 24-11, cont'd    Hereditary multiple exostoses. **C,** Same patient, AP view, ankle. Exostoses are seen along the medial aspect of the distal fibular diaphysis and the medial and lateral aspects of the tibial diaphysis. **D,** Different patient, adult. Involvement of the second through fourth metatarsals and third-toe proximal phalanx.

maturation of collagen occurs in both mineralized and nonmineralized tissues. Radiographic features include diffuse osteopenia (occasionally coarse trabeculae and a honeycomb appearance), diminished bone girth, and flared metaphyses (Figure 24-12). An obvious complication is fracture.

## THE SCLEROSING DYSPLASIAS

Four skeletal dysplasias are the result of abnormal metaphyseal and periosteal ossification caused by either excessive osteoid production or deficient osteolysis. The primary radiographic feature is increased bone density. They include osteopetrosis, melorheostosis, osteopoikilosis, and osteopathia striata.

*Osteopetrosis* (Albers-Schönberg disease) is an inherited, autosomal dominant (delayed type) condition presenting radiographically with diffuse bone sclerosis (Figure 24-13). Its characteristic feature has been described as a "bone within a bone" appearance.[11] These patients are relatively ymptomatic.[1]

*Melorheostosis* is a rare dysplasia that is not believed to be hereditary.[1] the patient may or may not have associated symptomatology.[9] The radiographic presentation is typically limited to a single limb and consists of hyperostosis along the bone's periphery, extending along its entire length in many cases (Figure 24-14). This picture simulates wax flowing down the side of a candle and has a wavy, sclerotic bony contour usually along the bone's endosteal surface.

*Osteopoikilosis* is an inherited skeletal dysplasia that is not associated with symptomatology. Numerous small, well-defined and homogeneous circular foci of increased density are seen radiographically, mimicking multiple bone islands (Figure 24-15). The distribution of these lesions is periarticular and symmetric, found at the ends of long bones.[1] They may also be found in tarsal bones.

*Osteopathia striata* is most likely inherited and is typically asymptomatic.[9] Radiographically, linear, regular bands of increased density extend from the metaphysis to the diaphysis, running parallel to the shaft (Figure 24-16).

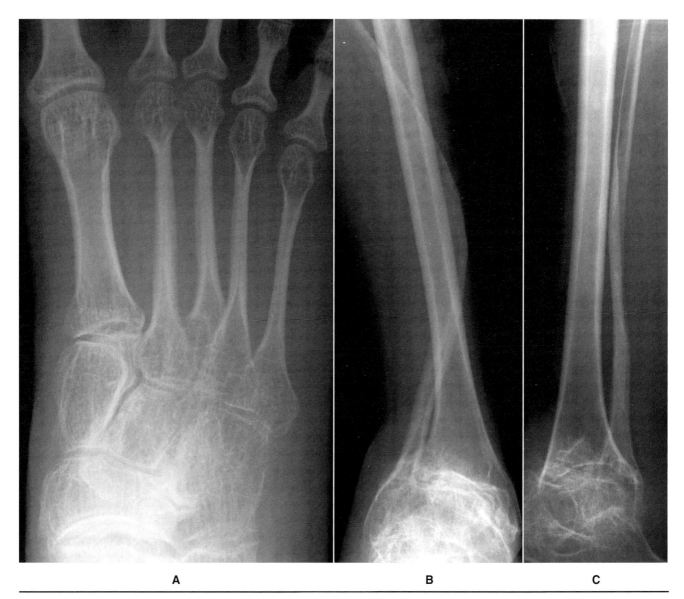

| A | B | C |

Figure 24-12    Osteogenesis imperfecta. **A,** DP view, foot. Characteristic features include narrowed girth of tubular bones and cancellous osteopenia. **B-D,** Different patient demonstrating severe osteoporosis and severe deformity of the fibula.

*Continued*

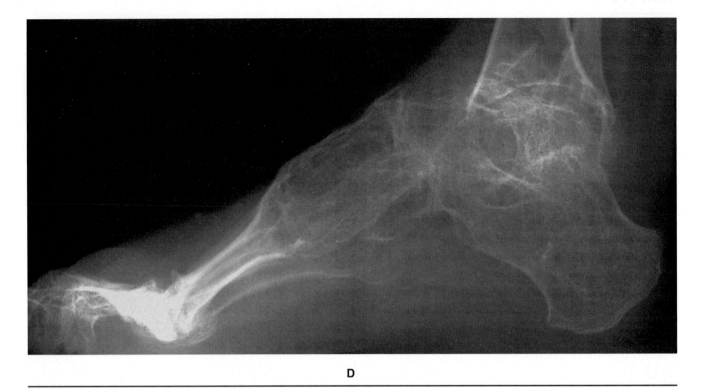

**D**

Figure 24-12, cont'd  Osteogenesis imperfecta. **A,** DP view, foot. Characteristic features include narrowed girth of tubular bones and cancellous osteopenia. **B-D,** Different patient demonstrating severe osteoporosis and severe deformity of the fibula.

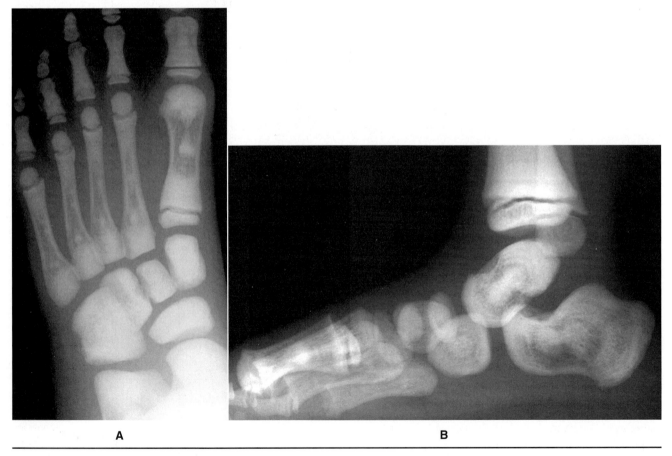

**A**

**B**

Figure 24-13   Osteopetrosis. **A,** DP view, 7-year-old; **B,** Lateral view, same patient at 3 years of age. Classic bone-within-bone appearance.

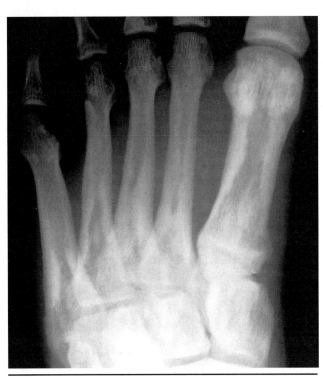

**Figure 24-14**  Melorheostosis. The wavy, thickened endosteal cortical surface simulates wax flowing down a candle. This patient also has osteopoikilosis, as demonstrated by the circular increased densities in periarticular regions.

## FIBROUS DYSPLASIA

Pathologically, normal bone undergoing physiologic resorption is replaced with fibrous tissue.[12] It may occur in one (monostotic) or many (polyostotic) bones. In tubular bones its location is intramedullary and diaphyseal, with only occasional epiphyseal involvement.[1] Radiographically the lesion is somewhat radiolucent with a hazy, ground glass (homogeneous) quality, and may appear expansile with endosteal scalloping (Figure 24-17).

## SOFT TISSUE MANIFESTATIONS OF SYSTEMIC DISORDERS

The primary radiographic soft tissue findings are calcification and ossification. *Calcification* appears as irregular punctate, circular, linear, or plaquelike radiodense areas with no cortical or trabecular structure.[1] *Ossification*, in contrast, demonstrates a trabecular pattern and a thin, cortexlike periphery. However, if the lesion is small, the distinction may be impossible to determine visually.

## Calcification

Conditions that lead to soft tissue calcification have been categorized as metastatic calcification, generalized calcinosis, and dystrophic calcification.[1] *Metastatic calcification* (Figure 24-18) results from a disturbance in calcium or phosphorus metabolism. Examples include hyperparathyroidism, hypoparathyroidism, renal osteodystrophy, hypervitaminosis D, and sarcoidosis. *Generalized calcinosis* (Figure 24-19) presents as calcium deposition in the skin and subcutaneous tissue in the presence of normal calcium metabolism. Examples include collagen vascular disorders (scleroderma, dermatomyositis), idiopathic tumoral calcinosis, and idiopathic calcinosis universalis. Tumoral calcinosis is rare in the foot but has been reported adjacent to a sesamoid[13] and a first-metatarsal-head medial eminence,[14] at the tip of digits,[15] and posterior to the ankle joint. With *dystrophic calcification* (Figure 24-20), calcium is deposited in damaged or devitalized tissue in the absence of a generalized metabolic derangement. Examples include neoplasm, inflammation, and trauma. Soft tissue calcification has been associated with local corticosteroid injection of the heel[16] and intra-articular corticosteroid injection of the small joints of the hand.[17] Extensive involvement of the foot suggests sarcoma.[18]

Vascular calcifications are frequently encountered in the foot and leg. *Phleboliths*, found in veins, are circular or elliptical in shape (Figure 24-21); they possess a thin calcific outline with a relatively lucent center. Phleboliths may be a solitary finding or multiple. Phleboliths have also been described associated with hemangioma of the foot.[19] Two types of arterial calcification have been described: Moenckeberg's sclerosis and atherosclerosis. *Moenckeberg's sclerosis* (Mönckeberg's arteriosclerosis, medial calcific sclerosis) is calcification of the vessel's tunica media layer. These lesions generally do not obstruct blood flow through the vessel. They are commonly seen in patients with diabetes. Radiographically, Moenckeberg's sclerosis has a characteristic appearance consisting of dual, curvilinear tubular calcifications running parallel to one another (Figure 24-22). They may be serpiginous and follow the anatomic course of the vessel. Not uncommonly the path of calcification is discontinuous. The term *atherosclerosis* refers to plaque formation along the tunica intima layer of the vessel. Progressive calcification at any particular site can lead to obstruction of the vessel. Radiographically, one notes patchy calcifications in the soft tissues that follow the path of vessels (Figure 24-23).

The site of soft tissue calcification may provide a clue to the underlying systemic disorder.[1] Periarticular calcification is associated with hyperparathyroidism, hypervitaminosis D, and collagen vascular disease. Calcifications of tendons and bursae are associated with calcium pyrophosphate dihydrate (CPPD) and calcium hydroxyapatite crystal deposition disease. Arterial calcification is frequently seen with diabetes

*Text continued on p. 566*

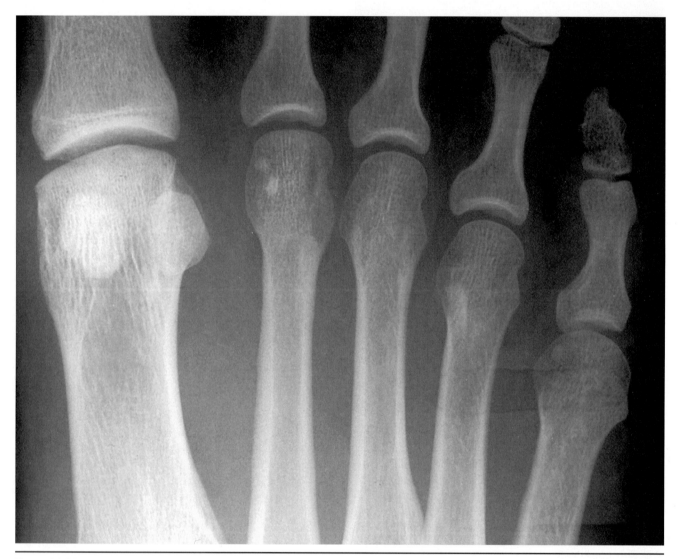

Figure 24-15    Osteopoikilosis. Multiple islands of cortical bone density are identified in the lesser-metatarsal heads.

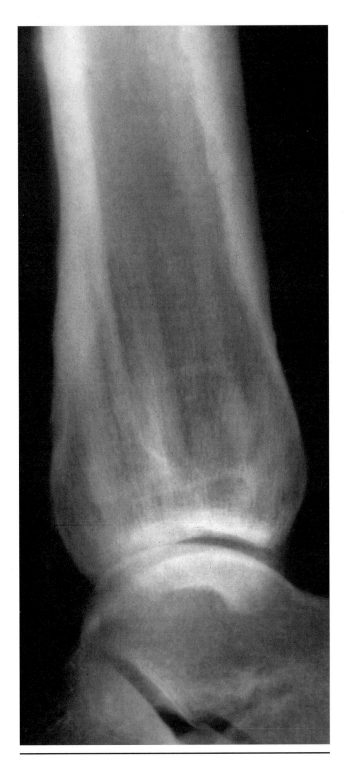

**Figure 24-16** Osteopathia striata. Lateral view, ankle. Mixed linear bands of increased and decreased density run through the metadiaphyseal region of the distal tibia, parallel to the bone's long axis.

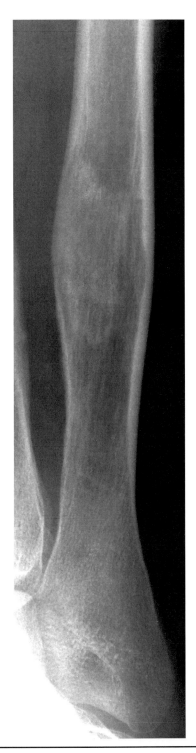

**Figure 24-17** Fibrous dysplasia. The geographic lesion in the distal fibular diaphysis demonstrates a hazy, ground glass appearance centrally. Notice its intramedullary location.

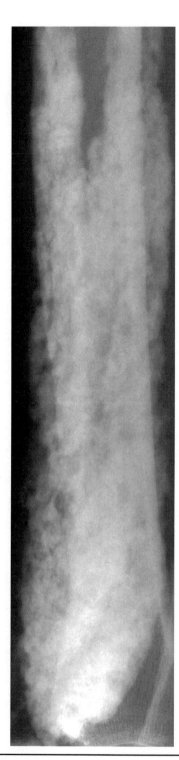

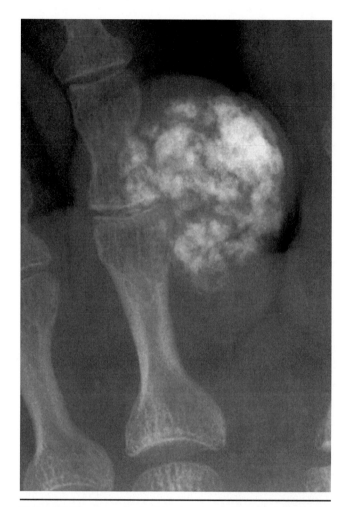

Figure 24-19    Generalized calcinosis: tumoral calcinosis. A large periarticular mass demonstrates calcification adjacent to the proximal interphalangeal joint of a toe.

Figure 24-18    Metastatic calcification: secondary hyperparathyroidism. The spectrum of radiographic abnormality may be seen in these patients. This example demonstrates significant soft tissue calcification in the distal leg.

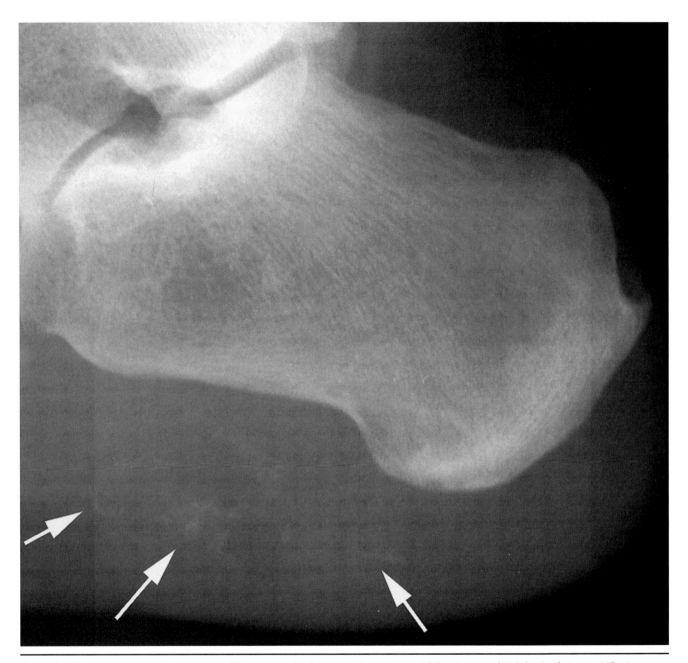

**Figure 24-20**  Dystrophic calcification: trauma. This patient related a recent injury to the heel. Multiple areas of ill-defined soft tissue calcification are identified *(arrows)*.

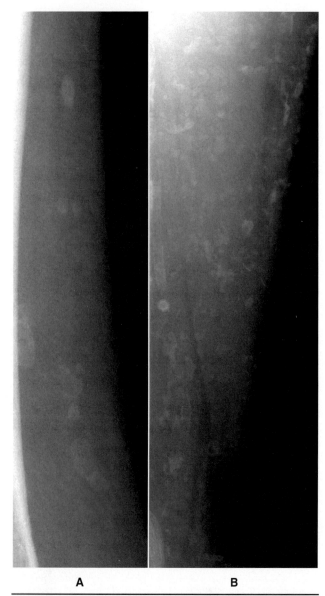

**Figure 24-21**   Vascular calcification: phleboliths. **A,** Phleboliths may be solitary or multiple, as demonstrated in this example of the distal leg. **B,** Numerous phleboliths are seen throughout the calf in this patient with chronic venous insufficiency.

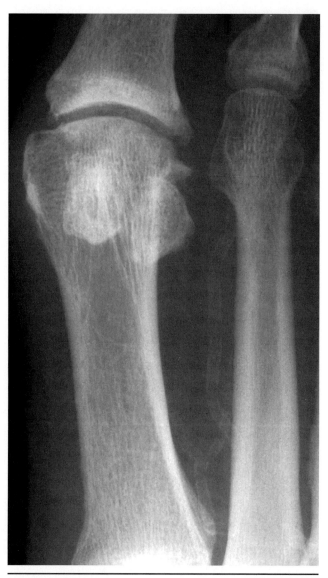

**Figure 24-22**   Vascular calcification: Moenckeberg's sclerosis. The classic presentation is shown in this diabetic patient (DP view). Tubular, serpiginous calcifications are easily identified in the first intermetatarsal space following the course of arterial vessels.

mellitus, hypervitaminosis D, and renal osteodystrophy. Calcification of cartilage (chondrocalcinosis) suggests CPPD deposition and hemochromatosis. Sheetlike collections in the lower leg are associated with tissue injury and compartment syndrome.

The term *calcific tendinitis* (Figure 24-24) has been used to describe tendon calcification resulting from the deposition of calcium hydroxyapatite crystals.[20] Its etiology is

closely associated with trauma, but injury is not prerequisite. Pain is the most common associated symptom. Holt and Keats illustrate examples involving the Achilles, peroneus, and forefoot flexor tendons.[20] Similar reports include examples involving the peroneal tendon,[21,22] although they are not identified specifically as calcific tendinitis. Radiographic evidence of adjacent bone erosion, mimicking malignancy, has been reported.[23]

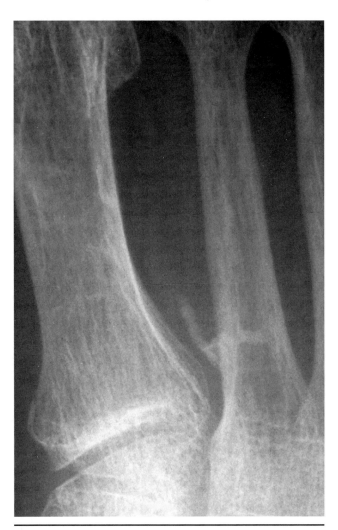

Figure 24-23   Vascular calcification: atherosclerosis. In contrast to Moenckeberg's sclerosis, the calcifications that follow the course of arterial vessels are patchy and solid.

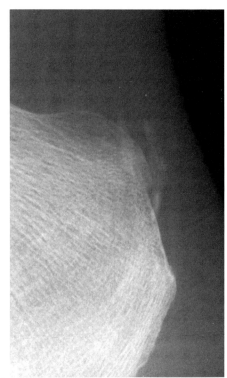

**A**

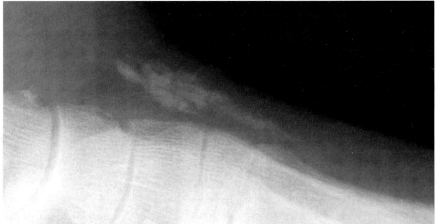

**B**

Figure 24-24   Calcific tendonitis. **A,** Achilles tendon calcification near its enthesis. **B,** Calcification of extensor tendons along the dorsum of the midfoot.

## Ossification

Causes of soft tissue ossification include neoplasm (sarcoma), trauma (myositis ossificans, ossifying hematoma), and venous insufficiency.

Achilles tendon ossification (Figure 24-25) is frequently associated with pain.[24,25,26] Interestingly, MRI analysis of several cases failed to demonstrate inflammatory changes, even with acute symptoms.[27] Morris and associates have presented a classification of Achilles tendon lesion based on anatomic location, including calcification and ossification.[28]

Generalized periostitis is associated with venous stasis (Figure 24-26), hypertrophic osteoarthropathy (primary and secondary), thyroid acropachy, and hypervitaminosis A.[1,11] Radiographically, varying degrees of periosteal new bone formation is possible, but typically it is thick and undulating (irregular).

The term *myositis ossificans* is used to describe non-neoplastic heterotopic soft tissue calcification. Four categories are described in the literature, relating to underlying etiology (or lack of):

1. Myositis ossificans progressiva is a rare genetic dysplasia with associated congenital osseous abnormalities.[7]
2. Myositis ossificans circumscripta, caused by localized trauma, is the most common form (Figure 24-27, *A*). Several cases in the foot have been described.[29-32]
3. Myositis ossificans associated with neurologic disease (Figure 24-27, *B*) may be due to a variety of neurologic causes.[7]
4. Pseudomalignant myositis ossificans is similar to the circumscripta form but without a history of antecedent trauma.[33]

Yochum and Rowe[34] warn that the early stages of myositis ossificans circumscripta may mimic sarcoma. It initially presents as a soft tissue swelling that proceeds to an ill-defined calcific density followed by ossification. A radiolucent zone may be seen between the lesion and adjacent bone, which helps to distinguish it from sarcomatous soft tissue extension.

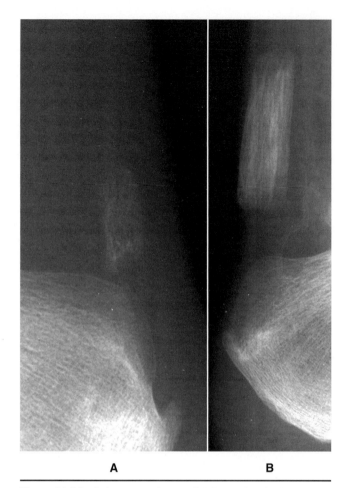

**A**        **B**

Figure 24-25    Soft tissue ossification: Achilles tendon. **A,** Notice the trabeculations in the lesion, which distinguish it from calcification. **B,** A much larger ossification; this image also demonstrates Moenckeberg's sclerosis.

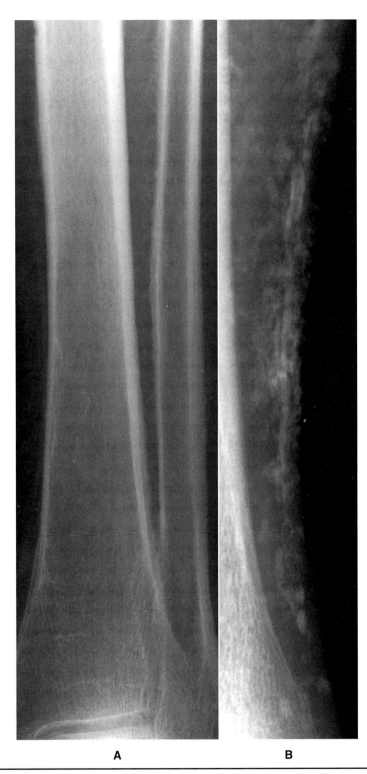

A          B

Figure 24-26   Generalized periostitis: venous stasis. **A,** Irregular, wavy periostitis is identified along the lateral and medial margins of the distal tibia and fibular diaphysis, respectively. **B,** This patient, with chronic venous insufficiency (AP view), demonstrates solid periostitis along the distal tibial diaphysis with diffuse soft tissue calcification (phleboliths).

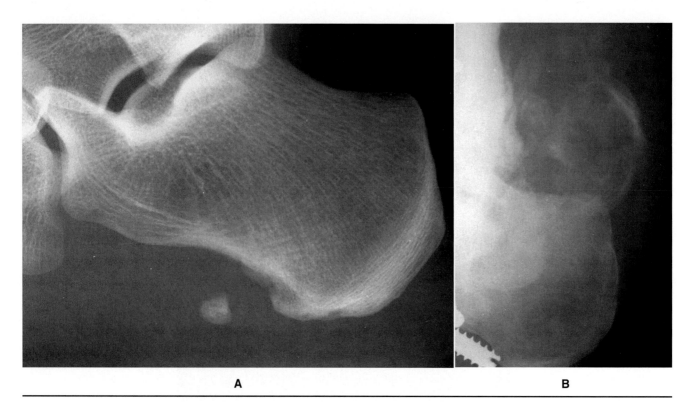

**A**                                                              **B**

Figure 24-27    Heterotopic soft tissue ossification. **A,** Myositis ossificans circumscripta. A lesion identified in the plantar fascia musculature. **B,** Myositis ossificans associated with neuropathic osteoarthropathy, posterior ankle.

## References

1. Resnick D: *Bone and joint imaging,* ed 2, Philadelphia, 1996, Saunders.

2. Bullough PG, Vigoria VJ: *Atlas of orthopaedic pathology with clinical and radiologic correlations,* Baltimore, 1984, University Park Press.

3. Christman RA: Misconceptions regarding use of the term "osteoporosis," *J Cur Podiatr Med* 35(10):11, 1986.

4. Genant HK, Vogler JB, Block JE: Radiology of osteoporosis. In Riggs BL, Melton LJ, editors: *Osteoporosis: etiology, diagnosis, and management,* New York, 1988, Raven Press.

5. Jhamaria NL, Lal KB, Udawat M et al: The trabecular pattern of the calcaneum as an index of osteoporosis, *J Bone Joint Surg* 65B(2):195, 1983.

6. Cockshott WP, Occleshaw CJ, Webber C et al: Can a calcaneal morphologic index determine the degree of osteoporosis? *Skeletal Radiol* 12:119, 1984.

7. Greenfield GB: *Radiology of bone diseases,* ed 4, Philadelphia, 1986, Lippincott.

8. Jaffe HL: *Metabolic, degenerative, and inflammatory diseases of bones and joints,* Philadelphia, 1972, Lea & Febiger.

9. Berquist TH: *Radiology of the foot and ankle,* ed 2, Philadelphia, 2000, Lippincott Williams & Wilkins.

10. Aegerter E, Kirkpatrick JA: *Orthopedic diseases,* ed 4, Philadelphia, 1975, Saunders.

11. Forrester DM, Kricun ME, Kerr R: *Imaging of the foot and ankle,* Rockville, Md, 1988, Aspen.

12. Yochum TR, Rowe LJ: *Essentials of skeletal radiology,* vol 2, Baltimore, 1987, Williams & Wilkins.

13. Slomowitz M, Nixon B, Mott RC: Tumoral calcinosis of the foot: case report and literature review, *JFS* 29(3):278, 1990.

14. Caspi I, Friedman B, Horoszovski H: Tumoral calcinosis simulating osteomyelitis, *JFS* 28(6):547, 1989.

15. Black JR, Sladek GD: Tumoral calcinosis in the foot and hand, *J Am Podiatr Assoc* 73(3):153, Mar 1983.

16. Conti RJ, Shinder M: Soft tissue calcifications induced by local corticosteroid injection, *JFS* 30(1):34, 1991.

17. Dalinka MK, Stewart V, Bomalaski JS et al: Periarticular calcifications in association with intra-articular corticosteroid injections, *Radiology* 153:615, 1984.

18. Wu KK: Tumoral calcinosis with extensive pedal involvement, *JFS* 29(4):388, 1990.

19. Miller SJ, Patton GW, Xenos D, Wulf MR: Multiple capillary hemangiomas of the foot with associated phleboliths, *J Am Podiatr Assoc* 70(7):364, 1980.

20. Holt PD, Keats TE: Calcific tendinitis: a review of the usual and unusual, *Skeletal Radiol* 22:1, 1993.

21. Wirtz PD, Long DH, Vito GR: Calcification within the peroneus brevis tendon, *J Am Podiatr Med Assoc* 77(6):292, 1987.

22. Lepow GM, Korfin DH: Calcification of an accessory peroneal tendon in an athlete, *J Am Podiatr Med Assoc* 75(6):323, 1985.

23. Hayes CW, Rosenthal DI, Plata MJ, Hudson TM: Calcific tendinitis in unusual sites associated with cortical bone erosion, *AJR* 149:967, 1987.

24. Lotke PA: Ossification of the Achilles tendon, *J Bone Joint Surg* 52A(1):157, 1970.

25. Raynor KJ, McDonald RJ, Edelman RD, Parkinson DE: Ossification of the Achilles tendon, *J Am Podiatr Med Assoc* 76(12):688, 1986.

26. Hatori M, Kita A, Hashimoto Y et al: Ossification of the Achilles tendon: a case report, *Foot & Ankle* 15(1):44, 1994.

27. Yu JS, Witte D, Resnick D, Pogue W: Ossification of the Achilles tendon: imaging abnormalities in 12 patients, *Skeletal Radiol* 23:127, 1994.

28. Morris KL, Giacopelli JA, Granoff D: Classification of radiopaque lesions of the tendo Achillis, *JFS* 29(6):533, 1990.

29. Kaminsky SL, Corcoran D, Chubb WF, Pulla RJ: Myositis ossificans: pedal manifestations, *JFS* 31(2):173, 1992.

30. Fuselier CO, Tlapek TA, Sowell RD: Heterotopic ossification (myositis ossificans) in the foot, *J Am Podiatr Med Assoc* 76(9):524, 1986.

31. Herring KM, Levine BD: Myositis ossificans of traumatic origin in the foot, *JFS* 31(1):30, 1992.

32. Mandracchia V, Mahan KT, Pruzansky J, Uricchio JN: Myositis ossificans: a report of a case in the foot, *J Am Podiatr Assoc* 73(1):31, 1983.

33. Ogilvie-Harris DJ, Hons CB, Fornasier VL: Pseudo-malignant myositis ossificans: heterotopic new-bone formation without a history of trauma, *J Bone Joint Surg* 62A(8):1274, 1980.

34. Yochum TR, Rowe LJ: *Essentials of skeletal radiology*, vol 1, Baltimore, 1987, Williams & Wilkins.